Software Development and Quality Assurance for the Healthcare Manufacturing Industries

Third Edition

Steven R. Mallory

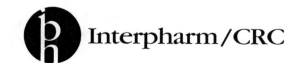
Interpharm/CRC

Boca Raton   London   New York   Washington, D.C.

Library of Congress Cataloging-in-Publication Data

Mallory, Steven R.
   Software development and quality assurance for the healthcare
manufacturing industries / Steven R. Mallory.— 3rd ed.
        p. cm.
   Includes bibliographical references and index.
   ISBN 1-57491-136-8
   1. Medical instruments and apparatus industry—Data processing. 2. Medical care—Data processing.
3. Medical supplies industry—Data processing. 4. Medical instruments and apparatus industry—Quality Control.
   [DNLM: 1. Software. 2. Industry. 3. Program Development. 4. Quality Assurance, Health Care. I. Title.
W 26.55.S6 M255s   2002]
R856.M285 2002
681'.761'0285—dc21   2002005716

Visit the CRC Press Web site at www.crcpress.com

© 1994, 1997, 2002 CRC Press LLC
Interpharm is an imprint of CRC Press

No claim to original U.S. Government works
International Standard Book Number 1-57491-136-8
Library of Congress Card Number 2002005716
Printed in the United States of America   1 2 3 4 5 6 7 8 9 0
Printed on acid-free paper

Contents

Preface to the Third Edition   ix

Preface to the Second Edition   xi

Preface to the First Edition   xiii

Acknowledgments   xv

Introduction   xvii

**1. How Did a Nice Discipline like Quality Get Mixed Up
     with Software Engineering?**   1

    Historical Perspectives of Software Quality Assurance   2

    The Need for Software Quality Assurance   4

    Complexity and Precision in Programming   5

    Hardware versus Software: Similar but Different   6

    Built-in Software Quality   7

    Is It Soup Yet?   9

    Software Quality Dimensions   14

2.   The Components of a Software Quality Assurance Program   17

Aspects of Quality   18

Overview of the System Design and Software Design Process   22

Software Standards and Procedures   25

Implementation of a Software Quality Assurance Program   31

Software Quality Assurance Education   35

**3.   The Software Quality Assurance Program:
       Foundations of Methodology and Process   37**

Software Methodology and Process Definition   38

Software Methodology and Process Documentation   53

Software Policy Guidelines   88

Software Quality Assurance in the Maintenance Cycle   95

**4.   The Software Quality Assurance Program:
       Project Software Estimations   105**

Software Project Estimation   108

Work Breakdown Structure   110

Software Team Characteristics, Organization, and Staffing   115

Reliable Estimations of Software Development   123

Estimation Models   127

Estimation Methods   132

Estimation Model and Methods: Conclusions   135

Function Point Analysis   135

**5.   The Software Quality Assurance Program:
       Project Software Documentation   145**

Software Planning Documents   146

Software Requirements and Design Documents   175

Software Testing and Verification and Validation Documents   196

Software Documentation Usage   201

6.   The Software Quality Assurance Program: Software Development Activities   **205**

Software Requirements Engineering   207

Quality Function Deployment in Software   214

Heuristics, Rigor, and Cost in Software Design   215

Software Requirements versus Software Design   217

The Software Life Cycle in Practice   223

Prototypes   229

Software Reviews   243

Software Reuse   249

The Software Postmortem   253

7.   The Software Quality Assurance Program: Software Testing Activities   **259**

Software Nodes and Paths   260

Stress and Boundary Tests   262

Software Testing Strategy   263

Selection of Orthogonal Array Testing   266

Unit and Module Testing   268

Static Testing   268

Integration Testing   270

Validation Testing   272

Device System Testing   274

Software Safety Testing   276

Allocation of Software Testing   279

Software Reliability Engineered Testing   280

Software Statistical-Based Testing   286

Designing an Integrated Corporate Test Strategy   290

When is "Good Enough" Good Enough Testing?   293

The Last Test   294

8.   The Software Quality Assurance Program: Software Verification and Validation Activities   **297**

Verification and Validation in the Software Life Cycle   299

Quality Assurance   303

Attributes of Quality Software   305

Attributes of Quality Software Specifications   306

Verification and Validation of Off-the-Shelf Software   309

Verification and Validation of Software Safety   310

Management Interface   312

**9. The Software Quality Assurance Program:
    Software Configuration Management Activities   315**

Baselines   318

Code Control   320

Firmware   321

Configuration Management   322

Control of Installed Variants   326

**10. The Software Quality Assurance Program:
     Software Hazards and Safety Activities   329**

Risk Management   330

Hazard Analysis   333

Hazard Analysis Models and Techniques   337

Hazard Analysis Difficulties   351

Safety   352

Reliability versus Safety   355

Software Safety   356

User Interface and Safety   365

**11. The Software Quality Assurance Program:
     Software User Interface Activities   375**

The Ubiquitous User Interface   375

What Is Usability?   376

Developing Human-Computer Interaction   377

Behavioral and Constructional Domains 377

Roles in User Interface Development 379

The Value of User-friendly Medical Device Interfaces 381

A Life Cycle for User Interaction Development 385

A Different Perspective of Noninterface Software Development 386

User Interface Development 391

Integration of Development Processes 391

12. The Software Quality Assurance Program: Software Metrics **395**

Software Metrics and Models 396

Software Size Metrics 401

Data Structure Metrics 409

Logic Structure Metrics 412

Composite Metrics 414

Software Defects 417

Software Defect Models 420

Software Reliability and Reliability Growth Models 425

Maintainability Metrics Models 428

Software Statistical Process Control 431

Decision Making with Metrics 433

13. The Software Quality Assurance Program: Productivity and Capability Maturity Measurement **435**

Overview of Software Process Improvement Measurement 435

Productivity Differentials in Software 438

Software Assessment Standards and Models 439

Software Metrics and Process Maturity 442

The Steps in Using Maturity Metrics 447

Identifying and Managing Risks for Software Process Improvement 448

Bibliography **459**

Index **499**

To Beth

for her understanding and, therefore, her patience.

Preface to the Third Edition

I am, again, very grateful for and flattered by the continuing favorable reception enjoyed by this work. In this third edition, I have reviewed the entire manuscript (again) and have made a large number of refinements, as well as including new material. The previous edition's Chapter 2 has been removed while Chapters 1 through 5 are fundamentally the same as the previous editions but new subject matter and clarification of topic discussions have been included.

The most substantial revision is the old Chapter 7 and the entirely new Chapter 11. Based on suggestions from readers, I have created new chapters for each of the major topics previously presented as software project activities in Chapter 7. In this edition the activities of software development (Chapter 6), testing (Chapter 7), verification and validation (Chapter 8), configuration management (Chapter 9), and hazards and safety (Chapter 10) now occupy their own chapters. Because of this organizational approach, I also moved material related to these topics from other chapters so that each chapter now contains all information germane to the chapter subject. For example, safety and hazard discussions found in Chapter 2 previously are now located in Chapter 10, testing that was originally spread throughout the manuscript is now located in Chapter 7, and V&V is now concentrated in Chapter 8. In addition, this material has been greatly expanded and clarified, and new subject matter and topics have been included. Chapter 11 is entirely new and discusses the topic of user interfaces. Chapters 12 and 13 in this edition are the previous Chapters 8 and 9 and have also undergone expansion with new material as well as additional, clarifying discussions. Last, the reference list has been brought up-to-date and reflects all of the new and revised material in this manuscript.

I wish to thank all of you who provided the comments to me that the information presented could be better organized and provide a more centralized approach for reference. I hope that this new organization satisfies your requirements.

Steven R. Mallory
September 2001

Preface to the Second Edition

I am very grateful for the favorable reception enjoyed by the first edition of this work. I have also enjoyed the stimulating comments, questions, discussions, and observations about the content of this manuscript that I have had with many of you on the telephone, as a medical device software consultant, and at conferences where I was an invited speaker. Each of you has contributed substantially to this new edition. In this second edition, I have reviewed the entire manuscript and have made a large number of refinements, as well as including new material. A casual reader will hardly notice any difference between this edition and the first except for the renumbering of figures and an entirely new chapter on software process maturity measurement.

The most substantial revisions occur in Chapters 5 and 7 and the entirely new Chapter 9. In these chapters, I have greatly expanded and clarified a great deal of this material, as well as included new subject matter and topics based, again, on conversations with and recommendations from readers. Chapters 1, 3, and 8 have also undergone expansion with new material as well as additional, clarifying discussions. Chapters 2, 4, and 6 have been revised, but not to the extent of the other chapters. Last, the reference list has been brought up-to-date and reflects all of the new and revised material in this manuscript. I wish to thank all of you who provided helpful and valued input to me, each in your own way, and especially Jane Steinmann of Interpharm Press who worked with me as editor, critic, and counselor with the first, and now second, manuscript.

Steven R. Mallory
January 1997

Preface to the First Edition

Software quality assurance is the mapping of managerial precepts and design disciplines of quality assurance onto the applicable management and technological space of software engineering. The familiar quality assurance approaches for improving control and performance metamorphose into the techniques and tools for software engineering, which are different from those of quality assurance. Although these new approaches to the construction and maintenance of software have been given new form and procedural efficiency, both the quality assurance community and the software development community can easily relate to the concepts of software quality assurance.

Although software quality assurance is more ingrained than it used to be, I tacitly admit that other views of software quality assurance do exist. There are proponents within the software industry who feel that better software will result through the increased commitment by software practitioners to the adoption of formalized and disciplined practices of software engineering. However, they seem to ignore the proven statistics related to benefits realized from the application of quality methodology. Conversely, there are proponents within the quality arena who feel that better software will result through the overseeing of software's conformance to its own development and maintenance standards. However, they frequently ignore the fact that the majority of companies lack software development and maintenance standards, as well as the understanding of the content of those standards.

Software quality assurance not only promises to be constructive, it has a proven track record of enormous benefit. Furthermore, software quality assurance can avoid being a bureaucratic impediment, but only by drawing on the fundamental concepts of both software engineering and quality assurance. It is essential to the success of any medical device company, helping to develop a more profitable and reliable product and create a more satisfied customer base. Software quality assurance reduces the risk of liability and builds confidence with regulatory agencies that the company can meet the requirements of their standards and regulations.

It is hoped that this text will assist medical device companies in the establishment, operation, and maintenance of a medical device software quality assurance program. There are no "silver bullets" in the software industry. When I first formulated the idea for this book, I felt that it should address software quality assurance as a pseudonym for software verification and validation. As this idea matured, it became apparent that the subject of software verification and validation required clarification on how software development performed its functions and activities in order to provide software verification and validation within the proper framework of task accomplishment. This lead me to the conclusion that even software development needs a discussion of software quality assurance. Ultimately, the need to provide the discussion about the quality assurance of software development lead to the logical conclusion that even ancillary and peripheral software development activities, such as estimating, scheduling, and team organization, were also a reflection of software quality. Consequently, software quality assurance is, in reality, a comprehensive, interrelated, and disciplined program. It is not a singular activity that occurs without foresight, thought, or planning.

The easiest analogy that I know of that conveys the software quality assurance concept is a comparison to those crystal balls that can be purchased at most gift shops or drugstores that have numerous facets on them. The crystal ball, with all of its facets, is software quality assurance. Although it is an entity that can be observed and understood conceptually, in order to be able to discuss it, you can view it through only one facet at a time. Through one facet, you can see the software design aspects of software quality assurance. Rotate the crystal ball and you get a different facet, which represents software development activities. Rotate it again and you see the software verification and validation aspects of software quality assurance. Each time the crystal ball is rotated, another aspect of software quality assurance comes into view, and each facet represents a subject that is an integral part of the whole.

Another difficulty with presenting a discussion related to a software quality assurance program is that some readers will have prior experience with some, or all, of the topics that are presented here. Consequently, they will take exception to what, how, and where some topics are presented because their experience and familiarity are different. For example, I tend to think of the software quality assurance function as the "software verification and validation group," whereas others view it as a splitting of the functions between the quality assurance group and the software test group. I have tried to account for such differences whenever possible.

Acknowledgments

I am deeply indebted to many people for their encouragement, help, support, and constructive criticism that led to the making of this book. I especially want to thank my wife, Beth, and daughter, Lauren, who constantly encouraged me, sacrificed time together, and tolerated my verbal dissertations about technical topics that they knew little or nothing about. I also want to thank my parents for the sacrifices they endured over the years so that they could send me to college to receive the education that has been rewarding and fulfilling to me.

I want to thank Russell Horres, who has worked within the medical products industry for years and recognized something in my background in the defense software contracting business and my software expertise that was applicable to medical device software development.

I want to thank Gary Stephenson, John McDaniel, and Kent Beckstrom of IVAC Corporation for imparting to me their years of experience and perspectives of the medical device industry and software development within that industry. They provided countless hours of stimulating and intriguing discussions relating to methods, practices, philosophies, and strategies that influence medical device hardware and software development. I want to thank Jenny Hankard, Mark Gordon, and David Doan of IVAC Corporation, who lent their point of view relative to dealing with regulatory agencies on a firsthand basis and for providing guidance on the standards and regulations dealing with software development, software reliability, and software safety. All of these individuals have provided special, key, and new insights on the technical materials that are presented in this book.

Lastly, I want to thank Gary Stephenson, John McDaniel, Kent Beckstrom, Mark Gordon, Jenny Hankard, David Doan, and Steve Rakitin of Ciba-Corning Diagnostics Corporation for providing the time and effort to review the draft manuscript. Their review, critique, commentary, and editorial comments have been valued, appreciated, and heard.

Steven R. Mallory
January 1994

Introduction

This book has not left the practical, "hands-on" and "soup-to-nuts" approach to the formation and operation of a medical device software quality assurance program. The reader searching for the software quality assurance "cookie cutter," the "quick fix," or the "right answer," will not find them here. Presented in this book is an interrelated and integrated program approach that can be used to implement a new or repair an existing software quality assurance program for medical device software development. The details of the approach, as well as how the various software quality assurance program elements interact, are presented through multiple alternative choices, in order to give the reader a feel for the manner and intent in which the various elements might be used. For those wishing to delve deeper, references are given at the end of the book.

In general, Chapters 1 and 2 present the philosophy, strategy, high-level mechanics, and implementation plans for a software quality assurance program. These chapters have been expanded to include ethical responsibility and refinement of the levels of concern and standards organizations. Chapter 3 presents the foundations and steps for implementation of the software quality assurance program as a process and methodology. This chapter was expanded with the addition of new material detailing standards and conventions, guidelines, and documentation responsibilities. Chapter 4 was expanded with the inclusion of new discussions relating to function points as a project estimation technique. Chapter 5 was expanded with clarifying information throughout the topic areas of document descriptions as well as new strategies with old and new documents.

The second edition's Chapter 7 has been divided into five new chapters, and material has been moved from several other chapters to the new topic chapters. Chapter 6 details the software development activities and has additional new material. Chapter 7 (extracted from the previous Chapter 7) encompasses software testing activities. New material has been added related to testing strategy, built-in testing, reliability testing, test planning, safety testing, and user interface testing. Chapter 8 (part of the old Chapter 7) details software verification and validation activities; new material was added. Chapter 9 (formed from the old Chapter 7) presents software configuration management activities. Chapter 10 (created from the old Chapter 7 and sections of the previous Chapter 2) discusses software hazard and safety activities; new material in it addresses risk management and user interfaces. Chapter 11 is entirely new and presents software user interface activities.

Chapter 12 (the previous Chapter 8) includes new topics relative to maintainability metrics, defect metrics, metrics capability evaluation, measurement of software maintenance, and predicting software reliability. Chapter 13 (the previous Chapter 9) presents new material and concepts detailing evaluation of software development capability and identifying and measuring risks for software process improvement.

The book concludes with an expanded list of references that will allow the reader to pursue in more detail any of the specific topics presented in the various sections of the manuscript. The references represent a broad spectrum of sources as well as a diverse source of information— books, periodicals, and journals relating to historical perspectives; software development methodology and process subjects; technical material; and future trends and predictions.

1

How Did a Nice Discipline like Quality Get Mixed Up with Software Engineering?

What's past is prologue.

—William Shakespeare

Software-based medical products have been at the forefront of healthcare innovation since the early 1980s. The breadth of medical products that are controlled by software is considerable, ranging from the sophisticated nuclear magnetic resonance (NMR) system to the simple electronic thermometer. Software has become an integral component of product function, competitiveness, and quality.

As important as software has become in product design, most of what is practiced in development applications of medical product software has been borrowed from other disciplines. This is particularly true in software quality assurance. The organized, systematic, and "scientific" approach to software development originated in the late 1960s as a result of the need to correct the deficiencies in the "code and fix" software development process that was in use at the time. However, the quality assurance of software development predates that by a decade. Given the rate at which innovative techniques are being introduced in software engineering, the organized and disciplined approach to software development and software quality assurance is far from an established and mature doctrine. Software development and software quality assurance will continue to evolve in the arena of medical device software as more individuals become intimately involved and familiar with all aspects of software engineering.

In the competitive environment of medical device development, management is continually faced with the challenge to organize and deploy resources in an optimal manner to satisfy customers with safe and effective products. The computer revolution has intensified this challenge by making new and major demands on personnel and their organizations. Unfortunately, senior management seldom has sufficient training, experience, or understanding needed to properly evaluate the methods that can be used to control software development and assure its quality. The result of this situation is that software development is all too often a chronicle of schedule and cost overruns that continue beyond the product's delivery and well into the product life cycle.

Historical Perspectives of Software Quality Assurance

Tracing the evolution of quality assurance from its primitive origins to its present reflection of today's technological society can help us to understand the development of parallels to software.

Quality Assurance in the Industrial World

In the pre–20th century industrial world, quality assurance was implemented as an inspection, and the responsibility for that inspection lay with the artisan who made the product. The inspection was not considered a separate and distinct action. It was made in order to ensure that the final product met the artisan's personal high standards of workmanship and that the product was precisely what the customer had ordered. As the industrial revolution took hold and products were commonly mass-produced, the artisan all but faded away, and the standardization of production and inspection methods became the rule. Eventually, this standardization was coupled with formal programs that were necessary to support, plan, and manage these production and inspection efforts.

Manufacturing operations became even more complex over time, and the volume of product output increased. To manage these increasingly more complex manufacturing operations, increased controls were implemented to assure the continuing uniformity of the products that were produced. This necessitated the establishment of acceptance and rejection criteria, because these higher product volumes made individual product inspections impractical. To economically control the higher manufacturing output and apply the acceptance and rejection criteria, statistical quality control of the manufacturing processes was instituted.

As the quality function became more sophisticated and its effectiveness in dealing with more complex problems and controls became obvious, enlightened production managers began to realize the importance of the quality function. This fertile and receptive attitude enabled the more progressive and innovative members of the quality assurance community to develop, and convince management to support, quality assurance programs. These programs eventually expanded and encompassed all facets of product design and development, as well as manufacturing operations. Ultimately, product liability, reliability, and safety led to the expansion of quality control into all industries.

In manufacturing organizations, product acceptance at the incoming, in-process, and final product levels is usually conducted by the quality department. Product acceptance activities include inspection, final test operations, and the necessary planning activities required to make it effective. For service organizations, the conformance of the service to requirements is usually determined by the quality department, using inspection, quality auditing, and other techniques. The results of these actions are reported in order to assure that corrective action will be taken to prevent repetitive defects and to provide management data.

Quality Assurance in the Software World

Early on, the same quality assurance approach was used for software as for goods production in the pre–20th century industrial world (see Table 1-1). The accuracy and effectiveness of software depended initially on the software developer's diligence, ability, and personal standards of quality. It was the widespread demand for software by the government and such related agencies as NASA, the Department of Defense, and military organizations that began to seriously tax the software developer's approach to quality.

Table 1-1 Evolution of Quality Control

Time Period	Quality Control Implementation			Remarks
	Sector	Characteristics		
Pre–20th century	Industry	Inspection by producer		Pride in workmanship
1916	Industry	Introduction of quality control		First formal programs
1920–1940	Industry	Standardization and inspection		Necessitated by mass production
1940–1950	Industry	Introduction of statistical quality control		To economically control complex and higher output manufacturing process
	Software	First uses of computers and software		Pride in workmanship
1950–1970	Industry	Formal programs encompassing all facets of design and development		Prevalent in defense organizations
	Software	Introduction of standardization		First formal development techniques; prevalent in defense organizations
1970–1980	Industry	Product liability and safety; management recognition		Expansion of quality control into all industries
	Software	Structured design and development; introduction of computers into products; introduction of formal quality assurance		Large software programs; prevalent in defense organizations; explosion of software development
1980–1990	Industry	Quality and customer focus become foremost		Shrinking economic markets and global competition
	Software	Product liability and safety; management recognition		Introduction of development tools; formal quality assurance and reliability efforts
1990–present	Industry	Quality, customer focus, and time to market become foremost		Quality award
	Software			Expansion of quality control

Reprinted with permission from "Building Quality into Medical Product Software Design," Steven R. Mallory, in *Biomedical Instrumentation and Technology*, Vol. 27, No. 1, page 118. Association for the Advancement of Medical Instrumentation, 1993.

The difficulty of using the pre–20th century approach for software quality assurance is that software is as much a product as are manufactured goods and services. Software engineering has grown from casual preparation of small programs affecting a few developers to the development and maintenance of complex software systems that involve the participation of a team of software engineers. As the size and complexity of software projects have escalated, new techniques have evolved within the software industry for accomplishing and controlling the software effort.

Medical devices are becoming more and more dependent on microprocessors that are, in turn, dependent upon the software that is resident and executed within them; quality assurance must address this change. Managers of medical product development face changing technologies in the types of products that are being produced; until recently, the changes in these products have been primarily in the hardware area, where classical quality assurance methods can be used. The expanding role of software in defining product capabilities compels managers of medical product development to face a fundamental and often radical change in the development process for medical device products.

However, this shift toward software is not nearly as straightforward for quality assurance as was the transition through the various hardware technology levels. Engineers working on medical device software development must recognize that software can no longer be developed and maintained in the informal, casual atmosphere of the past. Medical device companies need to recognize that a fundamental technological shift from an electromechanical base to a software base has occurred within the industry. It is senior management's responsibility to marshal all of its resources in the understanding and controlling of software development cost, schedule, and reliability. The more progressive companies have been able to meet this challenge by adapting their corporate philosophies, attitudes, and organizations. Those unwilling to recognize and adapt to this fundamental shift are destined to technical obsolescence.

The Need for Software Quality Assurance

Although software quality assurance is concerned with all types of software, nowhere is the need for software quality assurance more visibly demonstrated than in medical device software. Medical device software not only monitors sensors, controls mechanisms, keypads, and contact buttons, and drives display devices, but also indirectly controls the health and wellbeing of patients who are using the devices. Furthermore, software frequently must operate in a real-time environment, most often without the benefit of highly trained operators.

No interrelated system can be of greater quality than the quality of its individual components. When one of these components is a microprocessor, the quality of the software controlling the processing will affect the quality of the entire device. The difficulty associated with the code within the microprocessor is that the software can have latent design and logic defects. These defects could cause the performance of the device to degrade, at best, or could cause the device to fail catastrophically, at worst.

Microprocessors that are used in medical devices today have considerable logical and arithmetic power. The embedded software applications that drive the medical devices exert an influence on the performance of the device to an extent equal to or greater than that of the hardware; thus, the quality of the product is as much vested in the software as it is in the hardware. At present, the specific tasks that are related to software quality assurance and reliability are addressed principally by the engineers who develop the software. However, effective software quality assurance is a three-way challenge.

1. Software engineers must accept the philosophies and tenets of quality.

2. Senior management must recognize that their own goals of timely, cost-effective software will be best attained by understanding, funding, and committing to software quality and control.

3. Quality and reliability engineering disciplines must acclimate to the software development practices that are appropriate to and supportive of software quality.

Complexity and Precision in Programming

The microprocessor has introduced highly complex, precisely formulated, and logical systems on a vast scale. These systems may be large and highly complex, but if human beings and analog devices are components within them, then a wide spectrum of error tolerances must be present, and such components must adjust to, compensate for, and adapt to each of these tolerances. The microprocessor not only makes the idea of perfect precision possible but frequently requires perfect precision for satisfactory operation. Consequently, intolerance to the slightest logical error gives software a new dimension in its requirement for precision on a large scale.

The combination of the requirement for precision and the commercial demand for software on a broad scale has created many false values and distorted relationships in medical devices containing software. They arise from intense pressure to achieve complex and precise results in a practical way without adequate technical foundations on the part of the users. It is universally accepted that software development is an error-prone activity and any software system is presumed to have errors, yet the process of debugging software is mysterious and nearly an art form—more time is spent in debug and testing than in design and coding. Even though errors in program logic have long been around, software development is relatively young as a technical activity. Many of its past technical foundations have given way to new technical processes and methodology, while techniques and tools have permitted an entirely new level of precision in software development. This new level of precision has allowed the development and implementation of large, fast, and accurate software medical applications that have enormous mean times between detected errors, but this improvement has also required a new attitude toward software development, in users as well as developers.

A child can learn to play the game of tic-tac-toe perfectly, but a person cannot learn to saw a board exactly in half. Playing tic-tac-toe is a combinatorial problem where a single move is selected from a finite number of possible moves. Sawing a board exactly in half is a physical problem for which no discrete level of accuracy is sufficient. The tic-tac-toe player is capable of perfect play and does not usually make mistakes. Software development is a combinatorial activity, just like tic-tac-toe; it is not related to sawing a board in half. It does not require perfect resolution in measurement and control, but it does require correct choices out of finite sets of possibilities at every step.

The difference between tic-tac-toe and software development is complexity. The purpose of a formal software development doctrine is to control complexity through discipline, rigor, and the reduction of available choices and options at any given step. In learning to play tic-tac-toe, we develop theory and strategies that deal with "center squares," "corner squares," "side squares," and the self-discipline of blocking possible defeats before building threats of our own. In software development, theory and strategies are also critical. Software process and methodology are such theories and strategies, and they provide a systematic way of coping with the complexity in software requirements, design, and development.

Knowing how to play tic-tac-toe perfectly is not enough for our intellect; we must also understand that we know how. This knowledge is vital in understanding that we are capable of analyzing the playing board and making a conscious decision and that we do not need to guess and hope about the outcome. For software engineers it is the same; if they know what is correct, then committing it precisely to paper is just as important as the activities that directly create the final code. If software engineers think that the code is probably all right but are subconsciously counting on debugging and testing to ferret out logic and other errors, then the entire process of committing the application design to paper and ultimately into the computer suffers in small ways, which might later torment and haunt the development effort. Software process and methodology allow the software to be developed with unprecedented precision, but it is not enough to be able to program with precision. The capability for precision programming must be known, in order to supply the discipline to match the capabilities.

As another example, 500 years ago it was not known that air had weight and that at sea level it supports a column of water 34 feet high. Well-pump manufacturers operated on the theory that "nature abhors a vacuum"; their devices could raise well water through pipes by means of a plunger and by tightening the pipe seals. However, at 35 feet, frustration set in, because no matter how tight the seals are, the water cannot be raised. In medical device software development, complexity has weight, and it is not easily measured or described. Frequently, it is ignored. When this complexity exceeds certain unknown limits, then frustration ensues; the software becomes crippled in its logic and execution, maintenance is precarious, and modification becomes nearly, if not completely, impossible. Problems of storage, execution, and throughput can be fixed, but problems of complexity can seldom be adequately recognized, let alone fixed.

Hardware versus Software: Similar but Different

Being able to comprehend and accept software quality assurance requires some rethinking of the manner in which quality assurance can be effected. While the traditional hardware quality assurance and quality engineering approaches can capitalize on being independent from the hardware development process, the inherent differences between hardware and software that will affect the practices that quality engineering employs when dealing with software must be recognized. For example, much of the hardware quality assurance effort is related to the certain knowledge that hardware degrades with use over time. Software, on the other hand, tends to improve over time because once a software defect has been identified and corrected, it remains corrected. Although this example helps to illustrate that the hardware concept of mean time to failure (MTTF) is applicable to software, it also demonstrates that the concept must be interpreted in a new light.

The most prominent traditional quality assurance role has been related to the physical inspection of hardware. This effort is mainly directed at assuring that the original design is copied correctly into the production units. There is no such need in software quality assurance. After a program has been judged to be acceptable by the criteria that have been established for the software program, there is little concern for the ability to copy it precisely. However, for safety reasons, checksums and cyclic redundancy checks (CRCs) are used in order to validate that the replication remains correct while the device is in operation.

Another difference is that hardware can initiate a warning that a failure is likely to occur. For example, as part of hardware quality assurance, the periodic monitoring of pulse shapes, power supply, output voltages, or other physical characteristics can be made for evidence of impending malfunctions. Software, in general, will give no such warnings. However, in some real-time systems, measurements can be made that will give evidence of an impending malfunction—for example, as software processing overhead becomes too great for the device's real-time activities. Furthermore, hardware can be built from standardized, off-the-shelf components and complete subassemblies and, for each hardware component, its reliability can be determined for a given environment. Software, even though it can contain reused code, usually does not have prior experience of its components.

After a failure has occurred, hardware can be repaired and restored to its original condition, whereas the repair of software results in a new baseline condition. The consequence of this new software baseline is that the modified software requires testing as well as verification and validation, and any existing software documentation will potentially need updating in order to reflect those modifications. Furthermore, the entire software program will probably require some level of regression testing to ensure that the new modifications have not introduced an error in any of the nonmodified code sections. The long-term effect of this strategy goes beyond merely assuring the quality and reliability of the current software repair; it also helps to ensure that the success of future repairs is not jeopardized.

In general, medical device hardware can be tested over the entire spectrum of conditions in which it is expected to operate, implying that the performance aspects of the device's hardware may be completely verified by test. However, software failures can occur when diverse combinations of inputs cause either previously unused or differently used branch logic to execute, resulting in an unexpected output, device state, or failure. The sources of these inputs can vary from unanticipated hardware states to irrational and unforeseen operator inputs. Furthermore, the number of discrete states that software within a medical device of even modest capability can assume is usually so great that any exhaustive testing of software is not a practical consideration.

The last comparison between hardware and software deals with the perception of changes. Although hardware changes tend to be difficult and costly, it is easy to predict and measure the costs that are associated with those changes through reworking, layout, fabrication, testing, and so on. Software changes, however, are perceived as being easy to make and low in cost, but in reality they are probably more complex than the original task of creating the code. The difficulty with the costs associated with software changes is that they are not easy to predict or measure, because making a software change adds the risk of introducing new defects outside of the altered code areas. This, in turn, may require additional changes outside of the initial scope of changes, as well as more testing time. These activities cannot be accurately predicted, and they are not measured carefully if at all, in most companies.

Built-in Software Quality

The differences between hardware and software imply that while traditional quality assurance disciplines and methods may apply, implementation practices will vary. Specifically, software quality assurance practices need to emphasize the software concept of built-in quality, since software quality cannot be inspected, as is done for hardware, nor can software quality be added into the product as a final software development step. Software quality assurance is formulated on the notion that software quality is built in as the result of interdependent technical and managerial techniques and tools. The fundamental role of software quality assurance, then, is to focus attention on the establishment of software development standards that are conducive to quality and to audit the fidelity to which those standards are followed.

In keeping with the traditional hardware approach that quality is the conformance to requirements and the prevention of defects, it is the responsibility of the software quality assurance function to act as an independent instrument of management in auditing all of the various aspects of software development and maintenance. The concept and operation of the software quality assurance process is straightforward in theory, but intricate, complicated, and detailed in real life—it consists of verification and validation (V&V). Verification entails those activities and documents that assure that a project's software activities and end products have followed the documented software methodology, process, and standards. Validation entails those activities, tests, and documents that assure that the requirements at the software, system, and product levels have been satisfied.

In Figure 1-1, the top bubble represents a company's documented software methodology, process, and standards; the bottom left bubble represents the software project related activities and documentation; and the bottom right bubble represents the software project end products, such as code and the "as built" documents. The act of verification consists of three distinct functions:

1. Verify that the software project activities and documentation satisfy the documented software methodology, process, and standards.

2. Verify that the software end products satisfy the documented software methodology, process, and standards.

3. Verify that the software end products satisfy the software project activities and documentation and that the design as identified in the project documentation was, in fact, implemented.

Some of these verification activities will take place over the entire software development life cycle on a daily basis.

Validation (see Figure 1-1) consists of a series of formal, approved tests on the software end products that demonstrate that the software, system, and product requirements were satisfied. Validation usually consists of test information sheets that are signed and dated. They indicate what the test was and what the test results are. When all of the validation tests have been completed and pass the predefined test criteria, the software is deemed to satisfy the requirements. A report is then generated indicating that the software project has complied with all of the documented methodology, process, and standards and that the software satisfies the stated requirements. This report in effect certifies that the software is safe, efficacious, and reliable and satisfies all the requirements. The software can then be released and used in the medical device.

In addition to the creation and maintenance of in-house software, these software quality assurance precepts also apply to purchased software packages. Software quality assurance for medical instruments must also assume the responsibility for the surveillance of procured software. This encompasses the qualification and acceptance of all software that will be used in the medical device, as well as the certification of the tools that are used as a part of software development and testing, defect analysis, and quality improvement analysis. A natural reaction of medical device manufacturers is: "Why should we V&V procured software or software tools? We are not in the software V&V business; we are in the medical device business." This is true as far as it goes, but most companies have missed the reverse application of their software quality assurance program. If the supplier of a software package has an equivalent software quality assurance program, then their product does not necessarily require V&V by the purchaser's in-house personnel. In fact, a simple policy or standard operating procedure (SOP) statement conveying the criteria for not performing V&V on a software supplier's product is all that is

---

Figure 1-1 Software quality assurance program high-level concept and process activities

---

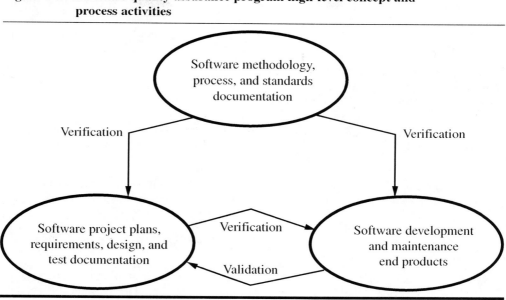

needed. However, due diligence must always be adhered to in order to assure the medical device software developer that the software supplier still conforms to their declared software quality assurance program.

Is It Soup Yet?

Perfect software for a complex system cannot be guaranteed (Cobb and Mills 1990), and new software is assumed to contain errors even after rigorous testing. Even though the software matches its specifications perfectly, it will contain errors because the specifications are not necessarily error free. Even if the software matches its specification perfectly and the specifications are perfect, the software may be used wrongly. The question "Is it soup yet?" relates to laying the foundation for the development of general engineering parallels to medical device software engineering. The concepts that make another engineering field an engineering discipline provide the basis for instituting similar concepts in software engineering. It is this engineering approach to software development that also allows and fosters software quality assurance.

Ethical Considerations

Medical device malfunctions, particularly in software, can have severe consequences. Substantiated cases have cost human life and have been responsible for multimillion dollar financial loses from software errors or misuse (Neumann 1989). The Therac-25 radiation therapy machine is an oft-cited example of the need for improved software quality assurance. This device could deliver two types of X-ray radiation therapy: a low-power beam aimed directly at the patient and a high-power beam that was reflected from a metal target at the patient. An error in the design of the control software caused patients to be exposed directly to the high-intensity X-ray radiation; as a result, they died. Although there were undoubtedly software errors, a mechanical interlock on the machine could have prevented the series of fatal accidents. Whether for economic reasons or by mere oversight, no such interlock was installed.

Some of the many articles about software quality have raised serious ethical questions (Parnas, Von Schowen, and Kwan 1990; Leveson 1991; McFarland 1991) about the way in which software is developed and the role that computers play in our society. The software process in general is a social process that involves human participants who want and need different results from the process. Assuming that humanity generally benefits from advanced technology and that people avoid harm more than they seek good of the same magnitude (Collins, et al. 1994; McFarland 1991) then, from an ethical standpoint, the following list describes the principles relative to medical device software and its development process:

1. Medical device software should not increase the degree of harm to patients and users already most vulnerable to that kind of harm because of their lack of knowledge about software.

2. Medical device software that is designed for a low-threat context should not be used in a higher-threat context.

3. Trade-offs of financial benefit to one group and nonfinancial harm to another group should be made on the basis of a cost-benefit ratio that, should it be made public, would not outrage most members of the public.

From these basic principles, more specific rules of conduct can be derived for the software process. For example, medical device software should not make a risky situation worse. The use of software intended to support or preserve life should not threaten life any more than its absence would, especially if the software should fail. Furthermore, life-preserving software should have control backups in case failure should occur, and these backups could consist of combinations of electrical, mechanical, software, and human monitoring. A medical software developer has obligations to set testing goals beforehand and then to meet them, to provide warnings about untested areas, to educate users about the limitations of the testing, and to provide testing information on demand from people who can be affected by the software.

Each of the participants in the software process has obligations to all of the other participants, and sometimes participants have ethical obligations to themselves. Software engineers are expected to make responsible decisions and judgments even when their own self-interest is involved in the issues decided. All of the participants in the software process have responsibilities to themselves to sustain a standard of work and behavior that upholds their personal and professional dignity. The software profession has been plagued by problems of quality since the beginning (Huskey and Huskey 1990). Contemporary quality approaches focus on professional standards for software engineers, documentation and development standards, standards for testing, and formal verification. Each of these approaches has made progress, but none is fully successful yet. The current state of practice in software quality assurance, an active area of research, occupies an increasingly important position in software development; ethical considerations can also contribute to the various efforts to improve and standardize software quality.

How sensitive should designers and software engineers be to the ethics of technology when they are trying to persuade an organization to adopt a way of doing business that is commonly antithetical to the idea of "just get product out"? The answer lies in the fact that the motivations underlying a persuasive act and the intent of that persuasive act are not the same. For example, consider three people trying to persuade a stranger to improve his or her personal health. One persuader might be motivated by a desire to increase the stranger's quality of life, the second persuader might wish to reduce healthcare costs, and the third might be malicious and hope the stranger will be severely injured. The persuasive intent is constant for the three persuaders, but the motivation varies in an ethically relevant way. The first is laudable, the third is problematic, and the second lies in a more neutral zone where cultural context, relative importance, and other factors come to bear. Furthermore, if a person were to convince a stranger to be healthier by using exaggerated facts or fears, then these methods might be judged unethical even if the motivations appeared laudable.

Research has shown (Fogg and Nass 1997) that computers can flatter just as well as humans can. However, technologies embed ethical motivation in new and compelling contexts, and the ultimate outcome of the persuasive intent must be evaluated. For example, if something is unethical for you to do of your own volition, it is equally unethical to do when someone persuades you to do it. What about unintended outcomes? Suppose one of the people above persuaded the stranger to eat more fruit to improve his or her health, and the stranger proved to be severely allergic to a specific fruit and died after ingesting it. This unfortunate but unintended outcome would not be considered reasonably predictable, and the persuader would not be held responsible for the outcome. However, if this was a common allergy and the ensuing reaction was reasonably predictable, the persuader would have to be called to account. Designers of persuasive technologies should be held responsible only for reasonably predictable and unethical outcomes, and Table 1-2 can be used as a guide to ethical responsibility.

Software engineers can create active persuasive agents and therefore are more accountable for the persuasive nature of their work and especially for the persuasive methods that these agents employ. Software engineers should never be reduced to the level of mercenaries, such that they perform work for hire without sharing in the responsibility for it. Certain acts of persuasion may not be practical without technology. For example, it would be difficult to persuade someone through conventional means to maintain the proper pulse rate during exercise, but a simple biofeedback monitor can intervene appropriately. The implementation of persuasive technologies in domains where conventional persuasive techniques are difficult at best calls for heightened ethical scrutiny.

Legal Considerations

The law also imposes standards on the quality of software. When software does not perform as expected, the software providers may be subject to suit under contract or tort theories. For

Table 1-2   Levels of Ethical Responsibility Associated with Predictable and Unpredictable Intended and Unintended Consequences

If the . . .	Outcome					
is . . .	**Intended**		**Unintended**			
and . . .			reasonably predictable		not reasonably predictable	
and . . .	ethical	unethical	ethical	unethical	ethical	unethical
then the designer is . . .	praiseworthy	responsible and at fault	not responsible	responsible and at fault	not responsible	not responsible

example, a purchaser could bring a breach of contract action against the producer of faulty software, claiming breach of express warranty or breach of implied warranty. Those harmed by faulty software may bring tort claim against the provider by means of four doctrines: negligence, misrepresentation, strict liability, and professional malpractice. If the claim is negligence, the cost to the provider of preventing the harm would be compared to the foreseeability and to the severity of the harm that materialized. That result would be a standard of care to the buyer or user of the software. If misrepresentation is claimed, the plaintiff would have to show that the developer either carelessly or intentionally made misrepresentations about the software. If the claim relates to strict liability, the developer must be found liable whether at fault or not. Finally, when software is considered a service rather than a good, software developers may be sued for professional malpractice; they are held to a standard that is not that of a professional programmer, but rather in the field of the purchaser.

William Norris, the chairman of Control Data Corporation, has said that the technological wheel is being wastefully reinvented every day (Breton 1981). Technical blindness has many costs; one of the most important is legal. When a medical device is improperly designed or constructed, there is a risk that somebody will get hurt. With the increasing use of technology, this risk has grown to the point where just about every engineer and scientist should be concerned. It has been estimated that 25 percent of all new-product litigation alleges engineering negligence and that most technical negligence is due to the designer's failure to use readily available information (Breton 1981).

With the continuing rapid advance of technology, product development grows more complex. Even as the design problems increase, products are being used in newer and more demanding applications. Computers on board the Boeing 777 jet airliner contain over 2 million lines of code (Sabbagh 1996). Television sets contain hundreds of thousands of microprogram instructions, automobiles are controlled by networks of interconnected computers and software, and medical devices are becoming ever more complicated. Design mistakes in such products can easily lead to costly manufacturing changes, embarrassing product recalls, product development delays, or even physical damage and death. The potential risks of poor-quality technical work are increasing every day.

Products get used in many ways, and each new application creates added liabilities. To be reasonably safe, software engineers should be aware of the latest advances in their fields and use this knowledge in their work. If they do not, their work may be deemed incompetent and costly to correct. It is both safer and cheaper to know the subject and use the knowledge than to face the risk of product liability.

The Software Crisis

It is a commonly held perception that there exists a "software crisis." Personal experiences with company software projects have contributed to this notion, and the U.S. General Accounting Office (GAO) has released data showing that a horrendous percentage of government software projects already in trouble were never successfully completed, adding to the perception that software is in trouble. The software crisis, however, has neither been proven to exist nor analyzed as to its root causes.

Suppose that there is a software crisis and that many medical device software projects are behind schedule, over budget, unreliable, and unsafe. If you subscribe to the scientific theory that says the simplest solution that covers all of the observed phenomena is correct, then the cause of the software crisis really is that we do a bad job of estimating how long it will take to develop software. Obviously, a poor estimation will lead to high cost and poor schedule performance because meeting cost and schedule goals were based on estimates that were never valid to begin with. This, in turn, will tend to contribute to unreliable software, because software projects workers, on finding that they are badly behind schedule, will tend to skimp, particularly on testing, and release software that inherently contains more errors. The software crisis is not about how we actually construct software but about how we think we build software. It is not the technology of software development that is the problem; it is the management of that technology. It is extremely unlikely that a management problem will be solved by technical solutions.

Suppose that the software crisis is a management problem. To solve it, better ways to estimate software project schedule and effort could be derived, but this solution relegates the problem to the technology arena. Better algorithms for software project estimations can be found; in fact, they have been known since the 1980s. We are better off using these algorithms even if they have not proved to be particularly accurate in their predictions. Estimation algorithms by themselves are not the entire solution to the crisis. Managers and organizations who understand the complexities and intricacies of software development are needed also.

Consider the environment in which the software engineer creates project estimates. Someone conceives of a medical product that requires software. Not only does this idea seem so good that everybody wanted the product yesterday, but marketing and sales are already pushing to have the product ready. Engineering in general pushes to have it available when its interface, prototype, or working model is to be available. In other cases, corporate management pushes because the product allows the company to dominate an important product arena. The schedule pressures become enormous, and the software group typically responds in one of three ways:

1. They give in to the desired schedule dates rather than holding firm to their own best estimates.

2. They give estimates at the start of the project and then attempt to manage it on that schedule even as they learn more about the magnitude of the product and its requirements.

3. They live and die by estimates that were generated before the requirements were fully defined or solidified. In reality, their estimates are given before the problem to be solved was understood.

We may not fully understand what caused the software crisis or even if there really is one, but software development cost and schedule performance are perceived as abysmal, and poor management, not poor technology, as the most likely culprit.

The Quality Characteristics of an Engineering Discipline

To comprehend software quality assurance, it is important to understand that software development is a technical activity called software engineering. It makes sense, then, to discuss the quality characteristics of an engineering discipline in general. The success or failure of many engineering efforts often assumes the attributes of luck, fate, or destiny. However, engineering generally is not based on any of these characteristics. The fundamental underpinning for all engineering disciplines is that an individual can systematically and predictably arrive at pragmatic, cost-effective, and timely solutions to real-world problems.

Engineers have a significant degree of control and influence over the outcome of their engineering effort because the best engineering practices and techniques have well-defined attributes and characteristics that can be described both quantitatively and qualitatively, and they can be used repeatedly in order to achieve similar results each time. The best engineering practices and techniques can be taught to other engineers in a reasonable time frame, and they can be applied by others with a reasonable level of confidence and success. The best such practices and techniques achieve significantly and consistently better results than any other techniques, and they are applicable in a large number of cases and applications.

True engineers are not magicians. When a good engineer discovers an apparently better way of doing a job, that individual attempts to inform others of the method. Magicians, on the other hand, must keep their techniques shrouded in mystery. A good engineer is not a "guru" or a "wizard." A good engineer is talented, gifted, and intuitive and can effectively communicate to others the techniques that were used in order to achieve a higher rate of success than was previously the norm.

Engineering is also different from science. Engineering uses science, mathematics, error analysis, configuration management, risk assessment, and reusability. Engineering also utilizes communication skills to develop pragmatic, cost-effective, and timely solutions to real-world problems. Although most scientists are not engineers, engineers must have a firm foundation in the sciences.

Software Quality Dimensions

The quality of a medical device containing software can be defined in three dimensions: feature set, schedule, and reliability. The feature set defines the product and represents the what and how of the device. Schedule means simply shipping the product on time. The third dimension, reliability, is the traditional focus of product quality. For a medical device, reliability assumes a wide gamut of characteristics, from dependable to safe, but underlying the reliable dimension is the concept of the rate at which an end user will encounter anomalies. Implementation of the product software through coding and testing is meant to maintain the product's reliability while new features are being added and to increase reliability until it is good enough for the product to be released.

Depending on the market and available technology, the relative importance of each of these quality dimensions may differ. For example, a low number of defects might be the most important factor in a mature market where the competing products are not otherwise differentiated. In another situation, being first to market may take precedence over reliability. At another time, product definition and schedule may be relatively more important than the number of defects. Features may be cut from a product in order to increase the amount of time that is available for testing or to increase the certainty of making the ship date.

While the relative importance of each quality dimension may change in proportion to the others, the absolute importance of each should be high within the product development group. A company cannot succeed unless the capability of the software group is very high. The cost of shipping a product with a recall-class defect can be fatal to the profitability of an organization. If a product is recalled, production units may have to be scrapped, inventory may have to be returned, and replacement products manufactured and distributed; recalling a product may require re-releasing foreign language versions as well. Even if the defects do not warrant a recall, they may incur higher support costs, which may be charged directly to the business unit that produces the product. If a product is late, it may never capture the market share that it has lost to the competition, and if it lacks imagination, features, and functionality, it will tend to have a short life in the market.

The important aspect of these quality dimensions is that they can be traded off against each other, but none can be expanded unilaterally without serious consequence to the others. As evidenced by the marketplace, medical devices and instruments are becoming more sophisticated and, therefore, more complicated. If the underlying technical approach to developing products remains unchanged, then the enormous effort required to program the product software is probably the way of the future. This means that both financial and resource commitments will increase significantly over each succeeding project. To offset this trend and assure that the overall product and specifically that the software development process stays under control, three basic approaches can be pursued:

1. Reduce product features.

2. Change the underlying technology base.

3. Allow software to complete product requirements and feature definitions before any hardware work is begun.

To achieve shorter development schedules, particularly in software, a combination of these approaches could be implemented. For example, the scope of the features per release can be reduced, thus reducing the software effort. This does imply more frequent product releases in order to deliver ultimately the entire feature set to the user.

The technology base can be shifted away from a monolithic technology architecture and toward a distributed system in which features and technologies are developed in parallel by small teams on stand-alone processors. Each individual processor could then report to a master processor, which would monitor the status and condition of the technologies resident on those other processors. A distributed system has several long-term effects:

- It is easier to develop stand-alone features on a single processor and then monitor the multiprocessor environment than it is to integrate all product features onto a single processor.

- Products that are developed in this manner can be shipped with "plug-compatible" features, such that clients or users can select the features (technologies) they want.

- If one technology (feature) is not maturing as fast as expected, it need not hold up the entire product.

- Regulatory agencies find that verifying the design, safety, and efficacy of an instrument is generally simplified with this type of architecture.

- This system allows an organization to direct and increase its core competencies, technologies, and features rather than merely managing products.

Starting the software development process earlier than development of the hardware counterpart would help to alleviate several inherent problems with software development. First, because software is usually on the schedule's critical path, starting it early would allow it to be the pacing effort on a project rather than the catch-up effort. Second, an early start would allow the gathering and solidifying of the feature set, which is what software development needs in order to begin in earnest. This, in turn, would allow the software group to document and define the requirements of the hardware before the hardware group begins conceptual design. Third, beginning software development first would help to alleviate the problem of memory having to be upgraded because the software cannot fit in the available memory. Increasing the memory of hardware that has already been developed can increase the cost of an instrument significantly.

The approach to product definition and software development must be carefully examined and altered in order to lessen the escalation of development schedules and development effort. While no one solution to this problem will be the elixir, various combinations will lead to success for product development in general and software in particular. Limiting the feature set of medical products in any given release will help software development because the quantity of features is directly proportional to the number of lines of code required to implement a feature, and the number of lines of code is directly proportional to the development effort and schedule. Adopting a technology base that is centered around independent processors holding the various features will allow manufacturers to return to small (one-, two-, or even five-person) software development teams, allow shorter and more manageable software development schedules, and allow manufacturers to manage their technology more intelligently. Letting the software group lead the way in product development would allow the most frequent critical-path activities to begin early, allow the requirements that are feature driven to mature and solidify earlier, and allow the hardware to be designed such that the software would have a reasonable growth margin.

2

The Components of a Software Quality Assurance Program

A bad beginning makes a bad ending.

—Euripides

In the 1970s, many quality managers and quality engineers felt that software quality assurance was an issue they would rather see just go away. Software quality assurance was a new world that embraced new and different technologies as well as foreign practices. To quality managers and engineers, it meant dealing with a new breed of technical people, some of whom had bizarre personalities, personal traits, and outlooks on the professional world. It meant that entirely new methods and ways of communicating would have to be learned, along with a new technical lexicon. The feeling among software managers about quality managers and quality engineers was the same. Some software managers were fond of intimating that quality was not what was really needed in software, and therefore, quality assurance could do nothing for software.

If the software quality assurance role in vogue then was restricted to the level of inspecting the holes that were punched into the Hollerith cards of the time, then these feelings would have been justified. However, what both quality engineers and software engineers learned was that the scope of software quality assurance extends over the entire life cycle of the product. It begins with the conceptual stage, in which the decision is made that software is needed to support the new product, and it ends with the removal of the device containing that software from the marketplace. The customers of software quality assurance include the device user, software engineers, upper management, and the software industry as a whole.

The fundamental purpose of the software quality assurance program is to ensure that medical device software is of high quality, that it is reliable, and that it is safe. The classic yardstick for assuring that a device works reliably has usually come at the end of the development process, when tests are conducted that yield some measure of reliability with some degree of confidence. However, since software is an intellectually created product, software engineering differs from other engineering disciplines; consequently, no test is sufficiently comprehensive to adequately test all aspects of software. With this in mind, software quality assurance embraces two fundamental philosophies:

1. It assures that the device software meets its intended requirements and implements its intended design.

2. It assures that the device software was constructed according to the device manufacturer's documented software development process.

Software quality assurance, then, is founded on a systematic approach that is documented and well defined, and it incorporates measurable milestones for the tasks and end products to be verified as consistent with the device's intended functions and operations, as well as with the constraints of the development environment. Because software quality assurance is a comprehensive, all-encompassing philosophy that embraces all of the software and device life cycle, all aspects of both life cycles must be covered in a systematic and rigorous fashion. After all, software quality cannot be ascertained nor assured if there is no documented process of assessment. There is more than one way to develop a systematic software quality assurance program, as this chapter shows.

Aspects of Quality

The term *quality* is usually defined as the degree of conformance to specifications and/or workmanship standards. However, although quality reflects this conformance at a particular instant of time, the traditional concept of quality does not really include any notion of time. For example, medical device quality is frequently assessed against a specification or a set of attributes and, assuming that the device has passed this assessment, it is then delivered to the customer, accompanied by a warranty. The customer is relieved of the cost implications of an early device failure by the warranty and believes that the device will not fail until sometime in the distant future. This way of doing business assumes two things:

1. No measure of the device's quality is provided outside of the warranty period.

2. The device's quality outside of the warranty period is the responsibility of the customer and not of the manufacturer.

The need for a time-based measure of quality is satisfied by the concept of reliability. Reliability is the estimation, control, and management of the probability that a device will fail over time. Medical device quality is assessed not only against a specification or a set of attributes, but also against a mean time between failures (MTBF), the metric by which reliability is designed into the product. This means that device manufacturers recognize that continuation of product success as well as a satisfied customer base is responsible for ensuring the quality of the device beyond the warranty period.

The Role of Quality

The keys to understanding the potential contributions of software quality assurance can be found in the historical examples of the distance between quality and the production of goods and services. Quality involves monitoring of the adherence to standards; any deviation or compromise of the established performance, methods, or acceptance criteria is viewed as just that. Quality is an impartial judgment that a deviation has occurred, without regard to the impact or relevancy of the compromise. This independent position has made quality the traditional instrument of management for the unbiased validation of product conformity to specified performance.

Additionally, quality involves both keeping and using records in the performance of the quality function. The software community has rarely been able to record its defect histories in a manner that would permit the use of past problems for the benefit of current projects. Although software metrics are becoming more prevalent, the vast majority of software practitioners still do not record defects meaningfully. Software industry studies have documented the fact that roughly half of all software activity is spent in the search for and the correction of defects.

In the absence of any objective software evaluation, the first hint that a software development project is in trouble usually appears at some point after the software testing has begun; under the worst of practices, it occurs after the customer receives the device. Reviews of the software requirements definition and of the software design material can provide keen insights into the software aspects of the project long before testing begins. This insight can also allow for the correction of deviations or compromises and the reduction of internal software complexities.

Because of the past track record of software development for overbudgeting and late deliveries, management in general has learned to be wary of software development projects. In many instances, management has sought reassurance by requiring software development personnel to report the software development status in a tedious battery of reports generated at frequent intervals. This is not only time-consuming, but it can also be counterproductive, especially when it diverts software management away from its task of managing software development or maintenance activities. From the software management standpoint, many of these reports are cursory and reflect the priorities of software management. In theory, the reports might be useful, but in practice they are probably unreliable. Management's fear that the current software development project might join the history of software cost, schedule, or performance disasters is understandable. However, required reports are not a solution to the problem, but a reaction to the circumstances. If software quality assurance did nothing more than provide a better window for management to glimpse impending software problems, its existence would be justified.

Software quality assurance provides not only this window, but much more. An effective software quality assurance program, paradoxically, reduces much of the need for these glimpses, by helping to prevent problems and by helping to solve many of the problems that do occur. The essence of software quality assurance is to prevent problems and to remove any defects from the software. Quality assurance also contributes to the reusability and maintainability of the code, improves the productivity of code generation, and makes software development generally more efficient.

The adoption of software practices and techniques is primarily the responsibility of the software group rather than of the quality group. The quality organization may encourage, support, and participate in the development of these standards, but software developers own the responsibility for setting their software standards. Management's participation involves understanding and approving the standards created by the software group. Whatever the defined software standards, it is quality's function to make certain that those standards are adhered to.

The intent of software standards is to establish uniform, consistent, and disciplined software practices and techniques that foster software productivity, efficiency, acceptable performance, predictability, and control. These standards are, of course, confining in numerous ways; at times, there will be pressure to circumvent or compromise these standards, usually when the standards are most needed. The function of the software quality assurance program is to maintain control during these times by acting to avoid such lapses.

The Role of Reliability

Reliability is an extensively used but greatly misunderstood term. Reliability in a medical device indicates the dependability of the device for performing a required function under stated conditions for a specified period of time. It is a characteristic that must be planned, designed, and then manufactured into the device. Reliability is a philosophy that dictates quantitatively just how good the medical device should be. To fully comprehend this concept, its opposite should be examined. Unreliability is the measure of the potential failure of the device, and it reflects lack of planning for the design and manufacturing activities.

The consequences of unreliability are antithetical to good engineering and business practices. Unreliability can lead to high development costs, which are usually passed to the customer in the form of higher sales prices. Another consequence of unreliability is squandered engineering and manufacturing time, which can also be equated to higher costs. Unreliability will cause customer inconvenience and will eventually guarantee a poor reputation.

To ensure the utmost reliability, processes that avoid the causes of unreliability should be installed and institutionalized. These processes should stress the elimination of improper designs and inappropriate materials. Reliable processes reduce manufacturing, assembly, and inspection errors. Processes that support reliability reduce and help to eliminate improper testing, packaging, and shipping. Finally, reliability processes help to ensure the proper device operations at start-up, help reduce the impact of misuse, and help prevent misapplication of the device.

Reliability encompasses three key requirements. First, the device must be fully specified as far as possible prior to design. It must ultimately perform the required functions specified through activities such as customer and market surveys. Second, the device must perform its functions without failure for a specified length of time. Normal operation of the device must be defined in order to understand what a failure is, as well as anticipating the misuse or abuse to which the device could be subjected. The life expectancy of the device as well as the expected daily usage for it are delineated. Third, the device must perform under a set of predefined conditions. The environment in which the device operates must be specified, including temperature ranges, humidity ranges, methods of shipping, shock and vibration, and electromagnetic and radio frequency interference and emission from associated or nearby equipment.

Developing a design to meet these reliability requirements will result in a product that is appropriate for its market. Reliability requires that fault-tolerant engineering design techniques, practices, processes, and principles were used. Another requirement is that the manufacturing processes will work with the development processes so that the reliability of the device will not be affected during production.

Reliability is a disciplined engineering practice that provides the tools needed to evaluate, with confidence, the functionality of the device or its components by forming a structured approach to its life cycle. To provide this functionality, reliability engineering relies on basic mathematics and statistics, current regulatory standards, and disciplined engineering design practices. It draws upon system interface principles, human factors such as ergonomics and common sense, and cost-benefit analysis. It depends on software quality assurance.

Device reliability can be defined for the system as a whole. However, within the different engineering disciplines, reliability has different characteristics. For example, the device's electronic reliability depends on the age of a component or assembly, for which the rate of failure is defined in terms of the number of malfunctions that occur during a given period of time. The electronic failure rate is initially very high, decreases rapidly, and then stabilizes. During this stable period, the failure rate of the components is typically constant; eventually, the failure rate increases rapidly. The device's mechanical reliability differs from electronic reliability in its reaction to aging. Mechanical failure begins at a rate of zero and then increases rapidly.

The device's software, however, is not subject to the physical constraints of its hardware counterparts. Software reliability is the probability that the device software will not cause the failure of the product for a specified time under specified conditions. Software reliability is a function of the inputs to and the usage of the device, as well as of faults within the software. The inputs to the device determine whether accidental conditions exist that may cause the software to fail to perform its required function. Once these errors or bugs are removed, the software itself will operate without that failure.

The Role of Device Reliability

The reliability bathtub-curve model (generically shown in Figure 2-1) represents the life cycle of a medical device. In this model, some of the device's components fail in the initial period of use, followed by a useful life of few or no failures, and finish with a period called wear-out. The bathtub curve is a graph of the device failure rate versus the age of the device. The device manufacturer's objective is to optimize the device life cycle over all three of these periods.

The major factors that influence and eventually degrade the device's operational reliability must be addressed during design, thus facilitating the control and maximization of the device's reliability. Early electronic life-cycle failures can be offset and even eliminated by a systematic and controlled process that screens and burns in the appropriate components and assemblies. Mechanical stress-related failures are minimized through the provision of adequate design margins, not only for each component, but also for the device as a whole. Wear-out failures may also be eliminated through the use of a judicious preventive maintenance program in which the affected components are replaced.

Subjecting a medical device to a reliability program provides a disciplined and structured approach to the product development process. It provides techniques that improve the quality of the device over time and that reduce development time and cost. The reliability program can provide data that quantify the success of the development process and at the same time predict

Figure 2-1   Reliability bathtub-curve model

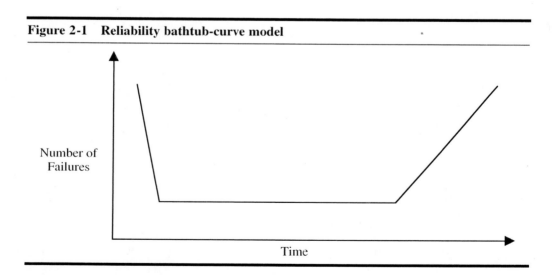

Number of
Failures

Time

the device's future performance. The program also assures that the device will meet regulatory requirements and gives confidence that subsequent regulatory audits and inspections will produce no major discrepancies. Use of the various reliability techniques in the hardware and software areas will result in decreased warranty costs and, therefore, help increase customer acceptance of the manufacturer and the device. Reliability techniques will also help to reduce liability risks by assuring that safety has been a primary concern during the design and development of the device.

Overview of the System Design and Software Design Process

The design of an electronics-based medical device can be divided into three major phases, and each of these can be subdivided into other stages of design definition and levels of refinement. The major design phases are system requirements and their associated specifications, component requirements and their specifications, and component design. The process of determining the system requirements and specifications identifies both the hardware and software components. Once the system specifications are reviewed and approved, the hardware and software design activities can proceed in parallel, but not independently of each other (see Figure 2-2).

System Design Process

The device's system requirements include user needs, operational and environmental conditions, and maintenance considerations. For a medical device, the system requirements phase begins with a set of inputs such as product goals, clinical approaches, market constraints, and safety factors. Analysis of these data in conjunction with hazard and risk analysis results in the system requirements that explicitly define the environmental conditions, physical limitations, and equipment capabilities of the system. The system requirements will also define the performance, safety, human-factor, and timing requirements.

Figure 2-2   Overview of system design and software design process

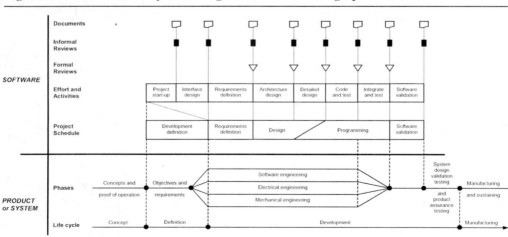

System specifications are an amplification of the system requirements in relation to the system architecture. The system requirements focus on components and interactions, such as device failure functions, user interface components, the isolation and propagation of error conditions, and mean time to failure of each component. The system specifications provide a model of the way the proposed system will interact with its environment. This model represents the breakdown of the system into its major hardware and software components. The model describes functions performed by each component, constraints imposed on each component, and the interfaces between each component. Systems analysis tools are available to support the development of the specification models.

For embedded systems, decisions must be made regarding the target microprocessor, the software operating system or executive for the device, and the software development environment. Each of these elements significantly affects which parts of the system will be implemented in hardware and which parts will be implemented in software. Consequently, it is imperative that the system specifications be completed before the software and hardware development efforts begin. Making changes to the system during the system requirements and specification phase is relatively straightforward and cost-effective. Changes to these specifications later in the process are often difficult to accommodate, can compromise the system reliability, and require unplanned efforts and resources.

Management attitudes toward the review process are important to the success of the design process. Reviews must be held at the conclusion of the systems requirements activities and following the generation of the system requirements specifications. Treating the reviews informally and documenting them poorly can be major contributors to inaccurate or incomplete specifications. Guidelines for the review process can provide an effective framework from which to develop a thorough review methodology.

During the second phase of the system design process, parallel development of the system's hardware and software begins. The initial steps in the software development phase are similar to those in the systems requirements and specifications phase. The software requirements are defined and a functional specification is produced. At this stage, techniques that employ mathematical notation, formal languages, and formal logic provide unambiguous and concise methods for establishing the software requirements. Techniques for determining the safety requirements and specifications for embedded systems include hazard analysis, fault-tree analysis, failure modes and effects analysis, and risk assessment. Because of the parallel development of the hardware and software components, the respective specifications will impose changes on each other. For example, timing studies or hazard analysis for a hardware specification might result in additional timing, safety, or functional requirements for a software component, and vice versa. To address these interdependencies, designers conduct trade-off studies to develop the best balance among the various components and to facilitate accurate and timely communications between the software and hardware development teams.

The software requirements and specifications steps conclude with a formal review to ascertain the correctness and assess the robustness of the specifications. Correctness distinguishes the correct system behavior and response from all possible behavior responses by the system; robustness determines that the specification addresses all possible conditions, constraints, and assumptions placed on the system. The review process includes personnel from the relevant engineering disciplines, such as system design, software architecture and design, hardware design, software quality assurance, software safety, and regulatory affairs. The selected reviewers need to have adequate experience and training to ensure that they bring the necessary expertise to the review process.

Software Design Process

The software requirements and specifications phase is followed by the software design phase. This is typically divided into the top-level architecture design and the detailed design phases. The architecture design phase is the conversion of the software requirements into the major components, modules, routines, functions, or tasks that will become the executable code. The architecture design delineates the control logic, data flows, function orientation, and global data structures. An architectural design document describes the responsibility of each module, discusses design alternatives, and provides the rationale for the chosen design. As a part of the architecture design, an interface design document provides a complete black-box description of each module's interface from the hardware and software standpoints.

In an embedded system, several factors can influence the architecture design and must be resolved before actual development can begin. The performance requirements of the software design must be weighed against the speed of the selected hardware, and the anticipated memory requirements of the program must be reviewed against the memory allocations that were made during the system design phase. The structure of the software modules can be affected by any number of issues. Among these are: Is the design maintainable? Can new features be added easily? Are like functions grouped together? Are the interfaces clear, distinct, and well defined? Are extraneous data being passed? Are inconsistent units being passed or used?

The detailed design phase entails the refinement of the architecture design, the definition of local data structures, algorithms, and development of the logical functions within each module. In the detailed design phase, the level of refinement, definition, and detail increases throughout the phase. For example, functional performance and memory data and management are reviewed by each of the individual module designers. Frequently, programming design languages or graphically oriented computer-aided software engineering (CASE) tools are used to facilitate and capture the design as it matures and to help with the generation of the design documentation.

Both the architecture and detailed design phases are formally reviewed before the next stage of software development. For architecture designs, the purpose of the review is to assess the structure, modularity, interface simplicity, interface precision, cohesiveness, and completeness of the design. The reviewers examine noncritical software interaction with identifiable critical sections of the structure and ensure that the design meets the software requirements and specifications. The review team is made up of individuals with strong software design experience and of safety and quality assurance specialists with strong software backgrounds. The detailed design reviews focus on verifying that the data structures, algorithms, and logic design are consistent with the architecture design and function specification. The review team is expanded to include algorithm specialists and configuration management personnel.

Causes of Software Errors

Even when system design includes the phases described above, problems and errors occur. The most insidious problems can often be tracked back to design flaws or to changes in the requirements and specifications that were not passed along to those involved at the software implementation phase. Errors are often located in relatively minor software algorithms and logic; they can go undetected during the many hours of testing of the software. Software problems of any kind can be disastrous. Safety-critical embedded systems in particular need a software development approach that emphasizes the quality assurance of the software development process.

Two important goals of the system design process are the management of the requirements and the prevention of design flaws. Requirements management traces the changes in the requirements and the impact those changes have on the system. These two goals require trained, experienced personnel as well as appropriate support tools, realistic schedules, and adequate finances. If reviews are an integral part of the development process, an inadequate design or specification will most likely be detected. Reviewers can only be effective, however, if they are properly qualified and function independently, and if their recommendations are implemented and tracked.

Effective communication of information is essential. Bad information management can result in reviewers and implementers working from different versions of the specifications. Failure to track reviewer recommendations is also a breakdown in communications and can lead to the inclusion of errors that were thought to be eradicated at the time of the review. Failure to review revised designs is another source of software errors. Changes implemented in one area of code can have repercussions in a seemingly unrelated area of the code. Incomplete, ambiguous, or out-of-date documentation causes errors and problems because it is the documents themselves that represent the system to be built, not the collective memory of the individual developers.

Software Standards and Procedures

Standards offer a starting point for the definition of document templates as well as guidelines for the development of software process models. The standards are not meant to suggest that there are no other ways to perform the practices addressed. Rather, the standards represent the consensus of the committee that developed the standard at the time that the standard was published. Nearly every standard is reviewed periodically; the Institute of Electrical and Electronic Engineers (IEEE) standards are reviewed at least once every five years for revision or reaffirmation.

Development of Standards In House

The effectiveness of the software quality assurance program depends on adherence to a well-defined set of documented software development standards. The software quality assurance personnel must actively participate in the development of these standards and sponsor their uniformity and consistency. The standards and procedures apply to both the software development group and the software quality assurance group.

If the software development function is concentrated within one group of the organization, that group may have a set of well-defined and documented standards. If there is no such set of well-documented software standards or if they are incomplete, then the software quality assurance personnel should urge the formalization and completion of these standards and their management. If the software development function is decentralized, which is the usual case, then there is probably no set of standards common to all of the various groups and probably one or more groups who have no standards at all. In this instance, the software quality assurance personnel should urge that all of the groups and their appropriate managers get together in order to establish documented standards. Not only should the documents be generated for each group, but also they should exhibit as much commonality as possible.

The software quality assurance function needs to operate with a given set of software development standards, but the quality assurance function also needs a documented standard of its own. This standard could be a single plan or a set of plans if the diversity of the software that is developed warrants it. The intent is that the software quality assurance standard will provide much of the background needed for project-specific software quality assurance activities and functions. A set of procedures should be assembled that outline the manner in which software quality assurance personnel carry out each activity. These plans and procedures will then reflect the quality assurance groups' approach to software development. These standards will be updated to reflect any changes that are implemented in the software development activities.

The need for direct cooperation between the software development group and the software quality assurance group may lead to the assumption that software quality assurance can be established on an informal basis. Real life has demonstrated that this does not work. The role of software quality assurance must be explicitly drawn and made clear to all individuals concerned. The proper instrument for documenting the software quality assurance function and activities is a policy on software quality assurance. This vehicle clearly demonstrates the corporation's commitment to the tenets of software quality assurance and encourages support of it. This level of commitment cannot necessarily be attained with a departmental directive or initiative. In addition to establishing the framework for software quality assurance activities, the policy should also clearly establish the software quality assurance group as the part of the corporation that is charged with the responsibility and empowered with the authority for assuring the quality of the software delivered to the customer. The policy is extended to cover all software purchased or procured from outside commercial vendors for use within the corporation and related to device development.

Industry Software Engineering Standards

The creation and generation of software quality assurance standards is not particularly difficult. Numerous industry standards have been published, supported, and maintained over the years by various organizations and professional societies (see Table 2-1). The concepts and approaches to the various aspects of software quality assurance are so similar that they can be used nearly interchangeably. Some of the standards may be implemented verbatim or modified to suit the business philosophies, culture, and environment of the company.

Several of the IEEE standards are referenced in the FDA's principal guidance documents, although the Food and Drug Administration (FDA) does not specifically require them. The *Standard for Software Quality Assurance Plans* (ANSI/IEEE Std 730-1989) provides a generic framework for defining quality assurance activities that are performed during the life cycle of a software development project. The plan identifies tasks including reviews and audits, quality measures, test activities, problem reporting, training requirements, supplier controls, and control of code and documentation. The standard can be augmented to reflect the conduct and review of hazard analysis. The *Standard for Software Test Documentation* (ANSI/IEEE Std 829-1983) provides a comprehensive set of documents that support the conduct and documentation of the software testing process. Templates, proposed outlines, and an explanation of purpose are provided for a test plan, test design specification, test case specification, test procedure specification, test item transmittal report, test log, and test incident report.

The *Standard for Software Requirements Specifications* (ANSI/IEEE Std 830-1984) provides an overview of the background and general characteristics of a quality software requirements specification and several examples of ways to construct this specification. The standard also provides candidate outlines for the principal section that defines specific requirements, and the developer can then select the outline that presents the medical device requirements in the most readable manner. This standard has been criticized because it defines the system from a functional perspective and is not particularly adaptable for object-oriented development methods.

Table 2-1   Partial List of Software Engineering Standards

Standard Number	Standard Title
ANSI/IEEE Std 730-1989	Software Quality Assurance Plan
ANSI/IEEE Std 828-1990	Software Configuration Management Plan
ANSI/IEEE Std 829-1983	Software Test Documentation
ANSI/IEEE Std 830-1984	Software Requirements Specifications
ANSI/IEEE Std 983-1986	Software Quality Assurance Planning
ANSI/IEEE Std 1002-1987	Taxonomy for Software Engineering Standards
ANSI/IEEE Std 1008-1987	Software Unit Testing
ANSI/IEEE Std 1012-1986	Software Verification and Validation Plans
ANSI/IEEE Std 1016-1986	Recommended Practice for Software Design Descriptions
ANSI/IEEE Std 1028-1988	Standard for Software Reviews and Audits
ANSI/IEEE Std 1042-1987	Guide to Software Configuration Management
ANSI/IEEE Std 1058-1987	Standard for Software Project Management Plans
ANSI/IEEE Std 1063	Standard for Software User Documentation
DOD-STD-2167	Defense Systems Software Development
DOD-STD-2168	Software Quality Evaluation
DOD-STD-7935	Automated Data Systems Documentation
FAA-STD-018	Computer Software Quality Program Requirements
IEC 601-4	Safety Requirements for Programmable Electronic Medical Systems
IEEE Std 610.12-1990	Standard Glossary of Software Engineering Terminology
IEEE Std 982.1-1988	Standard Dictionary of Measures to Produce Reliable Software
IEEE Std 982.2-1988	Guide for the Use of IEEE Standard Dictionary of Measures to Produce Reliable Software
IEEE Std 1016.1-1993	Guide to Software Design Descriptions
IEEE Std 1045-1992	Standard for Software Productivity Metrics
IEEE Std 1059-1993	Guide for Software Verification and Validation Plans
IEEE Std 1061-1992	Standard for a Software Quality Metrics Methodology
IEEE Std 1074-1991	Standard for Developing Software Life Cycle Processes
IEEE Std 1219-1992	Standard for Software Maintenance
ISO 9000-3	Software Guide to ISO 9001

Continued on next page.

Continued from previous page.

Standard Number	Standard Title
IEEE Std 1298-1992	Software Quality Management System, Part 1: Requirements
MIL-S-52779	Software Quality Assurance Program Requirements
MIL-STD-SQAM	Software Quality Assurance Assessment and Measurement
MIL-STD-470	Maintaining Program Requirements for Systems and Equipment
MIL-STD-480	Configuration Control—Engineering Changes, Deviations, and Waivers
MIL-STD-481	Configuration Control—Engineering Changes, Deviations, and Waivers (Short Form)
MIL-STD-482	Configuration Status Accounting Data Elements and Related Features
MIL-STD-483	Configuration Management Practices for Systems, Equipment, Munitions, and Computer Programs
MIL-STD-490	Specification Practices
MIL-STD-881	WBSs for Defense Material Items
MIL-STD-1521	Technical Reviews and Audits for Systems, Equipment, and Computer Programs
MIL-STD-1535	Supplier QA Program Requirements
MIL-STD-1679	Software Development
VDE 0801	Principles for Computers in Systems with Safety-Related Tasks

The standard could be augmented in two areas—the conduct and review of hazard analysis efforts and the validation activities that will be performed. The validation section could include a software requirements traceability matrix and requirements for testing at the unit, integration, and system levels.

The IEEE *Standard for Software Verification and Validation Plans* (ANSI/IEEE Std 1012-1986) provides a framework for defining the responsibilities of the developer and quality assurance personnel during the software development life cycle. It also provides a suggested outline and a description of each activity to be performed for a verification and validation plan. The standard includes a diagram that shows verification and validation activities that may be applied for various phases of the software development effort. The proposed tasks in this standard represent a comprehensive validation program that may not be applicable to every development effort. The standard can be augmented to support the definition of hazard analysis activities and the oversight of third-party software developers.

The IEEE *Recommended Practice for Software Design Descriptions* (ANSI/IEEE Std 1016-1987) defines a recommended practice for describing a software design and is meant to be independent of the design methodology. The standard provides a discussion of the organization of design documents and a sample table of contents. The major sections include decomposition description, dependency description, interface description, and detailed design. This standard has been criticized because it lacks a comprehensive description for all sections of the design document and is heavily oriented toward the use of functional design methods. Some of these weaknesses have been addressed in the IEEE *Guide to Software Design Descriptions* (IEEE Std 1016.1-1993). This standard provides much of the requested detail and also presents specific examples that reflect the major design methods not addressed in IEEE Std 1016. The latter standard is more consistent with the FDA 510(k) reviewer guidance requirements.

Another strategy is to tailor the standards to reflect the various types of medical devices that are produced by the company and as used by the customers. For example, instead of a single, monolithic set of standards being used on all software development projects, one complete set of standards could be defined for each level of concern related to a device produced by the organization. This means that the standards for each level of concern would be geared to support only the set of requirements needed to meet the expectations of the appropriate regulatory agency.

A possible advantage exists with adapting the military or government software standards for use by a corporation. Many of these standards provide ready-to-use, complete document outline templates that include written descriptions of the desired contents for each section of the document. Thus, the software staff would not need to develop document contents from scratch. This approach can easily provide the foundations for software development standards and their supporting documentation; suitable modifications can be made for use by medical instrument companies.

Software Staffing and Organizing

To implement an effective software quality assurance program, it is necessary to understand that software quality assurance is concerned with built-in quality, rather than with the quality that can be derived from inspections or any of the other after-the-fact techniques associated with hardware disciplines. Software quality assurance, therefore, is intimately involved with all phases of the software life cycle, particularly design. The software quality assurance function should be staffed by individuals who command a comprehensive understanding of software engineering. The best candidates are, of course, other software professionals.

This does not necessarily mean that the software department must be fully staffed with only software engineering professionals. With a viable software quality assurance program defined and implemented, quality engineers, for example, can be trained to augment the duties, responsibilities, assignments, and activities of software quality assurance engineering professionals. Quality engineers can then consult the appropriate software personnel concerning software quality assurance matters about which they are uncertain. The tacit assumption, however, is that explicit software quality assurance procedures are documented and available. Eventually, the quality engineer who is trained in software quality assurance will become reasonably proficient, competent, and independent; however, it should be obvious that at least one software engineer must be made available to provide guidance and serve as a trainer for the quality engineers.

There is a scarcity of competent software engineers, and software quality engineering is competing with software development in the open market for software quality assurance individuals. This competition is not on a particularly level playing field. Software development offers the opportunity to create software rather than to control it. For the majority of technically oriented software engineers, the intellectual satisfaction of building an object usually far outweighs that of monitoring and control of the object. Furthermore, software development usually offers a much stronger and well-defined career path than does software quality assurance. The opportunity to hire professional software engineers to perform software quality assurance activities does exist, however. Just as hardware engineers can have various specialties or areas of concentrations, software engineers also have areas of expertise, and software quality assurance is one of them. Hiring from outside the company will require an extremely aggressive recruitment program, a committed management group, and competitive salaries. The only factor outside the control of the hiring program is the size of the pool of available software quality assurance engineers.

However, the most effective means to obtain a software quality assurance engineer is to transfer a well-respected and competent individual from the existing in-house software development engineering group into the software quality assurance group. There are numerous advantages to this solution:

- The individual is already familiar with the type of software being generated.

- The individual has insight into known weaknesses of the current software development process and methodology.

- The individual has already established a working rapport not only with the other hardware development groups, but also with the regulatory affairs, reliability engineering, and quality engineering groups.

- The individual already knows how to operate within the corporate organization.

The need for the software quality assurance function to be independent from software development engineers cannot be stressed too much. Even where the disciplined approach to software engineering is in effect, a variety of events and circumstances conspire to try to defeat the interests of software quality assurance. At best, software is usually produced under the most aggressive of schedules. All too often, the completion of the system-level analysis and requirements that are needed to define the overall hardware-software configuration may slip, or the hardware does not become available when originally estimated, or the new support software may be delayed. Even though these events occur too frequently on too many projects, the end delivery date seldom changes; the most vulnerable of scheduled activities become targets for elimination. For software, this translates into trying to skip the test planning, skimping on the design documentation, passing over the test documentation, or circumventing configuration control. Only single-minded devotion to quality by a group that is independent of the software design and implementation group can realistically curb these attempts to recover schedule slippages or cost overruns at the expense of software quality. The software quality assurance group must be independent in order to achieve the highest possible quality and reliability results.

In addition to being independent of the software design and implementation group, the software quality assurance group and their activities should report to the same or even a higher level management than those groups it must evaluate and audit. The software quality assurance group must be autonomous, and its reporting management must have the same organizational status and access to management as the software development function. This means that the software quality assurance organizational structure and the individuals within it are of paramount importance in ensuring the implementation, direction, and control of the software quality assurance program.

Implementation of a Software Quality Assurance Program

The quality solution for medical device software rests on the foundation of these technological and managerial techniques and practices that support and encourage orderly, predictable, and controllable software development and maintenance. Medical device software quality cannot be assured in the same manner that adding a rib or a gusset strengthens the case or derating the power dissipation helps the hardware. Software quality must be built in, and the only way to do so is to ensure that all phases of software development and maintenance are organized toward that objective.

Software is the product of a reasoning process; all other engineering disciplines derive from the natural sciences, where their end products are realized in a physical sense and their success can be measured against physical observations. This luxury does not exist for software engineering. The contributions of software engineering are measurable in cost and schedule improvements throughout the entire software life cycle. An additional area of contribution for software engineering is in the cost associated with the reliability of the device over its own life cycle. The best measure of the extent to which software engineering is applied to the development of the device is qualitative. This measure is the degree to which the software development and maintenance are systematic.

As Table 2-2 illustrates, the implementation of a software quality assurance program consists of eight major steps. The first step in implementing the software quality assurance program is to create the software methodology and process infrastructure and document what it is. This infrastructure must address software development, software verification and validation (V&V), and software configuration management. The purpose of this step is to isolate the fundamentally different activities so that each area can be documented in a fashion that facilitates and accommodates ease of understanding and comprehension. These activities should be documented as policies, to give them the enforcement commitment they require.

To support their implementation, a corresponding set of standard operating procedures (SOPs) should be generated, to provide the support, explanation, and instructions relating to the "how" of the policies. The guidelines indicate how to interpret and successfully apply the SOPs and policies on a project. The guidelines also detail the software engineering standards and conventions that would be applied to each device project. In practice, the SOPs and the guidelines evolve as the projects are identified and the policies implemented. The standards and conventions could also be generated after the first project has been completed under the software quality assurance program, and they can be based on lessons learned and ideas tried.

To assess the quality of the software, certain important attributes of it, such as reliability, usability, and maintainability, must be measured. These external product attributes are assessed by observing the behavior of the software during the testing and operation of the product. These measures are derived indirectly from other, direct measures of process attributes. For example, reliability can be measured by an analysis of the failures over periods of operating times. Incidents, faults, defects, and changes are fundamental entities that are observed during software development and testing and the operation of the device. In order to have a sound basis for the derivation of the indirect product measures, the appropriate direct measures must be defined for the attributes of these basic entities. The last activity in creating the software quality assurance program infrastructure is to define the process metrics.

The second step in the software quality assurance program implementation is to target two pilot projects. This step can begin as the first step nears completion, or it can wait until the documents of the first step have been approved. Because of the complexities and intricacies associated with creating the infrastructure of the first step, the initial use of the new software quality

Table 2-2   Outline of Software Quality Assurance Program Implementation

Step Number	Step Description
1.0	Create Methodology and Process Infrastructure Documentation
1.1	Generate software development policies
1.2	Generate software V&V policies
1.3	Generate software configuration management policies
1.4	Generate supporting SOPs
1.5	Generate supporting guidelines
1.6	Generate programming standards and conventions
1.7	Define process metrics
2.0	Select a New Product and an Iterative Product as Pilot Projects
3.0	Software Analysis, Requirements, Design, and Code Generation Tools
4.0	Create the Appropriate Project Software Documents
4.1	Generate software planning documents
4.2	Generate software design documents
4.3	Generate software V&V documents
4.4	Generate software test documents
5.0	Implement the Product Software
5.1	Code, test, and V&V the software
5.2	Integrate, test, and V&V the software
5.3	Validation test the software
5.4	Place software under configuration management
5.5	Collect data related to process metrics
6.0	Project Software Postmortem and Lessons Learned
7.0	Make Updates as Necessary From the Postmortem to the Policies, SOPs, Guidelines and Process Metrics
8.0	Begin the SQA Process Again on the Next Project

Reprinted with permission from Steven R. Mallory, "Building Quality Into Medical Product Software Design," in *Biomedical Instrumentation and Technology*, Vol. 27, No. 1, p. 131, Association for the Advancement of Medical Instrumentation, 1993.

assurance program should be limited to one new family, new platform, or new generation device and one iterative, enhancement, or incremental device. The software quality assurance program is initially limited rather than corporate-wide because it represents a paradigm shift, from whatever the previous software development mentality was to a new, different point of reference. This is usually a transition from an unstructured, but possibly disciplined, approach to a structured and highly disciplined methodology and process; such paradigm shifts are best accomplished by a successful example. The reason for using projects related to both a new product and an iterative product is that the software development environments and techniques are usually sufficiently different from one another to allow the software quality assurance program to be applied in the unique conditions that each type of project represents. In effect, this allows the software quality assurance program to be empirically "tested."

The third step in the software quality assurance program implementation is the integration and use of software development tools. These tools run the gamut from analysis and requirement tools to standard text editors and software compilers and linker-loaders. Software tools are not always given the same managerial consideration as, say, a new tool or a machine that keeps production moving. Most of the available software development tools are oriented toward the improvement of software productivity; quality is usually considered a casual by-product of these tools. However, just as code-productivity tools also enhance software quality, most software quality–oriented tools also improve productivity.

The basic tools provide diagnostics, change tracking, file management, and comparator capability. A more complex class of software tools includes the definition and design processor tools. Figure 2-3 illustrates the type of integration environment that this class should and, in some

Figure 2-3   An example of an integrated CASE environment tool

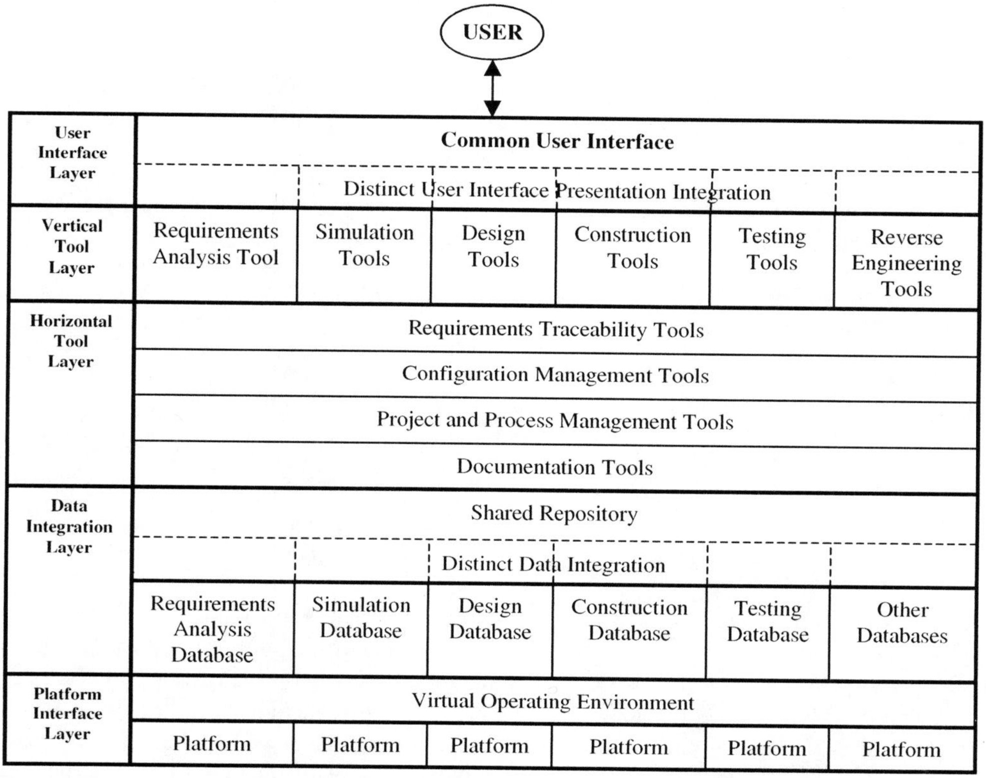

User Interface Layer	Common User Interface					
	Distinct User Interface Presentation Integration					
Vertical Tool Layer	Requirements Analysis Tool	Simulation Tools	Design Tools	Construction Tools	Testing Tools	Reverse Engineering Tools
Horizontal Tool Layer	Requirements Traceability Tools					
	Configuration Management Tools					
	Project and Process Management Tools					
	Documentation Tools					
Data Integration Layer	Shared Repository					
	Distinct Data Integration					
	Requirements Analysis Database	Simulation Database	Design Database	Construction Database	Testing Database	Other Databases
Platform Interface Layer	Virtual Operating Environment					
	Platform	Platform	Platform	Platform	Platform	Platform

Reprinted from Anthony I. Wasserman, "Tool Integration in Software Environments," in *Software Engineering Environments,* ed. F. W. Long, Berlin: Springer-Verlag, 1990, p. 137.

instances, can provide. These computer-aided software engineering (CASE) tools facilitate software requirements analysis, design, and construction activities so that these requirements and design descriptions can be converted directly into usable code. These tools can also provide automated tracking of requirements from initial definition to location within the design and ultimately to final location in the source code.

Regardless of type, software tools should already be in place prior to start-up of the project. However, they can be added to the repertory of tools while the project is ongoing, provided that the integration of the tool into daily use does not adversely disrupt the software development process or disrupt the overall product development schedule and deliverables.

The fourth step in the software quality assurance program implementation occurs after the projects that were identified in step two have begun. The fourth step is concerned with the generation of the appropriate software documents, the first of which are the planning documents. These documents capture the how, what, who, and when of software project activities, specify project software deliverables, and delineate criteria for acceptance of software end products. Software design documents, the next set of project documents generated, capture the design of the device software. The project documents are followed by the verification and validation (V&V) and testing documents, which delineate the V&V activities as well as the V&V testing strategy, the test acceptance criteria, and the testing procedures. Software testing consists of a suite of tests performed by software developers and an independent suite of tests conducted by the software V&V group. The order and intent of these software documents are controlled by the policies that were specified and created in step one. The format, content, and information in these documents are controlled by the SOPs; clarification or additional guidance are specified in the guidelines.

The fifth step in implementing the software quality assurance program is the implementation of the device's software. Although this step includes all of the myriad software development activities, tasks, and milestones, there are only five generic activities:

1. The software components must be developed, which involves the coding, testing, verification, and validation testing of the evolving code.

2. The component code then is integrated into a larger whole, tested, verified, and then validation tested.

3. After all of the components have been assembled and their integration has been completed, the software as a complete entity or system is then verified and validation tested.

4. While all of these activities are occurring, the software and its associated documentation are placed under configuration management and control.

5. The data related to the process metrics defined in step one are continuously collected and generated while the software is being implemented.

The sixth step in the software quality assurance program implementation is to begin project postmortems and determine the lessons learned. After each of the pilot projects has concluded, a software postmortem, an introspective examination of the project just concluded, is held. The intent of this examination is to identify the process metrics, activities, and experiences, both positive and negative, that can be used to calibrate, refine, and fine-tune the software quality assurance methodology, process, policies, SOPs, guidelines, and metrics. The most important concept to remember for a successful software postmortem is that it is an objective evaluation of the effects of the currently defined software quality assurance program. Therefore, only the elements of the software quality assurance program can be considered, not how well or poorly an individual or group performed. Ideas and metrics, not individuals, are scrutinized.

The seventh step in the software quality assurance program implementation is to incorporate the results from the postmortem into the policies, SOPs, guidelines, and process metrics. The results of the postmortem should be agreement on the modifications needed to improve the software quality assurance program. These modifications are then made to the appropriate software policy, SOP, and guideline documents, and these updated documents formally constitute the new software quality assurance program for all new software projects.

It is reasonable to expect that the degree of the modifications made to the policies, SOPs, and guidelines will vary. If these documents were initially well defined, then there will probably be few, if any, changes to the policies, perhaps some alterations to the SOPs, and most of the modifications applied to the guidelines. If these documents were adequately defined but not well integrated with each other, then there probably will be numerous changes necessary in all three sets of documents.

The last step in the software quality assurance program implementation is to begin the program on the next set of device projects. These next projects then commence within the newly modified software quality assurance program, and they implement and adhere to the updated software quality assurance life cycle. The entire software quality assurance cycle is then repeated for each new project, and the lessons learned are assimilated into the software quality assurance program. Each completed project's iteration of the software quality assurance life cycle contributes to the betterment of the overall process and allows the next product and project to be delivered in a more efficient and effective manner.

Software Quality Assurance Education

The software quality assurance program also has an educational aspect. The history of software development and maintenance includes many infamous examples of cost overruns and schedule delays. Although on the surface it appears that software development cannot be controlled, this is not true in the vast majority of cases. Management needs to be educated to understand that software projects can be managed and controlled just like any other engineering project.

The staged sequence of controlled development, estimating practices, configuration and revision control, and use of historical data that represents the software quality assurance program will provide and achieve the necessary software control. The historical record should include not only defects but also engineering time expenditures, software project costs, and user feedback. In organizations where the norm is to accept lesser standards and performance from the software group than from any of the hardware engineering groups or others, software quality assurance has the responsibility to educate and encourage management to take a top-down approach toward the responsiveness of software to the larger needs of the project.

Furthermore, management needs to be educated to understand that software is not constructed in the same manner as hardware products are. Management should not attempt to pressure the software group into producing code prematurely, and it should understand that software development requires capital, just as any manufacturing or production group needs capital equipment. The tools used by the software group are less imposing than 5-ton drill presses, 10-ton headers, or production tooling, but the software tools are no less necessary to the pursuit of effective and efficient production of software.

Management, and probably the organization in general, should also be educated about the software quality assurance program itself. Although this entails "presenting" the software quality assurance program to upper management, it is in reality "selling" the program and its implementation to management. A soft sell of the software quality assurance program is needed to raise the awareness of the organization about the ramifications and implications of the program. This should include the high-level details of each step as discussed above, as well as the responsibilities and commitment needed from the organization.

Additionally, management should be educated to understand that software development needs adequate lead time. The adding of more resources to a troubled project may be of no help in meeting an unrealistic schedule, and the managing of unrealistic plans can be counterproductive. Helping management to learn to enjoy life with software development is one of the educational roles of software quality assurance.

3

The Software Quality Assurance Program: Foundations of Methodology and Process

> As a result of structural complexity, it is notoriously difficult for someone unfamiliar with a large system to gain an understanding of it and notoriously easy to make a modification to a system that has unexpected and devastating consequences. These problems can be ameliorated by documentation that makes global structure visible and can thus impart an understanding of overall structure.
>
> —Harold Ossher

To an outside observer, software development can at times appear to resemble Brownian motion. Many software engineering project efforts are nearly indistinguishable from organized chaos. Both of these perspectives may be due in part to ignorance, poor management, lack of training, or numerous other reasons, but mostly they reflect a lack of understanding and comprehension concerning the foundations of software engineering methodology and process.

Some individuals have difficulty with the word *methodology* when used in the context of software engineering. Many know that the suffix *ology* means "the study of"; thus, they feel that the term *methodology* in a software context is more correctly interpreted as "the study of methods." No matter how logical this appears to be, most of what are commonly referred to as "methodologies" in software engineering are really "methods," a situation that is not unique to software. For example, the word *paradigm* has the dictionary definition of a pattern or example. However, paradigm has come to mean a way of viewing the world or an approach to solving a problem.

For the software engineering populace as a whole, "methodology" has come to mean an approach that reflects a specific software engineering process. Methodologies encompass step-by-step methods, graphical representations, documentation techniques, quality evaluation techniques, procedures, and strategies. In fact, a software process model and a software methodology are two separate and distinct entities. A software process model, usually called a "software process" or just "process," determines the tasks and phases involved in the development of software and the criteria for allowing the transition from one phase to the next. Software methodology defines the products or deliverables of each phase and describes how these products and deliverables should be achieved. The process guides the order in which tasks and phases are carried out, and the methodology describes what each task or phase should achieve and how to achieve it.

Software Methodology and Process Definition

The choice of which process model best fits a particular corporation's product development environment and culture is not easy, and any off-the-shelf process selected will most likely require modification. Regardless of where or how the process is selected, the fundamental activities of software development should fit an overall and integrated software quality assurance program. This includes not just the selection of methodology and process, but integration of the project's software development residual tools. For example, software test tools used on one project should be placed into a repository for test tools and become standards for future testing. Stand-alone documentation tools should become automated processors for subsequent projects. Software development tools should be recycled, to streamline and automate the next software project. Furthermore, measurements that are accumulated during the software development process should be used in conjunction with payroll and general ledger account information in order to refine the time, resource, and funding cost estimations of the next project. Several measures should be used to track and help improve software quality and productivity; these metrics can be used to quantify the presence or absence of quality in software.

Structured Programming

Until the mid-1950s, software development was chaotic, but simple; code was not particularly "developed" as much as it was "written," and resulting bugs were corrected. Although elegantly simple, this code-and-fix process had several major difficulties. First, as the code was fixed in an attempt to remove errors, it usually deteriorated by becoming poorly organized. This resulted in subsequent fixes becoming more and more difficult, complex, and expensive. Second, the code was neither configured nor organized for ease of testing and modification; this also contributed to an increase in the cost of subsequent fixes. Third, the software was such a poor match to the user's needs that it was not unusual for it to be rejected outright and redeveloped, often by using the same process. Among other things, this situation highlighted the need for a requirements phase prior to the software design.

The code-and-fix process was replaced by the stagewise process model in the middle to late 1950s (Bennington 1956). In this process, software evolved through a series of stages—operational plan and specification, coding specifications, coding, parameter testing, assembly testing, shakedown, and system evaluation. Although this resolved some of the code-and-fix problems, it introduced its own set of difficulties. First, the stagewise model did not recognize the value of limiting feedback between successive stages. Every stage was allowed to have feedback and, therefore, modify any previous stage, whether it was the immediate predecessor or the first stage. Second, the process did not allow nor incorporate any sort of prototype production step that could run in parallel with the requirements and design stages to take advantage of the early elimination of the invariable dead ends.

The early 1960s saw the arrival of a new and radical way of thinking. In 1962, Edsger Dijkstra made the observation that any piece of source code was essentially a series of mathematical statements. He proposed that any arbitrary program could be proven mathematically correct or incorrect and, thereby, provide a quality judgment as to whether the code had implemented the requirements correctly. By 1965, Dijkstra and others were aware of the major obstacles with this approach, one of which centered on the unconditional "GO TO" statement (Dijkstra 1965; Knuth 1974; Yourdon 1975). In 1967, the term *software engineering* was used for the first time, in advertisements for a 1968 North Atlantic Treaty Organization (NATO) conference. The purpose of the conference was to address and try to resolve many of the critical issues dealing with the development of software. One of those issues was to determine what "software engineering" was and what it entailed.

In 1968, Dijkstra published a paper that described in detail his successful efforts at developing an operating system (Dijkstra 1968b). He propounded the layers of abstraction approach that led to the publication of "Notes on Structured Programming" (Dijkstra 1969). In this article, he not only coined the term *structured programming,* but also emphasized the importance of error prevention rather than error removal, which was the previously accepted norm. Somewhat later, Niklaus Wirth (Wirth 1971) published an article that presented a systematic refinement of previous works by other authors.

During this time, software engineers also realized that "structured programming" was not sufficient. Remember that all of these process models were not just academic research and publications without any practical applications. Most large projects of the time, both commercial projects, such as the *New York Times* Project (Baker and Mills 1973), and government projects, such as Skylab, used these processes and developed other milestone results. Concepts such as the "chief programming team," "optimized programmers," and early versions of "structured design" emerged. Some software industry individuals began to wonder if there were dependable mechanisms for both avoiding bad designs from the start and recognizing potential problems before development began. Larry Constantine's 1965 article "Towards a Theory of Program Design" led to his formulation, in 1967, of both a graphical notation and a vocabulary for describing the structure of programs (Constantine 1967).

Waterfall Model

The stagewise model was eventually replaced by the waterfall model (Royce 1970). The waterfall model (Figure 3-1) represents two primary enhancements to the stagewise model:

- It recognized that feedback between stages was necessary, but it confined feedback to only successive stages, to minimize rework across several stages.

- It provided for a prototype step that ran in parallel with the requirements analysis and design, thus leading to a "build-it-twice" step.

In the pure waterfall model, as each stage progresses and the design is further refined and detailed, there is an iteration with the preceding and succeeding phases, but rarely with the more remote, completed phases. The virtue of this approach is that as the design proceeds, the change process is reduced to a manageable size and limit. This means that at any point in the design after the requirements analysis, there is an evolving baseline that can be returned to in the event that unforeseen difficulties arise. It effectively provides a fallback position that can maximize the extent of the earlier work. In addition, any phase may be planned and staffed for independent from any other phase, to achieve the best use of resources.

Figure 3-1   The waterfall software development life cycle shown with verification and validation

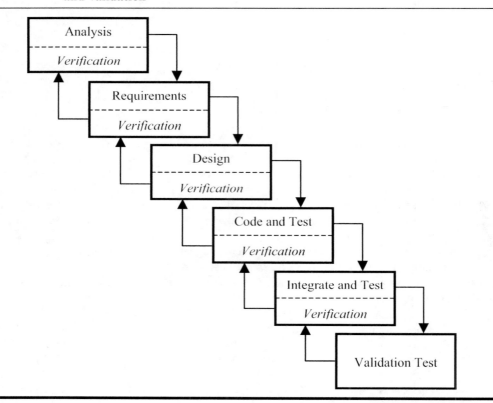

Although the waterfall approach was consistent with the top-down structured programming models defined by Dijkstra (Dijkstra 1970) and Mills (Mills 1971), when the various versions were applied to projects, they ran into several problems. First, the build-it-twice step was unnecessary in applications where design issues were well defined and well understood. This invariably led to unproductive situations, such as a second system that had been overloaded with embellishments from the first system (Brooks 1975). Second, pure top-down approaches must be tempered with some sort of look-ahead mechanism, so that high-risk, low-level elements, reusable code, and common software modules can be accommodated.

Around the mid-1970s, the waterfall model evolved into another form, based on Boehm's writings (Boehm 1975, 1976). In this variant, each step of the model is expanded to include verification and validation (V&V) activities to cover high-risk elements, reuse considerations, and prototype development. Other authors added further refinements, such as incremental development, information hiding, and distinguishing between pre- and post-specification activities. The successive phases used in the waterfall model helped to eliminate many of the difficulties that had previously been encountered in software projects.

The incremental model implements the waterfall model in overlapping repeated steps (see Figure 3-2) and attempts to compensate for the overall duration of the waterfall model project by producing functionality earlier. This may involve a complete up-front set of requirements that

Figure 3-2   The incremental software development life cycle

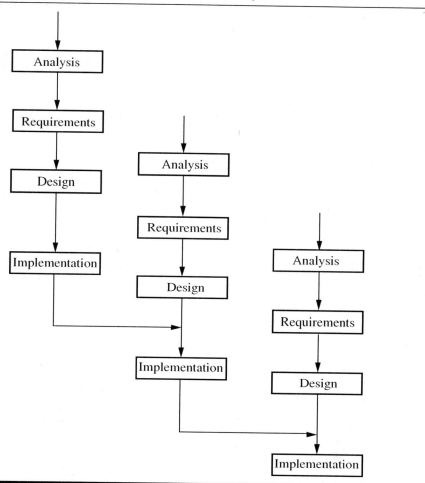

are implemented in a series of small but complete projects. As an alternative, some projects begin with gross, general objectives and some of these objectives are defined as requirements that are then implemented. This is followed by the next set of objectives and continues until all objectives have been implemented. A major drawback to this method is that the use of general objectives rather than completely specified requirements is difficult for some management and regulatory affairs groups to work with. Another drawback is that because some modules are completed long before others are, well-defined interfaces are an absolute necessity. Formal reviews and audits are more difficult to implement on incremental projects than on a completed system. Last, there is a tendency to postpone the more difficult problems to future implementation projects, to demonstrate early project success to management.

The V&V waterfall model has become the basis for most software acquisition standards in government and industry. However, even with extensive revisions and refinement, the basic scheme has encountered significant difficulties that have led to the formation of still other alternative process models. By the late 1970s, the number of software engineering method-ologies in general and the number of software development methodologies in particular had exploded. There were functional decomposition approaches (DeMarco 1978; Yourdon and Con-stantine 1979), data-driven and data-structured approaches (Warnier 1974; Jackson 1975), and formal mathematical approaches (Jones 1980).

A primary source of difficulty with the waterfall model has been its emphasis on fully elaborated documents as the completion criteria for the early requirements and design phases. Document-oriented standards have driven many projects to make documents more efficiently rather than to help with software development in general. These concerns led to the formulation of the evolutionary development model (McCracken and Jackson 1982). In this model, the stages consist of expanding increments of an operational software product. The direction of the prod-uct's expansion is set, or it is determined by operational experience with the results of the pre-vious stage. This model is ideally suited to a fourth-generation language application in which users are unsure about what the software should do, but they definitely know it when they see it. It gives users rapid initial operational capability and provides a realistic operational basis for determining the subsequent improvements. The primary difficulty of the evolutionary devel-opment model is that it is generally indistinguishable from the code-and-fix model of the 1950s, in which the spaghetti, hacker, or engineering code, as well as the general lack of planning, was the impetus and initial motivation toward the waterfall model.

To counter these difficulties and overcome other application shortcomings of the waterfall model, the transform model was formulated (Balzer, Cheatham, and Green 1983). In this model, the existence of a capability to transform automatically a formal specification of software directly into a program that satisfies the specification is assumed. The performance of the resulting code is then improved and optimized through the automatic transform system, and the product is then used under operating conditions. The specification is adjusted to reflect opera-tional experience, and then the product is rederived, reoptimized, and operated. The primary dif-ficulty of this model is that automatic transformation capabilities are available for only a few limited areas. The transform model also shares a disadvantage with the evolutionary model in that it assumes that the user's operational product will always be flexible enough to support unplanned evolutionary paths. Furthermore, dealing with the rapidly increasing and evolving supply of reusable software components and commercial software products requires a formi-dable knowledge base and can be a maintenance problem.

By the beginning of the 1980s, there were so many software development methodologies that keeping track of them became a full-time effort; several methodology surveys (Freeman and Wasserman 1982; Blank et al. 1983; Birrell and Ould 1985) were conducted, compared, and contrasted. In 1982, the U.S. Department of Defense attempted to investigate 48 different methodologies in use at the time. In the end, the effort was so exhausting that only 24 of the 48 were reported on, and of the 24, none was examined in any great detail. The 1980s also saw the expansion and increased importance of prototype development approaches, real-time appli-cations and issues (Ward and Mellor 1985), and computer-aided software engineering (CASE). CASE was envisioned as the integrated programming support environment that would automate all of these ideas, technologies, and methodologies.

Spiral Model

The spiral model (Boehm 1988a) (see Figure 3-3), is principally a risk management and assess-ment tool that relies heavily on the development of a prototype, but eventually it turns over its software end products to the more traditional software development processes. The spiral model

Figure 3-3   The spiral software development life cycle

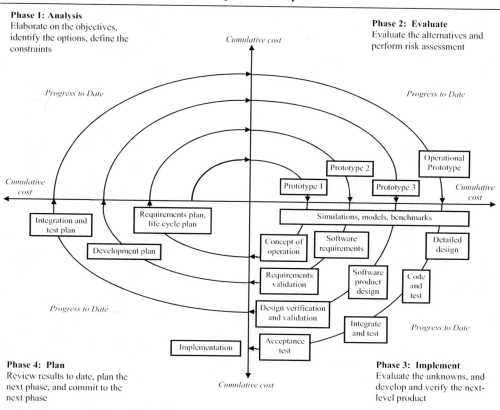

Phase 1: Analysis
Elaborate on the objectives, identify the options, define the constraints

Phase 2: Evaluate
Evaluate the alternatives and perform risk assessment

Cumulative cost

Progress to Date

Progress to Date

Cumulative cost

Cumulative cost

Operational Prototype

Prototype 2

Prototype 1

Prototype 3

Simulations, models, benchmarks

Integration and test plan

Requirements plan, life cycle plan

Concept of operation

Software requirements

Detailed design

Development plan

Requirements validation

Software product design

Code and test

Progress to Date

Design verification and validation

Integrate and test

Progress to Date

Implementation

Acceptance test

Phase 4: Plan
Review results to date, plan the next phase, and commit to the next phase

Cumulative cost

Phase 3: Implement
Evaluate the unknowns, and develop and verify the next-level product

Reprinted with permission from "A Spiral Model of Software Development and Enhancement," B. Boehm, in *Software Engineering Project Management,* R. H. Thayer, ed., p. 131, © 1988 IEEE.

assumes that each cycle of the product progresses through the same series of steps and that these steps are applied to each part of the product, from concept to detailed coding.

Each process cycle starts in the upper left-hand quadrant of the model illustration (Figure 3-3), initially closest to the origin. In this phase, the objectives of that part of the product being elaborated or investigated are identified. For example, the investigation may be in relation to performance, functionality, or accuracy. The alternative means of implementing this part of the product are also identified. For example, there may be differing candidate designs, the reuse of code may be an alternative, or the purchase of hardware or software might be an alternative. Last, the constraints on the application of each of the alternatives are identified. These could relate to cost, schedule, resources, or technical issues.

The next phase (upper right-hand quadrant) is evaluation of the alternatives with respect to the objectives and constraints identified in the first phase. The intent of this phase is to identify the areas of uncertainty that are significant sources of risk to the project. The evaluation and the risk assessment of the various alternatives are conducted using any of the traditional risk management techniques, such as prototype development, analytic modeling, simulations, user questionnaires, or any combination of these and other risk-resolution techniques.

Once the risks have been evaluated, the next phase (lower right-hand quadrant) is determined by the relative risks that still remain for the product. For example, if performance or user interface risks strongly dominate over software development or internal interface-control risks, then the next step might be one of evolutionary development. In this step, a minimal effort would be expended to specify the overall nature of the product, plan for the next level of prototype development, and produce a more detailed prototype. The detailed prototype would continue to help resolve the major risk issues. Eventually, if the detailed prototype became operationally useful and robust enough to serve as a low-risk platform for the further development of the product, then the subsequent risk-driven steps of the spiral would be merely the evolution of further operational prototypes.

However, if the previous prototypes have resolved the performance or user interface risks and software development or if internal interface-control risks dominate, then the next step would be the waterfall approach. This approach in the spiral model is modified as appropriate to incorporate the incremental development of the product that had already been accomplished. Each level of the software specification is then followed by a validation step and preparation of plans for the succeeding cycle.

At this juncture another cycle of the spiral process could begin, or the traditional software development process could begin. The decision of which process is next is a function of the risk assessment question, Can the product begin the normal development cycle, given everything that is not known? If the risks are unacceptable, then the product would begin another cycle around the spiral. If the risks are acceptable, the product and all of the information generated to date are then passed as input to the traditional software development cycle. This cycle would then begin with the product operational concept, software requirements, architecture design, and so on. Each of these software development steps is appropriately modified to accommodate any incremental software development, as well as being followed by a verification and validation step.

An important feature of the spiral model is that each cycle is completed by a review that involves the primary individuals or organizations concerned with the product. This review covers all of the end products that were developed during the cycle as well as the plans for the next cycle and the resources needed to execute those plans. The objective of this review is to ensure that all concerned parties are mutually committed to the approach that is to be taken during the next phase. The plans for the succeeding cycle may also include a partition of the product into increments for successive development or into components that will be developed by individual organizations or persons. The review and commitment step could conceivably range from an individual walk-through of the design of a single software component to a major requirements review that would potentially involve developers, customers, users, and maintenance organizations.

From an objective standpoint, we can make several observations about the spiral model. First, the model presents a very structured approach to prototype development. It dictates that all functional groups associated with the development of the product be mutually committed to the understanding and objectives of what the prototype is to accomplish. Second, the spiral life cycle model is a prototype development approach, but not every prototype development approach is an example of the spiral life cycle. A common problem is that programmers all prefer coding to almost any other software life cycle activity, and management and clients exacerbate this problem by continually asking when the code will be done. Third, the spiral model is much more appropriate as a research project and requirements definition tool than as a development model. If the software development effort is a project in which many options are available, the requirements and constraints are unknown at the beginning, and the organization is committed to taking the time to explore the alternatives, then the spiral life cycle approach is ideally suited. If the effort is a project in which the product, options, requirements, and constraints are fairly well understood, then the spiral model is not nearly as appropriate as some other software life cycle approaches.

Object-Oriented Model

The 1990s saw the advent and expansion of object-oriented methodologies. Although the focus of many object-oriented discussions and articles tends to be highly specific to programming language, many of the concepts covered have implications that go beyond their implementation in the programming language. Object-oriented software development is not the same as developing software in the C++ language, because C++ is a language that facilitates the implementation of code by means of object-oriented techniques. A software development process is object oriented if the organizing principle for the structuring of the system is based on an abstraction of the conceptual entities within the system. In object-oriented software development, the conceptual entities are the "things" (objects) in the system.

Object-oriented software development is a viable process and methodology for several reasons. First, the objects in a given type of system are relatively static over time. For example, the sensor technology in medical devices and the monitoring of these sensors are fundamentally the same as they were five years ago. Second, a system structure based on objects is more resilient. For example, an infusion device's object-oriented software that currently controls one channel is not readily affected by the adding of a second channel. If it is unaffected by the addition of another channel, then a multichannel version of the software is fundamentally nothing more than multiple extensions of the single-channel code. Third, a resilient system can be more easily maintained and reused.

Object-oriented technology methodologies also have a life cycle definition. Each phase of the object technology life cycle manifests itself differently during each phase, compared to the more traditional methodologies. For example, the traditional analysis phase is concerned with understanding the problem; the problem can be understood, by definition, when its requirements can be specified in a complete, consistent, reviewable, and verifiable manner. Traditionally, this phase delineates what is being done, what it is being done to, and when it is being done. Traditional analysis, then, is characterized by exposing information about the problem. Object-oriented analysis, on the other hand, specifies the requirements by defining the conceptual entities or objects in the problem, the attributes of these objects, the relationships between these objects, the behavior of the objects, and the operations that the objects perform.

The traditional design phases define the solution to the problem. A solution is defined when the components that are used to construct the system have been identified, on the basis of a given implementation technology. This phase identifies how the conceptual entities of the analysis will be realized, how they will be packaged or presented in the implementation technology, how system performance will be achieved, and how system construction will proceed. The traditional design is characterized by the hiding of information in the system in order to promote modularity. Object-oriented design, in contrast, identifies the components for constructing the system by packaging functions together with the data that they access. These classes are defined to encapsulate data and operations, to provide inheritance of data and operations, and to allow operations to be bound at run time.

Conceptually, object-oriented development is an iterative activity. Figure 3-4 illustrates this iteration through the use of a formal language syntax specification. Analysis consists of first "finding" any classes, objects, or methods that were defined, created, implemented, and then stored in a library from a previous application or project. As shown, finding a class, object, or method in the library may necessitate another find operation. If the find step did not turn up any

Figure 3-4   The iterative approach to object-oriented software development

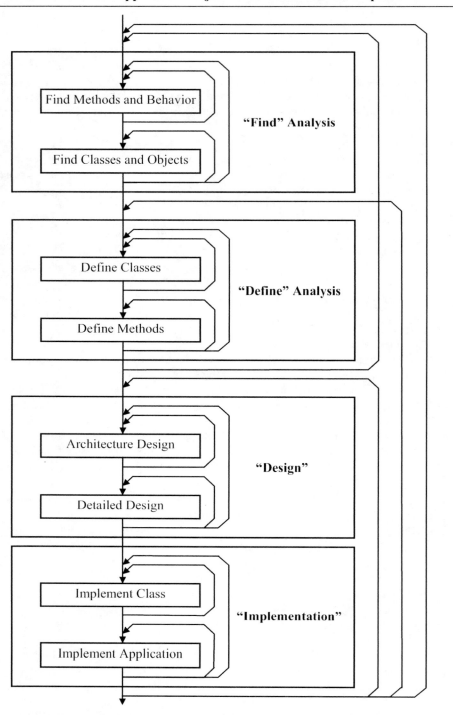

suitable classes, objects, or methods in the library, then the analysis phase allows for the "defining" of the class or method. This "defining" may, in turn, necessitate a new find operation.

Eventually, the analysis phase begins to wind down, and the architectural design phase begins to ramp up. In this phase, fundamental design decisions are made relative to the system as a whole. These decisions specify how to organize and access the data, how to manage the various threads of control, the structure of typical tasks, classes, and so on. These decisions are based on the available implementation technologies, such as the processor to be used, the operating system, the language, and perhaps the network or communication protocol(s). The architecture phase may necessitate a new find operation to locate any objects, classes, or methods needed to complete the architecture.

As the architecture design phase begins winding down, the detailed design phase begins. During this phase, the design of each object is based on the capabilities, requirements, and design structures specified by lower-level objects. The detailed design phase may also necessitate a new find operation or define operation, or a modification to the architecture. As the detailed design phase begins to wind down, the code construction, which consists of two fundamental steps, begins. First, the classes of the system are implemented through the use of object-oriented languages that help to facilitate the use of the unique features and capabilities of the object-oriented technology methodology. This may necessitate another iterative round through the life cycle. Second, after the application has been implemented, its new objects, classes, and methods are then added to the library for future use.

The advantages of object-oriented technology come from several areas. First, they are highly productive. Object-oriented languages, for example, promote and facilitate prototype development by reusing code and design from previous projects and instantiating them with new attributes and characteristics. Second, object-oriented technology expands the capabilities of the development staff through this same reuse feature. Third, object-oriented technologies will tend to provide smaller executable programs for large projects.

The disadvantages of object-oriented technology come from two areas. First, processing and implementation tend to be slow. Slow processing relates to the code execution of the object-oriented language within the device. However, this can be overcome just as in the traditional way, with the application of lower-level languages. Object-oriented technology is slow to implement because it is an emerging, viable technology and does not have a large experiential resource pool to draw on, as do some of the more traditional methodologies. Second, object-oriented technology will tend to produce larger executable code for smaller projects.

Cleanroom Model

Just like its physical world namesake, the cleanroom model attempts to keep the software bug contaminants out of the software. The concept is to control costs, schedule, development, and time to market by detecting software errors as early as possible and when they are less costly to remove. Rather than using natural languages such as English to convey the requirements and design, the cleanroom model uses more formal notations to produce specifications on which all software requirements and design validation are based. Off-line review techniques are used to develop an understanding of the software before it is executed. The cleanroom software model is intended to produce properly executing software the first time, and software engineers are not allowed to perform trial-and-error executions, although automated routines do check syntax, data flow, and variable typing. Testing uses statistical examination to focus on the detection of the errors most likely to cause operational failures. The cleanroom model is gaining acceptance particularly through inclusion in the software safety-related standards.

Cleanroom techniques have been used in military applications, and data have been provided to validate and judge the method. The general conclusion is that the resulting software programs are more reliable than programs developed with traditional life cycle models. The time required to produce a verified program has been shown to be less than or equal to the time necessary to design, code, and debug a program by means of the traditional approaches. Functional verification used in the cleanroom model has also been shown to be scalable up to large systems, which is not always the case with the more traditional development models. Statistical quality control testing has also proven to be superior to the time-honored technique of finding and removing bugs.

Cleanroom techniques can be used with the waterfall, incremental, or spiral models to produce software of arbitrary size and complexity. Although it has successfully demonstrated excellent results, particularly when the application requires safe and reliable software, such as in medical devices, the radical, nonintuitive approach of this model has blocked widespread acceptance. Cleanroom software development techniques provide higher quality software, rather than direct increases in productivity. An organization beginning to use cleanroom techniques needs to have in place systematic design methods, formal inspection procedures, documented requirements in a natural language, developer-performed testing, configuration management of software following its release to the independent testing group, and ad hoc functional testing.

The cleanroom process is based on developing and certifying a pipeline of software increments that accumulate into the final system. The increments are developed and certified by small, independent teams, and large projects are composed of a large number of these small teams. System integration is continual, and functionality grows with the addition of each successive increment. In the cleanroom approach, the operation of future increments at the next level of refinement is predefined by the increments that are already in operation; this helps to minimize interface and design errors and helps software developers maintain intellectual control. The cleanroom development process is intended to develop quickly and with high quality the right product for the user and then go on to the next version, to incorporate new requirements that arise from the user's experience of the previous version. In the cleanroom process, correctness is built in by the development team through formal specification, design, and verification. Correctness verification by the team takes the place of the traditional unit testing and debugging, and software enters system testing directly, with no execution by the development team. All errors are noted at the first execution, and no private debugging is permitted.

In the cleanroom model of incremental development and quality certification (Figure 3-5), the cleanroom team begins by analyzing and clarifying customer or user requirements outside of the formal process model. This stage is performed with substantial user interaction and feedback. If the requirements are ever in doubt, the team can develop cleanroom prototypes, to elicit feedback in an iterative manner. The cleanroom development process then begins formal activities that involve two cooperating teams and five major stages.

Cleanroom development begins with the development team and the certification team generating two specifications: functional and usage. Some large projects may employ a separate specifications team. The functional specification defines the required external system behavior in all circumstances of use, and the usage specification delineates scenarios and their probabilities for all possible system usage, both correct and incorrect. The functional specification becomes the foundation for incremental software development, and the usage specification provides the basis for generating test cases for incremental statistical testing and quality certification.

On the basis of these specifications, the development and certification teams together define an initial plan for developing the increments that will accumulate into the final system. For example, a system having 50 thousand lines of code (KLOC) might be developed in six

Figure 3-5 Cleanroom software process model

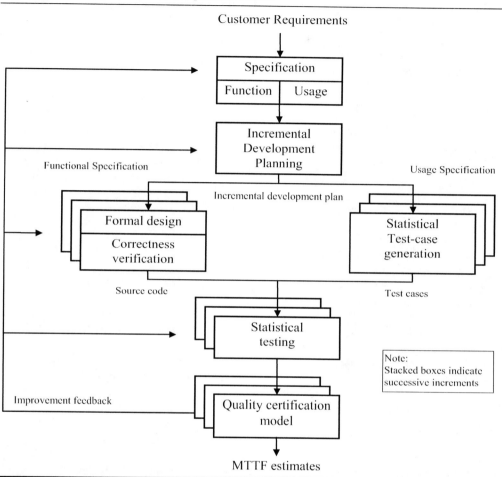

increments of roughly 8 KLOC each. The time it takes to design and verify the increments varies with the size and complexity of each individual increment, and long lead-time increments may call for parallel development. The development team then implements the design and correctness cycle for each increment, and the certification team proceeds in parallel and uses the usage specification to generate test cases that reflect the expected use of the accumulating increments.

Periodically, the development team integrates a completed increment with prior increments and delivers the result to the test team for execution of statistical tests. The test cases are run against the accumulated increments, and the results are checked for correctness against the functional specification. The elapsed times between failures are passed to a quality certification model that computes objective measures of quality. Of course, the quality certification model must employ a reliability growth estimator in order to derive the statistical measures. Certification is performed continuously over the life of the project. Higher level increments enter the certification pipeline before lower level increments. This means that major architectural and design decisions are validated in execution before the development team elaborates on them for the next increment. Because certification is performed for all increments as they accumulate, the higher level increments are subjected to more testing than the lower level increments, which implement the localized functions; errors uncovered during certification testing are returned to the development team for correction. If the software quality is low, managers and team members initiate process improvements to raise the quality through iteration and feedback that accommodates problems and solutions.

Fuzzy-Logic Model

It is difficult to decide whether fuzzy-logic technology is better than the traditional implementations. To determine whether fuzzy logic is applicable in the design, the first question to ask is whether the control variables are continuous. If the product has only *on* or *off* actions, then fuzzy logic is probably not the solution of choice, because fuzzy logic derives its response from the use of combinatorials of the product state space. A two-input product with only two states per input produces a maximum of four output possibilities. This output response is too small for fuzzy logic to be useful. However, if the product has a continuous number of states or a large number of discrete values, then fuzzy logic is a possibility.

The next determinant of whether fuzzy logic is applicable is the complexity of the product, and it is a very important issue. The real advantage of fuzzy logic over traditional controllers is its ability to deal with complex systems via the power of linguistics. The design of the product can make use of a system's imprecision as a function of the system's output. The linguistic nature of fuzzy logic enables it to control processes that traditional controllers have difficulty with. A system that opens a valve in response to a specific fluid height, for example, has low complexity. A system that opens a valve as a function of fluid height and temperature has more complexity. The addition of more variables makes the system more complex.

The next determinant to use in judging whether the product can use fuzzy-logic applications is how well the product is understood. Poorly understood systems are not easy to model mathematically. The easiest test for understanding is whether a designer initially understands the system. Is the lack of understanding caused by ignorance, or is the system inherently ambiguous from a mathematical standpoint? After further study, if the designer is still uncertain about the system operation, then it is possible that the system cannot be described using analytical techniques; fuzzy logic becomes a viable option. Another criteria for how well the system is understood is to determine how many measurements of the system can be made. If few measurements are available, human operators can probably control the process efficiently by monitoring the variables; therefore, fuzzy logic is probably not an option.

Linearity is the next characteristic to examine. Most real systems exhibit some degree of nonlinear behavior, and these are handled in one of two ways. Either the model is simplified so that any nonlinear components are factored out, or the irregularities are factored into the model's equations. The difficulty with the first technique is that it works best for simple systems or where the nonlinear component is so small that it is negligible. In systems in which the nonlinearity component plays a larger or more substantial role, the simplification approach does not work, and fuzzy logic becomes an option. The difficulty with the second technique is that it produces models that operate over a limited range of conditions, or it is too rigid to be of value. A way to tell if a system is nonlinear is to observe the input-to-output relationships on a scatter plot; if the plot does not look like a straight line, then the system is not linear. Another technique is to perform a curve fit on the scatter plot; if the resulting equation is not the general form for the equation of a straight line, then the system is not linear.

Another dimension to explore is whether the system contains any uncertainties or parameters that vary during the course of the system's operation. Determining the uncertainties consists of examining the physical components and determining if they change. For example, are there force and frictional components that vary over time such that the variation of parameters causes unpredictable responses in the form of overdamping, underdamping, and critical damping? In general, parameter uncertainties cause a system to be both nonlinear and complex because not enough information from direct measurements can be made. Modeling the system becomes difficult because relationships among intermediate variables cannot be derived; the only available information is the input-to-output relation, and that may not be enough, especially when intermediate variables are affected by unknown influences.

The last characteristic to examine is whether the system is probabilistic. In a probabilistic system, all parameters are known; if there are elements in the system that are random, then fuzzy logic can be used. If attempts to answer some of these questions do not clarify that fuzzy logic will aid the design, additional research might be called for. This can be accomplished by examining other fuzzy-logic applications and determining what criteria were used in their selection. Try to locate applications that closely match the product under consideration, or locate ones that have the same components.

When fuzzy logic has been determined to be a viable approach, the next step is to understand how the product should work. Known as *knowledge extraction*, this is very closely related to requirements definition. There are three ways to perform knowledge extraction and learn how the system works: by interview, by observation, or by trial and error. Interviewing a system expert, a popular method for determining how a product should work, is useful in situations that resist automation. This approach is typically less involved than analyzing the system, because operators can give enough feedback on the system to enable designers to narrow down the variables and parameters of the system. Possible drawbacks are difficulties in asking the right questions and in getting the expert to step through the control process in a logical, organized manner.

Extraction by observation is a form of system analysis that depends on a monolithic model approach. In this black-box analysis, the system is viewed as a box that has inputs and responds with a specific response that is a function of the input. It is assumed that the system is operational and observable. The analysis consists of quantitatively taking measurements and determining the input-to-output relations. The drawback is that this approach can fail at the system level if the system's inner workings are so complex that a top-level description is inadequate to specify all of the intricacies. A way around this limitation is to partition the system further into a group of interconnected, smaller black-box systems and intermediate relations that can be created to supply information to subsystems. This partitioning can lead to encoding the black box in terms of mathematical equations and thereby verifying results by calculating a response and comparing it to the actual response.

The use of trial-and-error extraction can be used if the first two knowledge extraction processes fail, or it can be used under several specific conditions. For example, if a physical system does not exist or if it is not understood well enough to describe its workings, then trial-and-error extraction can be employed. In this scenario, it is necessary to determine how the system works in terms of smaller, manageable pieces and then detailing the system from this perspective. The drawback is that this approach is iterative and time consuming and requires an educated guess about the approximation of the initial system and then adjustments to the system parameters until the system behavior matches the desired behavior.

Regardless of the knowledge extraction method, the result is a requirements document that is used to build and refine the model of the system. This document is used as input for the design and implementation of the model. Technically, the requirements are documented as informal, semiformal, and formal description notations. Informal description notation is the most familiar to software engineers; it includes enough text to describe complex problems. Although the length and details are up to the designer, it should include terms, definitions, assumptions, and the presumed level of knowledge of the reader. Language semantics might cause ambiguities and result in unclear, incomplete, or contradictory information; thus, the document should present system context within the scope of the requirements. Ambiguities can be partially offset by using semiformal notation such as programming constructs (e.g., IF-THEN conditionals and WHILE DO loops), but this generally requires more detailed information about the process. Another version of a semiformal notation, pseudocode, provides greater precision with less ambiguity and tends to allow as much or as little detail as warranted.

In the fuzzy-logic model (Figure 3-6), phases are similar to those of the spiral model of software development in that they allow for feedback at each phase. The fuzzy-logic development cycle consists of four phases: requirements, design, implementation, and integration. The first three phases are concerned with accurately capturing the model and the last with the integration of the model into hardware. The requirements phase involves accurately determining and describing the system's behavior. The design and implementation phases are concerned with model development and target implementation, respectively. The design phase is subdivided into four steps: determine the input-to-output relationships, identify membership sets, define system behavior, and select a defuzzing technique. The integration phase is concerned with the integration of the controller into the hardware.

When the system has been defined, designed, and implemented, it must be validated. Validation is the process of verifying that the model does exactly what the designers intended it to do. If it does not, then the parameters are adjusted until the model behaves as expected. For validation, both hardware and software methods are available. The hardware method consists of downloading the model to the target hardware and running it. For example, a state machine is downloaded to a programmable gate array and the hardware then executes the model. The software approach involves simulating the model in software. For example, the state machine is described as a program using a high-level language; it is compiled and executed on a PC. If the system must be altered, making adjustments in software is easier than doing so in hardware. Fine-tuning the system takes multiple iterations and commonly involves changing the membership sets, rules, or both to make the model operate properly. If the requirements are found to be incorrect or incomplete, then it is necessary to go back and correct the offending problem, and iteration continues until the operation of the system is satisfactory.

Figure 3-6   Fuzzy-logic software process model

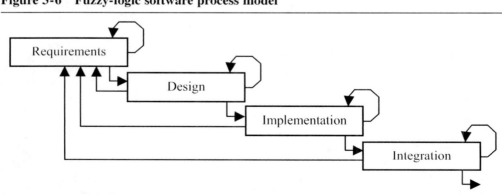

Software Methodology and Process Documentation

Engineering in general is not a rote discipline. Engineering practitioners must be aware of and continually make trade-offs among a number of differing and divergent items. While software methodology and process represent definite rules and guidelines, a good engineer can still achieve creativity and ingenuity and inject intuition into any given situation. In this regard, software engineering is no different from any other form of engineering; the documentation that captures and states the software engineering methodology and process must convey this concept throughout the software life cycle.

Reading any of the various standards and specifications that document a specific software methodology and process gives the impression that software development is a strictly sequential activity. Specifically, these documents convey the impression that one phase must be entirely completed before the next phase begins. In fact, this "think first and code later" mentality is fostered even by software engineers themselves, through such statements as "all design must be completed before any coding can begin." Although this appears to be a software reality, it is more akin to overseeing that helps to prevent the rushing into code development before the entire device is understood.

A good analogy is how people work jigsaw puzzles. Some people leave all of the pieces in the box that it came in and work out of there. Others leave the pieces in the box but locate all of the border pieces first. Others dump all the pieces out of the box and then begin. Still others dump the pieces out of the box, locate all of the border pieces, and then begin assembling the puzzle. Software engineers are typically like the latter. They want to know everything about the device as soon as possible, preferably before doing any work. They would be the first ones to dump the contents of the puzzle box onto the table, turn pieces over so that the picture side of each is up, find all of the border pieces, and then begin to assemble the border. At this point, the common methods used to assemble the puzzle begin to fade. Some will assemble all of the border pieces before continuing. Others will begin the border, but when similar puzzle patterns are found, they will begin to collect, in another location, all of those pieces for inclusion into the puzzle at a later time. Others will begin to assemble those components as a substep to creating the border, with the intent of integrating them later into the puzzle as a whole, and then return to assembling the border. It is not necessarily the individual and serialized steps that the software engineer takes to construct the software that are important, but rather it is the need to intellectualize the whole, to see what and where the common parts are, to understand where the patterns lend themselves to common processing, and to comprehend the larger picture.

In reality, any significant software engineering project will exhibit a great deal of iteration and overlap that seemingly contradict the methodology and process used to produce the software. The act of returning to a previously completed step, introducing a change there, and then propagating the effects of that change forward through the software and backward through higher level documents is normal for software engineers; however, it is not always done. Software engineering activities occur at varying levels of abstraction and detail simultaneously. Even though good software engineers may be functioning this way, there is often a noticeable top-down preference to the whole activity. The design phase of software development is not the only time during which software engineering activity will overlap and iterate on the software life cycle. Frequently, device or system-level changes require that the software engineer return to a previously completed step, introduce a change, and then carry the change forward.

Device or system-level requirements are also seldom at the same level of abstraction. Some requirements, such as "must be easy to use," "the user interface will consist of menus," or "all exceeded thresholds will be accompanied by an audible alarm," are very broad and high level.

Other requirements are very detailed, such as the specification of the number of digits of accuracy on displays, the number of analog to digital counts, or precision pressure readouts. Software engineers typically survey all of the requirements and note which requirements must be considered for the phase at hand and which ones may be delayed until later in the process. Software engineers continually practice cognitive dissonance, the simultaneous belief in two apparently contradicting ideas. Software engineers know that the ability to return to a previously completed phase and introduce a change or enhancement is possible, yet they make a good-faith effort to make each phase of the process as complete as possible. If a snapshot could be taken on any given day of a software project, it would show software activities throughout the entire software life cycle process—some will still be in requirements analysis, some in design, some in coding, and some in test, while still others would be completed.

Organization and Synergy of Software Methodology and Process Documentation

The proper point to begin the implementation of a software quality assurance program is with the establishment of formal methodology, process, and standards documentation. This documentation can take any form that seems appropriate, but the preferred form is usually a three-tiered, mutually supportive hierarchy. As shown in Figure 3-7, the top level should be in the form of policies that deal with the methodology and process of software development, verification and validation, and configuration management. Under these policies are the standard operating procedures (SOPs) that provide the support, explanation, and instructions to comply with and fulfill the policies. These are particularly useful, for example, in regard to the generation and completion of forms and reports, the activities of conducting reviews and audits, and how testing should be performed. The bottom tier is the software guidelines that deal with how to interpret and successfully apply the SOPs and policies, particularly when it comes to implementation and interpretation of them on a project. The guidelines also detail the software engineering standards and conventions that would be applied to each device project.

The rationale for this layering is straightforward. First, this document structure has an inherent enforcing attribute. For example, policies are more forceful and binding than SOPs,

Figure 3-7   Hierarchy of software quality assurance program documentation

SOFTWARE POLICIES					
Development	Verification and Validation	Configuration Management	Administration		

SOFTWARE STANDARD OPERATING PROCEDURES					
Development	Verification and Validation	Configuration Management	Administration	Other Software Procedures	

SOFTWARE GUIDELINES					
Development	Verification and Validation	Configuration Management	Administration	Other Software Guidelines	Standards and Conventions

which are more binding than guidelines, which are the least binding of all. Second, this document structure implies a strict change control structure. For example, policies normally cannot be changed without senior management approval. SOPs cannot be changed without department-level approvals, while guidelines may be changed by individual projects at the discretion of the lead software engineer. Because of this approval constraint, the software engineering methodology and process are not likely to change drastically or at the whim of any particular project.

Third, because of the binding characteristic of this document structure, the methods, practices, and processes can be documented experimentally for evaluation purposes. For example, suppose a new form for capturing metrics has been developed and will be used on a single project for the first time. Furthermore, assume that this new form proved to be useful on the project and that subsequently, at the project software postmortem, it was decided that it should become a standard way of conducting business. However, there was some doubt as to its full applicability for all projects in the software life cycle. The new form might then be documented in the guidelines as the form to use. After several other projects have tried the new form, it is decided, again through the postmortems, that the form should be integrated into the software development process as a standard reporting form. It is then included in the SOPs as the documented form to use, and the guidelines are modified in relation to the form's new status. Thus, the methods, practices, and processes can be captured at one level and then either elevated, demoted, or eliminated from the documentation, on the basis of project experiences of trying to meet the intent of the new method, practice, or process.

The individual policies deal with the methodology and processes associated with software development and are primarily organized around the phases that comprise the particular process model being implemented. For example, if the process model to be implemented were the top-down, structured methodology and process model, then the policies would deal with the subjects associated with the project start-up phase, the analysis and requirements phase, the design phase, the code and test phase, the integration and test phase, and the validation phase. The intent of this approach is to provide a convenient reference point as to their applicability at a particular time on a project.

Typical software engineering development methodology and process topics are varied but highly integrated. They deal with the content and intent of project software estimations, planning documents, design documents, and testing documents. The development policies should also cover the content, intent, and results of the project's software requirements reviews, design reviews, and walk-throughs. The policies should also lay the foundation for and give credence to software standards and conventions, and the type of software development process to be used.

The software engineering development methodology and process topics are also intimately tied to the verification and validation methodology and process policies. The V&V policies are the real crux of the software quality assurance program, and they are organized around the same software development phases as are reflected in software development policies. V&V deals with anomaly reporting and resolution, requirements tracking, and defect prevention and correction activities that are associated with each of the software development phases. V&V policies deal with the content and intent of project planning documents, reporting documents, and test procedures. Most important, they delineate the criteria for successful acceptance and release of the device software.

Associated with software engineering development policies and V&V methodology and process policies are configuration management policies. This set of policies details how changes are processed in order to control modifications to previously baselined software products. These policies deal with the content and the intent of audits and reviews, software end-product identification, and status accounting and reporting.

Finally, there is a set of software policies that completes the software quality assurance program. It deals with the non–project-related activities still required for a successful software quality assurance program. These policies deal with code and data integrity, security, and data retention periods. They discuss product-related support activities, such as simulations, throw-away software for breadboards, and prototype development. They also cover the aspects of how the software team is organized, who has what responsibilities, what software end products to release, and where the software end products will reside when the project concludes. These policies also deal with the management and administration of hardware platforms used for software development and maintenance activities.

The software development policies presented in the following sections are intended to be generic. However, in order to convey the entire framework of operation and to present them in a familiar context, they are arranged against the top-down, structured methodology and process model. Furthermore, they have been partitioned into arbitrary categories as an organizational aid for this discussion rather than for any implied reasons. Although no signature authorization or approval structure is presented here (that concept is related more to how an individual company organizes its projects), it is necessary to indicate for discussion purposes that a lead software engineer position is needed. It is assumed that appropriate positions by title or function can be found within any organization to satisfy appropriate signature requirements.

An additional point about the "policies" discussed in the following sections: Nearly every company has inherent distinctions among "policy," "SOP," and "guideline," as well as a preferred organization of these documents. For the sake of the discussion in the following sections, the distinction between policy, SOP, and guideline content, particularly as discussed above, has not been preserved. This was done in order to present all of the information needed relative to a specific software topic as a well-defined package; it is assumed that some of the details presented here as a component of "policy" would normally appear as information in an SOP or guideline. Furthermore, these "policies" may appear as a set of single, individually numbered policies or as a single policy with sections dealing with a specific software topic. It is assumed that the grouping of this policy information will support the corporate policy approach.

Software Governing Policy Topics

In some instances, depending on the complexity of the software processes and the desire of a company to recognize differing degrees of process within different departments, an overriding or governing software policy can be created. This document effectively states the philosophy or strategy of software development and software V&V. For example, this policy would delineate the differences among product, engineering, or development software and their counterparts in the business systems or information technology areas. Table 3-1 lists the topics in a typical governing policy of this type.

Section 1 conveys the purpose, scope, and overview of the policy. It lists the types of software that the policy applies to as well as the software that is excluded from the policy. The exclusion can be explicitly listed by department, product, or name of the process used to generated the excluded software. For example, it would indicate that the policy applies to all product software, computerized manufacturing process software, and quality assurance system software and does not apply to software developed under the information technology process or business system process. Section 2 lists the responsible parties for the policy. For example, it would list the areas or groups that the policy applies to as well as the responsibilities of the software development and software V&V groups under the policy.

Table 3-1   Typical Table of Contents for a Software Governing Policy Document

Section Number	Section Title
1	Introduction
1.1	Purpose
1.2	Scope
1.3	Overview
1.4	Reference Documents
1.5	Definition of Terms
2	Responsibilities
2.1	Software Project Responsibility
2.2	Software V&V Responsibility
2.3	Regulatory Affairs Responsibility
3	Software Procedures
3.1	Levels of Concern
3.2	Assignment of Software to Levels of Concern
3.3	Vendor-supplied Software and Commercial Equipment
3.4	Contractor Supplied Software
3.5	V&V Activities
3.6	V&V Implementation
3.7	V&V Certification
3.8	Documentation
4	Software Acceptance Criteria
4.1	V&V Philosophy
4.2	V&V Report
4.3	Compliance Audit

Section 3 details the procedures of the policy. This section would state that the policy is applicable to full-time permanent employees of the company as well as consultants and contractors assigned to company projects that the policy governs. For each type of software produced by the company, this section would describe the type of software and explicitly name the software or product and what category the software was assigned to. For example, it would indicate that infusion pump, magnetic resonance imaging, and heart-lung machine software is assigned to the major-concern category; vital signs and infrared thermometer software is assigned to the moderate-concern category; and quality assurance systems software used for tracing, tracking, or generating reports containing data used to make quality decisions, manufacturing equipment software, or bar code and labeling software is assigned to the minor-concern category.

Section 3 would also address the V&V of vendor-supplied software and commercial equipment with incorporated software. It is important to delineate the cases or situations in which V&V does not need to be performed and the acceptable documentation that can be used to substitute for rigorous V&V in-house testing. For example, software purchased from an established and reputable supplier does not require V&V if the supplier can provide evidence of at least one of the following:

- a product V&V certification,

- an error and bug tracking and reporting capability,

- maintenance, revision, and upgrade capabilities,

- or a software quality assurance program.

The rationale for this approach is that this type of software has V&V accepted by the computer software industry on the basis of validation through common usage and wide distribution. More important, if the vendor uses a software quality assurance program, then the type of V&V needed for the purchased software is most likely being used. However, it is still incumbent upon the purchaser to perform due diligence to ensure that the supplier is in fact following the system claimed to be in place. As another example, commercial equipment with incorporated software purchased from an established and reputable supplier and proven through use does not require V&V if the supplier can provide evidence of at least one of the following:

- a product V&V certification,

- an error and bug tracking and reporting capability,

- maintenance, revision, and upgrade capabilities,

- or test programs that may be used to assure that the equipment will appropriately and accurately perform all intended functions and operations before it is used for routine production.

It is still incumbent upon the purchaser to perform due diligence to ensure that the equipment is in fact operating in the manner claimed.

. Section 3 would also effectively state the conditions for assuring that contractors, consultants, and vendors will produce quality software. For example, the contracting department reserves the right to review the contractor, consultant, or vendor configuration management system prior to contract award and to periodically audit that system to assure that adequate methods are implemented for identifying and controlling each end product produced.

Section 3 would continue by effectively stating the V&V conditions for a project. For example, it would state that each software project, program, or task requires that V&V activities be performed to ensure an independent assessment and measurement of the correctness, accuracy, consistency, completeness, robustness, and testability of the software requirements, design, and implementation. It would also state that detailed specifics of V&V activities are documented in a separate policy. This section would indicate that the end result of V&V is a written affirmation stating that the software was developed in accordance with a documented software life cycle methodology, that good quality assurance procedures were followed, and that test results demonstrate that system specifications and functional requirements were met.

Section 3 concludes with a statement that details the documentation for software development, software V&V, and the software quality assurance system. For example, this section would indicate that the results of software development and related V&V activities are to be kept on file and where those files are located. It would also indicate that the software life cycle methodology, procedures, and practices be detailed in writing external to the product being developed. It would conclude with a generic description of the types of documents and their contents that are to be produced for each type of medical device produced by the company.

Section 4 delineates the acceptance criteria for the software. For example, it would effectively state that the company regulatory affairs or quality group will define and maintain the software governing policy philosophy, categorize how software is assigned to a level of concern, and assign specific software to a level of concern. In addition, this section would indicate that at the completion of all software development and V&V activities, a Software V&V Report (SVVR) will be generated. The SVVR summarizes the V&V tasks and results, including the status and disposition of anomalies. Furthermore, the SVVR provides an assessment of the overall software quality and recommendations for software and process improvements. Finally, Section 4 would indicate that the regulatory affairs or quality group will audit compliance to this policy.

Software Directory Policy Topics

Software development, software V&V, and software documentation are largely electronic in their representation and need a degree of control in how they are handled. In addition, most companies have several projects going simultaneously, which means that the directory structure organizing each project also needs a degree of control. It is possible to let each project group define its directory structure and place electronic documents within that structure as it sees fit, but that approach is usually not a viable solution. The reason is that as the project group arbitrarily creates and alters the directory structure and as resources are added to the project, an inordinate amount of time will be spent explaining the project's directory structure and where electronic documents are located. Consequently, a stable, predefined directory structure is invaluable in organizing the project and providing consistency between projects. Table 3-2 lists the topics in a typical electronic document control policy of this type. Table 3-3 shows the responsibility matrix for maintaining the policy.

Section 1 (Table 3-2) conveys the purpose, scope and overview of the policy. It would effectively state that the purpose of the policy is to provide a procedure for the control and maintenance of electronic documents created and stored in a project software directory and for the control and management of software project directory structures. For purposes of this discussion, an electronic document is one or more data files stored on a computer and includes any document, data, or software source code in the form of paper or electronic files that contains the source data used for creating the next revision and daughter document.

Section 2 states the responsible parties for the policy procedures (see Table 3-3). For example, it would indicate that the project software lead engineer is responsible for: determining naming conventions and maintenance procedures; providing a file administrator or configuration management engineer for the project; and that appropriate software directories are released to a build V&V directory. It would indicate that the project configuration management engineer is responsible for: naming conventions and maintenance procedures; software project directory generation; appropriate software document templates being loaded into appropriate directory locations; and initial document release of the appropriate software documents. The project software V&V lead is responsible for naming conventions and maintenance procedures and that

Table 3-2   Typical Table of Contents for a Software Electronic Document and Project Directory Management Policy

Section Number	Section Title
1	Introduction
1.1	Purpose
1.2	Scope
1.3	Overview
1.4	Reference Documents
1.5	Definition of Terms
2	Responsibilities
2.1	Software Lead Engineer
2.2	Software Configuration Management Engineer
2.3	Software V&V Lead Engineer
2.4	Software Team
3	Procedures
3.1	Project Directory Generation and Management
3.2	Managing Electronic Documents in the Development Directory
3.3	Managing Electronic Documents in the Build V&V Directory
3.4	Managing Electronic Documents in the Baseline V&V Directory

the appropriate software directories are released from the build V&V directory to the baseline V&V directory. Project team members are responsible for following all naming conventions and communicating with configuration management system for source documents when performing checkout, check-in, or release.

Section 3 details the procedures of the policy and would present the definition and usage of generic scripts and directory structures. A more detailed discussion of the scripts and directory structures and examples would be presented in the software configuration management guidelines, but this policy gives the requirements for the guidelines document. For example, Section 3.1 would delineate how the project directory would be generated at the beginning of a project and how it would be maintained throughout the project. It would describe users and the source file update privileges in the project directory, such as read, write, execute, and delete. This section would also indicate the use of a historical project subdirectory. For example, each product configuration would evolve through several baselines or prototype versions prior to achieving release status. The ongoing history subdirectory needs to be maintained, and the location of those directories needs to be specified. It would also indicate that data files representing

Table 3-3   Matrix for Software Directory Policy Responsibility

Document Title	CM[1]	SLE[2]	V&VLE[3]	Director
Software project directory procedures	Generate	Generate	Generate	Approve
Software project directory deviation	Generate	Generate	Generate	Approve
Software project directory waiver	Generate	Generate	Generate	Approve
Creation of project directory structure	Generate			
Change of project directory structure	Generate	Request	Request	Approve
Creation of project directory initial content	Generate			
Change of project directory labeling		Generate	Generate	

Notes: 1. The software configuration management engineer assigned to the project.
　　　　2. The software lead engineer assigned to the project.
　　　　3. The software V&V lead engineer assigned to the project.

key milestones in the product's development are to be archived off-line, as is the product development configuration just prior to software release.

Section 3.2 would effectively state the steps related to the first-time transfer of source documents to the project directories. It would also cover first-time creation of source documents, first-time generation of source documents, and the subsequent transfer of source documents and the directories that they transferred between. Section 3.3 would indicate the steps associated with the Build V&V directory and the uses of the directory. Section 3.4 would present the steps associated with the Baseline V&V directory and the uses of the directory.

Software Development Policy Topics

The software development policies (Table 3-4) have been divided into six major categories for discussion purposes: Project Preparation; Specifications; Reviews; Development Practices; Integration, Test, and Operations; and Product Management and Acceptance. Table 3-5 illustrates the software life cycle periods during which the software development policies are in effect. Table 3-6 shows the responsibility matrix for maintaining the policy and related documents.

The Project Preparation policy details the requirements for generating software development estimations; the software development schedule is the sole output of this activity. This policy should indicate who is responsible for generating and obtaining approval of the software development schedule, the proposed resource loading, and the software tasking. The software development schedule, resource loading, and tasking should be based on a bottom-up estimate of the required staffing levels for each work breakdown structure (see Chapter 4) item, on software estimation models based on size estimates of each software unit, and on historical data that relate to previous software development projects. The schedule estimates should include

Table 3-4   Typical Categories and Topics of Software Engineering Development Policy

Policy Category	Policy Topic Title
Project Preparation	Software Development Estimates
Specifications	Interface Design Specification (IDS) Software Requirements Specification (SRS) Architecture Design Specification (ADS) Detailed Design Specification (DDS)
Reviews	Software Requirements Review (SRR) Architecture Design Review (ADR) Detailed Design Review (DDR) Software Design Walk-Throughs Software Code Walk-Throughs
Development Practices	Programming Standards and Conventions Software Design Methodology Software Analysis Methodology
Integration, Test, and Operations	Software Tools Hardware Tools Development Test Information Sheets (DTIS) Software Development Test Plan (SDTP) Software User's Manual
Product Management and Acceptance	Software Quality Assurance Software Development Plan (SDP) Software Documentation Software End-Product Acceptance Plan (SEAP)

major milestones and the allocation of estimated time to each software development phase. The development estimates should be reviewed at the end of each development phase for accuracy and timeliness and should be adjusted to reflect any changes in the device's development plans, software requirements, or software design.

The Interface Design Specification (IDS) policy states that devices consisting of multiple components should be decomposed into autonomous elements or subsystems, and each subsystem should be developed in accordance with relevant policies. The intersubsystem interfaces should be defined and controlled, and an integration and test phase should be specified, to integrate the individual components into the complete device. The IDS completely specifies the interfaces among the subsystems and should be placed under configuration control at the time the software requirements are placed under control. The IDS should be updated at the end of the project to reflect the "as-built" software, to provide a basis for delivery and subsequent software maintenance.

The Software Requirements Specification (SRS) policy states that device software projects will have a written document to provide a controlled statement of the functional, performance, and external interface requirements for the software end products. The SRS should be generated prior to and is the subject of the Software Requirements Review (SRR). The SRS should identify the system-level functions and objectives that the software must support and should include functional and performance requirements. The SRS should define all of the interfaces

Table 3-5 Software Development Policies Throughout the Software Life Cycle

Procedure Topic Title	Software Life Cycle Phase							
	Project Start-up	Interface Design	Requirements	Architecture Design	Detailed Design	Code and Test	Integrate and Test	Software Validation
Software Development Estimates	DE		U	U	U			.
Interface Design Specification (IDS)		DE	U	U	U			U
Software Requirements Specification (SRS)			DE	U	U			U
Software Requirements Review (SRR)			D					
Software Architecture Design Specification (SADS)				DE				
Software Architecture Design Review (SADR)				D				
Software Detailed Design Specification (SDDS)					DE			U
Software Detailed Design Review (SDDR)					D			
Programming Standards and Conventions		E	E	E	E	E	E	E
Software Design Methodology		E	E	E	E			
System Analysis Methodology		E	E	E	E			
Software Design Walk-Throughs		E		E	E			
Software Code Walk-Throughs						E	E	
Software Tools	S	S	S	S	S	S	S	S
Hardware Tools	S	S	S	S	S	S	S	S
Development Test Information Sheet (DTIS)		S	S	S	DS	E	E	E
Software Development Test Plan (SDTP)		S	S	DS	UE	E	E	E
Software User's Manual		S	S	DS	UE	E	E	E
Software Quality Assurance	DS	E	E	E	E	E	E	E
Software Development Plan (SDP)	S	S	DS	U	U			
Software Documentation		E	E	E	E	E	E	E
Software End-Product Acceptance Plan (SEAP)		S	DS	UE	U			D

Notes: 1. D indicates that a deliverable or activity is required at that time.
  2. U indicates that an update of a previous deliverable occurs.
  3. E indicates that the procedure requirements are in effect for the entire phase.
  4. S indicates that the procedure requirements can start at any time.

Table 3-6 Matrix of Software Development Policy and Document Responsibility

Document Title	SE[1]	SLE[2]	EE[3]	ME[4]	System Engineer	Project Manager	Director
Software development procedures	Generate						Approve
Software development deviation		Generate			Review	Review	Approve
Software development waiver		Generate			Review	Review	Approve
Software Quality Assurance Plan (SQAP)		Generate					Approve
Software Development Plan (SDP)		Generate			Review		Approve
Development Test Information Sheet (DTIS)	Generate	Approve					
Software Test Plan (STP)		Generate			Approve		
Software End-product Acceptance Plan (SEAP)		Generate			Approve		
Interface Design Specification (IDS)		Generate	Review	Review	Approve	Review	Review
Software Requirements Specification (SRS)		Generate			Approve		Approve
Software Architecture Design Specification (SADS)		Generate			Approve		Approve
Software Detailed Design Specification (SDDS)		Generate			Approve		Approve

Notes: 1. Senior software engineer assigned to the project.
2. Software lead engineer assigned to the project.
3. Senior electrical engineer assigned to the project.
4. Senior mechanical engineer assigned to the project.

associated with the software to be developed, including hardware interfaces, software interfaces, external databases, facilities, and personnel with which the software must interact. Each unique requirement should also be assigned a unique identifier that will be used in subsequent project phases to trace the requirements to explicit parts of the software design, code, and test cases. The SRS should also specify the safety-critical parameters and critical indicators of the device that were identified in the hazards analysis and that are controlled or commanded by the software to be developed. Finally, the SRS should specify the criteria to be used for acceptance of the software to be developed. This should include the levels of test, the test objectives, and the methods. The SRS should be updated during the project in general; an end-of-project update should reflect the "as-built" software, to provide a basis for delivery and subsequent software maintenance.

The Architecture Design Specification (ADS) is an optional document that can be used to begin the early development of device software before detailed design has been completed. The ADS is generated for software products that are defined in the SRS to establish a documented design baseline from which the detailed design will be developed. The ADS contains design information needed to support the detailed definition of the individual software components. At the completion of the Architecture Design Review (ADR), the ADS becomes the design baseline for the development of the Detailed Design Specification (DDS), which is used in support of software construction. The ADS serves as a road map by assigning each unique requirement in the SRS to specific software components of the software design. The ADS also identifies and names all of the software components and levels of software hierarchy to be developed, as well as control interfaces, data interfaces, processing flows, and any existing software that is to be adapted for use within the device. The ADS would normally specify the processing resource budget in terms of timing, storage, and accuracy, as well as the bandwidths appropriate to this level of design. It would also identify all required major algorithms and their location in the software design. The ADS should delineate data names, engineering descriptions, units, default values, and size, as well as the dependencies and the relationships between the data and the software components. Finally, the ADS should address the methods chosen to meet the software testability requirements of the SRS and the Software Development Test Plan (SDTP), as well as the safety requirements of the SRS.

The DDS is an update to and an expansion of the ADS for the software products defined in the SRS. The DDS establishes the "build-to" design from which the software is actually developed. The DDS includes the ADS document as a subset and also includes a design description of the overall software operation and control and the use of common data; it emphasizes software timing, storage, and accuracy. The detailed design should be described down through the lowest level of software organization and the lowest logical level of the database organization. The detailed design should also adhere to the basic control structures allowed in the relevant programming standards and conventions guidelines. For each software component, the DDS should specify the component name, purpose, and assumptions; code and data sizing; calling sequence, arguments and definitions, define error exists, and return status; inputs, processing, and outputs; engineering descriptions of any equations, algorithms, and processing flows; and any restrictions and limitations. The DDS should contain a complete definition of the data down through the bit or field level. The DDS should be updated during the project; an end-of-project update should reflect the "as-built" software, to provide a basis for delivery and subsequent software maintenance.

After the SRS has been completed, the SRR should be held. The purpose of the SRR is to achieve written agreement on the provisions of the SRS, which will then serve as the basis for acceptance of the software to be developed. The SRS should be analyzed and evaluated for its technical acceptability, and a response should be prepared for each problem identified in the analysis. Specifically, the SRS should be analyzed for completeness, consistency, testability, and technical feasibility of the requirements from a flow-oriented and functional breakdown point of view. A description of the analysis techniques and tools that were used to perform the analysis should be prepared for the SRR. Any issues and problems identified in the requirements analysis and evaluation should be addressed at the SRR. Lastly, a review of the Software End-Product Acceptance Plan (SEAP) should be included. The result of the SRR is the acceptance of the SRS as the basis for software end product acceptance and its establishment as the formal baseline.

The ADR ends the design and planning activities that establish a preliminary design baseline as well as the implementation and test plans necessary to proceed into the detailed design and development. At the ADR, the architecture design, associated plans, and any technical issues are reviewed, to assess the adequacy of the design and plans, resolve and identify issues, and obtain mutual commitment to proceed into the detailed design phase. Specifically, the ADR should verify that every requirement has been properly accounted for in the design and that the design is complete, consistent, feasible, and testable from a flow-oriented and functional breakdown standpoint. In addition, the ADR should verify that the design budgets for storage, timing, accuracy, bandwidths, and so on are satisfied by the software components and do not exceed the limitations of the software's physical and functional environment or any margins for growth. Identification of issues or requirements not satisfied should also occur at the ADR level.

If done properly, one of the major advantages of conducting the ADR is that the resultant approved design can be used to begin software development activities. The ADR represents the acceptance of the ADS as the baseline design. As such, the ADS reflects the upper-level process control architecture for the device. The detailed design efforts use this upper-level process control as a given and merely augment the design contained in the ADS down to the algorithm level. Therefore, very little of the design in the ADS will radically change as a result of the detailed design; consequently, it represents a stable design.

The Detailed Design Review (DDR) terminates the design and planning activities that established the DDS, the detailed design, and the associated implementation and test plans as the necessary baselines for proceeding into the code and test phase. At the DDR, the detailed design, associated plans, and any critical technical issues are reviewed, to gain concurrence in the adequacy of the design and plans, resolve or identify issues, obtain mutual commitment to proceed into the code and test phase, and obtain commitment to a test program that supports the software acceptance. Specifically, the DDR should verify that every requirement has been properly accounted for by the design and that the design is complete, consistent, feasible, and testable from a device-inputs-to-device-outputs standpoint as well as a functional breakdown standpoint. In addition, the DDR should verify that the detailed design and critical parameter budgets for storage, timing, accuracy, bandwidths, and so on do not collectively exceed the limitations given in the SRS, exceed the physical and functional environments, or exceed any margins for growth. The DDR should review the current, detailed implementation and test plans; unresolved issues or requirements that are not satisfied should be identified. The result of the DDR should be an agreement to proceed with the code and test phase and an agreement on the test program that will support acceptance of the software end product.

The Software Design Walk-Throughs policy should indicate that software projects will conduct component design walk-throughs to facilitate the early detection of design errors. The design walk-throughs should be accomplished by having the component design reviewed by one or more individuals other than the actual designer. The technique to be used for the walk-through should consist of visual and oral presentations of the design by the originator(s) in the presence of the reviewer(s); the walk-through team should consist of at least one and probably not more than four people. The walk-through should include checks for responsiveness of the design, design completeness and consistency, data flow through interfaces, testability, procedures for recovery from error, modularity, simplicity, and adherence to the documented programming standards and conventions. The Software Code Walk-Throughs policy should mimic the methodology used for the design walk-throughs except that, obviously, it details the code rather than the design.

The Programming Standards and Conventions policy states that software projects should employ programming standards and conventions to promote uniformity, readability, understandability, reliability, maintainability, compatibility, and other quality characteristics of software products. Where applicable, these standards should contribute to the portability of software between hardware systems and compatibility with existing and future support software. These standards and conventions should include the standards to be followed during software design, development, and maintenance. This policy should also indicate that design and development should be periodically audited in progress, to assess adherence to programming standards and conventions. The frequency of audits of the design documentation and the code should be established in the project's Software Quality Assurance Plan (SQAP).

The Software Design Methodology policy should indicate, for example, that software projects will perform software design using a top-down approach, in which the design starts with the top-level device functions and proceeds through a downward allocation, evaluation, and iteration to successively lower levels of design. This design approach enhances design traceability, completeness, and comprehensiveness. The design process should be initiated by establishment of a functional design hierarchy, in which the top level of the design is the overall mission to be performed by the device as a whole. The lower levels are obtained by breaking down and partitioning the software into blocks with progressively greater functional detail; software requirements should then be allocated and mapped onto this design hierarchy. The lowest level of the design hierarchy should be defined such that its software components can be structured by the program control logic to implement all of the input-to-output paths in the requirements. The design should be a hierarchical structure of identifiable software components, where the highest-level of control logic resides at the top of the hierarchy, and the computational or algorithmic functions reside at the lower levels. The levels should be structured so that a lower level does not call upon a higher level. This policy should not preclude the use of prototypes, simulations, or the emulation of any critical components to an extent that is necessary to perform design verification. Furthermore, this policy should indicate that for software undergoing modification, the highest level of the software structure that encompasses all of the software elements to be modified should be considered the top of the design hierarchy.

The Software Analysis Methodology policy details the analysis methodology and establishes the requirement that the analysis is to be presented at the ADR and the DDR. This policy states that the system analysis must address the adequacy of the software design to fulfill software performance and safety requirements, and remain within the allocated design budgets for memory and other storage requirements, timing allocations, and communication bandwidths. Analytic analysis or simulation should be used to demonstrate the adequacy of the selected algorithms to meet the accuracy requirements. Acceptable analysis techniques should include functional simulation, manual static analysis, and walk-throughs. Not-to-exceed design budgets should be defined and validated for operational windows that are related to potential failure modes and system critical times. If a functional simulation is employed, this policy should denote that the requirements related to the simulation itself should be presented. For example, a design notebook should be made mandatory, and one section of that notebook should be set aside for simulator requirements.

The Software Tools policy addresses the tools used on software projects to analyze, design, and implement the code. This policy indicates that software projects should use software tools to support software development activities. It is the responsibility of software engineers to define the requirements for the software tools. This policy should indicate who is responsible for the development of tools when it is not possible to obtain existing software products to serve the required functions. It should also indicate that development of these tools is under the jurisdiction of these policies.

The Hardware Tools policy addresses the tools that are used on software projects to analyze, design, and implement the code. This policy indicates that software projects should use hardware tools to support software development activities and that it is the responsibility of software engineers to define the requirements for the hardware tools. This policy should indicate who is responsible for developing tools when it is not possible to obtain existing hardware products to serve the required functions. It should also indicate that development of these hardware tools should include a design review of engineering drawings, specifications, and test and maintenance plans. This policy should also assure the accuracy of hardware design and plans, resolve any identified issues, and obtain commitment to a program supporting hardware tool acceptance and subsequent maintenance.

The Development Test Information Sheet (DTIS) policy indicates that software projects should prepare and maintain a DTIS for each test conducted during software development. These sheets provide an organized, accessible collection of all software testing and test results, a means of tracking the progression and the status of the testing, and a means of test verification. A DTIS should be prepared for each test defined in the SDTP; it should be prepared prior to the DDR and maintained until end-product acceptance. The completed DTISs should be reviewed for completeness and technical adequacy of the testing and should be periodically audited to assess their compliance with relevant SOPs and guidelines. The DTIS should define the title of the test, the requirements to be tested, the specification containing the requirement, the objective and the success criteria, and the test approach to be used. In addition, the DTIS should specify the required test instrumentation; the expected duration of the test; and the data collection, reduction, and analysis requirements.

The Software Development Test Plan (SDTP) policy states that software project personnel will prepare an overall SDTP that defines the scope of software development testing to be successfully completed for each software component developed. The SDTP policy should specify how testing will be accomplished from the software development standpoint; how the testing and verification of all computations will be accomplished, using not only nominal data values but singular and extreme values; and how verification of all data input values, all data output options and formats, and error and message information will be accomplished. The SDTP policy should also indicate how all executable statements within a component will be exercised and tested, how all options at each branch point in each component will be tested, and how the software testing to assure compliance with the SDTP will be conducted and monitored. Finally, this policy should indicate that a completed, preliminary SDTP is due for review at the ADR and that an updated, final version is due for review and approval at the DDR.

The Software User's Manual policy, a companion to the software and hardware tools policies, addresses the generation of a user's manual for the software or hardware that is developed because it cannot be purchased commercially. This policy states that software projects should produce a User's Manual that contains the instructions necessary to operate any software system that was developed in-house. An outline of this document should be prepared for review at the ADR to obtain commitment to the design of the human-machine or user interface. The User's

Manual should be updated at the end of the project to reflect the "as-built" interface, to provide a basis for delivery and subsequent software maintenance.

The Software Quality Assurance Plan (SQAP) policy states that a software project will provide the independent assurance that its end products meet appropriate standards for software quality and that software quality will be achieved through ongoing review as well as by periodic software quality audits. This policy should require that each project's software quality assurance activities follow an SQAP that is to be prepared and approved within a specified time period of the project start-up. The degree of formality, control employed, and staff to be used on the project for software quality assurance should be contingent upon the size and complexity of the project, the significance of the project, and the investment risks.

The contents of the SQAP should direct all of the project's software quality assurance activities and address all requirements of the software quality assurance policy. These activities include identification, preparation, coordination, and maintenance of software development procedures for the control of critical steps that affect the quality of device software. The SQAP should direct the project personnel to schedule and conduct independent audits for consistent compliance with relevant software development procedures and that audit results are to be documented and reported. The SQAP should also direct project personnel to provide for the inspection of deliverable documents for compliance with software quality assurance provisions of the relevant software development procedures. Finally, the SQAP should direct project personnel to assure that the software discrepancy reporting system supports change control, forms a database for systematic problem resolution, performs periodic reviews of the problem reports, and makes recommendations as necessary.

The Software Development Plan (SDP) policy stipulates that the project will provide the means to coordinate schedules, control resources, initiate actions, and monitor progress of the software development effort. The plan for accomplishing these project management activities should be identified and described in the SDP, then prepared and approved prior to the SRR. The SDP should identify and describe the organizational structure, personnel, and resources to be used for software development, configuration management, and quality assurance efforts, as well as the development schedule and milestones. The SDP should indicate the methods and techniques to be used in the requirements definition and review, the design and design review, and the software testing, as well as indicate the methods to be used to ensure that the design requirements and requirements for device resources will be met.

If a Software Configuration Management Plan (SCMP) is prepared for the project, then a reference to that plan is sufficient to cover the configuration management requirements. If an SCMP is not prepared for the project, then the SDP should also describe the configuration control methods and organization for processing changes to the software and the associated documentation throughout the development life cycle. If an SQAP is prepared for the project, then a reference to that plan is sufficient to cover the quality assurance provisions of the project. If an SQAP is not prepared, then the SDP should also indicate the methods, techniques, and organization for assuring that the software end products meet the appropriate software standards for quality. The SDP should also identify the potential problem and high-risk areas of the software development effort in terms of schedule and technology risks and describe the means by which the software project may minimize the impact of the identified risk areas.

The Software Documentation policy states that projects will produce and maintain a set of software documents that satisfy the policies for the project, that the documents are necessary as design and planning tools for the disciplined and successful development of the software, and that they meet all regulatory requirements for the device being developed. Early in the project planning stage, project personnel should identify the set of software documents that satisfies the software policies, project needs, and regulatory requirements. This identification should include, for each document, the document's title, purpose, and schedule. The document content, format, and size should satisfy the relevant software procedures and guidelines, and be appropriate to user and project needs. The documents should also be grouped and bound into physical volumes that are consistent with user and project needs. This policy should also state the requirements for any documents required by the project but not specifically covered by the policies, procedures, or guidelines.

The Software End-Product Acceptance Plan (SEAP) policy states that projects will follow an orderly procedure and plan to prepare for and achieve approval of all end products related to software design, code, and test. The SEAP is prepared prior to the SRR. Although the SEAP is reviewed at the SRR and updated to reflect any modifications agreed to at the SRR, the SEAP can be approved at any time prior to the ADR. The SEAP should be prepared as a descriptive checklist for end products and services approved for the project. For each item, the SEAP should include the name or title, the format, the schedule for producing and delivering it, and the criteria for determining readiness for closeout. This policy should also direct that an acceptance audit be conducted near the end of the software project, with the purpose of reviewing the status of each item, achieving closeout of those items still open, and obtaining approval of each accepted item. The audit should be conducted in accordance with the agreements in the SEAP for the project.

Software Verification and Validation Policy Topics

The software V&V policies (Table 3-7) have been divided into four categories: Project Management, Phase Verification and Validation, Validation Test and Operations, and Verification and Validation Reporting. Table 3-8 illustrates the software life cycle periods during which the software V&V policies are in effect. Table 3-9 shows the responsibility matrix for maintaining the policy and related documents.

The Verification and Validation Management policy states that projects will provide the V&V required to ensure an independent assessment and measurement of the correctness, accuracy, consistency, completeness, robustness, and testability of the software requirements, design, and implementation. The methodology and procedures for achieving project-specific V&V activities should be described in the Software Verification and Validation Plan (SVVP). Management of the functions and tasks of V&V for each project should be assigned to an individual who is not associated with any of the software development aspects of the project. This person would be responsible for making decisions regarding the performance of all software V&V tasks, assigning task priorities, estimating the level of effort for V&V tasks, tracking the progress of V&V work, determining the need for V&V task iteration or for the initiation of new tasks, and assuring adherence to software V&V standards in all efforts. The authority for resolving any issues that are raised by the V&V tasks and the approval or disapproval of the V&V products should reside at the management level, preferably with the individual to whom the software V&V group reports.

The SVVP should describe the project's V&V organization, activities, schedule, inputs and outputs, and any planned deviations from the established policies that will be required in order to achieve effective management of the V&V tasks. The SVVP should be prepared and approved within a fixed time period of the project start-up. The requirement for the reperformance of any previous V&V task or the initiation of any new tasks that might be needed to address software

Table 3-7   Typical Topics in a Software Engineering Verification and Validation Policy

Policy Category	Policy Topic Title
Project Management	Verification and Validation Management Software Verification and Validation Plan (SVVP) Verification and Validation Task Iteration
Phase Verification and Validation	Interface Design Phase Verification and Validation Requirements Phase Verification and Validation Architecture Design Phase Verification and Validation Detailed Design Phase Verification and Validation Code and Test Phase Verification and Validation Integration and Test Phase Verification and Validation Software Validation Phase Verification and Validation
Validation Test and Operations	Requirements Traceability Matrix (RTM) Software Validation Test Plan (SVTP) Validation Test Information Sheet (VTIS) Software Validation Test Procedures (SVTPR)
Verification and Validation Reporting	Verification and Validation Reporting Anomaly Reporting and Resolution Software Configuration Audit Report (SCAR) Software Verification and Validation Report (SVVR)

Note: The Phase Verification and Validation policies match one-for-one to the software development phases documented in the software development policies.

changes should be determined through a continuous review of the ongoing V&V efforts, software technical accomplishments, resource utilization, future planning, and risk assessment.

Periodic reviews of the software V&V effort should be conducted, and an evaluation of the technical quality and results of the outputs from the V&V tasks should be made on the basis of these audits. These periodic audits are performed for several reasons. They provide independent information at the SRR, the ADR, and the DDR that is needed to support the decision to proceed or not to proceed with the next software development phase. They are also used to define alterations to the V&V tasks described in the SVVP to improve the V&V effort in support of the project.

The SVVP states that projects will prepare a V&V plan that identifies and describes the V&V of software end products produced by the software development effort. The SVVP should define the program to be applied throughout all phases of the software development; it should be prepared and approved within a specified time period of the project's start-up. The SVVP should specify the organization of the V&V effort, define the lines of communication within the V&V effort, and delineate the relationship of V&V to the other project efforts, such as development engineering, project management, product quality assurance, and reliability engineering. The SVVP should also present the schedule of the V&V tasks as well as the tools, techniques, and methodologies to be employed in the effort. The SVVP should also state the resources needed to perform the tasks, any special procedural requirements for these tasks, and the organizational elements of the responsible individuals. The SVVP should indicate the risks and the

Table 3-8   Software Verification and Validation Policies Throughout the Software Life Cycle

Procedure Topic Title	Software Life Cycle Phase							
	Project Start-up	Interface Design	Requirements	Architecture Design	Detailed Design	Code and Test	Integrate and Test	Software Validation
Verification and Validation Management	DS	E	E	E	E	E	E	E
Software Verification and Validation Plan (SVVP)	DS	E	E	E	E	E	E	E
Verification and Validation Task Iteration		E	E	E	E	E	E	E
Interface Design Phase Verification and Validation		DE						
Requirements Phase Verification and Validation			DE					
Architecture Design Phase Verification and Validation				DE				
Detailed Design Phase Verification and Validation					DE			
Code and Test Phase Verification and Validation						DE		
Integration and Test Phase Verification and Validation							DE	
Software Validation Phase Verification and Validation								DE
Requirements Traceability Matrix (RTM)				DE	U	U	U	U
Software Validation Test Plan (SVTP)				DE	U	E	E	E
Validation Test Information Sheet (VTIS)					S	DS	U	DE
Software Validation Test Procedures (SVTPR)					S	S	DS	E
Verification and Validation Reporting		DE	DE	DE	DE	DE	DE	DE
Anomaly Reporting and Resolution		E	E	E	E	E	E	DE
Software Configuration Audit Report (SCAR)								DE
Software Verification and Validation Report (SVVR)								DE

Notes: 1. D indicates that a deliverable or activity is required at that time.
        2. U indicates that an update of a previous deliverable occurs.
        3. E indicates that the procedure requirements are in effect for the entire phase.
        4. S indicates that the procedure requirements can start at any time.

Table 3-9 Software Verification and Validation Policy and Document Responsibility Matrix

Document Title	V&VE[1]	V&VLE[2]	SLE[3]	System Engineer	Project Engineer	Director
Software Verification and Validation Procedures		Generate				Review
Software Development Deviation		Generate		Review	Review	Approve
Software Development Waiver		Generate		Review	Review	Approve
Software Verification and Validation Plan (SVVP)		Generate	Review			Approve
Verification and Validation Reports		Generate	Review			Review
Interface Design Phase Task Summary Report		Generate	Review			Review
Requirements Phase Task Summary Report		Generate	Review			Review
Requirements Traceability Matrix (RTM)		G/U	Review			Review
Architecture Design Phase Task Summary Report		Generate	Review			Review
Software Validation Test Plan (SVTP)		Generate	Review			Approve
Verification Test Information Sheets (VTIS)	Generate	G/A	Review			Review
Software Validation Test Procedures (SVTPR)		Generate	Review			Approve
Detailed Design Phase Task Summary Report		Generate	Review			Review
Code and Test Phase Task Summary Report		Generate	Review			Review
Integrate and Test Phase Task Summary Report		Generate	Review			Review
Software Configuration Audit Report (SCAR)		Generate	Review			Review
Software Verification and Validation Report (SVVR)		Generate	Review			Approve

Notes: 1. Senior software V&V engineer assigned to the project.
2. Software V&V lead engineer assigned to the project.
3. Software lead engineer assigned to the project.
4. G/U means generate and update.
5. G/A means generate and approve.

assumptions associated with the V&V tasks and identify any planned deviations from the established software documents.

The Verification and Validation Task Iteration policy delineates the reperformance criteria for any completed V&V tasks. This policy states that the effects of any software change on any previously completed V&V tasks or on any future tasks should be analyzed to determine the necessity for the reperformance of previous tasks or the initiation of new tasks. The reperformance of completed software V&V tasks may become necessary in two situations:

1. The tasks themselves may uncover significant problems and/or tasks for which a significant part of the defined software development activity was not completed.

2. The source information that was originally supplied for the representation of the device or software requirements may have undergone significant changes.

In both of these cases, the associated V&V tasks are candidates for task iteration or reperformance. An iteration of the tasks should be determined through assessments of change, criticality, and quality effects. Any required iteration should also be documented as an update to the project's SVVP, and it should be made in accordance with the project's SCMP.

The Verification and Validation Phase policies present the software V&V tasks and activities that are to occur during each of the software development phases that were documented as a part of the software development policies. In addition, they present the testing tasks and activities associated with the final, completed software requirements validation testing.

The Interface Design Phase Verification and Validation policy states that software V&V tasks should be performed to ensure that the decomposition of the system into subsystems and the interfaces among those subsystems are completely specified. The V&V review of the IDS should be performed prior to its approval, to provide feedback to the project software development team and to support software project management. The IDS should be evaluated for its consistency, completeness, accuracy, and testability, as well as its compliance with the established software development policies and any relevant SOPs and guidelines. The results of the V&V tasks for this phase should be documented in a phase V&V task summary report. The summary report should document the tasks and activities that were performed and summarize the results of the V&V performance. This report provides an assessment of the software quality-of-progress, and it may also recommend initiation of any appropriate corrective action on the basis of those results.

The Requirements Phase Verification and Validation policy states that the Requirements Phase software tasks should ensure that both the problem to be solved and the constraints upon that problem solution are specified in a rigorous form. The evaluation and analysis of the SRS by the V&V group should ensure the correctness, consistency, completeness, accuracy, and testability of the functional, performance, and external interface requirements of the software end products. The results of the Requirements Phase V&V tasks are documented in a phase task summary report.

The device requirements document(s) that specify system performance, user interfaces, and critical system components should be reviewed by the V&V group and used for software planning as well as for defining the level of effort required to successfully verify and validate the software end products. During the review of these product requirements specifications, the software-related requirements should be documented in the Requirements Traceability Matrix (RTM), along with a reference to the document that specified them.

Analysis and evaluation of the SRS by the V&V group should ensure its compliance with the requirements that were defined in the SRS policy. Verification of the SRS should ensure the testability of all of the requirements that are specified as well as the compliance of the SRS content and format with the established software development policies and any relevant SOPs and guidelines. An assessment should also be made of how well the SRS satisfies the product objectives and safety considerations that were identified in the hazards analysis and that are controlled or commanded by the software. The RTM should then be updated to document the tracing of the software and interface requirements as specified in the SRS to the requirements that are defined in the product requirements documentation.

All V&V outputs generated during this phase should be provided to the project software development team prior to the SRR to support management in determining the adequacy, correctness, and testability of the stated software and interface requirements. The phase task summary report should document the software V&V tasks and activities that were performed and summarize the results. This report provides an assessment of the software quality-of-progress, and on the basis of those results, it may recommend appropriate corrective action.

The Architecture Design Phase Verification and Validation policy states that the Architecture Design Phase software V&V should ensure that the preliminary software design establishes the design baseline from which the detailed design will be developed. Evaluation and analysis of the ADS by the V&V group should ensure the internal consistency, completeness, correctness, and clarity of the information that is needed to support the detailed definition of the individual software components. Analysis and evaluation of the ADS should ensure its compliance with the requirements that are defined in the software development ADS policy and any relevant SOPs and guidelines. The verification should also ensure the robustness and testability of the software design and its compliance with established software development design SOPs and guidelines.

The Software Validation Test Plan (SVTP) governs the validation of software end products by the V&V group and is generated and approved before completion of the ADR; this plan can be generated concurrently with software development design analysis. The SDTP should be reviewed by the V&V group for completeness, correctness, and consistency of the software testing that will be required for each software component and for its compliance with policy requirements as specified in the software development policy and any relevant SOPs and guidelines. If a User's Manual is generated, evaluation of it should ensure compliance with the requirements defined for the User's Manual in the software development policy and any relevant SOPs and guidelines. The RTM should then be updated to document the tracing of the software design to the requirements as specified in the SRS and to provide a cross-reference of each software requirement to the test(s) described in the SDTP and the SVTP.

The results of the Architecture Design Phase V&V tasks are documented in a phase task summary report. All V&V outputs generated during this phase should be provided to the project software development team prior to the ADR to support management in determining the compatibility, reliability, and testability of the stated software and interface design. The phase task summary report should document the V&V tasks and activities that were performed and summarize the results. This report provides an assessment of the quality of progress of the software, and it may also recommend appropriate corrective action on the basis of those results.

The Detailed Design Phase Verification and Validation policy states that the Detailed Design Phase software V&V should ensure that the software detailed design satisfies the requirements and constraints specified in the SRS and that it augments the design specified in the ADS. Evaluation and analysis of the DDS by the V&V group should ensure the internal consistency, completeness, correctness, and clarity of the DDS; it should also verify that the design, when implemented, will satisfy the requirements specified in the SRS. Analysis and evaluation of the DDS should ensure its compliance with the requirements of the software development DDS policy and any relevant SOPs and guidelines. DDS verification should also ensure its consistency with the architecture design, its completeness in the allocation of the software end product functional capabilities to one or more software components, and identification of the relationships among the interfaces between all software components. Verification of the DDS should also ensure the correctness of the algorithms that are defined, as well as the robustness and testability of the design. The SVTP should be updated to incorporate the additional design details of the DDS.

The SDTP should be reviewed by the V&V group for completeness, correctness, and consistency of the software testing that will be required for each software component, as well as its compliance with the SDTP requirements as specified in the software development policies and any relevant SOPs and guidelines. The DTISs should be prepared prior to the DDR; analysis and evaluation of the adequacy of the software component testing is supported by the review of the DTISs. The SVTP should be updated to incorporate any additional design details of the DDS and should be approved before the DDR is completed.

Validation Test Information Sheets (VTISs) should be developed to define the objectives, approach, and requirements of each test defined in the SVTP. The generation of VTISs for each test defined in the SVTP can be accomplished concurrently with the software development design analysis. The VTISs should be provided prior to the DDR and should be used for assessing the adequacy of the test methods and limits defined for the software testing program. The preliminary version of the User's Manual (if one has been generated) should be reviewed, and the evaluation should ensure compliance of the manual with the User's Manual requirements as defined in the software development policy and any relevant SOPs and guidelines. The RTM should then be updated to document the tracing of the software detailed design to the requirements as specified in the SRS.

The results of the Detailed Design Phase V&V tasks and activities are documented in a phase task summary report. All software V&V outputs generated during this phase should be provided to the project software development team prior to the DDR to support management in establishing the compatibility, reliability, and testability of the stated software and interface design. The phase task summary report should document the V&V tasks and activities that were performed and summarize the results. This report provides an assessment of the software quality of progress; it may also recommend appropriate corrective action on the basis of those results.

The Code and Test Phase Verification and Validation policy states that Code and Test Phase software V&V will ensure the correctness, consistency, completeness, and accuracy of the implementation of the software design as defined in the DDS. The code for the software end products should be provided to the V&V group after successful completion of code compilation; audits should be performed as necessary to examine both the high-level and detailed properties of the code. These audits should verify the consistency of the code with the design as specified in the DDS, the adherence of the code to the relevant programming standards and conventions, and the correctness and efficiency of the code. Any anomalies detected during software V&V task performance should be documented in the Software Verification and Validation Anomaly Report. The RTM should then be updated to document the tracing of source code to the software design as described in the DDS and to the requirements as specified in the SRS. The results of the Code and Test Phase V&V tasks should be documented in a phase task summary report. The summary report should document the V&V tasks and activities that were performed and summarize the results. This report provides an assessment of the software quality of progress, and it may also recommend corrective action on the basis of those results.

The Integration and Test Phase Verification and Validation policy states that Integration and Test Phase software V&V should ensure the correctness, completeness, and accuracy of software component interactions and interfaces. Analysis and evaluation of software integration and testing by the V&V group should be accomplished through the review of the DTISs that document the successful completion of integration and testing for the designated software components. The DTISs and their associated test data should be provided in an incremental manner as each test is successfully completed. The DTISs should be analyzed to evaluate the adequacy of the test coverage, the adequacy of the test data, software behavior, and software reliability.

The Software Validation Test Procedures (SVTPR) are required to execute the tests defined in the SVTP; they are developed using the test information defined on the VTISs. The SVTPR should be generated and approved prior to test execution, and software validation testing should not be conducted without an approved SVTPR. Any anomalies that are detected during V&V task performance should be documented in a Software Verification and Validation Anomaly Report. The RTM should then be updated to document any changes that have occurred relative to the tracing of the source code to the software design as presented in the DDS and the requirements as specified in the SRS. The results of the Integrate and Test Phase software V&V tasks should be documented in a phase task summary report. The phase task summary report should document the V&V tasks and activities that were performed and summarize the results. This report provides an assessment of the software quality of progress, and it may also recommend corrective action on the basis of those results.

The Software Validation Phase Verification and Validation policy states that the V&V should verify that the software end products satisfy the requirements and the design specified in the SRS and the DDS. All software validation testing is performed in accordance with the SVTP, using the SVTPR. All procedures for the configuration management of software end products during and at the completion of validation testing are implemented in accordance with the project's SCMP. At the completion of all V&V activities, a Software Verification and Validation Report (SVVR) is generated.

The software validation should be performed using the most recent and controlled version of the software as determined and defined with the procedures in the project's SCMP. The software validation should be conducted in accordance with the SVTP, using the SVTPR; the results of software validation testing should be documented on the VTISs. The validation tests are analyzed to determine if the software end products satisfy the software requirements and design as specified in the SRS and DDS. Any approved changes to the software undergoing validation testing should be verified by regression testing to confirm that the redesign of the corrected software has been effective and has not introduced other errors. The RTM should then be updated to document the verification of each requirement in the SRS. Software Verification and Validation Anomaly Reports should be generated, to document any test failures and software faults.

A software configuration audit of the validated software should be conducted. The version description of all software end products is verified in order to demonstrate that the delivered software corresponds to the software that was subjected to the software validation. The completion of the software configuration audit is contingent on the closure of all outstanding software discrepancies and deficiencies. The Software Configuration Audit Report (SCAR) is used to document the final configuration of software end products. The SVVR is generated at the completion of all project software V&V tasks and approved.

The Requirements Traceability Matrix (RTM) policy delineates the requirements for the tracing of device requirements into the implemented code. This policy states that software projects will prepare an RTM that documents the development of software end products from requirements through software validation. The RTM should be generated during the Requirements Phase of software development and should be updated at each subsequent phase. All software requirements should be traced on the RTM from the SRS to the source code and into the subsequent software testing. The requirements for the software end products should be identified on the RTM and assigned a unique requirement number for reference. For each RTM requirement number, a description of the requirement as well as the higher level RTM number should be shown, if one exists. In addition, the paragraph number(s) and the requirement document name that specify the requirement, the paragraph number(s) and the name of the design document that specify the requirement, as well as the component name(s) that implement the requirement should be listed. The RTM should show the test(s) required to verify the requirement as well as the result(s) of the testing.

The RTM can be used for evaluating subsequent requirements and design documents, for developing test events and test data, and for documenting the validation of the software end products. The RTM should be reviewed by the V&V group for inconsistencies in the refinement of the software requirements, for incomplete definition of the software requirements in lower level specifications and code, and for incomplete specification of the software testing for requirements. Any discrepancies found in the RTM should be documented in the appropriate phase task summary report.

The Software Validation Test Plan (SVTP) policy states that software projects will prepare an SVTP that validates the required software testing for verifying that the software end products satisfy the requirements stated in the SRS. The SVTP should be generated by the V&V group and approved prior to completion of the ADR. The SVTP should define the methods for verifying the correct implementation of software requirements, the software system capabilities, and the throughput and timing requirements. In addition, the SVTP should define the methods for verifying the safety design requirements and the correct interface with the system environment. The SVTP should also specify the testing that will measure the compliance of the complete software product with all of the specified software functional requirements while operating in all system configurations and environments. The SVTP should also specify the testing that will measure the performance of the hardware, software, and user interfaces. It should specify the testing that will measure software performance at the software limits and under stress conditions, compliance with safety design requirements, and software performance in terms of accuracies, response times, storage, input and output rates, and margins for growth. The SVTP should also define the objectives, test methods, and system environments for each test to be performed during the Software Validation Phase. The SVTP should contain a test validation matrix that correlates the SRS requirements to the type of test verification method(s) to be used and the test level(s) in which the requirements will be tested. The SVTP should also define the procedures for collecting, reviewing, and evaluating the test results.

The Validation Test Information Sheet (VTIS) policy states that software projects will prepare and maintain VTISs for each test that will be conducted during the Software Validation Phase. The VTISs should provide an organized, accessible collection of all validation testing and test results, a means of tracking the progression and status of the validation testing, and a means of validation test verification. A VTIS should be prepared for each test defined in the SVTP. VTISs should be generated prior to the DDR, and they should be maintained until the tests are completed. Completed VTISs should be reviewed for completeness and technical adequacy of the testing conducted, periodically audited to assess their compliance with relevant V&V SOPs and guidelines, and formally approved upon completion of the test. Any problems detected during an audit should be identified in a written summary that should be attached to the VTIS. The VTISs should then be used as a basis for development of the SVTPR. The results of the validation testing that are described by the VTIS should be documented on the VTIS itself, and the test conductor should sign and date the completed VTIS. The overall results of VTIS testing should be reflected in summary report on the software validation phase tasks.

The VTIS should define the title of the test to be conducted, the objectives of the test, and the success criteria. The VTIS should also define the requirement(s) to be tested, including the requirement's unique identifier and the specification title where the requirement was defined. The VTIS should define the test approach to be taken down to the depth necessary to establish a baseline for resource requirements; the required test instrumentation; and the test phasing, scheduling, and duration. The VTIS should also define the data collection, reduction, and analysis requirements.

The Software Validation Test Procedures (SVTPR) policy states that software projects will prepare SVTPR that describe the detailed procedures for performing the validation testing defined in the SVTP. The SVTPR should be generated, maintained, and approved prior to execution of the validation test and should be developed using the test information defined in the VTIS. In addition, the SVTPR should specify the instructions for executing the set of tests defined in the SVTP, the requirements for logging test activities, the criteria for stopping or restarting the procedure, and the method for collecting and analyzing the test data.

The Verification and Validation Reporting policy states that the results of implementing software V&V should be documented in V&V reports and that such reporting should occur throughout all phases of the software development effort. At the conclusion of each software V&V phase, the appropriate phase task summary report should summarize the results of the software V&V tasks and activities performed during the corresponding software development phase. This summary report should contain, as a minimum, a description of the V&V tasks performed, a summary of the V&V task results, a summary of any anomalies and implemented resolutions, an assessment of software quality, and any recommendations. All of the inputs and outputs of the V&V effort for each project should be controlled and maintained in accordance with the procedures defined in the project's SCMP. Document change control and configuration status accounting for V&V should be implemented to ensure that the validity of the V&V results are protected from accidental or unauthorized alteration. All of the V&V inputs and outputs should be archived, to provide a project history for use in future software development project planning. The format, timing, and distribution of the reports should be made in accordance with the project's SVVP.

The Anomaly Reporting and Resolution policy states that all anomalies encountered while performing software V&V will be documented and reported on a Software Verification and Validation Anomaly Report, regardless of the perceived impact on the software development or on the severity of the anomaly with respect to operation of the device. Software Verification and Validation Anomaly Reports are reviewed for solution determination, implementation authorization, and signature closure. The report should be used to identify all problems detected during the V&V activities and can be initiated by software developers as well as the V&V personnel. The specific information that the report should contain includes the description and location of the anomaly, the severity of the anomaly, and the cause and method of identifying the anomalous behavior. In addition, the report should indicate the recommended action, as well as any actions taken to correct the anomalous behavior, and the impact of the problem on the capability of the product and on the continued conduct of V&V activities. Configuration identification, tracking, and status reporting of the Software Verification and Validation Anomaly Report should be made in accordance with the project's SCMP.

The projected impact of an anomaly should be determined by evaluating the severity of its effect on the operation of the device; the severity of the anomaly should be assigned a category of *high, medium,* or *low.* The anomaly is *high* if a change is required to correct a condition that prevents or seriously degrades a device objective, where no alternative exists, or to correct a safety-related problem. An anomaly is *medium* if a change is required to correct a condition that degrades a system objective, to provide for performance improvement, or to confirm that the user and/or system requirements can be met. An anomaly is *low* if the change is desirable to maintain the system, correct operator inconvenience, or for any other reason. This is not the only classification scheme; a classification that directly reflects the specific product development environment should be used. The report should be reviewed for anomaly validity, type, and severity by an appropriate project software engineer or by a software management person. Additional V&V can be directed, if required, to assess the validity of the anomaly or the proposed solution.

An anomaly solution that does not require a change to a baseline software configuration item may be approved by an appropriate project software engineer. However, if the anomaly does require a change to a baseline software configuration item, then the anomaly should be approved in accordance with the project's SCMP. Report closure includes documenting the corrective action(s) taken, verifying the incorporation of the authorized changes as described, and describing the status of the report.

The Software Configuration Audit Report (SCAR) policy states that software projects will prepare a SCAR that summarizes the results of the validated software configuration audit by reporting the final configuration of the software end products for the project. At the conclusion of validation testing during the Software Validation Phase, a software configuration audit should be conducted. At the completion of the software configuration audit, the SCAR should be generated to document the final configuration of the software end products. The SCAR is essentially a checklist that identifies and describes each item of software, verifies that the software configurations are what they were intended and proclaimed to be, and verifies that the configuration of each item of software is the same configuration that was validated during the Software Validation Phase. The SCAR should be completed and reviewed prior to completion of the Software Validation Phase.

The Software Verification and Validation Report (SVVR) policy states that the software project team will prepare a final report that summarizes the project's V&V tasks, activities, and results, and the status and disposition of any anomalies. An assessment of the overall software quality and any recommendations for improvements in software and/or product development processes should also be documented in the SVVR. The SVVR should be generated upon the completion of all software V&V tasks and activities during the Software Validation Phase. The SVVR should include, as a minimum, a summary of all of the project's V&V tasks that were performed, a summary of the task results, a summary of any anomalies and their resolutions, an assessment of the overall software quality, and any recommendations for improvements in software and/or product development processes. The SVVR should also include the results of validation testing performed by the V&V group. This document serves as the certification that the software was developed in a manner that was consistent with the set of software policies, SOPs, and guidelines and that the software implemented both the requirements and the specified design.

Software Configuration Management Policy Topics

The software configuration management policies (Table 3-10) have been divided into five categories: Software Configuration Identification, Project Management, Product Management and

Table 3-10 Typical Topics in Software Engineering Configuration Management Policy

Policy Category	Policy Topic Title
Software Configuration Identification	Software Configuration Item Identification
Project Management	Software Configuration Management Organization Software Configuration Management of Subcontractor and Vendor Products
Product Management and Acceptance	Software Configuration Management Plan (SCMP)
Configuration Change Control	Software Configuration Change Processing Change Request/Authorization (CRA) Form Software Change Review Board (SCRB)
Configuration Status	Software Configuration Status Accounting

Acceptance, Configuration Change Control, and Configuration Status Accounting. Table 3-11 illustrates the software life cycle periods during which the software configuration management policies are in effect. Table 3-12 shows the responsibility matrix for maintaining the policy and related documents.

The Software Configuration Item Identification policy states that software projects will provide configuration identification of the software end products developed in the project and that the configuration of each software end product will be identified by its technical documentation. Configuration baselines should be established at specific points during software development to further define the configuration of the items as they are developed. At a minimum, baselines should be established at the conclusion of each software development phase, as well as being established for the software project at appropriate development milestones. These baselines should define a formal departure point for control of future changes to the performance and/or design of the software end products. The items identified for configuration management at each configuration baseline are referred to as configuration items. The configuration items should be uniquely identified by a configuration identifier that is easily recognized and understood by the project's software personnel.

The Software Configuration Management Organization policy states that software projects will be responsible for the configuration management of the software end products developed in the project. The software configuration management activities to be performed for the project are those described in the project's SCMP. To achieve the successful configuration management of a software project, a product software development library should be established as the depository for the software end products that are placed under configuration management. The library should provide storage of and controlled access to the software and documentation in both human-readable and machine-readable form.

The management of the functions and tasks of software configuration management should include decisions regarding the performance of software configuration management, assigning priorities to software configuration management tasks, estimating the level of effort for a software configuration management task, tracking the progress of configuration management work,

Table 3-11   Software Configuration Management Policies Throughout the Software Life Cycle

Procedure Topic Title	Software Life Cycle Phase							
	Project Start-up	Interface Design	Requirements	Architecture Design	Detailed Design	Code and Test	Integrate and Test	Software Validation
Software Configuration Item Identification	DS	DE	DE	DE	DE	E	DE	DE
Software Configuration Management Organization	E	E	DE	E	E	E	E	E
Software Configuration Management of Subcontractor and Vendor Products	S	S	S	S	S	S	S	S
Software Configuration Management Plan (SCMP)	S	S	DS	E	E	E	E	E
Software Configuration Change Processing		S	S	S	S	S	S	S
Change Request/Approval (CRA) Form		S	S	S	S	S	S	S
Software Change Review Board (SCRB)		S	S	S	S	S	S	S
Software Configuration Status Accounting		E	E	E	E	E	E	E
Software Configuration Status Report (SCSR)		DE	DE	DE	DE	E	DE	DE

Notes: 1. D indicates that a deliverable or activity is required at that time.
2. E indicates that the procedure requirements are in effect for the entire phase.
3. S indicates that the procedure requirements can start at any time.

and assuring adherence to relevant configuration management standards in all efforts. The authority for resolving any issues raised by software configuration management tasks should reside at the management level. The project should prepare and maintain an SCMP that complies with the relevant software configuration management policies and any relevant SOPs and guidelines. The SCMP should describe the software configuration management requirements for the project and should be generated prior to the SRR.

The Software Configuration Management of Subcontractor and Vendor Products policy states that subcontractors and vendors who design and/or produce software delivered as a component of a software project and to be included in a medical device should comply with the same software configuration management requirements as those imposed on the project software. These requirements are imposed on the subcontractors and vendors through the procurement package that, after any source selection and negotiation, becomes the contract. The procurement package should assure the right to review the subcontractor's or vendor's configuration management system prior to procurement. Periodically, an audit should be conducted to ensure that

Table 3-12 Responsibility Matrix for Software Configuration Management Policy and Documents

Document Title	CM[1]	SLE[2]	V&VLE[3]	Director	Program Manager	SCRB[4]
Software Configuration Management Procedures	Generate			Approve		
Software Configuration Management Deviation	Generate			Approve	Review	
Software Configuration Management Waiver	Generate			Approve	Review	
Software Configuration Management Plan (SCMP)	Generate	Review	Review	Approve		
Software Change Request (SCR) Form (Class I and II)	Assigns	Review	Verify			Approve
Software Change Request (SCR) Form (Class III)	Assigns	Approve	Verify			
Configuration Status Accounting	E/M/A					
Software Configuration Status Report (SCSR)	Generate					

Notes: 1. Software configuration management engineer assigned to the project.
2. Software lead engineer assigned to the project.
3. Software V&V lead engineer assigned to the project.
4. Software Configuration Review Board.
5. E/M/A means establish, maintain, and archive.

the subcontractor or vendor has adequate methods in place for identifying and controlling each product to be delivered.

The Software Configuration Management Plan (SCMP) policy states that projects will perform configuration management functions that will establish a series of baselines and the methods for controlling changes to those baselines. The degree of formality, the control employed, and the personnel to be used for software configuration management should be contingent upon the size and complexity of the project, the significance of the project, and the investment risks. Software configuration management activities should follow an SCMP, which is prepared and approved prior to the SRR. The SCMP should address the requirements of this policy and any unique requirements of the project; it may be a separate document or a part of the SDP. The SCMP should specify the baselines to be used by the project and the configuration identification requirements of the project, including the types of products to be controlled and the rules for making, naming, or otherwise identifying those products. The SCMP should also specify the configuration control mechanisms, which include the definition of the changes as well as the approval and disapproval processes for the controlled products. The problem-reporting system, the configuration accounting system, and the configuration verification approach that will be used to assure that the products are developed and maintained according to the requirements of the policy should also be part of the SCMP.

The Software Configuration Change Processing policy states that software projects will provide for the systematic evaluation, coordination, approval or disapproval, and implementation of all changes to the configuration of a software item after the establishment of its configuration identification. The configuration change processing is described in the project's SCMP, and implementation and verification of the approved changes to baseline material should conform to the SCMP and SVVP. The software items that compose each configuration baseline should be provided to the appropriate configuration management person for software configuration management upon approval and/or completion of V&V related to the item. The current to-be-established baseline, the previous baseline material, and all changes to any baseline material that occurred during completion of the software development phases should be placed under configuration control.

Baseline material should be placed in the product software development library for version and access control. Version control should ensure the rapid, comprehensive, and accurate treatment of any approved changes to the items that are placed under configuration control. Access control should ensure restricted access to those configuration items that are undergoing change. Changes to baseline material should be documented on a Change Request/Approval (CRA) form and should be uniquely identified by a designator that combines the name of the software project, the initiator's identification, and a unique identification number.

The purpose of the CRA designator is to provide a historical record, naming the person who requested the change. The assignment of the identification number to the CRA is done in accordance with the relevant software configuration management SOPs and guidelines. The CRAs should be classified as Class I, Class II, or Class III, reflecting the potential impact of their change. Class I changes affect the performance, function, or technical requirements of the device. Class II changes require a change to any baseline materials that do not meet the criteria of Class I changes. Class III changes do not require alterations to any baseline material. Revised baseline material is verified in accordance with the project's SCMP and SVVP.

The Change Request/Approval (CRA) Form policy states that changes to baseline material should be documented in the CRA (see Figure 3-8) and that the format of the form itself is contained in the software configuration management SOPs. Each CRA should identify the affected

Figure 3-8 Typical Change Request/Approval (CRA) form

CHANGE REQUEST/APPROVAL (CRA) FORM

1. System name: _____   2. CRA Number: _____

3. Application Level: SOFTWARE ☐   DOCUMENT ☐   OTHER ☐

4.a. Originating Organization	5. Configuration Baseline Affected (highest level)	7. Configuration Items Affected
b. Initiator	6. Change Classification:	a. _____ b. _____
c. Telephone	Class I ☐	c. _____
	Class II ☐	d. _____
d. Date	Class III ☐	e. _____

8. Narrative: (If additional space is needed, indicate here — Page ___ of ___.)

   a. Description of change:

   b. Need for change:

   c. Estimated effects on other systems/software/equipment:

   d. Alternatives:

   e. Anomaly Number (if any) used to generate this CR/A: _____

9. Disposition: Additional Analysis   Approved   Disapproved

   DATE: [   ]   [   ]   [   ]

   Signature: _____

10. Change Verification Results:

11. V&V Signature: _____   12. Date: _____

13. Date Closed: _____   14. Signature: _____

software project name, the CRA number, the applicable level of the proposed change, and the initiator. In addition, the CRA should identify the configuration baseline(s) affected, the change classification, the document(s) affected, and the estimated impact of the proposed change on other systems, software, or equipment. The disposition of the proposed change(s) should be documented in the CRA, and it should include the date of disposition and the signature of the appropriate team member. The result(s) of the change verification should also be documented in the CRA. When change verification has been completed, the conductor of the CRA verification and validation activities should also sign and date the CRA. Closure of the CRA occurs when change implementation and verification are successful, or when a change is disapproved. When the CRA is closed, it should be signed and dated.

The Software Change Review Board (SCRB) policy describes the activities associated with CRA forms related to Class I and Class II changes. This policy states that software projects will establish an SCRB in order to coordinate, review, and decide the disposition of Class I and Class II changes to baseline material. The board should consist of an appropriate software management level individual, a person who is involved with the development of the baseline material to be changed, and a person who is involved with the V&V of the software project. The SCRB should analyze and identify the impact of the proposed CRA change and ensure that the change will either produce a substantial life cycle cost saving, significantly increase system effectiveness, correct software deficiencies, or prevent the slippage of the approved software development schedule. The SCRB should then direct the proposed CRA change disposition: additional problem analysis, a change different from that proposed in the change document, approval of the change as proposed, or disapproval of the change.

The Software Configuration Status Accounting policy states that software projects should establish and maintain configuration status accounting records for software end products developed in the project. Configuration status accounting should provide identification of the project's configuration baselines, traceability from the baselines resulting from approved changes, and a management tool for monitoring the accomplishment of all tasks that result from any approved changes. The results of this configuration management activity should be documented in the project's Software Configuration Status Report (SCSR). Configuration status accounting records should provide a list of the approved configuration identification, status of proposed changes to the configuration, and implementation status of approved changes. The types and formats of the configuration status accounting records should be in accordance with the project's SCMP. Configuration status accounting records should be maintained until all software end products developed in the project have been approved in accordance with relevant software development policies, any relevant SOPs and guidelines, and the project's SCMP. Upon acceptance of the end product, all configuration status accounting records should be archived in accordance with the project's SCMP, to provide software project history for use in future software development planning.

The SCSR policy states that software projects will document the results of configuration status accounting in the SCSR. The SCSR should be generated at the end of the software development phase associated with each configuration baseline. The SCSR should document the status of the configuration items being developed on the project, and the format of the SCSR should be defined in the relevant software configuration management SOPs and guidelines. The results of configuration status accounting for each configuration baseline should be reported in the SCSR. The SCSR should list the baseline configuration, all of the baselined material by current revision identification and referenced CRA Form number, and all CRAs, including current disposition or date of closure.

Software Nonproject Administration Policy Topics

The last set of software development policies, the nonproject-related administrative topics, are:

- Software End-Product Release

- Software Development Management

- Data Integrity and Retention

- System Management

- Data Security

- Software Development Support Activities

The Software End-Product Release policy states that the release of the software end products should be the responsibility of a single individual. The software end products to be released should be the IDS, the SRS, the DDS, the SVVR, read-only memory (ROM) if appropriate, and floppy disks that contain the validated device software and documents if appropriate. This policy would also indicate that the software end products should be delivered to the corporation's central repository of device information upon the completion of all software V&V tasks and activities for the project. Control numbers must also be assigned to each of the software end products placed into the central repository. Quantities and media for each of the end products to be released should also be noted. This policy should indicate that any further changes to the software end products should be implemented according to SOPs that govern changes to production-released device documentation.

The Software Development Management policy should delineate the software project management organization and who is responsible for the various tasks and activities related to management of software development, software V&V, and configuration management. It should also present the underlying rationale and approach to be used for generation of software project development schedules as well as the review criteria for those schedules.

The Data Integrity and Retention policy states that the data are to be duplicated in reliable media for storage in a secure area. For the purposes of this discussion, data should include, but not be limited to, systems software, application software, project software, files of collected data, and documents. This policy should also direct that all completed or suspended software project work be saved as a set of files that can be used to regenerate the work and that the storage media labels should indicate the time, date, and collection location for the data. Previously archived software project data should be catalogued and should be retrievable by specifying the data topic, the data title, the intended user or originator, the date, the document number, or the project account number.

The System Management policy would document the management and administration of the various hardware systems. This policy states that systems management is responsible for system security regulation, user account information, systems monitoring, system backup administration, computer room facilities, system utilities, and system selection and purchasing. In addition, this policy should indicate those actions and activities that should occur when an individual separates from the company or is no longer assigned to a specific software project.

The Data Security policy states that all confidential or copyrighted data must be physically secure. Confidential data should include, but are not limited to, project software, files of collected data, corporate written applications software, and project documents. Copyright data should include, but not be limited to, systems software, purchased application software, any software manuals, and purchased documents.

The last policy is the Software Development Support Activities policy. It states that software development is an integral part of product development activities and that the software development team is committed to supporting the overall product development process and administration, responding to product development needs, and providing technical software expertise to other areas. This policy should indicate that the software development team should actively support the safety and efficacy of the device through the generation of a hazards analysis, comply with corporate safety standards, and not knowingly release unsafe software.

Software Policy Guidelines

The implementation phase of software development is concerned with translating the physical model represented in the design specifications into the source code that then becomes the final software end product. The primary goal of implementation is to write the source code, and its embedded internal documentation, so that the conformance of the software to its specifications can be easily verified. This also facilitates the debugging, testing, modification, and maintenance efforts. This goal can be achieved by making the source code as clear and as straightforward as possible. Simplicity, clarity, and elegance are the hallmarks of good software, whereas obscurity, cleverness, and complexity are indications of inadequate design, misdirected thinking, and poor quality. Source code clarity is enhanced by many factors. Among them are structured coding techniques, good coding style, appropriate supporting documents, good internal comments, and the features provided in modern programming languages.

The production of high-quality software requires that the software team have a designated leader, a well-defined organizational structure, and a thorough understanding of the duties and responsibilities of each team member. The implementation team should be provided with a well-defined set of software requirements, an architectural design specification, and a detailed design description. Finally, each team member must understand the objectives of implementation. To facilitate these objectives, guideline documents are generated that augment the policy documents by providing explanatory information, instructions, or interpretation of implementation on projects.

Software Development Guideline

In general, style is the consistent pattern of choice among the alternative ways of achieving a desired effect. In software engineering, style is manifest in the patterns used by the software engineer to express a desired action or outcome; software engineers who work together soon come to recognize the coding styles of their colleagues. Software standards and conventions are the specifications for a preferred coding style where, given a choice of ways to achieve an effect, a preferred way is specified. Coding standards are often viewed by software engineers as mechanisms to constrict and devalue their creative problem-solving skills. This argument is usually made by software individuals who do not understand the spirit or intent of good coding style. Creativity has always occurred within a basic framework of standards. For example, artists follow the basic tenets of structure and composition. Poets adhere to the rhyme and meter of language, and musicians use fundamental chord progressions. In sports, aspiring professionals must learn and perfect the disciplines and techniques of their fields before they can be qualified to practice. Where health and public safety are concerned, qualifying boards administer rigorous examinations, and only those who can demonstrate competence receive a license to practice. Without a framework of standards to guide and channel an activity, creativity becomes meaningless chaos.

Although the necessity of standards in most software applications has gained widespread acceptance, standards and conventions are particularly crucial in the realm of software products developed in a multiprogramming environment, where a deliverable product will usually involve the successful integration of independent parts of programs developed by several different software engineers. In such an environment, there is a premium on software that is not only structured but also readily legible, comprehensible, and, if necessary, modifiable by any member of the software team. In this context, standards provide the critical set of common assumptions required for the intelligibility of the software. Standards are, furthermore, intended to establish software efficiency in a global, project-wide, and even corporate-wide sense. Because the greatest single obstacle to the success of a software project lies in the complexity of the development effort, attempts to optimize software development on a local, unstructured basis can be not only irrelevant to the overall software performance but even a hindrance to software development and project coordination. This emphasis on global rather than local efficiency is in keeping with both the principles of development methodologies and the growing differential between the cost of developing and maintaining complex software and the cost of a few extra executable instructions.

The software standards and conventions that are implemented should be derived from two sources: (1) the set of government and commercial or industry software standards and specifications that control software development, and (2) the experience of the software staff in actually developing software on different hardware platforms and for different target microprocessors.

Through use of these sources, software standards and conventions will continue to evolve as the experience of the software staff increases. Because of this evolution, an attempt should be made to formulate and justify the adoption of individual standards in terms that are, whenever possible, independent of any particular hardware platform, microprocessor, operating system, or programming language.

In software engineering, a standard is a definite rule or procedure established and imposed by authority. A convention is a customary or agreed-on rule or procedure that reflects a commonly accepted practice. Several conditions are necessary to obtain voluntary adherence to programming standards and conventions, as well as to ensure that they are followed.

- Software engineers must understand the value of programming standards and conventions.

- Software engineers must have the opportunity to participate in defining and establishing programming standards and conventions.

- Standards and conventions must be subject to review and revision when they become burdensome or obsolete.

- There must be a mechanism for allowing a deviation from the standards and conventions under special circumstances.

- Automated tools should be used to check adherence to programming standards and conventions.

The complete specification of a standard or convention should include, but not necessarily be limited to, a statement of the standard or convention, its purpose, implementation, and an example. This approach is intended to isolate those aspects of a standard or convention that can be stated in general, transportable terms from those that necessarily reflect the terminology and structure of a specific platform or microprocessor. However, many standards and conventions can only be meaningfully formulated in reference to their actual implementation. A typical table of contents for the standards and conventions document is shown in Table 3-13.

Section 1 introduces the standards and conventions document. In Section 2, the standards and conventions concerning the environment in which the software engineer works can be stated in terms of restrictions on the wide-ranging flexibility offered by the modern operating system and hardware platform environment. These restrictions are intended to increase the efficiency and facilitate the task of the software development effort by reducing the number of options, as well as the number of keystrokes required for the myriad software development activities. At the same time, the integrity and continuity of software development activities are ensured. The conventions stated in this section deal with the software programming environment relative to the use of the operating system, the use of system peripheral devices, and the use and organization of secondary file storage.

Section 3 relates to the software production process. These standards and conventions have evolved to facilitate the software development cycle of programming activities. During this cycle, system utilities and resources of the programming environment are coordinated in a logically consistent fashion toward the goal of more efficient software production. This cycle usually consists of a general-purpose, automated procedure that is invoked automatically at the beginning of a terminal session, which, in turn, invokes the appropriate sequence of system utilities to be used in software development activities.

Section 4 presents standards associated with the content, format, and style of software to be produced in a software project. Whenever possible, these standards should be illustrated with examples from existing validated and functional software. These standards should apply to high-level languages as well as to assembly language applications. In fact, this section should present the conditions under which assembly language is an acceptable alternative to higher level language. For clarity, this section is divided into standards for the specification of data structures, for acceptable control flow constructs, for code formatting, and for internal code documentation and comments. The standards that address the actual content of software are, by necessity, the most rigidly enforced. Standards concerning the format of code statements and routines are important for ensuring the legibility of software products. Standards that concern the programming style are generally suggested and illustrated by the examples given with the text.

Section 5 presents the standards and conventions that cover the content, format, and style of software documents produced by the software project team. For clarity of presentation, these standards have been divided arbitrarily into those for the specification of a user's manual, the specification of software documents, and for additional, automated, and supporting software documentation.

Section 6 presents the standards and conventions governing the use of the various platforms that software developers might use. These platform standards consist of administrative matters, directory construction, function key uses, application protocol, and control of the execution environment. For clarity of presentation and application, these standards have been divided arbitrarily into those for the PC, workstation, and platform operating environment.

Software Verification and Validation Guideline

The software V&V guideline document is intended to encompass the responsibilities of, methodologies used by, and testing to be performed by the V&V group. The goal is to provide

Table 3-13   Typical Table of Contents for a Software Development Guideline Document

Section Number	Section Title
1	Introduction
2	Software Production Environment Conventions
2.1	Overview
2.2	Conventions for the Development of Software
2.3	Conventions for the Use of System Devices
2.4	Conventions for the Use of File Storage
3	Software Production Process
3.1	The Programming Cycle
3.2	Source File Creation
3.3	Source File Editing
3.4	Language Processors
3.5	Linking and Loading Programs
3.6	Executing Programs
3.7	Command Procedures for Standardized Code Development
4	Software Product Standards and Conventions
4.1	Programming Standards
4.2	Data Specifications
4.3	Control Flow Constructs
4.4	Routine, Function, and Statement Formats
4.5	Formats for Internal Documentation and Comment
5	Software Documentation Standards
5.1	User's Manual Standards
5.2	Software Documentation Standards
5.3	Automatic Documentation Generator Listings
5.4	Additional, Support, and Miscellaneous Documentation Standards
6	Microprocessor Platform Standards
6.1	Overview
6.2	PC Standards and Conventions
6.3	Workstation Standards and Conventions
6.4	Operating Environment Standards and Conventions

commonality of V&V intent, tools, practices, procedures, and purpose for both the medical products and for equipment used in manufacturing or product development. A typical table of contents for the V&V guideline document is shown in Table 3-14.

Section 1 introduces the document. In Section 2, the tools, techniques, and methodologies of V&V are discussed. The intent of the tool subsection is to present the common test suite used to perform V&V testing for every processor, controller, and software language supported in the products manufactured by the company. The techniques subsection would present the approach to be used for each product, and the methodology subsection would delineate the test categories to be used for each product as a function of the product or equipment use.

Section 3 relates to the requirements to be fulfilled by the software V&V process. The subsection on software component level testing presents the definition of and the individual(s) responsible for accomplishing this testing. The subsection on software system level testing presents the definition of it, notes that the V&V group is responsible for it, and describes the approach of this type of testing. The remaining subsections specify the various testing techniques and types of testing.

Section 4 presents the high-level tasks that must be accomplished as part of V&V for each software life cycle phase. Section 5 presents the test documentation to be produced for reporting the results of V&V activities. For report forms, it would delineate the steps and information to be provided in each section of the form.

Software Configuration Management Guideline

The software configuration management guideline document defines consistent methods, standards, conventions, practices, and styles. The goal is to promote consistency in the configuration management of the software. This guideline is used primarily by the software configuration management engineer. A typical table of contents for the configuration management guideline document is shown in Table 3-15.

Section 1 introduces the document. Section 2 presents the documentation to be produced for managing the results of configuration management activities. For reporting forms, it would delineate the steps and information to be provided in each section of the form. Section 3 defines the electronic controls and standard directory structures defined for uniformity and consistency. It would present the directory path names that contain scripts, projects, and repository information. In addition, this section would discuss user, group, and superuser access rights and limitations.

Section 4 presents the responsibilities for software configuration management activities, including the determination of who is responsible for what activities and when. This section would also present any canned scripts that are used to move files around, perform routine configuration management activities, and provide configuration control. The appendices would present diagrams of the standard project directory structure and the department or group directory structure and a table indicating the execution permissions and responsibilities for the various configuration management scripts described in Section 4.

Software Metrics Guideline

The software metrics guideline document describes the set of industry standard software metrics that measure the quality of the software process and methodology, as well as the software end product, through each phase of the software development life cycle. The goal is to provide a continual assessment of an ongoing project to allow for timely adjustments and, at the end of the project, to establish baselines for making predictions about certain attributes of future

Table 3-14   Typical Table of Contents for a Software Verification and Validation Guideline Document

Section Number	Section Title
1	Introduction
2	Test Overview
2.1	Tools
2.2	Techniques
2.3	Methodologies
3	Test Requirements
3.1	Software Component Level Testing
3.2	Software System Level Testing
3.3	Functional Testing
3.4	Robustness Testing
3.5	Stress Testing
3.6	Safety Testing
3.7	Regression Testing
3.8	Sequence of Steps
4	Verification and Validation Phases
4.1	Requirements Phase
4.2	Architecture Phase
4.3	Detailed Design Phase
4.4	Implementation Phase
4.5	Software Validation Phase
5	V&V Reporting
5.1	Documentation Templates
5.2	510K Submittal
5.3	Test Logs
5.4	Requirements Traceability Matrix
5.5	Test Information Sheets
5.6	Anomaly Reporting
5.7	Task Reporting
5.8	Phase Summary Report
5.9	Software V&V Report

Table 3-15   Typical Table of Contents for a Software Configuration Management Guideline Document

Section Number	Section Title
1	Introduction
2	Configuration Management Reporting Practices
2.1	Anomaly Reporting
2.2	Configuration Management Deviation/Waiver
3	Project Directory Definition
3.1	Project Directory Scripts
3.2	Project Directory Source Depository
3.3	Project User and Group Identifications
4	Configuration Management Responsibilities
4.1	Integrator Responsibilities
4.2	Configuration Management Scripts
4.3	Script Execution Matrix
Appendix A	Project Directory Structure
Appendix B	Department Directory Structure
Appendix C	Matrix of Configuration Management Script Execution

projects. A typical table of contents for the software metrics guideline document is shown in Table 3-16.

The definition of terms in Section 1 is a fundamental section of this document, because it defines all the metrics to be generated for the project. For example, it would define the terms cyclomatic complexity, error estimate, essential complexity, module design complexity, process metric, product metric, program difficulty, program length, program level, program volume, programming effort, programming time, and Software Engineering Institute (SEI) Maturity Level. In Section 2, the process metrics might include SEI Maturity Level evaluation, a measure of completeness with regard to requirements implementation, a measure of software requirements stability, a measure of design stability, and the generation of fault profiles. The product metrics might include test coverage, program size, function size, logic structure, and composite metrics that reflect ease of software comprehension. Section 3 defines the metrics forms (in the appendices) that are used for reporting metrics and the allocation of the forms to the Section 2 metric categories (see Table 3-17). This section also maps the metrics into each software development life cycle phase (see Table 3-18).

The appendices of this document contain the metrics forms that are used to report the software development life cycle metrics. Although the forms presented here are examples, they do represent the metrics as discussed in later chapters. These forms would be completed at the conclusion of each life cycle phase, possibly following each milestone during the implementation

Table 3-16   Typical Table of Contents for a Software Metrics Guideline Document

Section Number	Section Title
1	Introduction
2	Description of Metrics
2.1	Process Metrics
2.2	Product Metrics
3	Collection and Reporting of Metrics
3.1	Forms
3.2	Collection
Appendix A	Software Engineering Metrics and Primary Characteristics
Appendix B	Software Development and Code Error Metrics
Appendix C	Software Development Code Metrics
Appendix D	Metric Collection by Software Development Phase

phases of Code and Test and Integrate and Test, and at the conclusion of the project. The results would then be entered into a database and become part of an ongoing repository of software metrics. Appendix A (Table 3-18) represents a count of the various errors, debugging, and anomalies generated during the project (see Figure 3-9). Two exceptions are the computed maturity level and complexity indices located in the Measurements column. These two values are computed on the basis of the SEI Maturity Level and McCabe complexities, for example. The maturity level would be determined at the time of the project postmortem, and the complexity numbers would be generated at each scheduled baseline and at the final release of the software. Appendix B (Table 3-18) contains the metrics form used for error metrics of software development and code (see Figure 3-10). The project name would be entered in the uppermost block on the left below the form title. The first section of this form represents calculated values generated from the scatter diagram produced by the McCabe complexity tool, for example. The remainder of the form is generated from simple counts of the anomalies, CRAs, and debug reports generated during the project. In Appendix C (Table 3-18), the code metrics (see Figure 3-11) are calculated by use of the Halstead metrics, for example. The metrics shown here are not the only set available, nor are they of any particular significance other than as examples. Any set of metrics can be collected, and any particular metrics generation tool can be used in place of those mentioned here.

Software Quality Assurance in the Maintenance Cycle

This lengthy discussion of policies indicates that the implementation of a software quality assurance program is a very significant undertaking. The policies must be mutually supportive and coordinate activities, document content, and reviews to fully achieve the built-in quality required for safe, effective, and efficacious medical device software. The approach outlined is directly

Table 3-17   Typical Allocation of Software Metric Forms to Metric Categories

Metric Category	Software Engineering Metrics and Primary Characteristics	Software Development and Code Error Metrics	Software Development Code Metrics
Traceability Coverage	x		
Requirements Stability	x		
Design Stability	x		
Fault Profiles	x	x	
Test Coverage	x		
Program Size			x
Function Size			x
Logic Structure			x
Composite Metrics		x	x

applicable to large-scale and new-generation types of software medical device projects. Now the question can be asked, What relevance, or degree of relevance, does this approach have in small-scale and iterative, maintenance, or sustaining types of software projects?

Conceptually, for smaller, multi-individual projects, software quality assurance program policies potentially represent a great deal of overhead that might not be needed or warranted. However, regulatory agency documents do not specify a difference between large and small projects dealing with medical devices. They specify differences in the application of medical

Table 3-18 Typical Software Metric Collection by Software Development Life Cycle

Software Metric			Requirements	Architecture Design	Detailed Design	Code and Test	Integrate and Test	Software Validation
Traceability Coverage	Percent requirements traced from:	System requirements document to SRS	×	×	×	×	×	×
		SRS to code						×
		SDDS to code						×
Requirements Stability	Number SRS anomalies resulting in Class I or II CRA		×	×	×	×	×	×
	Number Class I or II CRAs affecting SRS		×	×	×	×	×	×
Design Stability	Number SADS anomalies resulting in Class I or II CRA			×				
	Number Class I or II CRAs affecting SADS			×				
	Number SDDS anomalies resulting in Class I or II CRA				×			
	Number Class I or II CRAs affecting SDDS				×			
Fault Profiles	Number open and closed:	SRS anomalies	×	×	×	×	×	×
		Anomalies — Process violation	×	×	×	×	×	
		Anomalies — Methodology violation	×	×	×	×	×	
		SRS CRAs	×	×	×	×	×	×
		SADS — Anomalies		×				
		SADS — CRAs		×				
		SDDS — Anomalies			×	×	×	×
		SDDS — CRAs			×	×	×	×
		Code — Anomalies						×
		Code — CRAs						×
	Anomaly open age average		×	×	×	×	×	×

Continued on next page.

Continued from previous page.

Software Metric			Software Life Cycle Phase					
			Requirements	Architecture Design	Detailed Design	Code and Test	Integrate and Test	Software Validation
Test Coverage	Percent requirements:	Tested by development				X	X	X
		Passed component testing				X	X	X
		Tested by V&V						X
		Passed validation testing						X
	Degree of code testing					X	X	X
Program Size	Line counts							X
	Token counts							X
Function Size	Line count statistics							X
	Token count statistics							X
Logic Structure	Cyclomatic complexity statistics							X
	Essential complexity statistics							X
	Design complexity statistics							X
	Branch count statistics							X
Composite	Halstead metric statistics							X

devices, not in the effort to produce the devices. Therefore, regulatory agencies expect that a manufacturer's software quality assurance program will be the same for all devices of the same application, regardless of how the manufacturer organizes and staffs the project.

What is needed is a mechanism that allows the software quality assurance program to adapt to the size of the effort required for developing the medical device software. Two such mechanisms exist; one has already been discussed. In the policies that deal with the SCMP and the SQAP, the software project defines the degree of formality, the control employed, and the personnel to be used for software configuration management and quality assurance as a function of the size and complexity, significance, and investment risks of the project. Thus, smaller, iterative, and enhancement projects can have a lesser degree of configuration management and quality assurance than larger projects, but cannot eliminate them entirely.

Figure 3-9   Typical form for software engineering metrics and primary characteristics

Software Engineering Metrics and Primary Characteristics			Project:	
			Date:	
Category	**Metrics**	**Measurements**		**Value**
Management	Software engineering environment	Computed maturity level		
Requirements	Traceability	Percent requirements traced	System requirements to SRS	
			System requirements to code	
			SRS to code	
	Stability	Number of requirements changes	Anomalies	
			CRAs	
Quality	Design stability	Stability index	Number of anomalies	
			Number of CRAs	
	Complexity	Complexity indices		
	Breadth of testing	Percent requirements tested	By development	
			By V&V	
		Percent requirements passed	By development	
			By V&V	
	Depth of testing	Degree of code testing		
	Fault profiles	Documentation	Open	
			Closed	
		Software	Open	
			Closed	
		Process	Open	
			Closed	
		Methodology	Open	
			Closed	
		Other	Open	
			Closed	
		Average open age		
	Reliability			

Figure 3-10 Typical form for software development code and error metrics

Software Development Code and Error Metrics

Date:
Revision:
Number of files:
Number of functions:

Category	Description	Metrics			
		Number of Functions		Percent	
Scatter Diagram	Reliable and maintainable				
	Unreliable and unmaintainable				
	Reliable and unmaintainable				
	Unreliable and maintainable				
	Total				

Category	Phase Description	Metrics						Total
		Documentation		Software		Other		
		Open	Closed	Open	Closed	Open	Closed	
Anomalies, all	Requirements							
	Architecture design							
	Detailed design							
	Implementation							
	Total open							
	Total closed							

Continued on next page.

Continued from previous page.

Category	Phase Description	Metrics						
		Documentation		Software		Other		Total
		Open	Closed	Open	Closed	Open	Closed	
CRAs, all	Requirements							
	Architecture design							
	Detailed design							
	Implementation							
	Total open							
	Total closed							

Category	Phase Description	Metrics		
		Open	Closed	Total
Debug Report Entries	Requirements			
	Architecture design			
	Detailed design			
	Implementation			
	Total open			
	Total closed			

Category
Anomalies resulting in CRAs
Number of CRAs generated
Ratio of anomalies to CRAs

Figure 3-11   Typical form for software development code metrics

Software Development Code Metrics			Date:
			Revision:
			Number of files:
			Number of functions:

Category	Description	Metrics	Value
Program size	Number of lines	Total	
		Code	
		Comment	
		Blank	
		Code with comment	
	Token counts	Operators	
		Operands	
		Total operators	
		Total operands	

		Metrics				
Category	Description	Min.	Max.		Mean	Std. Dev.
Function size	Lines of code					
	Comment lines					
	Blank lines					
	Code with comment					
	Total					
	Number of operators					
	Number of operands					
	Number of tokens					
	Total operators					
	Total operands					
	Total token count					

		Metrics				
Category	Description	Min.	Max.	Total	Mean	Std. Dev.
Logic structure	Cyclomatic complexity					
	Essential complexity					

Continued on next page.

Continued from previous page.

Category	Description	Metrics				
		Min.	Max.	Total	Mean	Std. Dev.
Composite metrics	Design complexity					
	Branch count					
	Program length					
	Program volume					
	Program level					
	Program difficulty					
	Intelligent content					
	Programming effort					
	Error estimate					
	Programming time					

The second mechanism that can be used to tailor the software quality assurance program to the size and complexity of the device project is the inclusion of preambles in the software development, V&V, and configuration management policies. These preambles would state that some circumstances may require deviations from the stated policies. In these cases, a written authorization to depart from the documented policies should be required (see Figure 3-12). The written request for the authorization for departure should allow for two circumstances. First, a written deviation request should be required for any future software activity, event, or software product. The deviation request would allow management to be informed of a project's intention to employ a higher risk development approach that is not in direct support of the stated policies. Second, a written waiver request should be required for those software activities, events, or software end products that have already been started. This would allow management to be made aware of a project's intention to circumvent the established policies and employ a higher risk approach that is not in direct support of the stated policies.

In either case, a recommendation regarding the approval or disapproval of the written request should be made by a management-level individual who is intimately familiar with the ramifications and implications of such a request. The recommendation would then be forwarded, along with the request, to a senior management individual, who would then approve or disapprove of the request. Each request for deviation or waiver should explicitly identify each specific policy and the policy requirement to which it applies, the alternative approach to be taken by the project, and the impact of that approach on the project's schedule, performance, and/or risk. A copy of each approved deviation or waiver should be kept by the project team for inclusion in the product history file or master record file, and by the software quality assurance group for consideration during the postmortem of the software project as a potential improvement to be implemented in the software development policies, procedures, or guidelines.

Figure 3-12   Typical deviation/waiver form

Software Engineering Process Record of
Deviation/Waiver Approval

PROJECT:	TYPE: Deviation Waiver	PHASE:
		SOP Requirement Paragraph(s):

Initiated by: _____   Date: _____

     Signature   Title/Position

Reviewed by: _____   Date: _____

     Signature   Title/Position

Approved by: _____   Date: _____

     Signature   Title/Position

Reason/Rationale/Explanation:

Project schedule and performance impact:

Project risk:

Alternative approach to be used:

4

The Software Quality Assurance Program: Project Software Estimations

> More software projects have gone awry for lack of calendar time than for all other causes combined.
>
> —Frederick P. Brooks

When schedule slippage on a software project becomes known, the first thought is usually that some major calamities have befallen the project. In reality, however, the schedule has slipped imperceptibly but inexorably. The idea that major calamities and upheavals have occurred is easier to cope with because any number of solutions can be brought to bear on the problem. For example, new and major resources can be assigned to the project to alleviate the situation, a radical reorganization can be made to offset losses, or new approaches may be invented to recoup the lost time. These examples indicate that the entire organization recognizes the situation and rises to the occasion.

Day-to-day slippage, however, is harder to recognize, harder to prevent, and ultimately harder, if not impossible, to make up. For example, a key individual may be out for "only a day" because of illness, but a critical meeting could not be held and key decisions were postponed. The hardware system may go down and, consequently, the software development team cannot perform their normal activities. The expected shipment of new system parts does not arrive when promised, and time is lost waiting for their arrival from the factory. Jury duty, family crisis, unscheduled emergency meetings, and unplanned audits are the unforeseen, unforeseeable, and unaccounted-for activities that rob a software project of its most precious resource, time. Each event postpones some activity by "only" a half day or even a day, but the overall schedule slips one day at a time.

The control of projects, large or small, that are on tight delivery schedules is exercised through the mechanism of actually defining and having a schedule. The project schedule will have activities that lead to events called milestones that, in turn, have due dates associated with them. The selection of the milestone due date is an estimating problem that ultimately and crucially depends on experience, but the selection of the milestone itself involves only one rule.

Milestones must be concrete, specific, and measurable events that identify the vague phases of the project. Two studies (King and Wilson 1967; King, Witterrongel, and Hezel 1967) related to estimating behavior by government contractors on large-scale development projects illuminate three estimating characteristics:

1. Estimates of the length of an activity, made and revised carefully every two weeks before the activity started, did not significantly change as the start time drew near, regardless of how wrong the estimates turned out to be.

2. During the activity, overestimates of the duration steadily decreased as the development activity continued.

3. Underestimates did not change significantly during the development activity until about three weeks before the scheduled completion.

Let us consider an example (see Figure 4-1). Suppose that a project is estimated at 12 person-months of effort over a calendar period of four months and is assigned to three individuals. Four deliverables are scheduled for completion, one at the end of each calendar month (Estimate row of Figure 4-1). Suppose that the first deliverable scheduled at the end of the first month is actually delivered at the end of the second month. This then pushes the remaining three deliverables out by one month each, so that the project will now be completed at the end of five months instead of four months (Actual row of Figure 4-1). There are four possible alternatives to remedy this situation:

1. Assume that the project must still be completed by the end of the fourth month, that the effort estimates for the remaining deliverables are accurate, and that only the activities leading to the first deliverable were underestimated. With nine person-months of activities still to be done in the remaining two months, two additional individuals can be assigned to join the three currently on the project (Option 1 row of Figure 4-1).

Figure 4-1   Software development estimation for a mythical medical device

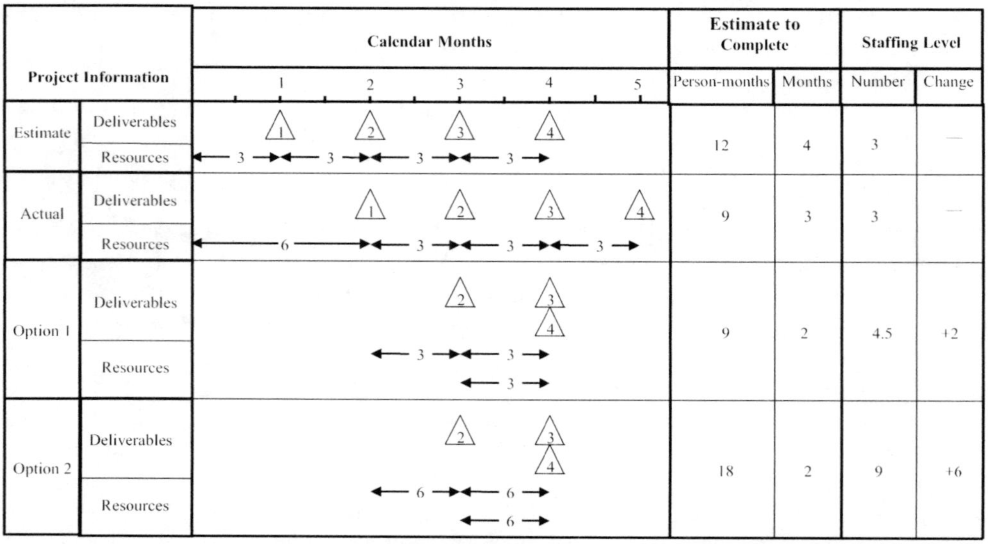

2. Assume that the project must still be completed by the end of the fourth month, that the whole project estimate was uniformly low, and that it was uniformly low by the same factor as the first delivery. Because the first deliverable took twice as long to complete as estimated, there are 18 person-months of activities still to be done in the remaining two calendar months, and six additional individuals can be assigned to join the three currently on the project (Option 2 row of Figure 4-1).

3. The project can be totally rescheduled in order to allow enough time for activities to be carefully and thoroughly done, so that rescheduling again will not be required.

4. The tasks, activities, and deliverables can be trimmed so that the project is completed on time, but with reduced scope.

Insisting that the project still be completed by the end of the fourth month without alteration (solutions one and two) is disastrous. The individuals who are added to the project, regardless of how competent, quickly recruited, and experienced they may be, will require orientation and training about the project status, objectives, deliverables, schedule, and so on by at least one of the existing project personnel. This represents additional time that was not originally estimated as a part of the project. For example, the project that was initially partitioned into activities for three must now be repartitioned into more parts. When this happens, some of the effort that already had been completed is lost, because the project must be reformed and retasked and activities reallocated. This will also consume additional time of both the current and newly assigned individuals. In either of the first two options, the product will be just as late, if not later, than if no new individuals had been assigned. If the additional project time consumed by training and reallocation of effort is taken into consideration, then even more resources must be assigned to the project, and this, in turn, would further exacerbate the situation—project activities would not have resumed any faster. Further, this discussion assumed that only the first milestone was underestimated. If each delivery was underestimated, then the recalculation, training, and repartitioning would repeat itself for each late deliverable, necessitating the addition of even more individuals.

This phenomenon was first described by Frederick Brooks (Brooks 1975), who stated it as a law of software development: "Adding manpower to a late software project makes it later." The period of performance for a project depends on its sequential constraints; the maximum number of resources depends on the number of independent subtasks needed to achieve project completion. When these two quantities are used, schedules requiring fewer resources and more months can be derived, but it is not possible to derive schedules requiring more resources and fewer months.

One of the fundamental difficulties of software project scheduling is the perception that all software activities occur in series, just as the waterfall model depicts them. For example, requirements analysis precedes only requirements definition, requirements definition must occur before software design, and software design must happen before coding can occur. However, this is not the situation in reality. As discussed in an earlier chapter, the phases of the software life cycle overlap; the challenge is how to represent this on a schedule correctly and explicitly, because this overlap of activities would produce a clumsy, awkward, and confusing schedule. However, if the waterfall model phases were used as the mechanism to collect and aggregate the total effort related to the generic software activities and the definition of the model was altered so that it was applicable to a schedule, then the waterfall activity effort can be thought of as the "area under the curve"; it indicates the total expenditure of software effort for that particular phase activity, even though it is spread across several schedule phases. The waterfall model represents a convenient way to gather all of the effort into a neat, concise category, but the expenditure of that effort is spread over the project and not strictly within the designated phase. It should be understood that the vast majority of the phase effort is expended within the phase, but some degree of residual activity does occur outside of the phase.

Software Project Estimation

Good software development estimation is not an end in itself. It is a means toward more effective software life cycle management that contributes to software quality. An estimate for a software project attempts to identify a plan that can be used to execute a specific job to successful completion. The success attributes of such a plan are the production of a working system that meets the user's expectations while being developed on time and within budget. An estimate involves three primary objectives:

1. It identifies the various tasks to be performed.

2. It lists the resources—personnel, equipment, and facilities—needed to carry out those tasks.

3. It associates a relative time span with each of those tasks and allocates a specific time duration to each resource to be used on those tasks.

Additionally, an estimate involves two secondary objectives:

1. A cost estimate of the accumulated monetary value for each resource multiplied by the time spent by each resource throughout the project. Consequently, a correct cost estimate can be made if accurate estimates for the tasks, resources, and resource time requirements are provided.

2. Good management practice calls for the identification of potential problem and risk areas and planning to avoid their disruptive effects.

Factors Affecting Software Development Estimations

Estimating software development is a complex task that requires a detailed understanding of the various factors that directly and indirectly impact the process. Several factors affect the software development effort directly. An incomplete, vague, and ambiguous requirements definition is a major contributor to inaccurate software estimation. A well-prepared and documented requirements definition forms the basis for a well-defined and well-understood software development estimation. The benefits gained through the availability of a well-prepared and well-documented requirements definition are greatly reduced, and even lost, if numerous changes are made to the requirements after the initial estimate. Other factors that directly affect the software development effort include the complexity of the hardware and software integration and the level of system testing required.

The major reason for the uncertainty in software development estimation is the large variance associated with the parameters used to compute the software development effort. The two most commonly used parameters are the size of the software to be developed and the programming productivity. The uncertainty inherent in the various estimation parameters can produce a relative range for the original software development estimate that may be four times as high as the actual prediction. As the size of the software increases, the resources needed to develop the software increase exponentially rather than linearly. The justification for this is related to the fact that as the number of individuals on a project increases, the interactions required between them also increases. Whereas the number of people increases arithmetically, the number of interactions increases geometrically. For n people, there are $n \times (n - 1)/2$ possible interactions. This increase in the number of interactions then forces the project people to spend substantial time and effort on human communications and less on productive work for the project. For example, the productivity level in terms of the number of instructions per person per year is about 10,000 when the interactions are very few. This decreases to about 5,000 instructions when interactions increase, and it drops dramatically, to 1,500 instructions per person per year for large numbers of interactions.

Another factor that adds to the large variance in software development estimates is the variation in programmer productivity when programmers perform the identical function and use different applications. In either case, productivity is also a function of the size of the project. Additional uncertainty in programmer productivity is related to the fact that during the project life cycle, personnel turnover is possible; the remaining project staff may take up the slack by working overtime until the empty position is filled. However, this may lead to stress and unhappiness, causing a resultant decrease in productivity. This drop in productivity does not necessarily end when a newly hired or replacement individual joins the team. Either type of person will most likely require some degree of training from the project personnel, further eroding productivity.

Variation in the estimate for error removal is another factor that may introduce uncertainty into the software development estimate. The estimate to remove software errors varies depending on the degree to which system testing and verification techniques are used. If the system testing and verification test plan follows a well-defined path and errors are removed at every step of the life cycle development, then the number of undetected errors will be minimized, and therefore the estimate to remove them will be small. If the bulk of the testing is left for the end of the life cycle, then the estimate to remove the errors will be high, for two reasons: (1) the errors will be difficult to detect, and (2) it will be difficult to isolate the root cause(s) from among the myriad routines, functions, and components that have been integrated into the system.

Most managers, despite the large variations in the level of programmer productivity, tend to treat programmers as a unified, common group when estimating software project resources. This produces another large degree of uncertainty in the software development estimation. When estimating resources to obtain an accurate productivity level, the manager should consider the type of application, the size of the project, and, where possible, the experience of the individuals who will perform the work. This type of data can be gleaned only from a good job-cost tracking and time-card system that allows software managers to capture the hours of effort for the various activities in each of the software life cycle phases, as well as by the feature set of the device. Because of the large variance in and the many factors associated with the original estimate, it is essential to be able to identify and capture the specific effort associated with each subtask to be carried out throughout the software development life cycle. The availability of these data allows the software development estimator to fine-tune the scope of the project productivity by directly matching the level of effort to the explicit resources that will be used in each of the phases of the project.

Numerous studies have shown that all medium and large software projects exhibit the same life cycle pattern, comprising a rise in resource loading, a peaking period, and a trailing off period (Putnam and Fitzsimmons 1979); this pattern follows the Rayleigh distribution function. The use of a resource curve and its corresponding equation can help to determine the number of resources required at any point of the project's schedule. The time of peak effort is associated with the development time when the system reaches full operational capability. The trailing part of the curve corresponds to the operation and maintenance phase of the software life cycle.

Putnam and Fitzsimmons also noted that resource and loading curves for smaller software projects tend to have a more rectangular pattern, rather than the Rayleigh distribution found in medium and large projects. This difference is attributed to the fact that many small projects are governed by level-of-effort activities, where the level of effort is predetermined by management, by contractual agreements, or simply by the fact that only one, two, or three programmers actually work on the project.

Generating Software Development Estimations

Once the software development estimator properly understands the product to be developed and the software pitfalls to avoid, the next logical step is to create an estimate for software development. It is always wise to generate multiple estimates before actually starting the software development phase. The first software development estimate should be generated during the product definition phase; as more information, knowledge, and understanding about the device and its related hardware are gained during the software life cycle and the uncertainties are reduced, the other software development estimates can be made.

During the product definition phase, only a broad estimate of the ultimate software size and development time is needed to establish the basic feasibility of the software development effort. Because there are few or no hard data about the system at this point, the estimation is in effect an educated guess at the range of the size of the software, based on past experience and what little is known about the system at this point.

The project's software team can develop the second estimate. This is particularly useful when the team members who actually formulated the early system definition are used and more information becomes available to them. The software development estimation uncertainty can be reduced at this point, because as the system is being decomposed into components, a software development estimate can be made for each requisite component.

A third and final estimate should be performed about midway through the functional design phase. This is an extremely informative estimate, because the preliminary specifications and system design should be, or are almost, complete. At this point the software functions are fairly well defined; the development estimate should reflect a low range in the estimate deviations and should represent only a few uncertainties.

The approach of using multiple estimates geared toward refinement of the software life cycle phase and increased system definition provides a powerful means of developing a creditable software development estimate. Although, depending on the particular circumstances of the project, the exact timing of each of the estimates may vary from project to project, this concept is extremely powerful. The following sections present a variety of techniques and methods that can be used for estimating software development.

Work Breakdown Structure

The work breakdown structure (WBS) is a means of dividing an engineering project into subprojects, tasks, subtasks, work packages, and so on. This important planning tool a links the project objectives with resources and activities in a logical framework of what must be accomplished. It can also be used as a status-monitoring device during the actual software implementation as completion of the subtasks is measured against the project plan. The WBS has been widely used in many other engineering applications and has been adapted successfully to software development and maintenance projects.

Theory and Justification

The WBS is an enumeration of all software activities in hierarchic refinements of detail that organizes the work to be done into short, manageable tasks. Quantifiable inputs, outputs, schedules, assigned resources, and resource responsibilities are attached to each task. The WBS can also be used for budgeting software development time and resources down to the individual task. It can also be used later in the project as a basis for reporting software development progress relative to meaningful management milestones. A software management plan based on a WBS contains the necessary tools to estimate costs and schedules accurately and to provide visibility and control during software construction. However, the knowledge of what a WBS is, what its goals and benefits are, and what its structure is supposed to be does not necessarily instruct a software estimator in how to apply that knowledge toward developing a WBS for a particular project.

For example, suppose that the task of developing a software program has been assigned and that the program is structured as illustrated in Figure 4-2. The goals of the WBS for this program (see Figure 4-3) are to identify the software tasks, needed resources, and implementation

Figure 4-2   Typical modular hierarchy of a program

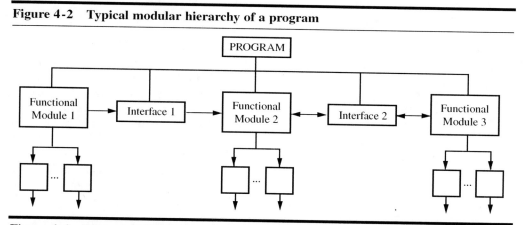

Figure 4-3   The work breakdown structure for the typical modular hierarchy of a program

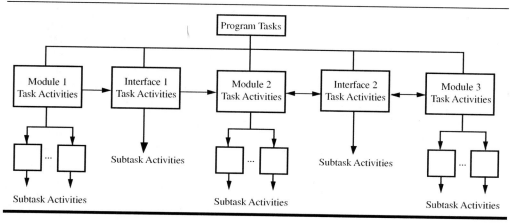

constraints to the level of detail that yields the development accuracy stipulated in the software development plan. An additional goal is to provide the means for the early calibration of this accuracy and for corrective replanning, if necessary, during actual software development.

If a software project has identified a specific number of equal-effort milestones to be achieved during the software development life cycle, then the number of milestones achieved by a certain date is an indicator of the progress toward that goal. A graph of the accumulated milestones as a function of time would permit certain predictions about any future completion date. Not only could such predictions be made easily, they also could be made with quantifiable accuracy if the milestones are chosen properly. For example, suppose that it is known a priori, as a result of generating the WBS, that a project will be completed after M milestones have been completed, that these milestones correspond to all of the tasks that must be accomplished on the project, and that some later activity does not reopen an already completed task. In reality, the number of milestones M may not be precisely known from the start of the project, and any uncertainty in M will certainly affect the accuracy of the estimated completion date. However, for our purposes, these uncertainties can be accounted for at a later date as secondary effects, when and if estimate accuracy refinement is needed. Suppose also that it has been possible to refine the overall project into these M milestones in such a way that each task is believed to require about the same amount of effort and time to accomplish. When viewed at regular intervals, a plot of the cumulative numbers of milestones that have been reached should rise linearly until the project has been completed.

Quantitatively, let m be the average number of tasks actually completed during each reporting period, let σ be the standard deviation of the actual number of milestones reached in each reporting period about this mean value, and assume that the values of m and σ are presumed to be constant over the project duration. The value of m is a reflection of the team average productivity, and σ is a measure of the ability to estimate the team's production rate. Furthermore, these values correspond to the team's ability to produce and their ability to create a work plan that adequately accounts for their time.

By definition, the mean behavior of the milestone attainment status is linear from the origin, with slope m. The project should require M/m reporting periods to complete, a number that should not depend on whether a WBS was created, M/m being a relatively constant value. If M is made large enough, then the tasks are smaller and shorter, and proportionately more of them are completed during each reporting period. The project schedule will assume some productivity or mean accomplishment rate, but actual performance values will generally be unknown until progress can be monitored for some period of time on the project itself.

However, although the numbers M and σ may not affect team productivity, they do directly influence the effectiveness with which a project team can monitor its progress and thus predict its future accomplishments. The generation of a WBS does estimate the parameter M and, while monitoring the attainment of milestones, provides estimates for m and σ. Projections of the end date and calculations for the accuracy of this prediction can then be made. On the basis of this information, the project team can divert or reallocate resources, to take corrective action if progress on the project is not suitable.

In this simplified model, a least-square-error, straight-line fit through the cumulative milestone progress over the first r reports of an expected $R = M/m$ reports at regular ΔT intervals will predict the time required to reach the final milestone. This will also provide an estimate of m and σ. The normalized completion date may be expected to deviate from the projected value as a one-sigma event by no more than

$$\sigma_M \leq 1.48 \times \sigma_1 \times (R/[r \times M])^{1/2} \tag{4.1}$$

(Tausworthe 1977a) within first-order effects. The value $\sigma_1 = \sigma/m^{1/2}$ represents the normalized standard deviation on an individual task milestone and is limited to values of less than unity in this model. The value σ_M represents the deviation in time to reach milestone M. The bound permits the specification of WBS characteristics that enable accurate and early predictions of future progress. High overall accuracy depends on a combination of low σ_1 and large M. Inaccurate appraisals of productivity can be compensated for only by the generation of a very detailed WBS.

As an example, suppose that a 10 percent end-date accuracy ($\sigma_1 = 0.1$) is required by the end of the first quarter ($r/R = 0.25$) of a project. Then, the trade-off figure is $M/\sigma_1^2 = 876$. Therefore, if the WBS is highly uncertain ($\sigma_1 = 1$), then the WBS should contain 876 milestones. If the project is confident that it can hold more closely to its average productivity and it has most contingencies provided for with an end-date accuracy of $\sigma_1 = 0.5$, then it needs only about 220 milestones. Conversely, a one person-year project with biweekly reporting of 26 reports and one milestone per report must demonstrate a $\sigma_1 = 0.17$ or 17 percent level of task prediction accuracy. This demonstrates that if accuracy in predicting the future progress of a project is of great importance, then it is necessary and important to generate a detailed WBS rather carefully and to monitor milestone achievement relative to this WBS very faithfully.

Although these examples are rather esoteric, let us explore the results of the first example project in a slightly different light. A project's lead software engineer on a two-year, ten-person task might be able to manage as many as 876 subtasks, where each subtask is formally assigned and reported on, since this amounts to about 1 subtask completion per week from each of the other nine project members. However, the generation of the WBS descriptions for the 876 tasks will require considerable effort, and it is unlikely that such a detailed plan would have a σ as large as one week. On the other hand, if the software lead engineer is able to break the software activities accurately into 876 week-long tasks, then task deviations can probably be estimated to within a week.

This discussion points out that the ability to generate a clear and accurate WBS will determine the level to which the WBS must be taken. Greater accuracy of the work breakdown definition produces greater understanding and clarity of the actions that are necessary in order to complete the task objectives. If the work is understood, readily identified, and achievable as discerned, then the confidence of reaching the objective is high. The further the subtask descriptions become defined, the better the development estimator is able to assess the individual subtask duration and uncertainties; the refinement ceases when the appropriate M/σ_1^2 is reached. In practical terms, a work plan with task times shorter than one week will usually require too much planning and management overhead to be worthwhile. On the other hand, a work plan with task times longer than one or two weeks will probably suffer from a large σ_1. Subjectively, a breakdown into one- or two-week subtasks is probably the most reasonable target for planning purposes.

A work year consists of about 47 actual weeks of work, if vacations, holidays, and sick leave are excluded. A project of w workers can reasonably accommodate only about $47 \times (w/d)$ tasks per year, d being the duration of each task. Spread over y years, the total number of milestones could reach $M = 47 \times (w \times [y/d])$, so that the practical accuracy limit that may be expected at the one-quarter point in a project ($r/R = 0.25$) is about

$$\sigma_M \leq 0.432 \times \sigma_1 \times (d/w \times y)^{1/2}. \tag{4.2}$$

This implies that the end-date accuracy is related to the total person-year effort on a project, other things being equal. A three person-year project completing one task per person-week can expect to have $\sigma_M \leq 0.21 \times \sigma_1$. A $\sigma_1 = 0.4$ represents ± 2 days per weekly task, and the end-date estimation accuracy is within 10 percent.

Generation

Individuals create WBSs all the time, although they may not realize it. Most of the activities that software engineers do as individuals are probably organized in their heads as a WBS; for small undertakings, this works fine. For more complex tasks, especially involving the coordination of other individuals, it becomes necessary to plan, organize, document, and review in a more formal fashion the project WBS. With this in mind, the generation of a WBS is generally a five-step algorithm:

1. The project statement of work is a TASK and is placed on the top of a "working stack."

2. Consider the TASK at the top of the working stack. For that TASK, define the technical performance objectives, end-item objectives, reliability and quality objectives, schedule constraints, and any other factors that are appropriate; inputs and materials required to start the TASK; accomplishments and outputs that indicate completion of TASK; known precedent tasks or milestones; known interfacing tasks; and required resources. Then determine if the TASK can be accomplished within the duration accuracy goal.

3. If the goal can be achieved, then continue with step four. Otherwise, partition the TASK into a small number of comprehensive, component subtasks, and include any interfacing tasks and those tasks for which the output is a decision regarding the substructuring of other subtasks. Mark the current TASK as a "milestone," move its description from the working stack to a "finished stack," and place each of its subtask descriptions onto the working stack.

4. Repeat steps two and three until the working stack is empty.

5. Sequence through all items in the finished stack and accumulate the durations into the proper milestones.

The steps created for this algorithm are not always simple to perform and cannot always be done correctly the first time, or without referring to and possibly removing items from the finished list. The WBS process is one of creation and requires judgment, experience, identification of alternatives, trade-offs, decisions, and iterations. Iteration is required because as the project requirements are refined, the implementation of the device software itself appears as one of the subtasks to be refined. When the software subtask is divided into its component parts, the work descriptions begin to follow the influences of the software architecture, organizational matters, chronological constraints, work locations, and the usual software development activities.

Relationships

Formation of the WBS, detailed planning, and software architectural design activities are all mutually supportive. Software architecture indicates how to structure tasks; the WBS goals indicate when the architectural phase of software activity has proceeded far enough. Scheduling makes use of the WBS as a tool and, in turn, influences the WBS generation by resolving resource conflicts. However, many subtasks within a software project are not connected directly with software architecture. These subtasks include requirements analysis, project administration and management, and preparations for demonstrations and deliverables. The structure of these subtasks, being independent of software architecture, can also be run through the WBS algorithm and added to the overall project software WBS.

To simplify and continuously improve the WBS concept, standard WBS outlines and checklists can be made that will facilitate software WBS generation. The standard WBS checklist (Table 4-1) includes those factors that are gained from previous project successes, as well as items that avert some of the identified shortcomings. The supporting and detailed task descriptions and guidelines for a WBS checklist that instruct individuals in the WBS method, approach, and practice are also necessary.

The WBS presents and defines the tasks for a software project at lower and lower levels of detail. This structure defines what must be accomplished to complete the project; time, however, is not a criterion of the WBS. A task network shows how a package of work that was developed in the WBS is to be accomplished by a specific team member or members, in what sequence the tasks are to be performed, and what resources will be required. The WBS is typically generated by the team management or team leaders and indicates the work or work packages to be completed. The task network, commonly called the Program Evaluation Report Technique (PERT), is typically generated by the individuals responsible for accomplishing the work packages. Consequently, the task network or PERT is a finer, more detailed planning tool and it represents the activity, job, or task controlling level used for start and completion dates and milestones for the project. Figure 4-4 shows the relationship between the WBS decomposition and the task network. Tasks A, C, and D have already been assigned; when Task B gets assigned, the PERT network will be expanded appropriately. The network will grow as the work packages are assigned and/or as the WBS grows.

Software Team Characteristics, Organization, and Staffing

The widespread ranges of medical device software applications, as well as their associated specific requirements, make it difficult to pinpoint a common software project team approach. However, in general, it is safe to assume that the great majority of medical device applications will require more than one software engineer. Microprocessor-based products very rarely require just one individual to write a single, small program. Commonly, medical device software is a coordinated effort of several people working together to produce a complete, usable software end product that controls the medical device. The types of expertise needed on microprocessor-based software projects for medical devices include digital design, knowledge of computer architecture, system interfacing, programming knowledge, specific knowledge related to the particular application to be implemented, and project management experience. Such a broad spectrum of expertise and knowledge is neither easy to find nor easy to assemble cohesively. Because of the relatively short duration of medical device projects, it is essential to use the best possible people; there will probably not be enough time to take advantage of the averaging effect that cancels out the very good and the very bad performance by individuals.

The Hardware Engineer as a Software Engineer

The software talent shortage often forces various organizations to recruit electrical engineering people with software background experience or computer science engineers with data processing experience. However, the typical hardware engineer, who is familiar with the hardware

Table 4-1   Typical Outline of a Detailed WBS

Outline Number	Activity
1	Analyze Software Requirements
1.1	Understand functional and software requirements
1.2	Identify missing, vague, ambiguous, conflicting requirements
1.3	Clarify stated requirements
1.4	Verify that stated requirements fulfill requested goals
1.5	Assess technology for supplying required software
1.6	Propose alternate requirements or capability
1.7	Document revised requirements
2	Develop Functional Specifications
2.1	Formalize external environment and interface specifications
2.2	Refine, formalize, and document the external operational view of the software
2.3	Define functional acceptance tests
2.4	Verify compliance of the external view with requirements
3	Produce and Deliver Software End Products
3.1	Formalize internal environment and interface specifications
3.2	Obtain support tools
3.3	Refine and formalize the internal design
3.4	Define testing specification to demonstrate required performance
3.5	Define quality assurance specification
3.6	Code and test the software
3.7	Integrate and test the software
3.8	Perform validation testing
3.9	Demonstrate software acceptability and deliver software
4	Perform Project Software Management Functions
4.1	Define project goals and objectives
4.2	Scope and plan the project
4.3	Administer the implementation
4.4	Evaluate the performance and product
4.5	Terminate the project

Figure 4-4　Relationship between the WBS decomposition and the task network

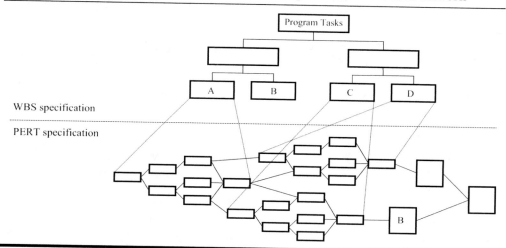

implementations of real-time systems, tends to experience difficulties when dealing with the large quantity of software that must be developed on a team project. Inadequate education in the software development field generally is reflected in the quality of the software and documentation produced and in the various software development estimates that are needed to implement real-time software. On the other hand, computer science graduates who have data processing backgrounds experience difficulty in working closely with other software engineers and generally have only a superficial knowledge of real-time software control requirements.

The ideal candidate for real-time process control applications is the software engineer who has a hardware and software background in terms of both education and work-related experience. Personnel with hardware and software experience are still scarce, and some engineering colleges and universities are adapting their programs to accommodate this duality. Consequently, it will probably be necessary to use several people with relevant experience in one of the areas of the project and, through good communication and organization, carry out the task of system software development. Good software engineers are hard to find, but they are very important to the success of the project; their guidance, ability to comprehend how the device hardware and software work with each other, and ability to solve difficult problems rapidly are critical. It is a major mistake to let a project proceed with only junior software engineers assigned to the project.

Programming Productivity

Major companies that develop software for microprocessor-based software projects have made numerous studies to determine programming productivity. In general, these studies show that data processing types of applications written in high-order languages will typically be produced at a rate of 15–20 lines per day. Productivity rates for real-time control programs written in assembly language will generally be 8–12 lines of code per day. Real-time control programs written for a bit-slice microprocessor that must be microprogrammed will be produced at an average rate of 2–5 lines per day.

Various factors directly affect daily productivity. These include vague and ambiguous hardware specifications as well as changing hardware designs. Experience has a key influence on software productivity. Lack of experience with the application and little or no previous experience with the microprocessor are major negative influences on productivity. Other negative factors include low-quality or no software development tools and inadequate time allocation for software design, testing, and documentation. Furthermore, some of the single-chip microcomputers have fixed amounts of memory; underestimating the actual memory that the application requires leads to decreased productivity. The number of lines of code per day that can be produced drops off sharply as the memory fills up. It is usually advisable to double the size of the initial estimate for memory and to work down from there, if necessary, as the software requirements become better understood.

Two factors can increase programming productivity. The first of these is the use of a high-level language. The use of a high-order language should be carefully evaluated for each individual microprocessor-based project. It is not so much a matter of *whether* a high-order language should be used as it is *which* high-order language to use. The software team must evaluate the application and verify which, if any, language is suitable for the particular application and whether its use will enhance the overall programming productivity. There are two major concerns associated with the application of a high-order language to microcontroller-type applications. First, the language must manipulate the hardware so that the developed code can meet the real-time requirements of the application. In general, high-order language compilers generate slower running code than hand-optimized assembly language programs. Second, the generated code must be able to fit within the allocated memory for the system. In general, high-order language compilers produce code that requires more memory than well-defined assembly language programs.

Care should be exercised to avoid arbitrarily dismissing use of a high-order language in microprocessor programming. High-order languages reduce development costs by improving programmer productivity; they reduce maintenance costs by improving software reliability and documentation. In order to benefit from these types of improvements and meet the critical timing and limited memory requirements of process control applications, a combination of both high-order and assembly language programming can be used. In most applications, the time-critical parts of the code account for only about 20 percent of the total code. Therefore, the time-critical part of the code could be implemented in assembly language; the rest of the code could be implemented in the high-order language. The number of lines of code that must be written to review a given software task in assembly language is seven to ten times more than that required by a high-order language (Barnes 1983). In addition, the number of software errors and faults tends to be proportional to the number of lines of code that are generated, regardless of the programming language that is used. Therefore, coding a particular task in assembly language may be worthwhile for real-time speed or code compactness, but the software programmer will have seven to ten times more faults to debug.

Use of microprocessor development tools also has the potential to help reduce the total software development effort, because of the increase in productivity of hardware and software. Such tools come in many varieties and combinations, and they are tightly coupled to a given microprocessor family. Therefore, as a separate and distinct step of the project's design phase, it is necessary to select the microprocessor on the basis of its particular characteristics as well as on the availability and maturity of good software and hardware development tools for that microprocessor. Once microprocessor development tools are purchased, they can be used in the software development phases to facilitate the generation of code as well as in the debugging processes for both hardware and software modules.

Software Development Effort and Difficulty

The day-to-day practice of developing software is a very involved process that requires the cooperation of the various software team members to ensure success. Several problems tend to complicate this already burdened and difficult process. The first of these is the almost universal underestimation of the complexity of software development. Many management people still appear to have the misconception that software development is a simple programming chore. However, historical experience in many companies has shown that the development of software is often the longest and least comprehensible element in the project's schedule, and commonly it is not only on the critical path, but it *is* the critical path. Because good programmers and good managers are rare, project software management is often assigned to personnel with hardware engineering backgrounds. These engineering managers often lack the necessary education and insight into microprocessor technology, as well as modern software technology and methodology.

Another factor that tends to complicate the software development effort is the confusion created by terminology. Many basic terms in engineering disciplines have different meanings for the various functional groups. Even in software, basic terms have multiple definitions and they tend to be associated with a given vendor and its specific products. Consequently, there is no set of standards for software products and, commonly, software from different vendors uses different names to describe the same functions or processes.

The lack of comprehensive integrated support tools also creates development difficulty. Although different manufacturers and software developers produce various software development tools, in a great majority of cases, those tools cannot be integrated to produce a comprehensive software development environment. In certain cases, this is exacerbated by management's misconceptions about the usefulness of the software development tool; thus, management will not provide all of the necessary tools to make software development more efficient. This, in turn, leads to excessive expenditures in personnel time, higher development costs, and ultimately to a longer time to market for the product.

The lack of standards for microprocessor language implementation also contributes to the difficulty of software development. Each of the various vendors has its own assembly language and specific versions of high-order languages that are frequently closely related to hardware architecture. To evaluate objectively these languages prior to their being used in a medical device, each project must perform independent evaluation tests of the high-order language; these tests take time and therefore contribute to higher project costs. However, the increased capabilities of 16- and 32-bit microprocessors are permitting the software to perform larger and more complex functions associated with more sophisticated applications. This implies that larger amounts of software can be written for microprocessors to perform these applications.

To be successful in developing medical device software, medical device manufacturers need to employ many of the techniques and methodologies used to aid in the development of software for the minicomputer and for mainframe applications. Rather than import such techniques and methodologies completely, manufacturers must scale them down appropriately and adjust them as necessary.

Software Engineering Functional Organization

Organization encompasses the structure and philosophy of the company as a whole and that of the individual software project in particular. The organizations must be compatible with each other to ensure the smooth operation of both. The two major issues (Thayer, Pyster, and Wood 1980) related to organizing software projects are type and accountability. The organizational type issue refers to the absence of decision rules used for selecting the proper organizational structure. The accountability issue refers to the poor accountability structure in many software engineering projects; this leads to questions and ambiguities about who is responsible for the various software project functions. The rule of thumb is to select and define the best organizational structure for the project environment and techniques.

Choosing a proper software organization for the project must fit within the overall company structure. The key requirement, usually, is that it must be flexible enough to accommodate the project environment. Although organizational structures impact software productivity, too little attention has been given to the effects that an organization and its ingrained methodologies have on software development rates. Companies can affect software development by the structure used to organize the programs, by the system used to plan and control the software development, and by the management and technical methodologies employed (Daly 1979). To reflect an organization's effectiveness in promoting software productivity, the term *organizational efficiency* is used to define the intrinsic ability of the company to generate quality software in minimal time with minimal resources. By identifying a company's individual organizational efficiency, its impact on software productivity can be determined. The most effective organization can develop high-quality commercial software at rates that are 12 times better than organizations that do not have the necessary talent to properly manage their software development activities.

Several traditional management principles are associated with an organization's internal structure:

- Each subordinate should have no more than one boss.

- Effort must be concentrated on urgent and important matters, and all routine matters should be delegated to lower levels of the organization.

- A single manager should be given only a limited number of subordinates to supervise.

- Similar activities should be grouped under a common category and allocated to a special department.

- Authority and responsibility should flow in a well-defined path from upper levels to lower levels.

In the implementation of these management principles for software, there are three predominant internal organizational structures: the functional organization, the project organization, and the matrix organization.

The functional organization has a hierarchical structure that attempts to integrate and follow the various traditional principles of organizational structure quite closely. It is based on the specialization of tasks, where all common activities are grouped under the supervision of a single manager. The manager-specialist has authority over specific processes or functions and does supervise subordinates within several different departments or groups, but only on matters in a specific functional area. Examples are the electrical engineering manager supervising the electrical development group and the printed circuit board group, or the software manager managing the software development group and the software verification and validation group. The responsibility of functional management in this type of organization is to provide an adequately trained staff that is responsive to the changing technology that drives the business; this includes guidance and direction of individuals in their career growth. Furthermore, given the equipment, facilities, and personnel necessary to perform the tasks and activities, the functional manager is responsible for accomplishing the assigned area of specialized work within the allocated cost and schedule constraints. Finally, the functional manager provides both the functional development policy and its interpretation and is prepared to implement and execute it.

The major advantage of the functional organization is its ability to establish company-wide policies and standards regarding items such as documentation, validation, verification, tools, development methods and processes, testing procedures, and training. The major criticism of the functional organization is that it tends to spread responsibility, and this tends to cause gaps in communication and accomplishment among the various functional groups. The spread of responsibility also tends to generate rivalries among the specialists in a group, which can then cause dysfunctional conflicts.

The project organization deviates from the classical principles of organizational structure in the area of departments. Rather than forming a large, homogeneous group that performs similar activities and functions, the project organization promotes the formation of a large number of small, heterogeneous groups, each of which is responsible for the majority of activities associated with a single project. Each project, for example, is assigned a project or program manager who is given the resources and control to carry out the tasks related to the project. All project problems are thus resolved with the most direct path by the individuals who are closest to the problem area. Project-oriented organizations tend to promote loyalty among project personnel. This tends to increase productivity of software development groups, which in turn tend to complete projects on time and within budget. The major drawback of this type of organization is its inability to share expensive and specialized software resources among various projects. In addition, it suffers from the difficulty of establishing and verifying that common software standards are being adhered to by all projects.

The matrix organization attempts to combine the best characteristics of the functional and project organizations. This is usually described as a horizontal project organization overlaid on a vertical functional structure. Matrix organization, a complex structure, tends to be more appropriate for large companies that have larger projects and can afford to carry the management overhead associated with this type of structure. In the matrix management organization, a certain percentage of the total personnel working on various projects will report to both a project manager and a functional manager. The major advantage of the matrix organization is its ability to promote both long-term organizational objectives (such as company-wide software standards and procedures) and project-oriented objectives (such as completion of the software on time and within budget) with a product that meets the user's requirements.

One of the characteristics of the more successful software development companies is the attention they pay to the overall structure of the company and that of the individual projects. Organizational structures in efficient companies are optimized for the project being developed; consequently, a project structure and a matrix structure are used. In addition, the organizational hierarchy includes a lead software engineer and a lead verification and validation engineer assigned to the project, as well as a thoroughly documented and enforced design and implementation methodology.

Software Engineering Team Organization

Two distinct types of software engineering teams are the chief programmer team and the egoless programming team. Conceptually, the former can be categorized as a centralized control approach and the latter as a democratic, decentralized approach. There are almost as many permutations and combinations of these two team types as there are projects in which they can be used.

In its most basic form, the chief programmer team features a highly structured group that consists of at least three individuals: the chief programmer, a senior-level programmer, and a program librarian. Additional personnel can be added to the team on a temporary basis to meet the specific, immediate needs of the project. The chief programmer manages all the technical aspects of the project and reports, horizontally, to the project manager who performs the administrative duties of the project. Software design and task assignments are initiated at the top levels of the team, and communication occurs through a programming library system that contains all of the latest information on the code that has been developed to date. The program librarian maintains the library and performs clerical support for the project. Rigid programming standards are upheld by the chief programmer.

In general, communication is limited in this structure and is usually directed toward the manager. As a result, the software team's morale and goal motivation are low. The chief programmer structure is not particularly well suited for multiple tasks that require multiple inputs for solution or unstructured tasks that require substantial cooperation. The chief programmer team is well suited for a simple, structured, and well-defined programming task that has rigid completion deadlines and little individual interface with the ultimate client or user.

In its most basic form, the egoless team structure promotes the notion of consensus management. The egoless team would consist of ten or fewer programmers, who exchange their code with other team members for error examination. The team's goals are set by group consensus, and the group's management is a rotating function. In this approach, the leadership of the software group migrates to the individual already on the team who has the abilities that are currently needed. This approach does not work well on projects that have severe time constraints, simple solutions, large information exchange requirements, or unusual approaches. It does work well with difficult projects of considerable duration and which demand personnel interaction with the customer or user of the software.

In a third software development team organization (Figure 4-5) the software management and quality assurance functions remain in place for the duration of the project. The software team is assembled, and the project is decomposed by features, functions, components, or subsystems, or by a combination of these characteristics, in such a way as to form small software development subteams. Each subteam is then responsible for the analysis, design, coding, testing, documentation, and evaluation of the assigned feature, function, or component for the entire duration of the project. If a subteam's part of the project is completed early, the team may be given another piece of the software to be implemented, and it would then also be responsible for the new assignment during the duration of the software effort. Verification and validation of the software occurs on a team-by-team basis and is then performed on the final integrated software, by the software verification and validating group that was initially set up for the project. This approach works well with projects that have severe time constraints and simple to moderate solutions, with structured and well-defined tasks. It does not work well with projects that have restricted or limited resources, unusual technical approaches, or poorly defined requirements.

These three approaches effectively represent the vertices of a triangle that reflects the possible philosophic approaches to software team organization. There are many variations on these approaches. The selection, creation, and implementation of a specific software team structure must be done individually for each situation and project. Factors that should be considered in the organizational selection should include the size and complexity of the code to be developed and the inherent difficulty of the application to be implemented. The chosen team structure must be compatible with and able to fit into the overall company structure.

In any kind of team structure, software engineers are disturbed by an environment in which they must work without knowing all of the rules by which they must function. When software

Figure 4-5   Typical software team and subteam organization

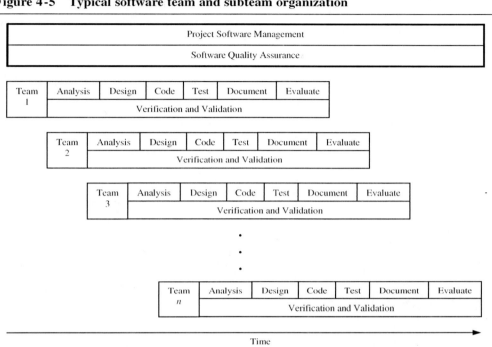

engineers know that their work and structure are governed by rules and that some of those rules are not stated, most of them will work harder, to discover the hidden rules. However, if they know that there are no rules or that the rules can be arbitrarily changed, then they tend to get hostile and belligerent and mentally disengage from their work. Psychologists indicate that this behavior demonstrates a strong need for a feeling of control; in fact, this behavior influences the types of jobs that software engineers seek and keep. Their desire or lack of desire to assume management responsibilities, their entire attitude toward management styles, their feelings about team programming and technical reviews, and many other aspects of the software engineering lifestyle are embodied in this behavior.

One reason software engineers like to engage in rule-bound situations is that they are good at it; people who are not successful in such situations do not usually become software engineers. Consequently, in order to keep software engineering teams happy and productive, an environment must be established in which the rules are clear and known to everyone. The rules for software development teams must be well defined, well-understood, and communicated to all individuals. The rules are, of course, the standards, conventions, methodology, and process used in the software life cycle, but they also encompass the rules of how the teams are organized, how they function, and what the responsibilities of the team are.

Reliable Estimations of Software Development

Without doubt, the most difficult and complicated of all software activities is software development estimation. Possessing a good and reliable model of software development estimation does not guarantee good and reliable estimates. As with any other model, a software development estimation model is highly dependent on the quality of the data used for the estimate. If poor sizing data and attribute-rating data are provided for the model, then poor estimates will be generated. This implies two critical observations:

1. A methodology, process, or algorithm is needed to use a software development estimation model, because it can usually lead to the generation of an appropriate set of model inputs that can be correlated to the desired estimation objectives.

2. Several different estimating methods and techniques should be used to check and confirm the results of the algorithmic software development estimation.

Reliable software estimates consist of more than simply plugging numbers into a formula and accepting the results. Software estimation can also be accomplished through the use of rote methods or procedures as well as relatively sophisticated estimation models. Regardless of the methods, procedures, or devices used to estimate software development, it should be understood that software estimation activities are in fact a mini-project. They should be planned, the results should be reviewed, and at the completion of the project the actuals should be compared to the predicted values.

One rote method for software development estimation is a seven-step process:

1. Establish estimation objectives.

2. Plan for required data and their sources.

3. Stabilize software requirements.

4. Work out as much software detail as is feasible.

5. Use several different and independent techniques and sources to make the estimate.

6. Compare the estimates and iterate on their results.

7. Follow up on the results in order to refine the estimation techniques.

The principal factor that helps to establish the estimate objectives is the current project phase of the software life cycle. The software phase correlates directly with the level of understanding of the software being estimated and with the level of confidence or commitment that will be made as a result of the estimate. When alternative concepts for a new software application are being evaluated, the relative range of the software development estimation can vary by roughly a factor of 4 on either the high or the low side (Boehm 1981a), as shown in Table 4-2. This spread reflects the wide range of uncertainties that apply to the product during the feasibility phase. Once the feasibility issues have been resolved and an operational concept has been delineated, the range of estimates fluctuates by a factor of 2 in either direction. This range is reasonable from the project standpoint, because issues such as the specific functions to be performed within the microprocessor have not been resolved at this point of the project. These types of issues will be resolved, however, by the time the software requirements specification is generated; the estimate at that time will be within a range of 1.5 in either direction. By the time the product design specification has been completed and validated, the software estimate should be accurate to within a factor of 1.25. This factor could apply because, for example, the data structures, processing techniques, and device drivers have been determined, but discrepancies related to specific algorithms, error handling, and safety could still remain. These issues would normally be resolved by the end of the detailed design phase, but a residual uncertainty of 10

Table 4-2   Example of Relative versus Absolute Estimation of a Software Project

Project Phase		Relative Range Multiplier		Estimated Completion (months)	Actual Project Duration Range (months)	
Phase	**Milestone**	**Min.**	**Max.**		**Min.**	**Max.**
Product idea	Estimation guess	0.25	4	12	3	48
Feasibility	Concept of operation	0.5	2	12	6	24
Plans and requirements	Requirements specification	0.67	1.5	12	8	18
Product design	Product design specification	0.8	1.25	12	9.6	15
Detailed design	Detailed design specification	0.1	0.1	12	10.8	13.2
Development and test	Released software	n/a	n/a	done	0	0

percent will still remain. This uncertainty relates to how well the software team really understands the specifications they are to implement.

In more practical terms, let us examine these range factors in an example. Suppose that an initial software development estimate assumes a software development period of 1 year (Table 4-2). Using Boehm's (1981a) relative estimation ranges, this estimate could actually be for a project that ranges from a low of 3 months to a high of 4 years if estimated during product conceptualization. At the end of the concept-of-operation phase, assuming again that it is still estimated to be a 1-year project, the actual development effort could range from 6 months to 2 years. After the requirements specification has been generated, the same 1-year project could, in reality, be a project that lasts from 8 months to 1.5 years. The product design phase estimation could actually represent a development project range of 9 months to 16 months, and the detailed design phase estimate range could be realized within 11 months to 13 months.

The fundamental software estimating implication of this example is that the estimating objectives for the various phases of the software product need to be consistent. In general, a balanced set of estimating objectives would make the absolute magnitude of the uncertainty range for each phase roughly equal. Another estimating implication of this example is that software development estimates should include an indication of the degree of uncertainty.

As a mini-project, software development estimation activities need to be scheduled and resources allotted to it to be effective. The software estimation mini-project should conceptually be thought of as the plan that delineates the responsible individual(s), what is to be produced, and by when the estimate end products are to be produced. The estimation end products could be a schedule, Gantt charts, PERT analysis, milestone lists with due dates, or even a WBS as presented above.

Software engineers are extremely adept at producing software if they understand what it is that they are producing. If what is to be produced is unknown or unclear, then it is difficult, if not impossible, to estimate the time needed to develop the software. This means that it is extremely important to have a set of software specifications that are as unambiguous as possible, especially when they might be relevant to any qualifications that relate to the estimating objectives. The best way to determine to what extent a software specification is estimable is to determine to what extent it is testable; a software specification is testable to the extent that a definitive pass-fail test can determine whether the developed software will satisfy the specification. From this, it follows that in order to be testable, software specifications must be specific, unambiguous, and quantitative wherever possible.

For example, suppose a software specification contains the following two requirements: "The software shall provide accuracy sufficient to prevent overinfusion," and "The software shall provide real-time response to user input." These statements are good goals and objectives for the device, but they are not precise enough to serve as the basis of a pass-fail acceptance test. Consequently, they cannot serve as the basis of a software development estimate. A more testable version of these two statements might be the following: "The software shall provide accuracy sufficient to prevent overinfusion by 10 milliliters," and "The software shall provide real-time response to user inputs within 0.2 seconds." Even when the specifications are quantifiable, they may not be sufficiently testable without further amplification. For example, does "overinfusion by 10 milliliters" and "within 0.2 seconds" mean root mean square performance, 90 percent confidence limits, or never-to-exceed constraints? Does "real-time response" include key debounce time, bus communication time, or strict processing time?

Often a good deal of added effort is required to eliminate the vagueness and ambiguity in a software specification in order to make it testable, but such efforts are usually worthwhile. In the long run, the clarification will have to be resolved anyway, to complete the testing phase; clearing up these types of issues early reduces expense, controversy, and possible bitterness in later software project phases. Clarification at this stage will also lead to better estimates for the current phase, as well as more accurate estimates during later software phases. However, it is impossible and impractical to ensure that all of the software requirements are testable. In these cases, it is valuable to document any assumptions that were made in estimating the software development.

In general, the more detail the estimating activities encompass, the more accuracy will be reflected in the estimates. The more detail that is explored, the more thorough the understanding and comprehension of the technical aspects of the software to be developed. The more detail is examined, the more distinct the pieces of software being estimated; the law of large numbers begins to work to reduce the estimation variance. For example, if the software is estimated in one large piece and its development is overestimated by 20 percent, then the project inherits a 20 percent error. If the software is decomposed into ten smaller pieces, then chances are that some pieces will be overestimated and some will be underestimated; the net effect is that the project will inherit a considerably smaller estimating error. Furthermore, the more the functions of the software that are considered, the less likely it will be that pieces will be missed, particularly the unobtrusive and ubiquitous components; therefore, a greater percentage of the software will be included in the estimation. There is a powerful tendency in software estimation activities to focus on the highly visible components of the software and to underestimate or completely miss the low-level components.

Several major classes of techniques are available for software estimating; it is important to understand that none of the alternatives is any better than the others, in all aspects. In fact, for some techniques, their strengths and weaknesses are complementary. It is important to use a combination of techniques in order to avoid the weaknesses of any single method and to capitalize on their joint strengths.

The most valuable aspect of using several independent estimating techniques is the opportunity to investigate why they give different estimation results. For example, if a bottom-up technique estimated a 1-year effort and a top-down technique estimated 1 year and 9 months, then the reasons for the differences should be identified, and a more detailed analysis of those differences could be undertaken. Following this analysis, an iteration of these two estimates may then converge toward a more realistic estimate, rather than making an arbitrary compromise of the 12-month and 21-month estimates without any analysis. The need to investigate the differences that will exist between the estimates leads to the fundamental constructive characteristic of development estimation models. Constructive estimate models make it clear to reviewers why the model gave the estimates that it did. Otherwise, there is very little objective evidence with which to compare the model's results.

There is an additional rationale for iterating the development estimates. In estimates involving multiple software components, it is not unusual to find components that are similar in function but yield radically different development estimations. This frequently results from one estimator being pessimistic about the component and a second estimator being optimistic about the same component. Commonly, there are several components whose estimates contain the majority of the development time; these estimates follow Pareto's law, in which, in this case, 80 percent of the estimate is contained in 20 percent of the components. In such instances, it is particularly important to examine and iterate these components in greater detail than the other components because these components tend to be the larger sized ones that are frequently overestimated with respect to their complexity.

People have a tendency to equate software size with complexity, whereas the estimating models tend to define complexity as an inherent attribute of the code that is independent of the code size. People also have a tendency to rate the complexity of a software component as the complexity of the hardest software segment within that component. Commonly, large software components have many simple housekeeping functions embedded in them, and these easily become overestimated relative to the component's overall complexity.

Once the software project has begun, it is essential to gather data on its actual progress and compare this to the original estimates, because the software estimating inputs as well as the estimating techniques are imperfect. If a project team finds a difference between the estimated and actual data that can be explained by improved knowledge about the estimate inputs, it is important to update the estimate with that new knowledge. This, in turn, provides a more realistic basis for future estimates, as well as for the current project management. Another reason to capture the estimation differences is to ascertain whether the project really fits the estimating model that was used. If the project does not fit the model, then it is based on assumptions that have no bearing on reality, and similar future projects should use a different estimation model. In addition, software projects tend to be volatile, as new components are added and the original, estimated components are added to, split up, rescoped, and combined in unforeseeable and unpredictable ways as the project progresses. The software project must identify these types of changes and generate a more realistic update for the estimated upcoming deliverables.

Estimation Models

A simple but effective technique for comparing project actuals to project estimates is the schedule-milestone chart. The format for this chart displays the schedule months along the x-axis and the resource-months of effort along the y-axis; it graphs the intersection of the estimated number of months and resource-months that are required to achieve the salient software development milestones and deliverables. Starting with these estimates, the software project can subsequently plot the actual date and effort associated with the achievement of the particular milestones. If there is a significant difference between the estimates and the actuals, then there is a basis for investigating and taking any necessary corrective action.

A variety of classes for categorizing the estimating methods have been created to further software development estimation. The algorithmic model methods provide one or more algorithms that produce a software development estimate as a function of variables that are considered to be the major drivers of the development effort.

Algorithmic Estimation Models

The algorithmic software development estimate models provide one or more mathematical algorithms that produce a software development estimate as a function of several variables that are the major drivers of the development effort. The most common forms of the algorithmic models used for software development estimation are linear, multiplicative, analytic, tabular, and composite.

Linear development estimating models have the form

$$\text{Effort} = a_0 + a_1 x_1 + \ldots + a_n x_n, \tag{4.3}$$

where $x_1, \ldots, x_n$ are the development driver variables and $a_0, \ldots, a_n$ are a set of coefficients chosen to provide the statistical best fit to a set of observed data points. This type of model was used primarily during the mid-1960s, when software development estimation was in its infancy. It might still be a usable approach for companies that maintain extensive and exhaustive databases of metrics for software development projects, because it can be used to generate an estimating model that is explicitly tailored to the company's experience. However, because this model is based on a linear best fit algorithm and software contains an inordinate number of nonlinear interactions, it is questionable whether this approach is viable anymore.

Multiplicative development estimating models have the form

$$\text{Effort} = a_0 \, a_1^{x_1} \, a_2^{x_2} \ldots a_n^{x_n} \tag{4.4}$$

where $x_1, \ldots, x_n$ are the development driver variables and $a_0, \ldots, a_n$ are a set of coefficients chosen to best fit observational data. This model was used during the mid-1970s. The development driver variables are constrained to the discrete values of 1, 0, and -1. The multiplicative model usually works reasonably well if the variables chosen from the company database are reasonably independent. If they are not, then the effects of the interaction activities are doubly accounted for. The constraint on this model, that the development driver variables can assume only these discrete values, tends to generate unstable models, because the development estimates can change only in large steps. For example, suppose that one of the coefficients is 1.83 and that one of the development driver variables represents the concurrent development of the hardware with the software. Then, if concurrency is present in the project, the estimate is multiplied by $1.83^1 = 1.83$ and by $1.83^0 = 1.0$ if it is not. There are no intermediate multipliers.

Analytic development estimating models take the more general mathematical form

$$\text{Effort} = f(x_1, \ldots, x_n), \tag{4.5}$$

where $x_1, \ldots, x_n$ are the development driver variables and f is some mathematical function other than a linear or multiplicative function. Of the many such models derived over the years, most contain only a small number of variables. They are, therefore, insensitive to key development driver factors, such as hardware constraints, that are often critical determinants of software development. The Halstead model (Halstead 1977) takes the particular form

$$\text{Effort} = (\eta_1 \times N_2 \times N \times \log_2[\eta_1 + \eta_2])/(2 \times S \times \eta_2), \qquad (4.6)$$

where η_1 is the number of distinct operators in the program, η_2 is the number of distinct operands in the program, N_2 is the total usage of all operands in the program, N is the total usage of all operators and operands, and S is a constant that is dependent on the programming language to be used. Another example is the Putnam model (Putnam 1978), which takes the form

$$S_s = C_k \times K^{1/3} \times t_d^{4/3}, \qquad (4.7)$$

where S_s is the software product size, C_k is a "technology constant" that reflects current best practices, K is the development effort in person-years, and t_d is the development time in years.

Tabular development estimating models contain tables that relate the values of development driver variables either to distinct parts of the software development effort or to multipliers that are used to adjust the effort estimate. For example, the Aron model (Aron 1969) consists of a 3×3 table that relates development effort to project duration and difficulty. The Wolverton model (Wolverton 1974) estimates development effort as a tabular function of the software type, software difficulty, and software novelty. The Boeing model (Black et al. 1977) estimates a basic productivity rate as a tabular function of the type of software and then modifies the productivity rate by multipliers obtained as another tabular function of other development drivers. The tabular models are generally easy to understand, implement, and modify on the basis of new development driver insights. They also create some difficulties related to the number of development driver variables that can be used in the tables. For example, if only a few variables are used, then the model may be insensitive to some of the more important development drivers. If many variables are used, then the model will probably have an even greater number of table values to be calibrated; this would probably necessitate a large database for thorough model calibration and validation.

Composite Estimation Models

Composite models incorporate varying combinations of linear, multiplicative, analytic, and tabular functions to estimate the software development effort as a function of development driver variables. Composite models have the advantage of using the most appropriate functional form for each component of the software development estimate. Their main difficulties are that they are more complicated to learn and to use by hand, although some are available as commercial products; they also require more data and effort to calibrate and validate.

The composite algorithmic Constructive Cost Model (COCOMO) is probably the best known of all standard estimator models in the software industry. It is used for estimating the size of the effort and the duration of software projects by means of a hierarchy of increasingly detailed and accurate forms. The top-level model, called Basic COCOMO, is applicable to most small- to medium-sized software projects that are developed in a familiar, in-house software development environment. Basic COCOMO is good for quick, early, and rough order-of-magnitude estimates for software projects, but its accuracy is limited because the Basic COCOMO factors do not account for the differences in hardware constraints, personnel quality and experience, use of tools and techniques, and other software project attributes known to have a significant influence on software development. Intermediate COCOMO extends and refines the estimate generated by Basic COCOMO by incorporating 15 predictor variables that account for much of the variation in software development estimation not addressed by Basic COCOMO. Detailed

COCOMO provides two main capabilities that address the limitations of Intermediate COCOMO: for each development driver attribute, a set of software phase-sensitive effort multipliers are used to determine the amount of effort required to complete each phase, and (2) a three-level product hierarchy addresses effects that occur at the module, subsystem, and system levels.

The fundamental metric used to drive COCOMO is the number of thousands of source instructions to be delivered (KDSI) by the project. The count of delivered source instructions does not include support software, but it does include all lines of code, any job control language statements, format statements, data declarations, and procedurals. The development period covered by COCOMO estimates starts with the beginning of the product design phase that correlates closely with the end of the software requirements review phase in the waterfall model. COCOMO estimates end with the integration and test phase that ends the software acceptance phase in the waterfall model. The COCOMO assumes that a person-month consists of 152 working hours. It also assumes that the requirement specification(s) are not substantially changed after the software planning and requirements phase. It does allow for requirement refinements and reinterpretations, but any significant requirement modifications or additions should be addressed by a revised estimate. The COCOMO does include documentation time in its estimate, but not verification and validation time. The following technical discussion is about the Basic COCOMO, not to Intermediate or Detailed COCOMO, because the latter two are refinements and extensions of the Basic COCOMO.

The Basic COCOMO provides basic effort and schedule estimates for the most common mode of software development, the small- to medium-sized project developed in an in-house, familiar, and organic software development environment. However, several distinct types of software development modes are recognized by the model. These different modes have estimating relationships that are similar in form but yield significantly different estimates for software products of the same size. The two additional development modes are the tightly constrained embedded mode and an intermediate mode between organic and embedded, the semidetached mode. The Basic COCOMO provides an estimate for the organic, semidetached, and embedded projects for each of the standard product sizes; a linear interpolation technique can be used to ascertain project estimates for projects that are between the standard-size ones.

To use the COCOMO, an estimate of the number of thousands of delivered source instructions (KDSI) must be known. One technique that can help with this estimation is the PERT sizing technique (Putnam and Fitzsimmons 1979); the simplest version of this technique involves the estimation of two quantities. For the sake of the following discussion, let a represent the lowest possible size of the software in delivered source instructions, let b represent the highest possible size of the software in delivered source instructions, and let these low and high estimates represent three standard deviation limits on the probability distribution of the actual software size. This means that the actual software size would lie between the a and b sizes 99.7 percent of the time. The PERT statistical equations estimate that the expected size of the software is given as

$$E = (a + b)/2, \tag{4.8}$$

and the standard deviation of the estimate is given as

$$\sigma = (b - a)/6. \tag{4.9}$$

For example, suppose the lowest possible size was 22 KDSI and the highest possible size was 64 KDSI. Then, the expected software size is 43 KDSI with a standard deviation of 7 KDSI. This means that 68 percent of the time, the actual size of the software should fall between 36 and 50 KDSI. It also means that 16 percent of the time it will fall between the ranges 22–36 KDSI and 50–64 KDSI. These formulas, however, are based on the assumption of a normal distribution of software sizes between the two extremes *a* and *b*. If the upper limit *b* is the maximum amount of code that will fit in the processor, then there is probably a much better chance than 16 percent that the final size of the software will be between 50 KDSI and 64 KDSI.

An improved PERT sizing technique is also discussed by Putnam and Fitzsimmons (1979). This version is based on a beta distribution of the software sizes and on a separate estimation for each of the individual software components. For each software component *i*, the lowest possible size of the software is represented by *a*, the most likely size of the component is given by *m*, and the highest possible size of the component is specified by *b*, where *a*, *m*, and *b* are expressed in thousands of words. The PERT equations estimate the expected size E_i and standard deviation σ_i of each component as

$$E_i = (a_i + 4 \times m_i + b_i)/6 \tag{4.10}$$

and

$$\sigma_i = (b_i - a_i)/6. \tag{4.11}$$

The estimated total software size E and the standard deviation σ_E are then given by

$$E = \Sigma^n E_i \tag{4.12}$$

and

$$\sigma_E = (\Sigma^n \sigma_i^2)^{1/2}. \tag{4.13}$$

This sizing technique is somewhat better than the previous version in that it requires more thought to decompose the software into components and to estimate the most likely sizes for each resulting component. However, the calculation for σ_E is highly misleading because it assumes that the estimates are unbiased in relation to underestimation and overestimation.

In practice, the "most likely" size estimates tend to cluster more toward the lower limit than the upper limit, while actual product sizes tend to cluster more toward the upper limit. The rationale for this is that most individuals tend to follow a geometric progression in making "most likely" size estimates rather than an arithmetic progression. For example, given the low and high limits of 16 KDSI and 64 KDSI, people are more likely to choose the geometric mean of 32 KDSI as their "most likely" size rather than the arithmetic mean of 40 KDSI, and they very rarely choose a "most likely" size estimate of 48 KDSI or higher. The net result of this is a significant underestimation bias in the PERT estimation results.

Estimation Model Comparison

Software undersizing is probably the most critical obstacle to accurate software development estimations. There are no magic formulas that can be used to overcome this problem. In the absence of any such formula, it is important to understand the major sources of the software undersizing problem. There are three main reasons why software engineers underestimate software size:

1. They are basically optimistic and want to please. Software engineers want the software to be small and easy because high estimates tend to lead to confrontations and the potential for cancellation of the software project.

2. Software engineers tend to have incomplete recall of their previous project experience. They tend to have a strong recollection of the primary application software functions

that were developed and a weaker recollection of the large amount of user interface and housekeeping software that was developed.

3.   Software engineers are generally not familiar with the entire software job to be performed on the project to be estimated. This factor tends to interact with the recall issue to produce underestimates of the more obscure software end products to be developed as well as the more obscure parts of each product.

In summary, there is no easy way to perform software sizing. There is no substitute for a thorough understanding of the job to be done and the tendencies to underestimate software size, and for a thoughtful, realistic application of this understanding to medical device software development.

Compared to other estimation methods, algorithmic models tend to have several strengths:

*   They are entirely objective in how they manipulate the data they use. Algorithmic models are not influenced by factors such as the desire to please, a distaste for the project, or the desire to reach the marketplace faster than is truly possible.

*   These types of models are repeatable. Given the same data at two different points in time, they will generate the same results.

*   They are efficient and able to support a wide variety of parametric estimations and sensitivity analysis.

*   They can be objectively calibrated to previous experience.

Algorithmic models also have weaknesses:

*   Because they are calibrated to previous experience, they are always vulnerable to the subjective inquiry that questions the extent to which those previous projects are representative of future projects. This is particularly acute when new techniques, new processor architectures, new application areas, and new development tools are constantly being sought, integrated, and used on the newer projects.

*   They are unable to deal with the exceptional conditions that tend to arise among personnel, in teamwork, and around the personalities and the job to be done.

*   There is no practical way that the model can compensate for poor sizing inputs and inaccurate development driver ratings.

Estimation Methods

A variety of classes for categorizing estimation methods have been created in order to further software development estimation. Expert judgment methods involve consulting one or more experts to gather their opinions on the software development effort. The analogy method involves reasoning by analogy from one or more completed projects to relate their actual development schedules and resources to an estimate of a similar project. The Parkinson methods use the Parkinson principle, that work expands to fill the available volume, to equate the development estimate to the available resources. In price-to-win methods, the estimate that is developed is equated to the schedule believed necessary for the company to be first in the marketplace with the new product. Top-down methods generate an overall estimate for the project that is derived from the global properties of the product; the estimate is then broken into its various components.

In bottom-up methods, each component of the software is estimated separately, and the results are aggregated to produce an estimate for the overall software development.

Expert Judgment Methods

The human intellect is capable of compensating for some of the drawbacks associated with the algorithmic models. For example, expert judgment techniques involve consulting with one or more experts who use their experience and understanding of the proposed software development project to arrive at an estimate of its development effort. The strengths and weaknesses of this method tend to be highly complementary to the strengths and weaknesses of the algorithmic models. An expert is able to factor in the differences between past project experiences and the new techniques, architectures, or applications that are involved in the project to be estimated. The expert can also factor in the exceptional personnel characteristics and interactions, as well as any other project-unique considerations. However, expert judgment is no better than the expertise and objectivity of the estimator. Experts may be biased, optimistic, pessimistic, or unfamiliar with the key aspects of the project. Because of the possible bias in an individual expert, it is preferable to obtain estimates from more than one expert.

If estimates are obtained from several experts, there are several ways to combine their opinions into a single estimate. One such way is to compute the mean or median estimate of all of the individual estimates. Although this method is quick and simple, it is subject to adverse bias by one or two extreme estimates. Another method is to conduct a group meeting for as long as is necessary to get the experts to reach a consensus about a single estimate. This will at least filter out any uninformed estimates in general, but it has two distinct difficulties. First, some group members may be overly influenced by the more glib and assertive group members. Second, some group members may be overly influenced by any figures of authority who may be present or by political considerations.

One technique that has been used to avoid the drawbacks of the expert group meeting and take advantage of the group estimation process is the Delphi technique (Helmer 1966), which originated at the Rand Corporation in the late 1940s as a means of predicting future events. The standard Delphi technique, an expert-consensus method for estimating software development, consists of five steps:

1. A coordinator presents each expert with the appropriate project specifications and a form on which the expert's software development estimate is recorded.

2. The experts fill out the forms anonymously. They may ask clarifying and qualifying questions of the coordinator but not of each other.

3. The coordinator prepares a summary of the experts' responses on another form that shows their estimate along with the group's median estimate.

4. The coordinator distributes a copy of the summary form to each expert and requests an iteration of that expert's previous estimate along with the rationale behind the new estimate.

5. The experts fill out the summary forms anonymously, and the process is iterated for as many rounds as appropriate.

The standard Delphi technique shows an impressive convergence of some initially very diverse estimates, but the results are less accurate than if the expert group is allowed to arrive at a joint estimate. The standard Delphi technique can be modified to facilitate the estimation process in any number of ways.

Analogy Methods

Estimation by analogy involves reasoning by analogy to relate actual development effort of completed projects to an estimate of the development effort of a similar, new product. Estimating by analogy can be done at the project level or at the subsystem level. The advantage of estimating at the project level is that all components of the development effort will be considered; subsystem-level estimating has the advantage of providing a more detailed assessment of the similarities and differences between completed projects and the new project. The main strength of estimation by analogy is that the estimate is based on an actual experience that can be studied to determine specific differences from the new project and, therefore, their likely impact. The main weakness of the analogy estimation is that it is not clear to what degree the previous projects are representative of the constraints, techniques, personnel, and functions in the new project.

In top-down estimating, an overall development estimate is derived from the global properties and expected characteristics of the software project. The major advantage of this method is its system-level focus. To the extent that the estimate is based on previous experience with entirely completed projects, it will usually encompass system-level activities such as integration, user's manuals, and configuration management. The major disadvantages of top-down estimates are that they do not identify the traditionally difficult low-level technical problems that drive up the actual development effort. Top-down estimates provide neither a detailed basis for the estimated development effort nor iteration feedback. Finally, top-down estimates are less stable than a multicomponent estimate in which estimation errors in the components have a chance to balance each other out.

In the bottom-up estimating method, an individual, usually the person who will be responsible for developing the particular software component, estimates the development effort of each software component. The development effort for each component is then summed up, to arrive at the development effort estimate for the entire project. Bottom-up estimating is directly complementary to top-down estimating in that the strength of one is the other's weakness. Making a bottom-up estimate also requires more effort than a top-down approach, but this can also be an advantage. For example, having each part of the development effort estimated by the person responsible for its success is helpful in two ways: (1) each estimate is based on a more thorough and detailed understanding of the activities to be performed, and (2) each estimate receives the personal endorsement and commitment of the individual who will be responsible for the end product. The bottom-up estimate also tends to be more stable in that all of the estimation errors for each component have a chance to balance out.

The most effective way to ensure that system-level considerations are included in a bottom-up estimate is to organize the project into a WBS. The WBS includes not only the product's hierarchy of software components, but also the activity hierarchy of the project tasks to be done. This ensures that the development efforts for activities such as integration, configuration management, and low-level technical tasks are accounted for. However, unless these estimates can be delayed until the estimates for the product's components are established, they may be inaccurate. For example, it would be difficult to estimate the integration effort without a good understanding and idea of the size, complexity, and nature of the components to be integrated.

The traditional approach to software development estimation and the one used most frequently for bottom-up estimation is the task-unit approach. In this approach, the job of developing a software component is broken into task units. The effort required for each task unit is estimated by the component developer, and the resulting estimates are then summed to produce the overall effort estimate for the software component. The main advantages of this approach are generally the same as those of the bottom-up method. In addition, the task estimates provide a sound foundation for overall project planning and control. One main difficulty with the task-unit approach is overlooking the system-level efforts. In particular, it glosses over the incidental software project activities that add to the amount of effort really needed to produce the software end products. This includes software development activities such as reading and reviewing specifications, attending meetings, and performing analyses to determine the best approach to fixing errors. Another main difficulty with the task-unit approach is that of overlooking the incidental, nonproject activities. This includes training, personnel business, nonproject communication, and other company-related activities that do not contribute directly to software development but must, nonetheless, be attended to. These difficulties should not be considered as fundamental drawbacks that would preclude use of the task-unit approach as a viable estimation method. They are noted as considerations to be covered in reviewing the task-unit estimates for completeness. On the whole, the task-unit method is an extremely valuable approach, particularly for estimating software development effort for small projects.

Estimation Model and Methods: Conclusions

Conclusions that can be drawn from this discussion of software development effort estimation models and methods include these:

- None of the alternatives is any better than any other, in all aspects.

- The strengths and weaknesses of the techniques are basically complementary. For example, the algorithmic model complements expert judgment and the top-down estimate complements the bottom-up estimate.

- It is important to use a combination of techniques and then compare, contrast, and iterate the estimates obtained from each method.

- The particular combination of methods should be driven by estimation objectives, such as using the top-down method for early estimates and the bottom-up method for detailed planning estimates.

- The current state of the art for software development estimation is a long way from being uniform, standard, and consistent.

In general, an effective combination for estimating the software development effort is this: A top-down estimate using the judgment of more than one expert should be coupled with analogy estimation when a comparable previous project is available. A bottom-up estimate using an algorithmic model should be coupled with inputs and component-level estimates provided by the responsible developers. The results of both should then be compared and iterated.

Function Point Analysis

An alternative to the estimation models and methods is to use function points. Function point metrics can be used as a foundation for the measurement of productivity, development time, and defect rate. Function point measures are unique in that they can be used to compare different software applications. Function point analysis (FPA) represents a shift from estimating the number of lines of code to be created or reused to using function point counts to size software projects. Analysis shows (Bernstein 1995) that productivity as measured by function points per staff month varies as a function of the type of software being built, and the complexity of the software accounts for a 10:1 difference in software productivity. In addition, operating system or real-time software that is sensitive to the peculiarities of its environment is ten times more difficult to produce than administrative or information technology software. Productivity of projects based on FPA can be four times higher than projects not based on FPA. To achieve these results requires an investment in people to establish real expertise in FPA, but when fully developed the experts can make important contributions to a project's architecture. The expert often finds opportunities for reuse that are missed by the developers and discovers redundancies, especially in large projects. In effect, an additional systems view is possible through FPA.

Non–Real-time FPA

Many software organizations are more comfortable with estimation based on previous experience or with counting lines of code. However, early estimations of the size and effort of projects using source lines of code or past experience are inaccurate and often lead to significant cost and schedule overruns. Function points, however, are a logical unit of measure of the software functions of a system as seen by the user. They define the essential value of what the software is and what it does with data from a user's point of view; FPA, therefore, is a count of the number of internal logical files, external interface files, external inputs, external outputs, and external inquiries. The FPA emphasis is on the external point of view, and because the effort and cost estimation based on FPA does not depend on language and technology, counts are available in early stages of development. Function points can be counted directly from the product or software requirements, and this has led to widespread acceptance of the technique.

Data functions comprise *internal logical files* and *external interface files*. Transactional functions consist of external inputs, external outputs, and external inquiries. *Internal logical files* are a data function that allows users to utilize data that they are responsible for maintaining. For example, a user may enter infusion data through a display or touch pad on the medical device. The data are stored in an internal file for use and can be modified during the infusion. Logical groupings of data that are maintained by the end-user are referred to as internal logical files (ILFs). *External interface files* are a data function that allows users to utilize data that the user is not responsible for maintaining. The data usually reside in another system and are maintained by another user or system, and the system being estimated requires these data for reference purposes only. For example, it may be necessary for a medical device to reference data from the facility during use. Groupings of data from another system that are used only for reference purposes are defined as external interface files (EIFs).

The transactional functions address the user's capability to access the data contained in ILFs and EIFs; this capability includes maintaining, inquiring of, displaying, and outputting data. The *external input transactional function* allows a user to maintain ILFs through the ability to add, change, and delete the data. For example, a user can add, change, and delete device information prior to and during use of the medical device. In this case the user is utilizing a transaction referred to as an *external input* (EI). An external input gives the user the capability to maintain the data in ILFs through adding, changing, and deleting contents. The *external output transactional function* gives the user the ability to produce outputs. For example, the user has the ability to display speeds, volumes, and doses. The results displayed are derived using data that are maintained and data that are referenced; in function point terminology, the resulting display is called an *external output* (EO). The *external inquiries transactional function* addresses the requirement to select and display specific data from files. To accomplish this, a user inputs selection information that is used to retrieve data that meet the specific criteria. In this situation there is no manipulation of the data, because it is a direct retrieval of information contained in the files. For example, if a user requests the display of rate data that were previously set, the resulting output is the direct retrieval of stored information. These transactions are referred to as *external inquiries* (EQ).

In addition to the five functional components, two adjustment factors need to be considered in FPA. *Functional complexity,* the first adjustment factor, is applied to each unique function and is based on the combination of data groupings and data elements of a particular function. The numbers of data elements and unique groupings are counted and compared to a complexity matrix that will rate the function as low, average, or high complexity. Each of the five functional components (ILF, EIF, EI, EO, and EQ) has a unique complexity matrix. Functional complexity for data functions is based on record element types and data element types. *Data complexity* for transactional functions is based on the data element types and the file types referenced. All of the functional components are analyzed and yield an *unadjusted function point* count.

The individual unadjusted function points are summed to produce a *total unadjusted function point* count, which is multiplied by a second adjustment factor, the *value adjustment factor.* This factor considers the system's technical and operational characteristics. The value adjustment factor is a function of 14 characteristics of the system. The factors include data communications, distributed data processing, performance, a heavily used operational configuration, transaction rate, on-line data entry, end-user efficiency, on-line update, complex processing, reusability, installation ease, operational ease, multiple sites, and ease of change. Each of these factors is scored on the basis of their influence on the system being estimated; the resulting score will increase or decrease the unadjusted function point count by 35 percent. The result of this calculation provides the *adjusted function point* count.

In estimating projects, two key data points are essential: (1) the size of the deliverable and (2) how much of the deliverable can be produced within a defined period. The size can be derived from function points as described above. The second requirement for estimating is to determine how long it takes to produce a function point. This delivery rate can be calculated on the basis of past project performance or by using industry benchmarks. The delivery rate is expressed in function points per hour (FP/hr) and can be applied to similar proposed projects to estimate effort where project hours are calculated as the estimated project function points times FP/hr. Productivity measurement is a natural output of FPA because function points are technology independent and can be used to compare productivity across dissimilar applications, tools, and platforms. More important, they can be used to establish a productivity rate for a specific application, tool set, and platform. Once productivity rates are established, they can be used for project estimating as described above and tracked over time to determine the impact that continuous process improvement initiatives have on productivity.

Real-time FPA

An interesting extension of FPA is to real-time applications. The principal operating characteristic of a real-time system is that the software must execute almost instantly, at the boundary of the processing limits of the processor. The real-time system is an on-line, continuously available, critically timed system that generates event-driven outputs almost simultaneously with their corresponding inputs. These inputs could occur at either fixed or variable intervals, selectively or continuously, and they could require interruption to process inputs of a higher priority, often using a buffer area or queue to determine processing priorities. Data are commonly, but not always, stored in memory. Real-time systems have some characteristics that function points do not fully support. These characteristics must be evaluated separately, because they ultimately will impact the software development time or the enhancement and maintenance productivity.

These characteristics include mathematical and logical algorithms, memory constraints, timing constraints, interruptions, execution speeds, communication constraints, continuous availability, and processor event-driven processing.

The function point counting process is fundamentally the same for real-time systems and information systems; however, the frame of reference changes to address the characteristics of real-time systems. As an example of the similarity, data displayed to a user on the real-time device display are counted in the same way as data displayed on an office computer screen. In addition to the traditional characteristics evaluated by FPA, other application characteristics that are not addressed using function points must also be evaluated. Examples of the dissimilarity include security, communications process, network transaction rate, functional domain, performance, algorithmic complexity, memory constraints, data relationships, and system interfaces.

New development projects represent the functionality of the initial system; consequently, the function point count serves as both the project size and the initial size of the system. Any changes after the initial delivery or release of the product can be considered as enhancements. From an FPA standpoint, such projects deliver changes in functionality by adding new transactional functions (inputs, outputs, or inquiries); changing existing transactional functions by adding or deleting fields or changing the processing (different edits, validations, algorithms, and calculations, or files read, referenced, or updated); adding new logical database files; or changing existing logical database files (different fields or different sizes or structure of fields). Changes in functionality might result from any number of sources, but enhancements are changes to the processing within a system rather than fixes of the existing functionality, and enhancement function point counts describe the size of a software project. However, function points may also be added to or subtracted from the total subsystem size for an existing system to give an indication of the total size of a system that will need maintenance activities. Maintenance projects include the effort to maintain existing systems and exclude changes defined as enhancements. From the FPA standpoint, maintenance refers to the effort to fix bugs and defects, respond to issues about existing functionality, start, restart, or install existing systems, and change text on screens and reports. The function point count for a system undergoing maintenance includes the initial development count plus the counts, as modified by past enhancements, that compose the current subsystem.

Typically, real-time FPA follows specific steps once a new development or enhancement project has been selected for counting. These steps are: establish the system boundaries, identify the data functions (ILFs and EIFs), identify transactional functions (EI, EO, and EQ), calculate the unadjusted function point count, determine the value adjustment factor, using general system characteristics, and calculate the adjusted function point count. A project may include one or more applications or systems, and each should be measured as a distinct individual entity on the basis of how they will ultimately be used. Once the system boundaries are established, the process for real-time function point counting of each system begins. The first step is to identify logical data stores that are maintained or held in memory within the system. External data, transactions, messages, or controls will populate, revise, update, change, or add to the logical data stores, and these stores will be used within the system to support external outputs (EOs) or external inquiries (EQs). A data group should not be dependent upon or attributive to another data group for its existence.

Data groups classified as an ILF are counted once per subsystem. Examples of ILFs include usage information, alarm data, user profiles, customer data, parameter values and processing history. The key to their identification is that the data actually exist or may exist when the software is in use and that the data are dynamic, not hard-coded. Each identified ILF must be assigned a functional complexity of low, average, or high on the basis of the number of *data element types* (DETs) and *record element types* (RETs) associated with that ILF. DETs are unique, user-recognizable, nonrepeating fields or attributes and include foreign key attributes that are maintained on the ILF. RETs are optional or mandatory user-recognizable subgroups of data elements contained within an ILF. Subgroups are typically represented in an entity relationship diagram as entity subtypes or attributive entities, commonly called parent-child relationships. DETs and RETs are applied as shown in Table 4-3 to determine the functional complexity of each ILF. In terms of function points, ILFs receive the highest weights or values when compared to the other functions.

Data files extracted or read from another system's ILFs that do not directly update an ILF within the system but are read or referenced only and are used in processing are EIFs. An EIF is counted only once per system. Common examples are help, security, parameters, system tables and directories, and operating system or product status. The rule of thumb for an EIF in a system is that it is an ILF in another system and only read or referenced by the system being counted. RETs and DETs are counted in the same way as ILFs to determine the complexity of each EIF. Table 4-3 is also used to determine the complexity of each EIF.

Data elements received from outside the system boundary that add, change, maintain, populate, or delete data in an ILF or provide control functions are identified as EIs. Examples of data EIs include alarms, analog data, transactional data, incoming messages and parameter selections. Examples of control EIs include commands or messages from other systems, users, sensors, equipment or hardware that might contain warnings, processing instructions, firing commands, setup or shutdown commands, or speaker volume controls. Data elements with unique processing requirements are counted as separate EIs; these inputs could arrive via data packets or files, control panels, screens, button controls, and so on. Each identified EI must be assigned a functional complexity of low, average, or high, based upon the number of DETs and *file types referenced* (FTRs) associated with the EI. DETs are usually unique, user-recognizable, nonrepeating fields or attributes that enter the boundary of the system. FTRs are equal to the number of ILFs maintained, read, or referenced plus the EIFs read or referenced by the transaction. DETs and FTRs are applied as shown in Table 4-4 to determine the functional complexity of each EI.

Table 4-3   Complexity Matrix of ILF and EIF Data Functions

Number of RETs	Number of DETs		
	1–19	20–50	51+
2 or fewer	Low	Low	Average
2–5	Low	Average	High
More than 5	Average	High	High

Table 4-4   Complexity Matrix of EI Transactional Functions

Number of FTRs	Number of DETs		
	1–4	5–15	16+
0–1	Low	Low	Average
2	Low	Average	High
More than 2	Average	High	High

Data elements generated within the system that exit the system boundary are counted as EOs. Outgoing data, commands, alarms, processing instructions, printed information, and screen displays of information could all be EOs. One exception to this is that all operator-requested retrievals of information from any combination of ILFs or EIFs that do not contain any derived or calculated information are counted as EQs and not as EOs. Each identified EO is assigned a functional complexity of low, average, or high based on the number of DETs and FTRs associated with the EO. DETs are usually unique, user-recognizable, nonrepeating fields or attributes that exit the boundary of the system. The FTR count is the total number of ILFs read or referenced and the EIFs read or referenced by the EO transaction. DETs and FTRs are applied as shown in Table 4-5 to determine the functional complexity of each EO.

External inquiries identify unique operator trigger or response combinations that retrieve stored data without any mathematical calculation. EOs are usually common retrieve, view, extract, display, browse, or print functions. Typical examples might include an event report or log, a display of a user profile or current operational settings, diagnostic data, help messages, parameter settings, or system status. Retrievals of data by operator request from any combination of ILFs or EIFs that contain any derived or calculated information are counted as EOs, not as EQs. FTRs and DETs are counted separately for both the input and output sides of each EQ. The higher of the two complexities from either the EI matrix (Table 4-4) or the EO matrix (Table 4-5) determines the value of the EQ.

Table 4-6 shows the weighting applied to each type of function point element. The number of low, average, and high ILFs, EIFs, EIs, EOs, and EQs are entered into the matrix, and values for each data and transaction category are calculated to determine the total unadjusted function points

Table 4-5   Complexity Matrix of EO Transactional Functions

Number of FTRs	Number of DETs		
	1–5	6–19	20+
0–1	Low	Low	Average
2–3	Low	Average	High
More than 3	Average	High	High

Table 4-6   Weighting of Function Point Elements

Elements	Count Weights		
	Low + Average + High = Total		
Internal logical files (ILF)	__ × 7 + __ × 10 + __ × 15 = __		
External interface files (EIF)	__ × 5 + __ × 7 + __ × 10 = __		
External inputs (EI)	__ × 3 + __ × 4 + __ × 6 = __		
External outputs (EO)	__ × 4 + __ × 5 + __ × 7 = __		
External inquiry (EQ)	__ × 3 + __ × 4 + __ × 6 = __		
Total Unadjusted Function Points	__		

for the system. Determining the value adjustment factor using general system characteristics then modifies the total unadjusted function points. The *degree of influence* (DI), a value ranging from 0 to 5 (see Table 4-7 for definitions), is determined for each of 14 *general system characteristics* (GSCs) listed in Table 4-8. To calculate the *value adjustment factor* (VAF), the

Table 4-7   Degree of Influence Definitions

DI Rating	Definition
0	Not present or no influence
1	Incidental influence
2	Moderate influence
3	Average influence
4	Significant influence
5	Strong influence throughout

Table 4-8   General System Characteristics

Factor	System Technical and Operational Characteristic
Data communications	Data and control information used are sent or received over communications facilities
Distributed data processing	Distributed data or processing functions are characteristic within the system boundary
Performance	Performance objectives in response or throughout influence the design, development, installation, and support
Heavily-used configuration	Heavy operational usage requires special design consideration
Transaction rate	Transaction rate is high and influences design, development, installation, and support
On-line data entry	Data entry is on-line and controls information functions
End-user efficiency	On-line functions emphasize end-user efficiency design
On-line update	On-line update of internal logical files provided
Complex processing	Complex processing is characteristic
Reusability	System and code are designed, developed, and supported to be usable in or with other systems
Installation ease	Conversion and installation ease are characteristic; conversion and installation plan or tools tested during system test phase
Operational ease	Operational ease is characteristic; start-up, backup, and recovery procedures tested during system test phase
Multiple sites	System specifically designed, developed, and supported to be installed at multiple sites for multiple organizations
Facilitation of change	Facilitation of change is specifically designed, developed and supported

DI score for all 14 GSCs is totaled and multiplied by 0.01, and that value is added to 0.65. The resulting VAF will be within a range of 0.65 to 1.35. All that is left is to calculate the *adjusted function point* count, which is the VAF multiplied by the unadjusted function point count, to determine the final function point count.

Figure 4-6 depicts the identification of files and transactions that could be used in a function point count. As shown in the figure, several EOs, EIs, EQs, and EIFs must be recognized in the function point count. Table 4-9 is representative of a function point count for the device illustrated in Figure 4-6.

Figure 4-6   Function point analysis for a mythical medical device

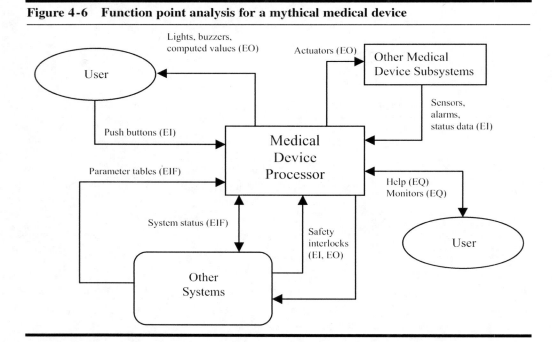

Table 4-9 Function Point Count by Function for Mythical Medical Device

Function Name	Function Type	RETs	DETs	FTRs	Count Weights			Unadjusted Function Points
					Low	Average	High	
N/A	ILF	N/A	N/A	N/A	0×7	0×10	0×15	0
Parameter tables	EIF	1	3	N/A	1×5	0×7	0×10	5
Push buttons	EI	N/A	36	1	0×3	1×4	0×6	4
Safety interlocks	EI	N/A	36	1	0×3	1×4	0×6	4
Alarms	EI	N/A	36	1	0×3	1×4	0×6	4
Safety interlocks	EO	N/A	3	20	0×4	0×5	1×7	7
Buzzer	EO	N/A	3	20	0×4	0×5	1×7	7
Computed values	EO	N/A	3	20	0×4	0×5	1×7	7
Monitors	EQ	N/A	1	1	1×3	0×4	0×6	3
Total Unadjusted Function Points								41

5

The Software Quality
Assurance Program:
Project Software Documentation

Failing to prepare is preparation to fail.

—John Wooden

If there is one item on which all software experts agree, it is the necessity to establish the correctness of the software to meet customer requirements. Medical device software may have untold, unknown, and unobservable attributes of quality. It may be efficient, robust, portable, easy to operate, and even easy to modify to suit a changed application request; but if it is incorrect, then its value is nil. Every software program performs some task correctly, but what is of interest to the computer scientist, software engineer, and ultimately the user, is whether the program performs its intended tasks. To determine this, a precise and independent description of the software's desired behavior is needed. Software specifications provide such a description.

Several types of software specifications are usually distinguished. In the software life cycle, the first phase usually consists of an analysis of the requirements that the software is to satisfy. The result of this phase and of the analysis in general is a software requirements specification (SRS). The requirements specification is an informal description of the software's intended behavior, detailing tasks that the software should perform, presenting any constraints on the behavior of the software, and specifying software resource utilization and control. After the requirements analysis phase comes a design phase (or phases) during which the software structure that will be used to meet the requirements specification is defined. In reality, large software projects are not constructed as a single, monolithic entity, but rather as several interconnected components or modules. Nearly all of these modules are organized in a hierarchical fashion, the modules higher in the hierarchy being implemented in terms of "calls" to the modules lower in the hierarchy. The result of the design phase is identification of the modules and graphical representations of their interrelationships. As more design phases occur, the previous design phase's resulting modules are expanded and elaborated, evolving into their final design form.

A common difficulty in the construction of such a software system is that the type of behavior expected by the user of a lower-level module may not be the same behavior that the module actually provides. This problem can be greatly reduced if the design phase also provides specifications related to the lower-level module. The module specification serves to document the intended behavior of the module and communicates this behavior to the module's implementer and to other programmers who will use that module in implementing their code. Two types of module specifications exist:

1. Functional specifications describe the effect of the module on its external environment.

2. Performance specifications describe constraints on the module.

In this discussion, software project documents are divided arbitrarily into three categories: planning documents; analysis, requirements, and design documents; and testing and V&V documents. Although each document discussed below was presented previously in the section relating to the policy requirements for the document, the discussion presented here will help readers to understand the high-level contents and organization of the documents relative to the project so that insight is gained into their generation and uses.

Software Planning Documents

Software development planning documents (Table 5-1) are normally generated during the product definition phase while the project is being organized, the product objectives are being defined, and the system requirements are being determined. Although the content and format of these documents may vary on the first project or two, the documents can quickly become templates in which perhaps 75–80 percent of the textual descriptions remain unaltered from project to project, and only 20–25 percent of the content is specific to the project. The initial project will bear the burden of achieving these document templates, but all subsequent projects will benefit greatly. Software planning documents are presented and discussed in alphabetical order, not in implementation order. Determination of the implementation sequence was discussed previously as a function of software policies.

The intent of the planning documents is threefold. First, they provide a uniform and consistent method for communicating the overall scope of the project, not only to personnel initially assigned to the project, but also to those who join the project in progress. Each team member is presented with the same description of the project in the same verbiage, with no embellishments and nothing omitted. Second, the planning documents convey to management not only the scope of the project, how the deliverables will be accomplished, and the strategy to be used in developing the software, but also the areas of risk and how those risks will be managed. This set of documents provides management insight about where additional resources might be needed, when additional equipment or materials might be needed, and when additional funds might be required. Third, the planning documents provide the prediction of what the project is supposed to accomplish, how it is to achieve those milestones, and the sequence of events that will lead to those deliverables. This perspective is vital for the project's software postmortem, because the planning documents represent the historical record of what was supposed to be done, not what actually happened. Because the postmortem is the review of the actual project activities and accomplishments, the project results that were realized can be compared to the intended results that were generated before the project was started. Thus, a meaningful baseline comparison can be achieved.

Table 5-1   Typical Software Development Planning Documents

Document Title	Acronym	Document Description
Software Configuration Management Plan	SCMP	Specifies the methods and planning employed to implement software configuration management activities
Software Development Plan	SDP	Identifies and describes the procedures employed to implement the management activities that coordinate schedules, control resources, initiate actions, and monitor progress of the software development effort
Software Development Test Plan	SDTP	Defines the scope of software testing that must be successfully completed for each software component
Software End-Product Acceptance Plan	SEAP	Serves as a descriptive checklist of the end products and services required for approval and acceptance
Software Quality Assurance Plan	SQAP	States the software quality objectives of the project as conditioned by the product requirements and the significance of the intended application
Software Validation Test Plan	SVTP	Defines the testing required to verify that the software end products satisfy the requirements of the SRS
Software Verification and Validation Plan	SVVP	Describes the project's unique V&V organization, activities, schedule, inputs/outputs, and any deviations from policies required for effective management of the V&V tasks

Configuration Management Plan

The Software Configuration Management Plan (SCMP) describes the planning and procedures needed to accomplish the configuration management of all software end products that are developed for the device (Table 5-2). Section 1 of the plan conveys the purpose, scope, and overview for the project's software configuration management. It lists the generic items that make up the software end products, what groups are responsible for the various aspects of the software configuration management, and the objectives of the project's software configuration management.

The objectives to be achieved by the project for the device software as specified by this document include the assurance that the software end products meet the requirements established in the requirements, design, and implementation documentation; provide visibility to the software development process and the software configuration management of that process; provide traceability between the "as-designed" and the "as-built" device software; and support the definition and verification of software configurations. Other objectives specified by the SCMP

Table 5-2   Typical Table of Contents for a Software Configuration Management Plan

Section Number	Section Title
1	Introduction
1.1	Purpose
1.2	Scope
1.3	Overview
1.4	Reference Documents
1.5	Definition of Terms
2	Management
2.1	Organization
2.2	Software Configuration Management Responsibilities
2.3	Software Configuration Management Plan Implementation
3	Software Configuration Management Activities
3.1	Software Configuration Identification
3.2	Software Configuration Control
3.3	Software Configuration Status Accounting
3.4	Audits and Reviews
4	Tools, Techniques, and Methodologies
4.1	Automated Tools
4.2	Manual Tools
5	Records Collection and Retention
6	Configuration Management Activities for Purchased Software

are to control changes to software end products; monitor the implementation of those changes; track the various configurations of the software end products; and provide a consistent approach to the project's software configuration management. This section also includes a listing of all project reference documents, by document numbers if possible, for the hardware and software, the product-level specifications, and any other specifications and documents applicable to software configuration management on the project. This section concludes with a list of the terms and definitions that appear in the document.

Section 2 presents the administrative aspects of software configuration management. Section 2.1 discusses how the software team is organized to accomplish all of the project's software tasks. This includes how the software project team was defined and organized, as well as the representatives and their functions on the team. This organization should also indicate the composition of the software development team members as well as the verification and validation members. For each of the generic software member types, statements should be included that indicate how each member will support the software configuration management for the project. Section 2.2 delineates the various software configuration management activities and who is responsible for ensuring their implementation and enforcement in the project. Section 2.3, concerning implementation, delineates the various activities of software configuration management, including presentation of the software projects relationship to the system development effort, milestones and baselines associated with software development activities, and management of the configuration information. This section also presents the schema for the review, approval, and scheduling of changes to baselined configuration items.

Section 3 describes the procedures and methods for configuration management activities related to development of the device software. Section 3.1 outlines the materials to be identified and baselined at each major milestone during the development of the software. This section also establishes how to identify each software item to be accounted for, controlled, and assigned a status. Section 3.2 presents the mechanisms to be used in controlling the development, interaction, and suitability of software configuration items relative to each baseline. Software configuration management not only monitors changes to the software, but also monitors the specific implementation of the already-approved system design. The implementation of software configuration control is discussed here in terms of managing software baselines, change classifications, mechanisms for baseline change, responsibilities for the review of the software changes, and use of software libraries.

The objective of software configuration status accounting (Section 3.3) is to identify the project's baselines and provide traceability of approved changes to those baselines. It also provides a management tool for monitoring the accomplishment of all related tasks that result from each approved change. The results of configuration management activities are then documented in a status report as described in this section. Section 3.4 delineates the requirements for audits and reviews to be performed during the development of project software.

Section 4, on tools, techniques, and methodologies, reiterates that software baseline management, software configuration identification, software configuration control, and software configuration status accounting will accomplish software configuration management. Software end-product configuration should include the identification of all components that make up the software, a description of each component in the system, a description of the interdependencies of the system components, and a description of how the components fit together to form the system. In addition, the configuration includes identification of the proper revision of each component that makes up a version or software baseline, the documentation of the changes that might be made to each component, and an accurate building of the desired version of the system. Section 4.1 presents the specific tools, by name and version number if necessary, to be used for the automated control of the software baseline information. Section 4.2 presents the manual techniques that will be used to perform the manual audits of the software material. The objectives of the manual audits are to assure the following:

- The technical and administrative integrity of the "to-be-established" software baseline;

- That each element in the "to-be-established" baseline maps either directly or indirectly through parents to preceding baselines;

- That the system and software requirements are fulfilled through the software configuration specified in the "to-be-established" baseline;

- That the changes to a baseline that result in an update or version are implemented as intended.

Section 5 presents the software end products that would be collected, who is responsible for their collection, and where these products will be archived for future reference. It is also appropriate to relate how this collection and retention fits into any corporate disaster contingency or recovery plans that are formally documented.

Section 6 states the provisions for assuring that any vendor-provided or subcontractor-developed software will meet the requirements specified within the SCMP. This section describes the proposed methods for controlling any subcontractors and vendors when their services and products affect the execution of the SCMP. This description should explain the methods that will be used to determine the software configuration management capability of subcontractors and vendors, and the methods that will be used to monitor their adherence to the requirements of the SCMP. At a minimum, the subcontractor and vendor should be required to prepare and implement a software configuration management plan that is in accordance with the SCMP.

Development Plan

The Software Development Plan (SDP) describes the approach, environment, processes, and stages of product software development (Table 5-3). Section 1 of the plan presents the identification, purpose, and introduction to the development of the product software. It outlines how the software will proceed from initial concepts to end-product acceptance. This section describes the resource requirements, resource loading, schedule milestones, and risk management issues related to developing the product software. It also describes the support that will be needed for other activities so that proper V&V of the software can be performed. Section 2 is a listing of all project reference documents, by document numbers if possible, for the hardware and software, the product-level specifications, and any other specifications and documents that are applicable to project software development.

Section 3 deals with software resources and team organization. Section 3.1 describes the project resources in relation to any special-purpose hardware and software. This includes a description of any specialized tools needed to support the development of the software, such as font generators, an operating system or executive, data protocol software, debugging tools, and emulators. This section also lists any outside services, software, tools, or equipment that might be needed to support software development. It delineates the project software personnel required, in terms of their various software responsibilities and their expected average resource loading.

Section 3.2 describes the project-specific software development methods intended for use in development of the product software. This section includes organization of the software team and its relationship to the project team in general, as well as the responsibilities of the software team. This section covers the phases of the software development effort, the high-level activities to occur during each phase, the development schedule, and the milestones associated with that development schedule. Finally, this section presents the anticipated resource loading by each of the high-level activities for each phase of the software development, as well as the software development tools to be used for each software phase.

Section 3.3 states that the organization of software configuration management is contained in the SCMP and refers the reader to that document. However, as discussed in the Software Development Policy Topics section of Chapter 3, the project may decide not to produce an SCMP; in this case, Section 3.3 would be greatly expanded to include the appropriate and pertinent sections from the SCMP. Typically, this would entail all of Section 3 and sufficient detail from Sections 2, 4, 5, and 6 (Table 5-2) to provide guidance and understanding of software

Table 5-3   Typical Table of Contents for a Software Development Plan

Section Number	Section Title
1	Scope
1.1	Identification
1.2	Purpose
1.3	Introduction
2	Reference Documents
3	Resources and Organization
3.1	Project Resources
3.2	Software Development
3.3	Software Configuration Management
3.4	Software Quality Evaluation
3.5	Software Verification and Validation
3.6	Other Software Development Functions
4	Development Schedule and Milestones
4.1	Activities
4.2	Activity Network
4.3	Procedures for Risk Management
4.4	Identification of High Risk Areas
5	Software Development Procedures
5.1	Software Standards and Procedures
5.2	Software Configuration Management
5.3	Software Quality Evaluation
5.4	Software Verification and Validation
5.5	Additional Software Development Procedures
5.6	Commercially Available and Reusable Software
5.7	Deliverable Software, Data, and Documentation
5.8	Nondeliverable Software, Data, and Documentation
5.9	Software Developed for Hardware Configurations
5.10	Installation and Checkout
5.11	Interface Management
6	Notes

configuration management for the project. Section 3.4 of the SDP states that the organization of the software quality evaluation is presented in the Software Quality Assurance Plan (SQAP) and refers the reader to that document. As with the SCMP, the project may decide not to produce an SQAP; consequently, this section would be expanded to include the appropriate and pertinent sections from the SQAP (see Table 5-6; typically, this would entail all of Section 3 and sufficient detail from Section 2 to provide guidance and understanding of software quality assurance for the project). Section 3.5 of the SDP indicates that the organization for software V&V is contained in the Software Verification and Validation Plan (SVVP), and refers the reader to that document. Section 3.6 describes any software development activities that may be provided by other organizations.

Section 4 describes the software development schedule and milestones for the project. Section 4.1 presents the anticipated schedule, resource loading, and task assignment for the software development, as well as an indication of how the estimates were derived. For example, if a best engineering judgment estimation was used, then the method of determining the estimates should be presented. If an estimation model was used to generate the development estimates or if a model was used to verify the best engineering judgment estimation, then the assumptions and input data used for the model should be presented. In addition to showing the estimation of the software activity schedule, the milestones should also be presented, along with their expected beginning and ending dates.

Section 4.2 presents those software development activities and scheduled milestones that are to occur in parallel and what their prerequisites are, if any. Section 4.3 includes risk management statements that relate to the fundamental approach to be used on the project. It also presents the areas of high technology or innovation that will be used either to help develop the software or that will be integrated into the product.

In Section 4.4, the items to be discussed include any risk areas directly associated with the device's software, with the development of the software, or with any ancillary areas that are related to the software being developed. For example, the implementation of a new display device and user interface design might be presented, the use of a new development tool might be discussed, or the implementation of a new real-time operating system might be documented here.

Section 5 presents the procedures to be used in the development of device software. Section 5.1 states that the standards and conventions to be used during software development are encompassed by the software development policies, procedures, and guidelines. Section 5.2 states that the software configuration management activities and procedures are documented in the SCMP. If the project did not produce an SCMP, then Section 5.2 would be expanded to include the appropriate and pertinent SCMP sections as discussed above. Section 5.3 states that the software quality evaluation activities and procedures are contained in the SQAP. If the project did not produce an SQAP, then this section would be expanded to include the appropriate and pertinent SQAP sections as discussed above. Section 5.4 states that the software V&V activities and procedures are covered in the SVVP. Section 5.5 details any additional or new techniques or procedures that will be used by the software development team in any of the areas mentioned in Section 4. Section 5.6 presents any reusable or commercially purchased software that will be used and integrated into the product software. For example, if the C language is to be used for implementing the code, then Section 5.6 would state that Microsoft C version 5.1 and its associated libraries will be used. If a commercially purchased mathematical library, such as US Software, is to be used, then the purchased software would be specified here by name, version number, and release date.

Sections 5.7 through 5.9 delineate software data and documentation rights. For example, Section 5.7 states that all software, data, documents, and libraries actually used in the device will become the property of the documentation control group and will be integrated into the corporation's engineering change order system. Section 5.8 specifies that all software, data, documents, and libraries not used in the device will reside with the software development department and become integrated into the department's software library and its version control system. Section 5.9 specifies that all hardware, firmware, and hardware control support software will reside with the appropriate hardware group or with the software development department, as appropriate.

Section 5.10 describes how software installation and checkout will support the verification and validation of the developed software. Section 5.11 states that the software development group will manage the hardware and software interface compatibility through the generation of the Interface Design Specification (IDS), as well as maintaining it according to the software development policies, procedures, and guidelines.

Section 6 contains any explanatory information that might be useful or necessary to clarify, expand, explain, or illuminate any of the topics presented in the SDP. For example, definitions of terms might appear in this section, or a technical discussion concerning any algorithms that will be implemented as a part of the software could be documented here.

Development Test Plan

The Software Development Test Plan (SDTP) defines the test plans that are to be used during development of the product software (Table 5-4). The SDTP should describe how software testing will proceed from the beginning phase through the final testing phase and should be consistent with and follow the appropriate software development policies, procedures, and guidelines. The SDTP describes the detailed approach, environment, processes, and stages of software testing that will be employed for the software developed as a part of the project. It should be understood that this test plan refers only to software development testing and not to software validation testing, which is covered in the Software Validation Test Plan (SVTP).

Section 1 of the SDTP presents the identification, purpose, and introduction to software test plans. This section should delineate the organization that will be developing the software and performing the software tests. Section 2 presents a list of all project reference documents, by document numbers if possible, for the hardware and software, the product-level specifications, and any other specifications and documents that are applicable to the testing of the project software.

Section 3 describes the testing to be performed by the software development engineers to verify the design and functionality of the software components. The testing described in this section should encompass the tests of individual modules as well as tests of integrated modules. This section also indicates that the development team is responsible for the implementation of testing methods that are consistent with the appropriate software development policies, to ensure the development of quality software.

Qualification of the software, as described in Section 3.1, for delivery to the project as a whole to begin system design validation testing is established by the successful completion of the testing described in the SVTP, as well as the testing described in this document. The SDTP should also describe the scope of software testing that must be successfully completed for each software module and for module integration. The scope of software testing should reflect the test requirements, the levels of testing, and the test category.

The categories include functional, robustness, stress, safety, growth, and regression testing. Functional testing, which verifies that all of the functional requirements have been satisfied, is

Table 5-4   Typical Table of Contents for a Software Development Test Plan

Section Number	Section Title
1	Scope
1.1	Identification
1.2	Purpose
1.3	Introduction
2	Reference Documents
3	Plans for Testing
3.1	Qualification Methodology
3.2	Test Philosophy
3.3	Module Testing
3.4	Integration Testing
3.5	Resources Required for Testing
4	Plans for Validation Testing
5	Test Planning Assumptions and Constraints
5.1	Assumptions
5.2	Identification of High-Risk Areas
5.3	Contingencies
6	Notes

success-oriented, because the tests are expected to produce successful results. Robustness testing evaluates the software performance with unexpected inputs. These tests are failure-oriented because the inputs are designed to cause the product to fail, given foreseeable and reasonably unforeseeable misuse of the product. Stress testing evaluates software performance in a stress condition in which the amount or rate of data exceeds the amount or rate that is reasonably anticipated. Safety testing verifies that the software performs in a safe manner and that a complete assessment of the safety design has been accomplished. Growth testing verifies that the margins of growth as specified for any particular component, or the product software as a whole, are supported by the software. Regression testing is the reperformance of any completed test deemed necessary whenever a software change occurs, to correct detected faults that were introduced during software construction, to verify that the modifications have not caused any unintended adverse effects, and to verify the software still meets its specified requirements.

Verification methods for the developed software should include inspection, analysis, demonstration, and physical testing. Inspection is visual examination of an item. Analysis is evaluation of theoretical or empirical data. Demonstration is the operational movement or adjustment of an item. Physical testing is operation of an item and recording and evaluation of quantitative data based on the item's response to the operation.

The test philosophy for the software (Section 3.2) should include those actions needed to detect software deficiencies with the minimum amount of testing. These test requirements will depend on the previous actions of software engineers during component construction and debugging that detected and reduced the deficiencies prior to application of this test method. The methods to be applied should be formulated to support the software development effort and to provide support for the V&V of the software development effort. The test philosophy should reflect the tasks, modules, and subroutines and functions described in the software design documents, as well as reflect the details of the integration plan and strategy. This section should also present the test specification objective—to be able to identify that any given test will verify the performance of the software component in any one of several areas.

For example, the verification of the software interface would include transfer of control, parameters received and sent, interactions with data tables, use of adaptive parameters, and interaction with hardware components that can be covered by functional and robustness testing. The verification of all computations using singular, extreme, out-of-range, and normal values can be covered by robustness and safety testing. The exercising of all routines for interrupt handling, interrupt lockout, data write lockout, and reentry handling can be covered by robustness, stress, and safety testing. Section 3.2 should also present the code prerequisites for testing, including the completion of the routine's preamble or preface documentation, the completion of walk-throughs, and the conformance to the documented programming standards and conventions. Satisfying the prerequisites prior to testing can be left to the individual code author.

To facilitate testing, a software Development Test Information Sheet (DTIS) should be generated for each software development test specified in the SDTP (Figure 5-1). Each DTIS should be completed in a way that allows the test to be repeatable, so that the objective, approach, and success criteria of the test are known, the complete test setup is defined, the test can migrate from module-level testing into integration-level testing, and a record of the test results is generated into the DTIS. Once all of the code within a task or the integration of tasks has been tested and accepted, the task should be delivered to the responsible configuration management person for configuration control and insertion into the project software library for the V&V activities. The standard DTIS inputs are defined by the code requirements.

All of the code of a module will have already passed low-level development debugging by the code author prior to the beginning of module-level testing (Section 3.3). Each module and the functions that the module encompasses should be defined in the Detailed Design Specification (DDS). Module-level testing requirements should include out-of-bounds, extreme value, branching and logic control, interrupt and reentry, and component failure testing. Section 3.3 should also include a description of how module-level testing will be performed, the responsibilities for module testing, the module test category, and the module test schedule.

Software integration consists of several levels of integration that start with stand-alone code generation, the integration of code into modules, the integration of modules into tasks, and ultimately the integration of tasks into the final working system. Integration testing (Section 3.4) relates to the integrated modules within an executable task. Testing requirements should include out-of-bounds, extreme value, branching and logic control, interrupt and reentry, and component failure testing. A description of how integration testing will be performed should be included, and it should be understood that some degree of module-level regression testing must be conducted to assure that the modules still work within their new and larger working environment.

Once the constituent modules have been fully integrated into their respective tasks, detailed integration testing should begin. When all of the tasks have been mutually integrated, detailed system integration testing can begin on the individual tasks and on the software system as a

Figure 5-1   Typical Software Development Test Information Sheet (DTIS)

SOFTWARE DEVELOPMENT TEST INFORMATION SHEET

Test Category	Title of Test
Component Name	Requirement Number Satisfied

1. Component objectives and component success criteria

2. Test objectives and success criteria

3. Test approach

4. Test instrumentation

5. Test duration

6. Input data and format

7. Output data and format

8. Data collection, reduction, and analysis requirements

9. Test script

10. Test drivers

11. Test stubs

12. Test data stream

13. Test control flow stream

14. Pretest comments

15. Post-test comments

16. Component build description (and subordinate DTISs)

17. Signatures:

Test Conductor	Date
Software Lead Engineer	Date

whole. All of these testing levels should include the functionality of the instrument per the stated requirements, and several random tests should be performed by seeding errors into the code and recording how the software responds.

Section 3.4 should also present the integration test responsibilities, the integration test classes by categories, the integration test schedule, and the anticipated task integration order. The team should remember that this is merely a test plan and is generated early in the software development life cycle. The order of any particular task completion within the overall integration stage will be defined during the Detailed Design Phase and, therefore, integration testing referenced here may, in fact, become mixed with module build-up development.

The required resources for software testing (Section 3.5) should include facilities and any special equipment in them, the personnel required to perform the testing, and the anticipated hardware platforms. Section 3.5 should also indicate the interfacing support software and hardware that might be needed; this can include any operating system, real-time executive, communication protocols, and tools—display font generators; emulators; and language-specific compilers, linkers, loaders, and libraries. Section 3.5 should indicate the required target platform test configurations (target level) that will be needed for software coding, integration, and testing, and also the test bed hardware and software configurations.

Section 4 includes a statement that the testing oriented toward the validation of software requirements is covered in the SVVP. This section should also address how the software development group will help and facilitate V&V testing. Section 5 documents the testing assumptions and constraints, identifies high-risk and potential problem area testing, and presents the planned contingencies that will help to mitigate these concerns. Section 6 presents any explanations that might be needed to expand the understanding of the testing that is to be performed. This section might also include definitions of any terms that are used in the SDTP related to testing.

End-Product Acceptance Plan

The Software End-Product Acceptance Plan (SEAP) describes the plans for the acceptance of the design, code, and testing of the software developed for the device (Table 5-5). Section 1 presents the identification, purpose, introduction, and definition of terms related to the acceptance of the end-product software. The term "end product" as used in this plan refers to all software deliverables generated for and used directly in the device. Section 1 states that the SEAP is generated in accordance with relevant software development policies, procedures, and guidelines. It also describes the end products and services required by the software development team and the product's system engineer or system architect. In particular, it presents the criteria that will be met in order to obtain written approval for acceptance of the developed software end products. For example, the SEAP would describe the end products, services required, and acceptance criteria at the software project level as well as listing the specific acceptance criteria, reviews, audits, and approval schedules by which individual end products and services will be judged complete.

Section 1 states that the SEAP will be implemented by the software development team and will be in effect for the entire set of tasks described in the SDP. It also states that support will be provided by the software development team to other project-related activities so that those activities can be successfully performed. Section 2 is a listing of all project reference documents, by document numbers where possible, for the hardware and software, the product-level specifications, and any other specifications and documents applicable to project software development.

Each end product produced by the software development team requires a level of concurrence by the system engineer or system architect that relates to the receipt, acceptance, and content of the end product (Section 3). For example, it is fairly straightforward for the system engineer to acknowledge receipt of the end product and that the end product has met its acceptance criteria. However, the system engineer's concurrence on end-product content is assigned a rating of high, medium, or low. A high level of concurrence indicates that the system engineer or architect agrees with the content of that particular end product. A medium level of concurrence indicates that the system engineer or architect at least understands the content of the end product. A low level of concurrence indicates that the system engineer or architect is familiar with the content of the end product.

Table 5-5   Typical Table of Contents for a Software End-Product Acceptance Plan

Section Number	Section Title
1	Scope
1.1	Identification
1.2	Purpose
1.3	Introduction
1.4	Definition of Terms
2	Reference Documents
3	End-product Acceptance Checklist
3.1	Software Development Estimates
3.2	Software Planning Documents
3.3	Software Walk-Throughs
3.4	Software Requirements and Design Documents
3.5	Software Reviews
3.6	End-product Closures
3.7	Released and Support Software
3.8	End-product Acceptance Audit
4	Methods for Accumulating Acceptance-related Data

For each end product identified in Section 3, several identifying items are presented. First, the required format for the end product is specified—content, media, or the source document that governs the format of the end product. Second, the number of deliverables is stated in terms of the maximum number of distinct versions that should be produced, including the original. Third, the beginning and ending dates are shown. The beginning date is the expected date when the end-product activity will begin, and the ending date is the anticipated date by which the end product is scheduled to be delivered to the system engineer or system architect. Fourth, the review and acceptance schedule is presented. These are the anticipated dates when the end product will be reviewed and accepted by the system engineer or architect. Fifth, the end product's acceptance criteria are presented; these are the criteria that will be used to actually accept the particular software end product. Last, the concurrence level is specified; this represents the level to which the system engineer or system architect must agree with the end-product content.

A list of the software development end products is then presented, showing all six of the above identifying items and including an area for signature and date sign-off. The types of end products to be accepted include software development estimates; software planning, require-ments, and design documents; design and code walk-throughs; requirements and design reviews; the closure on all test information sheets and anomaly reports; released product software and hardware support software; and the audit on all software end-product acceptance.

Section 4 delineates the media that will be used to establish, maintain, and accumulate the end-product acceptance data for each end product. These data include the physical evidence that the product, subproduct, or end product has been produced or performed, the necessary written approvals have been obtained, and any other supporting documentation has been collected.

Quality Assurance Plan

The SQAP defines the quality evaluation plan and procedures to be used to assure that the software developed for the product complies with the appropriate software development policies, procedures, and guidelines (Table 5-6). The SQAP applies to the items that are produced and used during software development, and to those items under the direct control of the software development team. The SQAP provides the basis for the software quality evaluation activities to be applied to the software developed by the software development team, defines the software products and processes to be evaluated, and describes or references the procedures that implement evaluation activities throughout the software development process.

The concepts to be addressed by the SQAP are introduced in Section 1, which presents the purpose, scope, overview, reference documents, and definitions of terms related to the quality evaluation of the end-product software. The SQAP describes the quality assurance methods necessary to minimize the incorporation of software deficiencies, detect any introduced software deficiencies, and effect corrective action when deficiencies occur. Section 1 of the SQAP also describes the responsibility for the implementation of the quality assurance plan and that the

Table 5-6   Typical Table of Contents for a Software Quality Assurance Plan

Section Number	Section Title
1	Introduction
1.1	Purpose
1.2	Scope
1.3	Overview
1.4	Reference Documents
1.5	Definition of Terms
2	Management
2.1	Organization
2.2	Software Quality Assurance Responsibilities
2.3	Software Quality Assurance Implementation
3	Software Quality Evaluation Procedures
3.1	Evaluation Procedures, Methods, and Tools
3.2	Phase-independent Evaluation Procedures
3.3	Phase-dependent Evaluation Procedures

quality assurance plan will be in effect for the full set of tasks described in the SDP. Section 1 presents a listing of all project reference documents, by document numbers if possible, for the hardware and software, the product-level specifications, and any other specifications and documents applicable to project software development. Section 1 also presents a definition of all terms used in the discussion of the quality assurance activities.

Section 2 presents the organization, responsibilities, and implementation plans for the quality evaluation of developed software. Section 2.1 discusses how the software team is organized to accomplish all of the project's software quality assurance tasks. This includes who and how the project team was defined and organized, as well as the representatives and their responsibilities on the team. This organization should indicate the composition of the software development members as well as the V&V members.

Section 2.2 presents the quality evaluation functions that will be performed on the developed software. These include the generation, maintenance, and approval of the SQAP itself; the monitoring of software activities for the proper use of the tools, techniques, and records used to aid the production of quality software; and assuring the identification, preparation, coordination, and maintenance of, and compliance with the appropriate software development policies and procedures that relate to control of critical steps that affect software quality. In addition, Section 2.2 assures the compliance of the software project documentation and code with programming standards and conventions; assures monitoring of software library procedures and controls that are used to manipulate source code, object code, and related data; and assures the conduct of reviews and audits in accordance with the appropriate software development policies, procedures, and any relevant guidelines.

Section 2.2 also provides for the independent audit of the requirements definition, design, documentation, code production, testing, and software configuration management for consistent compliance with software development procedures; ensures the development and update of a requirements traceability matrix that is used to track requirements flow-down; and assures that software testing produces verifiable results traceable to the requirements specifications. Section 2.2 assures the prompt detection, identification, correction, documentation, and reporting of software end-product anomalies and deficiencies; preparation and maintenance of quality evaluation records and reports; and coordination with support groups on matters pertaining to the software quality assurance of the developed software.

Section 2.3 includes the delineation of when software quality assurance begins and ends, that the milestones and activities associated with the development process are presented in the SDP, and that the milestones are the specific times at which software quality assurance activities are applied. The products of each major milestone are reviewed, audited, and/or tested before advancement to the next phase of software development. A matrix should be provided that identifies the specific software quality assurance activities that will be applied at each major milestone of software development as well as their relationship to the software development activities, documents generated, and review(s) and/or audit(s) to be performed.

Section 3 presents the various software quality evaluation procedures. Section 3.1 describes the evaluation procedures, methods, and tools used to perform the software quality evaluation and that are applicable to the project in general and its various phases in particular. Section 3.1 states that the software development policies contain the requirements for the development of quality software and for performing software quality assurance activities. The procedures and methods governing software quality assurance activities for the project as specified in this section must be consistent and in compliance with software development policies. This section then presents the specific software quality assurance items and activities that will be used in the performance of software quality evaluation tasks.

Section 3.2 describes the evaluation procedures, methods, and tools that will be used to perform the phase-independent software quality evaluation procedures that are applicable to the project, but not specifically addressed by software development policies, procedures, or guidelines. The subjects encompass procedures such as evaluation of development plans, procedures, and tools; evaluation of configuration management practices; evaluation of any software development library; evaluation of records and memos; and evaluation of any corrective action related to discrepancies, deficiencies, and anomalies. Section 3.2 also specifies documentation reviews, reviews and audits specified in the SDP, and review of all test-related plans, procedures, and results.

Section 3.3 describes the evaluation procedures, methods, and tools that will be used to perform the phase-dependent software quality evaluation procedures that are applicable to the project but not specifically addressed by software development policies, procedures, or guidelines. The subjects encompass procedures such as the evaluation of phase activities, procedures, and processes and the evaluation of the documents produced during each development phase. In each of these discussions, the governing document(s) should be specifically referenced in order to clarify the source input information for the evaluation.

Validation Test Plan

The SVTP identifies and describes the plan for the validation testing of the software constructed by the software development team (Table 5-7). The intent of the SVTP is to define software validation testing and any information necessary to manage and perform the testing. Software validation testing is necessary to verify that the fully integrated software end products satisfy the requirements specified in the Software Requirements Specification (SRS) as well as any other, higher level requirements documents. The testing program described in the SVTP will be performed by the project's software V&V engineers during the Software Validation Phase of the software development life cycle.

The qualification of the software for delivery to the system- or product-level design validation testing is established by the successful completion of the testing described in both the SDTP and the SVTP. As discussed above, the SDTP defines the software component-level testing conducted by software developers for each software component defined in the DDS. The review and analysis of the recorded results of the testing described in the SDTP by the V&V engineers are prerequisites to the tests described in the SVTP.

In addition to presenting the purpose, scope, overview, reference documents, and definitions of terms related to the software validation test plan, Section 1 describes the test organization, activities, schedule, reporting, and administration required for validating the developed software. This section presents a list of all project reference documents, by document numbers if possible, for the hardware and software, the product-level specifications, and any other specifications and documents that are applicable to the validation testing of the project software.

Section 2 describes the organization, schedule, responsibilities, and tools, techniques, and methodologies associated with the validation testing of the software. Section 2.1 states that the software test program is organized and conducted independently by both the software development group and the software V&V engineering group. Software component testing is conducted by the software development group in accordance with the SDTP in order to verify that the input, processing, and output requirements of each software component as defined in the DDS was met. Software validation testing is conducted by the software V&V engineers in accordance with the SVTP to verify that the fully integrated software satisfies the requirements stated in the SRS.

Table 5-7   Typical Table of Contents for a Software Validation Test Plan

Section Number	Section Title
1	Introduction
1.1	Purpose
1.2	Scope
1.3	Overview
1.4	Reference Documents
1.5	Definition of Terms
2	Test Overview
2.1	Organization
2.2	Master Schedule
2.3	Responsibilities
2.4	Tools, Techniques, and Methodologies
3	Test Requirements
3.1	Software Validation Testing
3.2	Resource Requirements
3.3	Risks and Contingencies
4	Test Reporting
4.1	Test Recording
4.2	Anomaly Reporting
5	Test Administration Procedures
5.1	Tasks
5.2	Intertask Dependencies
5.3	Special Skills
5.4	Test Administration

This layered approach to testing provides assurance that software errors are detected early in the code development cycle and that the software end products are verified by personnel independent of the software developers. The software V&V engineers will make written recommendations to the software development group and to the responsible software management based on their testing and analysis of the software. These engineers will receive functional direction from and report to the responsible software management to accomplish an independent assessment of software quality.

Section 2.2 presents both the validation testing schedule and a validation test documentation schedule. This section refers to the SDP and the SCMP documents that contain the detailed description of the software development phases noted in the project, and to the SDP and SVVP documents that contain detailed schedules of testing. The SVTP governs the testing to be conducted during the Software Validation Phase, testing that occurs after the code has been completely implemented and integrated. It is important to take a larger look at the software activities before discussing the details of the software validation test schedules.

The development activities of the Code and Test Phase, the Integration and Test Phase, and the Software Validation Phase are not necessarily performed sequentially. During these three phases of software development, the software components are developed and tested independently. The individually tested software components are then integrated incrementally and tested as a group to ensure the integrity of software interfaces. This process is repeated until multiple software components have been integrated into functional capabilities or tasks. Multiple software components that have successfully completed the testing as defined in the SDTP should then be placed into the project's software library, at the request of the project's lead software engineer, by the individual responsible for software configuration management. Software validation testing will be done only on those software components that successfully complete the testing defined in the SDTP and that have been baselined in accordance with the SCMP. Software validation testing, consequently, begins only when baselined software is available from the library and continues until the end of the Software Validation Phase. The order in which the validation testing occurs is a function of the order in which the software developers complete the software modules.

The validation test documentation schedule refers not only to the various testing documents, but also to the SVTP itself, because of the composition and use of the SVTP. Remember that the SVTP and its testing plan should be completed and approved prior to the Architecture Design Review (ADR), because Validation Test Information Sheets (VTISs) are generated for each validation test defined in the SVTP. The VTISs must be prepared prior to the Detailed Design Review (DDR). The Software Validation Test Procedures (SVTPR) are the procedures used to perform the validation testing described in the SVTP. The SVTPR should be generated and approved prior to actual validation testing. At the conclusion of validation testing, a record of it will be provided in the Software Validation Test Report.

Section 2.3 delineates the responsibilities for accomplishing validation testing on the software. Software developers will obviously be responsible for the generation of the software as well as some degree of software validation test support. Specifically, they are responsible for generating the SDTP (with some help and support from the V&V group), generation of the associated software DTISs, and performance of software component testing in accordance with the SDTP. In addition, software developers are responsible for implementing any corrective action required by an approved Software Verification and Validation Anomaly Report, as well as implementing any corrective action required by an approved Change Request/Approval (CRA) form. Software developers are also responsible for directly supporting the conduct of software validation testing as required, and as specified in the SDTP and in Section 2.3.

The performance of software validation testing is the responsibility of software V&V engineers, although validation testing is usually separated into several distinct functional activities and associated functional positions, to organize the details of the testing. The functional positions are Test Administrator, Test Conductor, Test Team, and Data Analyst. These positions need not necessarily refer to organizational positions within the software V&V group. They are merely a convenient way to group the various types of software validation activities and the responsibilities for some or all of these positions. The duties of the positions may, in fact, be performed by the same individual, particularly if the software development project effort is of a relatively limited or small scale.

The Test Administrator is responsible for the development and administration of software validation testing as described in the SVTP; this includes planning, organizing, monitoring, and controlling the validation test activities for the project. In addition, the Test Administrator is responsible for scheduling support personnel as required during testing, monitoring the conduct of the testing, preparing and maintaining the Software Validation Test Log (SVTL), and generating the test result report.

The conduct of the testing performed in accordance with the SVTP and the detailed test procedures are the responsibility of the Test Conductor. Specifically, the Test Conductor prepares and coordinates the SVTPR, prepares and maintains the SVTP software VTISs, and reviews the results of the software component testing conducted by software development engineers. The collection and analysis performed in accordance with the SVTP and the detailed test procedures are the responsibility of the Data Analyst. The Data Analyst is responsible for data requirements definition, data reduction, and data analysis.

The actual execution of software validation testing is the responsibility of the Test Team. Team members are responsible for executing approved test procedures; for preparing Software Verification and Validation Anomaly Reports based on problems observed during test conduct; and for preparing daily updates to the test log that indicate accomplishments, recommendations, and/or results as appropriate. In addition, they are responsible for the operation of any equipment used during the testing, and for advising the Test Administrator of recommended changes in test conduct, data extraction, and emulation operation and/or debugging activities.

The Configuration Manager is responsible for configuration control and management of software end products, but also for impounding the source code in the software development library on request by the project lead software engineer. This ensures that only approved changes to baselined source code are allowed. The Configuration Manager also reports the revision, as well as the version of source code checkout to the software V&V engineers for software validation testing. In addition, the Configuration Manager is responsible for ensuring that only one user at a time is allowed access to the baselined materials to modify the files that are stored in the software library, and for the distribution of modified baseline materials to the V&V group for assessment of regression testing requirements.

Section 2.4 presents the tools, techniques, and methodologies associated with software validation testing. The testing performed in accordance with the SVTP will verify that the fully integrated software end products satisfy the requirements of the SRS. Software validation testing will also ensure that only the software that has been impounded into the project's software development library is used during testing. At the beginning of software validation testing, the software is checked out of the software library, and an executable version of the software is built by the software V&V group. The successful completion of this executable build is required before any further validation testing of the software may begin. This build activity is repeated each time a revision to the software is impounded into the library, and as required by the software V&V group, to ensure the proper configuration management of the software during validation.

The types of validation testing can be grouped into several categories: functional testing, robustness testing, stress testing, safety testing, growth testing, and regression testing. Functional testing consists of tests that are designed to verify that all of the functional requirements for the software have been satisfied. This is success-oriented testing, because the tests are expected to produce successful results. Robustness testing, designed to evaluate the software performance given unexpected inputs, is failure-oriented, because the test inputs are designed to cause the software to fail given foreseeable, and reasonably unforeseeable, misuse of the product. Stress testing is designed to evaluate software performance under a stress condition in which the amount or rate of data exceeds the amount or rate expected. Safety testing verifies that the software performs in a safe manner and that a complete assessment of the safety design has been accomplished. Growth testing verifies that the margins for software growth that are specified for any particular component, or the product software as a whole, are supported by the software. Regression testing is retesting deemed necessary whenever a software change occurs, to correct detected faults introduced during software construction, to verify that the software modifications have not caused any unintended adverse effects, and to verify that the software still meets its specified requirements.

The validation test verification methods for the developed software should include inspection, analysis, demonstration, and physical testing. Inspection is accomplished by visual examination of an item, and analysis is accomplished by evaluation of theoretical or empirical data. Demonstration is accomplished by the operational movement or adjustment of an item. Physical testing is accomplished by the operation of an item and the recording and evaluation of quantitative data based on the item's response to the operation. The detailed pass-fail criteria for the software is documented in the SVTPR, and the source of that pass-fail criteria is the validation criteria for the requirements of the SRS. The validation criteria for each software requirement of the SRS are defined by one or more test categories and test verification methods.

Software validation testing should verify that the requirements as specified in the SRS for all of the operational modes and functions that are commanded and/or controlled by the device software have been satisfied (Section 3). The objectives of functional testing are to define and detect specified classes of faults by executing each functional capability of the software against fault-revealing test data and to detect failures of the software that correspond to the wrong sequences of functional invocation or to the wrong transmission of data between functions. Tests should be conducted that will demonstrate that each function is fully operational and conforms to the requirements of the SRS. A list of all possible functions to be performed by the device software is presented in Section 3 for functional testing.

Section 3.1 lists each type of validation testing to be performed. Robustness testing determines the performance of the software given any foreseeable and reasonably unforeseeable misuse of the device. It measures the compliance of the software with the requirements of the SRS and the design with the DDS, while operating within its expected environment as defined in the product-level requirements document and given unexpected and/or invalid inputs. A list of all possible functions to be performed by the device software should be presented for robustness testing.

Stress testing verifies the compliance of the software with the SRS under operating conditions in which the amount or rate of data exceeds the amount or rate expected. A list of all possible functions to be performed by the device software should be presented for stress testing.

Safety testing verifies that the software performs in accordance with the safety requirements of the SRS and that a complete assessment of the safety design has been accomplished. A list of all possible functions that are to be performed by the device software should be presented for safety testing.

Growth testing verifies that the margins of growth as specified in the SRS are, in fact, supported by the software. At the time in the software development life cycle when the SVTP is generated, the growth margins may not be known; therefore, the definition of the tests needed to verify that the growth margins of the software have been met may be completed at the conclusion of the Detailed Design Phase.

Regression testing detects faults that might have been introduced during code modifications and verifies that those modifications have not caused unintended adverse effects and that the software still meets its specified requirements. Tests that have been previously performed during validation testing may be repeated as required in order to ensure the integrity of software revisions. The degree of validation retesting required is a function of the impact of software modifications on the safety and functionality of the software. All regression testing performed on the software should be documented prior to completion of the Software Validation Phase, as updates to the SVTPR.

Section 3.2 describes personnel, hardware, and support software needed. It includes allocation, to an individual or individuals by title, of the functional responsibilities for the positions discussed as part of SVTP (Section 2.2). The size and skill level of the software test team should also be presented. A representative of the software development team who is actively involved in the coding and integration of the software end products will be required to aid in the validation test setup and operation, as well as in the initial determination of the cause, severity, and solution set of the detected problems.

Section 3.2 includes the hardware required to support the development of the SVTPR, the actual conduct of the testing, and the data analysis performed on the test data. Because the software validation testing requires the actual device, Section 3.2 should include a description of the final hardware configuration of the device, as well as any prototype hardware that may be required if the final hardware configuration is not available. Also listed in this section is the support software required for development and maintenance of the test documentation, test preparation, test conduct, and data analysis.

Section 3.3 presents the risks and their contingencies associated with the assumptions of software validation testing. Risk management for software validation testing will be performed by the software V&V engineers at each software development milestone in order to identify any areas of uncertainty that are significant sources of risk. The engineers will formulate a cost-effective strategy for resolving the sources of risk. Updates to the SVTP and to the SVVP, if required, should be generated to document any modifications that are required as a result of risk analysis.

Section 4 describes the reporting of the validation test information. Test recording (Section 4.1) is accomplished through the development and maintenance of the SVTP VTISs, the SVTL, and the Software Validation Test Report. A VTIS is generated for each validation test described in the SVTP (Figure 5-2). Each VTIS describes the test purpose and success criteria, approach, and environment; this information is used in conjunction with the SVTP to develop the SVTPR. During validation testing, the VTIS for each test is updated to document the test conductor, the test results and associated comments, and the test completion signatures. The SVTP VTISs will be retained by the software V&V engineers in a central location for review by the software developers, software management personnel, and any quality assurance representatives.

The SVTL is used to record all of the chronological events that are relevant to the conduct of the software validation testing (Figure 5-3). The Software Validation Test Report, generated at the conclusion of all validation testing, represents a record of the validation testing that was performed on the software. The report may be in any format that is appropriate for technical disclosure, as delineated by the V&V SOPs. The report consists of a summary of the software validation testing, the SVTL, the SVTP VTISs, a summary of the analysis and an evaluation of the test results, and any recommendations.

Section 4.2 describes the reporting of anomalies. All software deficiencies discovered during software validation testing are reported on a Software Verification and Validation Anomaly Report; a description of the information required on the anomaly report is presented in the SVVP. Any Software Verification and Validation Anomaly Report generated during software testing is distributed to the project's lead software engineer for review and initiation of any corrective

Figure 5-2   Typical Software Validation Test Information Sheet (VTIS)

SOFTWARE VALIDATION TEST INFORMATION SHEET

Test Category	Test Number

Requirement	Requirement Number

1. Objectives and success criteria

2. Test approach

3. Test instrumentation

4. Test duration

5. Data collection, reduction, and analysis requirements

6. Comments

7. Results

8. Signatures:

Test Conductor	Date

V&V Lead Engineer	Date

action. A copy of the Software Verification and Validation Anomaly Report is given to the software Configuration Management individual, in accordance with the SCMP.

Section 5 presents the software validation test procedures. Section 5.1 lists tasks that are necessary to prepare for and perform the software validation testing; Section 5.2 describes any intertask dependencies. For example, the DDS must be approved prior to beginning the development of the SVTPR, the SVTP and VTISs will be approved prior to completion of the Detailed Design Phase, and the real-time executive will be validated before software validation testing begins. Section 5.3 delineates any special skills that might be required to complete validation testing—for example, the need for experience with data protocol analyzers or bus bandwidth and resource contention analyzers.

Section 5.4, details of test administration, would, for example, indicate that software validation testing should be suspended whenever a failure, an unexpected result, or an anomaly that is salient to the specific function being examined or to the software safety analysis occurs. Another example is that whenever the observed anomaly involves integrated software where more than one module is in memory, some form of regression testing will be performed on the

Figure 5-3   Typical Software Validation Test Log (SVTL)

SOFTWARE VALIDATION TEST LOG

LOCATION	SOFTWARE PROJECT	DATE

Time	Test Number	Entry	References	Engineer

Page _____ of _____

corrected software, including execution of the original test that detected the anomaly. To limit the scope of regression testing that may be required and to ensure efficient utilization of limited test resources, tools such as set-use matrices should be used to trace the effects of software changes through the system.

Verification and Validation Plan

The SVVP identifies and describes the plan for the V&V of software constructed by the software development team (Table 5-8). The V&V program defined in the SVVP will be applied

Table 5-8 Typical Table of Contents for a Software Verification and Validation Plan

Section Number	Section Title
1	Introduction
1.1	Purpose
1.2	Scope
1.3	Overview
1.4	Reference Documents
1.5	Definition of Terms
2	Overview
2.1	Organization
2.2	Master Schedule
2.3	Resources
2.4	Responsibilities
2.5	Tools, Techniques, and Methodologies
3	Requirements
3.1	Management
3.2	Requirements Phase Verification and Validation
3.3	Architecture Design Phase Verification and Validation
3.4	Detailed Design Phase Verification and Validation
3.5	Implementation Phase Verification and Validation
3.6	Software Validation Phase Verification and Validation
4	Reporting
4.1	Task Reporting
4.2	Phase Summary Report
4.3	Anomaly Report
4.4	Software Configuration Audit Report
4.5	Software Verification and Validation Report
5	Administration Procedures
5.1	Anomaly Reporting and Resolution
5.2	Task Iteration Policy
5.3	Control Procedures

throughout all phases of the software development effort as defined in the SDP. The scope is defined to be those tasks and the information necessary to manage and perform those tasks that are required to ensure the development of quality software for a medical device. The V&V program described in the SVVP is tailored to assure that an appropriate level of V&V is applied to all phases of software development and that it also supports the market strategy and product launch schedule.

Section 1 of the SVVP describes the organization, activities, schedule, and inputs and outputs required for an effective V&V program. The scope of participation by the various associated organizations in the V&V of software is also identified. For each phase of software development defined in the SDP, the SVVP presents the V&V tasks, as well as methods and evaluation criteria, inputs and outputs, schedule and resources, risks and assumptions, and roles and responsibilities. Section 1 gives an overview of the product and states that the V&V of software is an independent assessment and measurement of the correctness, accuracy, consistency, completeness, robustness, and testability of the software requirements, design, and implementation.

The goals of the V&V program are to verify that the products of each development phase comply with requirements and products of the previous phase; to address all safety-related requirements for critical components and functions; to satisfy the standards, practices, and conventions of the current phase; and to establish the proper basis for beginning the next software development phase. The goals include validating that the completed software end product complies with established software and system requirements, documenting the results of V&V tasks in support of software and management planning activities, and facilitating the accomplishments of product-level quality goals.

Section 1 also lists all project reference documents, by document numbers if possible, for the hardware and software, the product-level specifications, and any other specifications and documents applicable to the V&V of project software. It includes the definition of any terms used in the SVVP and that are related to the V&V of software.

Section 2 includes the organization; the master schedule; the resources and their responsibilities; and the tools, techniques, and methodologies of the V&V of software. Section 2.1 presents the organization of the project team and places the software development team and the V&V team within the context of the project. In addition, it indicates how the tasks, policies, and procedures are administrated and approved; where the authority resides for resolving issues raised by the tasks; and who has the approval authority for all V&V products. Section 2.1 also indicates that the V&V organization comprises personnel who have not been involved with the development of the software being verified and have not established the criteria against which the software is to be validated.

The functional responsibilities of the V&V organization are separated into two positions, the V&V project lead engineer and the V&V project engineer. These two positions need not necessarily refer to distinct organizational positions within the project; the responsibilities of both positions may be performed by the same individual, particularly if the project is small enough to warrant it. The development and administration of the V&V program described in the SVVP is the responsibility of the V&V project lead engineer, who is ultimately responsible for planning, organizing, monitoring, and controlling the V&V tasks on the project. The application of these tasks to each phase of software development is also the responsibility of the V&V project lead engineer. Section 2.1 also indicates that the V&V organization will comply with all approved configuration management requirements and procedures as described in the SCMP, relative to the development and submittal of the products defined in the SVVP.

Section 2.2 presents the master plan for the V&V of the developed software, an integral part of each phase of the software development life cycle. At the completion of each development phase, a project milestone is attained, and the V&V tasks are integrated into the project schedule, to provide feedback to the development process and to support management functions. The schedule for these V&V tasks and the relationship of each task to the appropriate phases of software development are presented in Section 2.2.

Management of the V&V tasks and the personnel required to support the management and technical reviews requires scheduling V&V tasks to correspond to and meet project milestones. As these tasks are completed, the results are documented in task reports that are correlated at the completion of each software development phase into a Phase Verification and Validation Task Summary Report. The exchange of the V&V data and results with the software development group effort is also provided through the Software Verification and Validation Anomaly Reports. The anomaly reports, task reports, and task summary reports provide the necessary feedback to the software development process regarding the technical quality of the software products. Resolution of all identified critical anomalies is required before the V&V effort can allow the project to proceed to the next software development phase.

Section 2.3 describes the personnel and material resources required to perform the V&V of software, along with the factors that are considered in analyzing the resource requirements. The responsibilities for performing the V&V tasks are defined in Section 2.4. The personnel selected to perform the V&V of software should have the technical credibility to understand the source of problems related to software quality, follow through with recommended corrective actions to the development process, and abort the delivery of defective software end products. Section 2.4 should indicate that the V&V personnel will not be assigned to the development of the software to be produced nor will they establish the criteria against which the software is validated. It also describes the specific roles and responsibilities of the V&V organization during each phase of the software development.

The V&V of software is accomplished by reviewing, inspecting, testing, checking, auditing, or otherwise establishing and documenting the conformance of the software to its documented, specified requirements (Section 2.5). These tasks are performed manually, as well as by means of automated tools and techniques. Examples of automated tools include traceability analyzers, static analyzers, dynamic analyzers, comparators, test result analyzers, and change trackers. Manual tools include inspections, walk-throughs, code audits, formal reviews, cause-and-effect graphing, and algorithm analysis. Support tools and techniques for software testing include general system utilities and text-processing tools for test preparation, organization, and modification; data reduction and report generation tools; library support systems that consist of database management systems and configuration control systems; and test drivers and languages. Selection of the tools to be used for the V&V tasks is based on the objectives and goals for each phase of the software development. The list of those tools and their usage by phase should be presented in this Section 2.5.

Section 3 describes the V&V requirements. The management of the V&V program described in the SVVP spans all phases of the software development life cycle, and the V&V project lead engineer is responsible for performing the V&V management tasks for the program (Section 3.1). The V&V project lead engineer is responsible for making decisions regarding V&V performance, assigning priorities to the tasks, estimating the level of effort for a task, tracking the progress of work, determining the need for task iteration or initiation of new tasks, and assuring adherence to the software standards in all phases of the program.

Management tasks to be performed for the V&V program include the generation and maintenance of the SVVP itself; assessment of software baseline changes for their effects on previously completed tasks; and periodic review of the V&V effort, technical accomplishments, resource utilization, future planning, and risk assessment. Daily management of phase activities and the technical quality of interim and final reports are also included, as are reviews and evaluations of V&V results to determine when to proceed to the next phase of the software development life cycle; to define changes to tasks that will improve the V&V effort; and to maintain good communication with all software team members and quality assurance personnel, to ensure the accomplishment of quality assurance goals and objectives.

At each phase of software development, the V&V tasks and associated inputs and outputs, schedule, resource requirements, risks and assumptions, and personnel responsible for performing the tasks are evaluated. This evaluation establishes the criteria for updating the SVVP and is necessary to ensure the completeness of the SVVP and consistency with changes in the developed software. A management-level individual should be assigned to support the management of the software V&V and to provide periodic reviews of the effort, technical accomplishments, resource utilization, future planning, and risk assessment. The technical quality and results of the outputs of each V&V phase should be evaluated by this manager, to provide management support for the V&V project lead engineer's recommendation to proceed or not to proceed to the next software development phase, and to define changes to the tasks, to improve the V&V effort. Updates to the SVVP during software development activities will also be reviewed and approved by this manager prior to implementation.

The rest of Section 3 describes the phase V&V activities and tasks for each software development phase specified in the SDP. Although the specific, related details will vary by project, the top-level tasks can be specified for each phase. These top-level tasks and activities are the V&V tasks, the inputs and outputs, and the risks and assumptions for accomplishing the tasks and activities.

Section 4 describes the V&V reporting for the project. Section 4.1 concerns the reporting of the tasks themselves. The results of the individual tasks are documented in a report that identifies the V&V phase at which the task was conducted, the responsible software V&V engineer(s), the responsible software development team member(s), interim results and status, and any recommended corrective actions. The report may be in any format that is appropriate for technical disclosure; it is governed by the software V&V procedures. The task reports are given to the project's software lead engineer and to the appointed software management individual in a timely manner, to aid in detection and resolution of problems before the start of the next software development phase. The reports are ultimately delivered to the responsible software configuration manager for archiving.

Section 4.2 presents the details related to the Verification and Validation Phase Summary Report. At the conclusion of each V&V phase, a Verification and Validation Phase Summary Report summarizes the results of the V&V performed during the applicable software development phase. The summary report contains a description of the tasks that were performed, a summary of the task results, a summary of any anomalies and their implemented resolutions, an assessment of the software quality, and recommendations, if any. The Verification and Validation Phase Summary Report may be in a format appropriate for technical disclosure and is governed by the software V&V procedures. The Verification and Validation Phase Summary Reports are delivered to the responsible software configuration manager for archiving.

Section 4.3 describes problem reporting initiated by the project engineer(s) through a Software Verification and Validation Anomaly Report. The anomaly report identifies any problem detected during the V&V activities. An anomaly report identifies how, when, and where the problem occurred and the perceived impact of the problem on the system capability of the product and on the continued conduct of V&V phase activities. Each report contains a description and location of the anomaly, the severity of the anomaly if it can be determined, the cause and method of identifying the anomalous behavior, and the recommended action, as well as any actions taken to correct the anomalous behavior (Figure 5-4). Anomaly report numbers are supplied by the responsible software Configuration Manager. When the anomaly report is completed, it is delivered to the Configuration Manager for configuration identification, tracking, and status reporting.

Section 4.4 presents the details of the Software Configuration Audit Report (SCAR), a checklist that documents the results of the software configuration audit. The SCAR identifies

Figure 5-4   Typical Software Anomaly Report

SOFTWARE ANOMALY REPORT

1. Date:	2. Severity: H M L	3. Anomaly Report Number:

4. Tile (briefly describe the problem):

5. System:	6. Component:	7. Version:

8. Originator:	9. Organization:	10. Telephone:	11. Approval:

12. Verification and Validation Task:	13. Reference Document(s):

14. System Configuration:

15. Anomaly Description:

16. Problem Duplication:	17. Source of Anomaly:	TYPE

		PHASE	
During run	Y N N/A		☐ Documentation
After restart	Y N N/A	☐ Requirements	☐ Software
After reload	Y N N/A	☐ Architecture Design	☐ Process
18. Investigation Time:		☐ Detailed Design	☐ Methodology
		☐ Implementation	☐ Other
		☐ Undetermined	☐ Undetermined

19. Proposed Solution:

20. Corrective Action Taken:	Date:

21. Closure Sign-off:

_____   _____

Software Lead Engineer   Date

and describes each software item, verifies that the software configurations are what they were intended and proclaimed to be, and verifies that the configuration of each item is the same configuration that was validated during testing in the Software Validation Phase. The SCAR may be in a format appropriate for technical disclosure, which is governed by the software V&V procedures. It is delivered to the responsible software Configuration Manager for archiving.

Section 4.5 discusses the V&V final report. The SVVR is issued after the completion of all V&V tasks during the software development life cycle. It contains a summary of all tasks performed, a summary of task results, a summary of anomalies and resolutions, an assessment of the overall software quality, and any recommendations. The SVVR may be in a format appropriate for technical disclosure, which is governed by the software V&V procedures. It is delivered to the responsible software Configuration Manager for archiving.

Section 5 describes the V&V administrative procedures. The V&V project lead engineer is responsible for the proper documentation and reporting of Software Verification and Validation Anomaly Reports (Section 5.1). All anomalies are reported, regardless of the perceived impact on software development or on the severity level relative to the device operation, because unreported and unresolved software problems can have a significant adverse impact during the later stages of the software development life cycle, when there may be little time for resolution. The Software Verification and Validation Anomaly Reports are reviewed by the software lead engineer for anomaly validity, type, and severity. The software lead engineer can direct that additional V&V should be performed if it is required to assess the validity of the anomaly or the proposed solution. All anomaly reports are submitted to the responsible software Configuration Manager for configuration management and control.

The impact of an anomaly is determined by evaluating the severity of its effect on the operation of the software and the device. The impact is deemed to be high if a software change is required to correct a condition that prevents or seriously degrades a system objective, where no alternative exists, or to correct a safety-related problem. The impact is rated medium if a software change is required to correct a condition that degrades a system objective, to provide for performance improvement, or to confirm that the user and/or system requirements can be met. The impact is classified as low if the software change is desirable to maintain the system, correct operator inconvenience, or for any reason not deemed high or medium. The resolution of critical anomalies rated high is required before the V&V effort can proceed to the next software development phase.

When an anomaly solution is approved and the personnel responsible for performing the corrective action are indicated, the software lead engineer will authorize implementation of the corrective action. The V&V project lead engineer is responsible for the anomaly report closure, which includes documenting that the corrective action(s) were taken and verifying that the authorized changes as described in the anomaly report were made. If the anomaly requires a change to a baselined configuration item, then a CRA is prepared by a member of the software development team for the item(s) to be changed, and a reference to any applicable anomaly reports should be included as part of the CRA. All CRAs are processed in accordance with the SCMP.

Section 5.2 deals with V&V task iteration. A distinct part of the software life cycle is the need for anomaly corrections, performance enhancements, and requirement changes and clarifications. Management of the effects of these changes on previously completed V&V software tasks as well as future tasks is required. Requirements for reperformance of previous tasks or initiation of new tasks to address these types of software changes are established by the V&V project lead engineer and approved by the appropriate software manager.

Continuous review of V&V efforts, technical accomplishments, resource utilization, future planning, and risk assessment is required for effective management. Tasks that uncover significant problems and/or tasks for which a significant part of the defined activity was not completed are candidates for V&V task iteration, once corrections to outstanding problems are implemented. Other opportunities for task iteration are found when the inputs to the task have undergone significant changes to the representation of the system and/or the software requirements. Required iteration of tasks is determined by the V&V project lead engineer through assessments of change, criticality, and quality effects.

Section 5.3 presents the V&V control procedures. All inputs and outputs of the V&V effort for each project are delivered to the responsible Configuration Manager for configuration management and archiving. All software development material used in any V&V task is configured, protected, and assigned a status on task completion by its delivery to the responsible software configuration manager. The procedures for document change control and configuration status accounting are implemented in accordance with the SCMP, to ensure that the validity of V&V results is protected from accidental or unauthorized alteration. All inputs and outputs are retained in accordance with appropriate retention policies, to provide project history for use in future planning of software development and analysis of life cycle requirements.

Software Requirements and Design Documents

The software development analysis, requirements, and design documents (Table 5-9) are normally generated after the product definition phase, when the product objectives have been defined and the system requirements have been determined. Although the content and format of these documents will vary greatly in the first project or two, they will tend to become templates in which perhaps 25–30 percent of the textual descriptions remain unaltered from project to project and only 70–75 percent of the documents are specific to the project. This is the core group of documents that must be updated at the conclusion of the software development activities to reflect the "as-built" code within the device.

Before the contents of these documents are examined, they should be placed in context with each other as well as with the type of information they contain. Figure 5-5 represents the conceptual environment in which these documents exist. When the product-level objectives and requirements have been determined and resolved in sufficient detail, software analysis can begin, to convert the high-level system requirements into their software equivalent, which constitutes a logical model of the product. Within the logical model, software engineers will derive an environmental model and a behavioral model, neither of which will exist in a physical sense. They represent an intellectual way to capture how the external environment influences the software and how the software will behave in response to external stimuli. These models are usually documented through the use of context diagrams, event lists, data-flow diagrams, state transition diagrams, and entity relationship diagrams. The User Interface Specification (UIS) and the IDS encapsulate information from both of these models, the UIS from the user's perspective and the IDS from the hardware-to-software and the software-to-software perspective. The SRS captures primarily behavioral model information that is specific or peculiar to the software as an entity, although it may need to reflect some data found in the UIS and IDS. In addition to using the same types of diagrams and lists as the UIS and IDS, the SRS also utilizes transform specifications, data composition specifications, data element specifications, object specifications, relationship specifications, and implementation constraint specifications.

Once the logical model has been constructed, the software engineering group then converts the logical model information into a physical model that represents the components of the software to be implemented. In the physical model, software engineers will derive a processor

Table 5-9   Typical Software Development Design Documents

Document Title	Acronym	Document Description
Architecture Design Specification	ADS	Establishes the design baseline as a description of the overall software operation and control, and the use of common data
Detailed Design Specification	DDS[1]	Constitutes an update to and an expansion of the design baseline established as the ADS, including a description of the overall software operation and control, and the use of common data. The detailed design is described through the lowest component level of the software organization and the lowest logical level of database organization
Interface Design Specification	IDS[1]	Completely specifies the interfaces among the product components, subsystems, or modules for both hardware and software
Software Requirements Specification	SRS[1]	Provides a controlled statement of the functional, performance, and external interface requirements for the software end products
Requirements Traceability Matrix	RTM[2]	Traces the software requirements from system specification through software validation
User Interface Specification	UIS[3]	Completely specifies the user interface to the product components, subsystems, and Graphical User Interface for both hardware and software

Notes: 1. The IDS, SRS, and DDS are updated at the end of the software project to reflect the "as-built" software.
2. The RTM may appear as an appendix in the SRS and DDS or as a stand-alone document.
3. A system-level document used for software development.

environment model, a software environment model, and a code organization model. None of these models will exist as a tangible entity. They are a convenient nomenclature used to capture the essence of the design activities, to convert the results and findings of the logical model into their physically implementable counterparts. The physical model uses the context diagrams, event lists, data-flow diagrams, state transition diagrams, and entity relationship diagrams of the logical models, as well as the transform specifications, data composition specifications, data element specifications, object specifications, relationship specifications, and implementation constraint specifications. It then allocates these materials into processor diagrams, task diagrams, and control flow diagrams as part of the Architecture Design Specification (ADS). The ADS then augments this information by generating database design information and by determining a resource and processing budget.

The DDS then captures all of the information contained in the ADS and expands and augments this information. The task diagrams, flow diagrams, and transform specifications are

Figure 5-5   Environment of information on software development design documentation

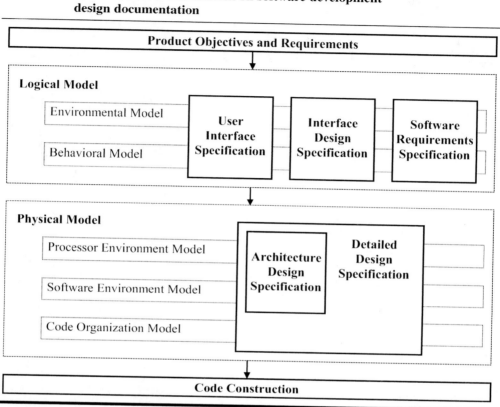

converted into processing modules, which are converted into structure charts. The structure chart is the lowest level of the design used to create device software. These charts are used to generate module specifications, module data composition specifications, and module data element specifications. The result of the physical model is the DDS used by software engineers as the blueprint for implementing the device software.

Software Design Specifications

As discussed above, the software design evolves through two distinct documents, the ADS and the DDS. The intent of the ADS is to serve as a design baseline for beginning top-level code development prior to formal approval of the entire, detailed software design. The ADS therefore represents a placeholder within the DDS and does not formally exist at any time outside of its own software life cycle phase; thus, it is not maintained beyond its delivery milestone. Another way to visualize the ADS and DDS relationship is through the following example. Assume that the design and architecture of software has been completed and is represented by the context diagram and the hierarchy diagram shown in Figure 5-6. The design continues down several more layers than presented in the figure. The ADS would capture the design down to an arbitrary level, in this case Level Three, and the DDS would capture the ADS design and continue to expand and augment this design information down to another arbitrary level.

Figure 5-6   **Relationships among the Architecture Design Specification, the Detailed Design Specification, and the software structure**

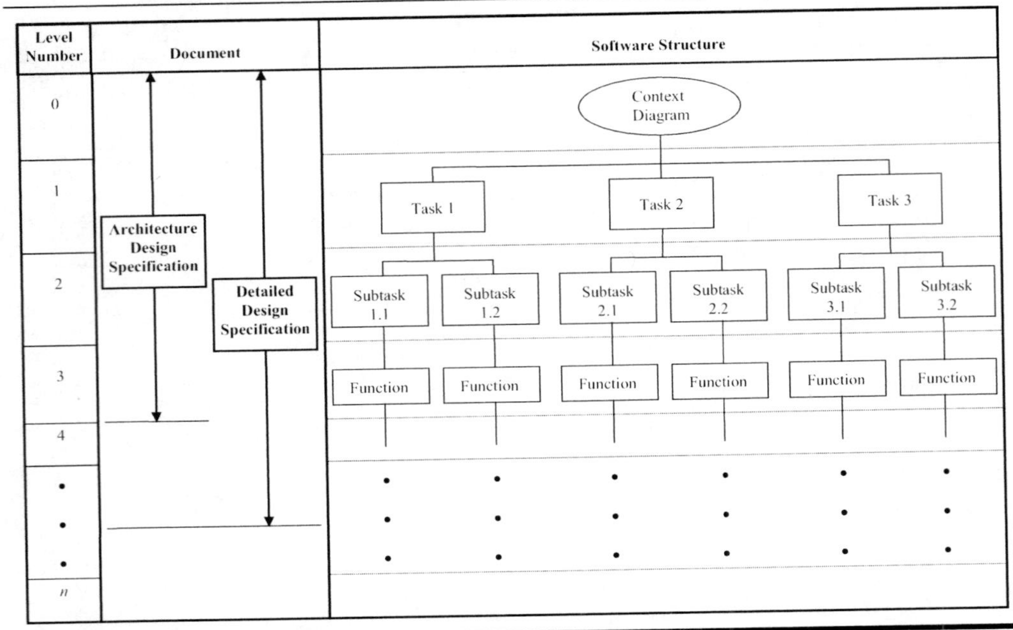

A cursory examination of the tables of contents in Tables 5-10 and 5-11 shows that the ADS document information is contained in total within one section of the DDS. For the purposes of this discussion, the description of the ADS document contents is the same as what would appear in the DDS, and so the ADS description will not be repeated as a part of the DDS description.

Section 1 of the ADS presents the identification, purpose, and introduction of the software architecture design. This section states that the ADS describes the top-level, physical model of the software design and the type of software to be developed for the device; it may list some of the key features or capabilities that the software is expected to control. For example, the code could be described as embedded software for a syringe pump whose features include variable pressure limit, pressure monitoring, purge function, nurse call function, and implementation of an RS-232 data communications protocol. Section 1 indicates those features that the software is responsible for implementing. For example, it could state that the embedded software is responsible for the device's functionality, including user interface, safety checks, and performance accuracy. Section 1 also presents the analysis, requirements, and design methodology used to generate the documented design. For example, it could state that the ADS specifies the segregation of the device software into tasks that execute under a multitasking, real-time executive and that the tasks, data flows, and control flows are described using the Yourdon (1989) methodology. Section 2 of the ADS is a list of all project reference documents, by document numbers if possible, for the hardware and software, the product-level specifications, and any other specifications and documents applicable to the design and implementation of the project software.

Section 3 of the ADS presents the decomposition of the top-level design into the physical tasks that will be implemented, the algorithms to be employed, and the flow of data and control

Table 5-10   Typical Table of Contents for an Architecture Design Specification

Section Number	Section Title
1	Scope
1.1	Identification
1.2	Purpose
1.3	Introduction
2	Reference Documents
3	Design Requirements
3.1	Architecture
3.2	Functional Allocation
3.3	Memory and Processing Time Allocation
3.4	Functional Control and Data Flow
3.5	Global Data
3.6	Top-level Design
4	Notes
Appendix I	Allocation of Requirements
Appendix II	Data Dictionary

between the tasks. Section 3.1 defines the software architecture through the use of a context diagram and processor diagram for the software design. It presents, for the first time, the high-level, logical task packages used to execute within the device. Within each task package are the individual tasks that will execute as software modules. Also included are the data and control flows to be employed to control the software execution.

Section 3.2 of the ADS presents the functional allocation of the software requirements to the various tasks presented in Section 3.1. This allocation can be accomplished by a statement that refers the reader to Appendix I of the ADS. Section 3.3, delineating the memory and processing timeline allocations for the software, might reference the total RAM and ROM and the total memory of nonvolatile erasable electronically programmable read-only memory (EEPROM) and specify any system critical times, volumes, or exposure amounts. The packaged task functional control and data flows (Section 3.4) can be presented by a statement that refers the reader to the data dictionary contained in Appendix II of the ADS.

Section 3.5 of the ADS identifies, states the purpose of, and describes data common to two or more of the tasks in the software design that are not presented in any other document or specification. It presents the data format, tasks using the data, and all other characteristics of the global data that are needed to satisfy the global data requirements. For example, global data value limits or ranges are given, as well as their accuracy and precision. For the convenience of document generation and maintenance, this information may also be provided in a data dictionary in Appendix II of the ADS. If files or a database are part of the global data, Section 3.5 also presents the details related to the purpose of each file or database, the structure of each

Table 5-11   Typical Table of Contents for a Detailed Design Specification

Section Number	Section Title
1	Scope
1.1	Identification
1.2	Purpose
1.3	Introduction
2	Reference Documents
3	Design Requirements
3.1	Architecture
3.2	Functional Allocation
3.3	Memory and Processing Time Allocation
3.4	Functional Control and Data Flow
3.5	Global Data
3.6	Top-level Design
4	Detailed Design
4.1	Design Conventions and Directives
4.2	Mailbox Design
4.3	Global Data
4.4	Detailed Task Design
4.5	Libraries Used
4.6	Macros Used
5	Notes
Appendix I	Allocation of Requirements
Appendix II	Data Dictionary

Note: The Allocation of Requirements may appear as an appendix in the DDS or in the Requirements Traceability
        Matrix document

in terms of contents and size, and the access methods or procedures, such as sequential or random access.

Section 3.6 of the ADS describes the function of each of the task packages presented previously. For each task package, a brief statement of the processing responsibilities of the task is made, including its related control and data flows. Each task package is described in terms of the constituent physical tasks that will be implemented as code within the device. This information can be augmented by the inclusion of any state transition diagrams, process specifications, or any other information that describes each physical task, along with an appropriate reference to the data dictionary (Appendix II of the ADS).

For each task package, a description of its inputs, local data, interrupts, timing and sequencing, processing, and outputs is presented. The inputs to each task are identified, along with their stated purpose. The input data may include data transmitted as global data, direct I/O, passed parameters, or through shared memory. The data identification should include the source(s), format(s), units of measure, and any other characteristics needed to satisfy the input requirements for the task package.

Local task data are any data that originate within the task and are not used by any other task. These data are identified by name, along with a stated purpose. This identification should include the format and any other characteristics needed to satisfy the local data requirements for the task. This information may be provided in a local data table or included as part of the data dictionary (Appendix II of the ADS). If files or a database are a part of the local data, Section 3.6 also presents the details related to the purpose of each file or database, the contents and size of each, and the access methods or procedures.

The task package interrupt describes the generation of and response to signal and interrupt control requirements by the task package. Where applicable, this should include the source, purpose, and priority of the signal or interrupt, as well as the required response time and the minimum, maximum, and probable frequency of the signal or interrupt.

The processing description of the task should address the various aspects of task functionality. It should include the conditions under which the task receives and passes control to interfacing tasks and the algorithms incorporated into the execution of the task. The mathematical description of the algorithm may be documented elsewhere, but its processing should be described in terms of its manipulation of the input and local data as well as the generation of outputs. Any special control features of the task that do not affect the main functions performs should be described, such as line-printer control, console displays, system loop tests for on-line maintenance, or program device checkouts.

Error detection and recovery features of the task should also be presented. These would include the handling of erroneous input data and any other conditions that affect the execution of the task. Section 3.6 should include any additional processing related to data conversion operations performed by the task to implement the interface between the tasks, or related to the interface features, such as synchronization and sequencing, that implement the required communication interfaces. The processing should describe the task's utilization of other elements, components, or system resources as well as any special limitations or unusual features that restrict the performance of the task.

The functional task's outputs should identify and state the purpose of the output data generated by the task. The output data may be transmitted as global data, direct input/output (I/O), or passed parameters, or through shared memory. The data should include the source(s), format(s), units of measure, and any other characteristics of the data needed to satisfy the output requirements for the task package.

Section 4 of the ADS could contain any general information that aids in the understanding of the document, any background information and formula derivations, and a list of any acronyms and abbreviations (and their meaning) used in the ADS.

The appendices should contain any supplemental information that can be published separately for the convenience of generation and maintenance of the ADS. The appendices could be bound as separate documents and referenced in the main body of the ADS where their data would normally have been provided. The appendices could present a wide range of ADS information, such as the mapping of the SRS requirements into the ADS, the data dictionary, or any other ancillary software analysis, requirements, or design information. When approved, the ADS represents a design baseline that can be used to begin the coding of the device software in parallel with the development of the DDS. It should be understood that this approach is at risk if the detailed design should require an alteration to the high-level architecture as presented in the ADS. However, the risk is usually minimal.

As mentioned above, the ADS is included in the DDS as Section 3, and only minor changes to the ADS text are made to convert the ADS into the DDS. Section 1 of the DDS presents the identification, purpose, and introduction of the software detailed design, just as Section 1 of the ADS does. However, this section reflects that the DDS describes the low-level, physical model of the software design and the type of software to be developed for the device, and it may list some of the key features the software is expected to control. It indicates those features the software is responsible for implementing. Section 1 of the DDS also presents the analysis, requirements, and design methodology used to generate the documented design. For example, it could state that the DDS specifies the total software design, from top-level task segregation of the device software down into the tasks, modules, utilities, and shared interfaces that execute in a multitasking, real-time environment and that the tasks, data flows, and control flows are described using the Yourdon (1989) methodology.

Section 2 of the DDS presents a listing of all project reference documents, by document numbers if possible, for the hardware and software, the product-level specifications, and any other specifications and documents applicable to the design and implementation of the project software. Section 3 of the DDS is the direct inclusion of the same section from the ADS without any fundamental changes, except modifications or alterations dictated and captured as a result of the detailed design activities.

Section 4 of the DDS presents the detailed design of the software, as well as for each of the functional tasks that were discussed in Section 3. Section 4.1 presents the naming conventions and directives that will be used in the development of the software, listing the global naming conventions and any pre- and postfix data, routine, function, or file extension abbreviations. Section 4.1 also presents any deviations from the published programming standards and conventions necessitated by the results of the software analysis and detailed design. In addition, this section would describe the conditions for using any development, support, or utility tool directives or templates.

Section 4.2 of the DDS presents the detailed design of any mailboxes, semaphores, signals, or event flags that will be used by the various functional tasks. This design should include the name(s), source(s), format(s), default value(s), and any other characteristics of the data needed to satisfy the processing requirements of the functional tasks. If files or a database, such as scratch files or temporary storage areas, are part of these data, this section also presents the details related to each file or database, such as the contents and size, as well as the file or database access methods or procedures.

Section 4.3 of the DDS identifies, states the purpose of, and describes data common to two or more functional tasks that are not presented in any other document or specification. It includes the data format, the tasks using the data, and all other characteristics of the global data needed to satisfy the global data requirements processing by the functional tasks. For example, global data value limits or ranges are described in detail, as well as their accuracy and precision. This section may be duplicated from the ADS and updated with the minor modifications necessitated by the detailed design activities.

In Section 4.4 of the DDS, the detailed design of the functional tasks described in Section 3, each functional task is a subsection. For each functional task, the inputs are identified, along with a stated purpose for those inputs. The input data may be transmitted as global data, direct I/O, passed parameters, or through shared memory. The data description should include the name(s), source(s), format(s), units of measure, and any other characteristics of the data that are needed to satisfy the input and processing requirements for the task.

Local task data are any data that originate within the task and are not used by any other task. These data are identified by name, along with a stated purpose, and should include the format and all other characteristics needed to satisfy the data and processing requirements for the task. For the convenience of document generation and maintenance, this information may be provided as an appendix and referenced appropriately. If files or a database are part of the local data, this section also describes the purpose of each file or database, the structure of each in terms of its contents and size, and the access method or procedures.

The functional task interrupts describe the generation of and response to signal and interrupt control. Where applicable, this should include the source, purpose, and priority of the signal or interrupt as well as the required response time and the minimum, maximum, and probable frequency of the signal or interrupt.

The processing description of the functional task should include the conditions under which the task receives and passes control to interfacing tasks, as well as the algorithms incorporated into the execution of the task during normal operation. The mathematical description of any implemented algorithm may be documented elsewhere, but its processing should be described here in terms of its manipulation of the input data, the local data, and the generation of outputs. Any special control features, including processing, of the task that do not affect the main functions performed should be described, such as line-printer control, console displays, system loop tests for on-line maintenance, and program device checkouts. The error detection and recovery features of the task should also be presented, including the handling of erroneous input data and any other conditions that affect the execution of the task. Section 4.4 should describe any additional processing related to data conversion operations performed by the task to implement the interface between the tasks, or to interface features such as synchronization and sequencing that implement the required communication interfaces. The processing should describe the task's utilization of other elements, components, or system resources, as well as any special limitations or unusual features that restrict the performance of the task.

The functional task's outputs should identify and state the purpose of the output data generated by the task. The output data may be transmitted as global data, direct I/O, or passed parameters, or through shared memory. The data identification should include the name(s), source(s), format(s), units of measure, and any other characteristics of the data needed to satisfy the output requirements for the task.

Section 4.5 of the DDS presents the details related to any code libraries used as an inherent part of the device software, such as reentrant mathematical functions or floating-point library functions. Each library to be included in the device software should appear as a separate subsection and should present a library-level function or processing summary and the inputs and outputs associated with the library. Section 4.6 presents the same type of information as in the library subsection, except that it addresses the use of macros or assembly-level code that will be used in the software.

Section 5 of the DDS will contain any general information that aids in the understanding of the document, any background information, a glossary, formula derivations, or an alphabetical listing of acronyms and abbreviations (and their meaning) that were used in the DDS.

The appendices should contain any supplemental information that can be published separately for convenience of generation and maintenance of the DDS. The appendices can also be bound as separate documents, explicitly referenced in the main body of the DDS where their data would normally have been provided. The appendices could present information such as the mapping of the SRS requirements into the DDS, the data dictionary, or any other ancillary software analysis, requirements, or design information. When approved, the DDS represents the agreed-upon design baseline that will be implemented as the device software.

Interface Design Specification

The IDS specifies the hardware-to-software interfaces and the software-to-software interfaces to be implemented as a part of device development. The intent of the IDS is to document the decisions that are made regarding how the functionality of the device will be implemented relative to hardware and software. As an example, let us consider the control of a motor in a medical device. There are several implementation strategies for motor control, from simplistic to more complex. One way might be to implement a motor control circuit and algorithm such that the software instructs the motor to turn on and turn off without any feedback. Another implementation strategy might be that the software instructs the motor to turn on and turn off and requests the motor to acknowledge that it did so. Still another strategy is for the software to instruct the motor to turn on and specify the rate, have the motor respond with the actual rate at which it is running, and respond when it is asked to turn off. The purpose of the IDS, then, is to capture this implementation strategy and specify explicitly the functions, communications, channels, number of bits, and discrete pin assignments of the information that would flow between the hardware and software to control the motor.

When properly documented, the IDS allows the electrical and software groups to develop their respective parts of the device in a more parallel fashion, by decoupling their direct dependence on each other until the time when the two disciplines must integrate their components. The definition of the hardware and software interface is a necessary prelude to the orderly specification of both the hardware and software requirements. Toward that end, the IDS provides the common definition and reference for the electrical and software groups. The IDS also provides for a documented, controlled, and approved vehicle for stabilizing the interface between the hardware and software. Table 5-12 shows a typical table of contents for the IDS.

Section 1 states the scope, purpose, and overview for the device's internal interfaces. The purpose of the IDS is to specify the interfaces between the software and the hardware platform on which it will operate. The interfaces to the hardware functions are specific to the device being developed, and they are presented in detail. The requirements and design specified in the IDS apply to the software development group and the electrical engineering group, and the information that the IDS contains is associated with a specific hardware and software configuration.

Section 2 lists the reference documents that are associated with the device interfaces. If the references include hardware documents, specifications, or catalogs that provide options, then the options selected for inclusion in the device being developed are described in detail in the IDS. Section 2 also lists all project reference documents, by document numbers if possible, for the hardware and software, the product-level specifications, and any other specifications and documents applicable to the specific configurations of the hardware and software.

Section 3 delineates the requirements necessary for the development of the interfaces that are presented later in the IDS document. The requirements to be included should be derived or allocated from requirements established by higher level documents and specifications. Section 3.1 describes the relationship of the individual hardware and software components for which the interface is specified. This interface may be provided by an interface block diagram to facilitate the understanding of the relationship.

Section 3.2 of the IDS describes the software-to-software interface requirements, and each interface is assigned to its own subsection. For each software-to-software interface identified in Section 3.1, the interface name is specified, along with a discussion of its purpose and a summary of the information communicated via the interface. In addition, a discussion of the sequential or serial execution should be presented; if the execution is serial, the method of synchronization should also be described. When the information is transmitted, the receiving component

Table 5-12   Typical Table of Contents for an Interface Design Specification

Section Number	Section Title
1	Scope
1.1	Purpose
1.2	Overview
1.3	Introduction
2	Reference Documents
3	Interface Requirements
3.1	Interface Relationships
3.2	Software-to-Software Interfaces
3.3	Hardware-to-Software Interfaces
4	Qualification Requirements
4.1	General Qualification Requirements
4.2	Special Qualification Requirements
5	Interface Design
6	Notes
Appendix I	Interface Reference Tables
Appendix II	Interface Format Tables

should be described relative to the data received and the communication protocol used. The format and, when applicable, the units of measure, scaling, and conventions of the data communicated via the interface should also be specified. Interfaces through shared memory, if any, and the purpose of the shared memory should be discussed. The conditions for initiating each data transfer should be presented, along with the frequency of the transfer, if it is a cyclical initiation. The expected response to each data transfer should be presented, and it should include the maximum time allowed for receiving and acquiring the data, as well as the effects of not receiving the data.

Section 3.3 describes the hardware-to-software interface requirements, and each interface is assigned to its own subsection. For each hardware-to-software interface identified in Section 3.1, the interface name is specified, along with a discussion of its purpose and a summary of the information communicated via the interface. Section 3.3 should discuss the direction of each signal, along with the format and, when applicable, the units of measure, scaling, and conventions of each signal communicated via the interface. The memory buffer requirements and the memory locations used by the hardware and software should be presented, if applicable. Section 3.3 includes the transfer protocol used for the interface, such as blocking, message switching, or handshaking, along with the conditions for initiating each signal and, if cyclic, the frequency of the signal. The priority level of the interface and of each signal, if applicable, should be discussed. Section 3.3

should describe the expected response to each signal, including the maximum time allowed for responding to each signal, as well as the effects of not responding within the allocated time interval. Any error control and alternate paths should be included.

Section 4 specifies the methods, techniques, tools, facilities, and acceptance tolerance limits necessary to establish that each interface satisfies the requirements in Section 3. Section 4.1 specifies the general qualification methods to be used to ensure that each of the requirements of the interfaces has been satisfied. These methods typically include demonstration, test, analysis, and inspection. For example, demonstration is carried out by the operation of the interface and relies on observable functional operation. It does not require the use of elaborate instrumentation or special test equipment. Testing is carried out by the operation of the interface and relies on collection and examination of data. Analysis is carried out by the processing of accumulated data compiled from other qualification methods, and it relies on interpretations and extrapolations. Inspection is by visual examination. Any additional qualification methods used to show that the interface requirements have been satisfied should also be presented. Section 4.2 specifies any special requirements associated with the qualification of the requirements presented in Section 3. These requirements may consist of special tools, techniques, facilities, acceptance limits, and test formulas or algorithms.

Section 5 presents the design of the interfaces that are presented in Section 3; all information passed across each interface is completely specified. Each interface presented in Section 3 appears as its own subsection in Section 5, and for each interface this description includes the interface name, a summary description, and data formats. The information passed across the interface should be listed and its purpose described; if the interface is bidirectional, then each direction should be addressed separately. The initiation criteria for and the response to each interface item of information that is moved should be specified. For each interface item of information, the data, messages, or control information associated with the item should be discussed. In addition, the format of the item should be completely described, including the information contained in the item field; first and last bit positions of the field and word number(s), if applicable; the name of the field if it is a variable; the value of the field if it is a fixed number; and the scaling, units of measure, and any conventions associated with the field. Any of the above data can be placed into a summary interface reference table and an interface item format table with appropriate references.

Section 6 presents any general information that aids in the understanding of the IDS. This could include, for example, background information, a glossary, and formula and algorithm derivations. Section 6 should include an alphabetical listing of all acronyms, abbreviations, and their meanings as used in the IDS. Appendices may contain any supplemental information that can be published separately, to facilitate maintenance of the document. The appendices may be bound as separate volumes or included as a physical part of the IDS. As applicable, each appendix should be referenced in the text of the IDS where the data would normally have been provided.

Software Requirements Specification

The SRS establishes the requirements for the software in the device (Table 5-13). Section 1 describes the software requirements of the device and states that the requirements are traceable to higher, product-level requirements and documents; it may also list some of the key features or capabilities that the software is expected to control. For example, the code could be described as embedded software for a syringe pump whose features include variable pressure limit, pressure monitoring, purge function, nurse call function, and implementation of an RS-232 data communications protocol. Section 1 could state that the embedded software is responsible for

Table 5-13   Typical Table of Contents for the Software Requirements Specification

Section Number	Section Title
1	Scope
1.1	Identification
1.2	Purpose
1.3	Introduction
2	Reference Documents
2.1	Specifications
2.2	Standards
2.3	Other Documents
3	Requirements
3.1	Programming Requirements
3.2	Design Requirements
3.3	Interface Requirements
3.4	Detailed Functional and Performance Requirements
3.5	Adaptation Requirements
3.6	Traceability
4	Qualification Requirements
4.1	General Qualification Requirements
4.2	Special Qualification Requirements
5	Preparation for Delivery
5.1	Instrument EPROM
5.2	Archive Documents
Appendix I	Requirements Traceability Matrix
Appendix II	Requirements Qualification Criteria
Appendix III	Additional Device Requirement Information

Note: The Requirements Traceability Matrix may appear as Appendix I in the SRS or as a stand-alone document.

the device's functionality, including user interface, safety checks, and performance accuracy. This section shows the correlation of the software requirements in the SRS to the requirements in previous and higher level documents parenthetically, in italic type.

Section 2 presents a listing of all of the project reference documents, by document numbers if possible, for the hardware and software, the product-level specifications, and any other specifications and documents applicable to the requirements of the project software. In the event of a conflict between the documents referenced in this section and the actual contents of the SRS, the contents of the SRS are considered to be superseding requirements.

Section 3 presents the requirements that are to be met by the device software. Section 3.1 specifies the programming language that will be used and allows the use of assembly language where necessary to achieve execution speed or close coupling of the software to the hardware that is not attainable with the high-order programming language of choice. It should be expected that I/O primitives, interrupt handlers, and processor diagnostics will be written in assembly language. Section 3.1 also states the compiler and assembler by manufacturer and version number and selects those compiler and assembler options that will be compatible with the processor of choice. This section should also state the programming standards that are not currently documented in the software development policies, procedures, and guidelines. Section 3.1 should specify the content of embedded ASCII strings that will be used to identify the software module, revision number, and standard copyright notice.

Section 3.2 discusses the design requirements for the software, including sizing and timing requirements, design standards, and design constraints. Section 3.3 includes the interface relationships, shown via a context diagram, the interface identification and documentation, and the detailed interface requirements.

The detailed functional and performance requirements listed in Section 3.4 include operational modes, user interface functions, data entry functions, display functions, indicator functions, audio functions, command flow control functions, instrument-specific functions, power-up test functions, and any hardware monitoring functions. In this section, each function's input(s), processing, and output(s) should be discussed. Additional information might include transition rules, menu operation and navigation rules, state transition diagrams, data flow diagrams, and control flow diagrams. Any foreign languages and special characters might be included, as well as device communications protocol, manufacturing test communications, and any other device-specific requirements that must be satisfied.

Section 3.5 presents any adaptation requirements related to the device software. For example, if the device was developed in a PC environment using a cross compiler that required in-line or embedded special commands or directives that must be removed prior to integration testing on the final hardware platform, these conditions should be presented here. If look-up tables are to be used to avoid hard-coding parameters, then the use of these tables should be described. Section 3.5 should document that the table information must be captured and entered at some point during the software development effort; a discussion of the source(s) of the data along with the associated resource(s) skill set needed to compile the table data should also be included.

Traceability of the requirements (Section 3.6.) is usually referred to as the Requirements Traceability Matrix (RTM); it represents the mapping of the product-level objectives and requirements, the UIS requirements, and the IDS requirements into the appropriate SRS paragraph numbers. This mapping can be accomplished through the use of a table that is included as Appendix I, to facilitate the generation and maintenance of the RTM. In a typical RTM (Figure 5-7), each requirement is assigned a sequential number and a general description. It is cross-referenced to a higher level requirement number, the SRS document paragraph number, and the DDS document paragraph number. The RTM then references the software component name where the requirement is satisfied, the number of the VTIS or DTIS test that verified the requirement, the verification test method, and the test result (as pass or fail).

As an alternative, the RTM can be produced as a stand-alone document. In this case, Section 3.6 would refer the reader to the RTM document, and the appendix would list only the first four columns of Figure 5-7. The RTM document would encompass the format shown in Figure 5-7. The advantage of generating the RTM as a separate document is that the RTM will be revised many times during the software development life cycle; making changes to an independent

Figure 5-7   Typical Requirements Traceability Matrix (RTM)

REQUIREMENTS TRACEABILITY MATRIX								
Reqm't Number	Requirement Description	Higher Level Reqm't Number	SRS Para. Number	DDS Para. Number	Software Component(s)	Test Number(s)	Verification Method(s)	Test Results Pass / Fail
								Pass / Fail
								Pass / Fail
								Pass / Fail
								Pass / Fail
								Pass / Fail
								Pass / Fail
								Pass / Fail

document is usually easier and preferable to modifying an SRS in its entirety. Generating a separate RTM has another advantage: it can act as a secondary check on the accuracy of the requirement trace. For example, the software developers would generate the version that appears in the SRS and demonstrate requirements traceability from the SRS to higher level documents and specifications. While that version was being developed, the software V&V engineers would generate the stand-alone RTM document by working from the higher level documents and specifications down to the SRS. Toward the end of the requirements phase, the two documents would be compared for disconnects from two standpoints. First, this would point to where the V&V group felt that a higher level requirement was specified but not addressed by the developers, because there was not an entry in the SRS version of the RTM. Second, there would be an entry in the SRS version generated by the development group but no corresponding entry in the stand-alone RTM. In either case, the discrepancy would need to be rectified and reconciled by the developers and the V&V engineers, and the documents would be revised.

Section 4 describes the qualification requirements of the software. Section 4.1 states that the software development team will implement a program that utilizes reviews, walk-throughs, audits, static and dynamic analysis, testing, and any other methods consistent with development policies, procedures, and guidelines, to ensure the development of quality software for the device.

In addition, this section indicates that the qualification of the software for delivery to the system design validation phase is established by successful completion of the testing described in the SDTP and the SVTP. The SDTP describes the scope of the software testing that must be successfully completed for each software component, whereas the SVTP describes the software testing required to verify that the fully integrated software product satisfies the requirements specified in the SRS. The success criteria for each test to be conducted on the software are identified in the test information sheets, and an appropriate test information sheet is generated for each test described in the SDTP and the SVTP. The DTISs are used as a guide for test setup and conduct, and the VTISs are baselines for development of the SVTPR, which are used to conduct the testing described in the SVTP.

Section 4.1 should also describe the scope of software testing that must be successfully completed, as well as the software test requirements in terms of levels of testing, test categories, and test verification methods. The qualification of the software is established by successful completion of the two levels of software testing, software component testing and software validation testing. Software component testing will verify the correct operation of each software component as described in the DDS. Software validation testing will verify that the fully integrated software product satisfies the requirements specified in the SRS.

The test categories for software component testing and software validation testing should include functional, robustness, stress, safety, growth, and regression testing. Functional testing is the set of tests designed to verify that all of the functional requirements have been satisfied—a test category that is success oriented because the tests are expected to produce successful results. Robustness testing consists of the set of tests designed to evaluate software performance given unexpected inputs. These tests are failure oriented because the test inputs are designed to cause the product to fail given foreseeable and reasonably unforeseeable misuse of the product. Stress testing is designed to evaluate software performance when the amount or rate of data exceeds the amount or rate expected. Safety testing verifies that the software performs in a safe manner and that a complete assessment of the safety design has been accomplished. Growth testing verifies that the margins of growth specified for any particular component, or the product software as a whole, are supported by the software. Regression testing is the reperformance of any completed test that is deemed necessary whenever a software change occurs because of detected faults that were introduced during software construction, to verify that modifications have not caused any unintended adverse effects, and to verify that the software still meets its specified requirements.

The test verification methods for software component testing and software validation testing should include inspection, analysis, demonstration, and physical testing. Inspection is accomplished by visual examination of an item; analysis is accomplished by the evaluation of theoretical or empirical data. Demonstration is accomplished by operational movement or adjustment of an item. Physical testing is accomplished by the operation of an item and recording and evaluation of quantitative data, on the basis of the item's response to the operation. The qualification criteria of each software requirement, as specified in the SRS, are defined by one or more levels of testing, test category, and test method. A matrix identifying the qualification criteria for the software requirements, as specified in the SRS, should be provided as Appendix II and be referenced in Section 4.1.

Special qualification requirements (Section 4.2) for the software might include qualification of the software through the use of special tools, techniques, facilities, or acceptance limits. For example, the software might be examined by a commercially available software complexity tool; any parts or segments of the code that exceed an arbitrary complexity index as defined by that tool would have to be reworked to reduce complexity. If no special qualification requirements exist, that should be stated in Section 4.2.

Section 5 describes preparation of the software for delivery. All software deliverables should conform to the standards set forth in the software development policies and procedures and the SEAP. This section should indicate any additional requirements that must be satisfied to deliver the software to system design validation testing. For example, it might address the inclusion of a copyright notice, device model number, compatible hardware revision numbers, and software revision numbers in any electronically programmable read-only memory (EPROM). The software revision numbers might further include those for the device software revision, the real-time executive or operating system revision, and the communication protocol software revision. The copyright notice, instrument number, and software revision number should also be included in the reference section of each document and in the appropriate electronic files.

For the convenience of document generation and maintenance, additional SRS information may be provided in Appendix III and referenced appropriately in the sections in which the data would have appeared. The appendices should definitely contain the RTM and the software requirements qualification criteria. The appendix information might also include conceptual menu descriptions for the user interface menus, technician menus, diagnostic menus, or configuration menus, as well as navigation among the various menus.

Software Requirements Traceability Matrix

As previously discussed, the Requirements Traceability Matrix (RTM) represents the mapping of the product-level objectives and requirements, the UIS requirements, and the IDS requirements into the appropriate SRS paragraph numbers. This can be accomplished in one of two ways. The first is to include the RTM (see Figure 5-7) as Appendix I of the SRS; the second is to produce the RTM as a stand-alone document and not include it in the SRS. If the RTM is to be a stand-alone document, then the SRS would refer the reader to that document, and Appendix I of the SRS defaults to the first four columns of Figure 5-7. The RTM document would encompass the format shown in Figure 5-7.

There are several advantages of generating the RTM as a separate document. First, the RTM will be updated and released many times during the software development life cycle; making changes to an independent document is usually easier and preferable to modifying the SRS and then having the SRS reviewed and approved. Second, the manner in which the stand-alone RTM document is created can act as a secondary check on the accuracy of the requirement trace. For example, the software developers would generate the version that appears in the SRS and demonstrate requirements traceability from the SRS to higher level documents and specifications. While this version is being developed, the software V&V engineers would generate the stand-alone RTM document by working from the higher level documents and specifications down to the SRS. At some point toward the end of the requirements phase, the two documents would be compared for consistency and coverage. Because the RTM document was assembled from the higher to lower requirement level, this comparison would point to where the V&V group felt that a higher level requirement was specified but not addressed by the developers because there was not an entry in the SRS version of the RTM. Because the SRS version was assembled from the lower to higher requirement level, there would be an entry in the SRS version by the development group but no corresponding entry in the stand-alone RTM. In either case, the discrepancy would need to be rectified and reconciled by the developers and the V&V engineers. Both the SRS and RTM would then be revised appropriately.

The RTM provides a trace of the software requirements into the implemented software. To accomplish this, each requirement is assigned a sequential number and a general description based on the detailed text entered into the SRS. This is then cross-referenced to a higher level requirement number in one of two ways. First, if the SRS requirement was generated to satisfy a requirement in a higher level document, for example, the RTM higher level requirement column would indicate something like "IDS 3.4.5," meaning that the SRS requirement satisfied the requirement in Section 3.4.5 of the IDS document. The same practice would be used for satisfying any higher level document or specification such as system performance specifications or system requirement specifications. Second, a software requirement may be created to satisfy a previous software requirement. For example, it may be decided that an alarm is needed when the motor speed of the device falls below a threshold value. The motor requirement is present because a motor was specified at the higher document level, and assume it was assigned RTM sequential number 010. The fact that an alarm was needed came through the software requirement analysis activities related to the motor requirement. Assume that the motor alarm was assigned RTM sequential requirement number 023. For this example, the higher level requirement column of the RTM for the motor alarm requirement would have the assigned sequential number of the motor requirement as its entry, or 010 in this example.

The last column to be completed during the requirements phase activities is the SRS document reference, which represents the location in the SRS where the details of the requirement can be found. There are several ways to mark or flag the requirements in the SRS, but the most efficient and effective is to structure the requirements text such that each requirement has its own paragraph number. This removes the burden of developing a separate numbering schema and provides an automated update as requirements are added or deleted. At the close of the requirements phase, the first four columns of the RTM have been completed.

During the design phases, the RTM is again updated to reflect the trace of requirements into the design. The DDS column is updated to reflect the location in the DDS of the design detail that satisfies the requirement. Usually this is accomplished by entering the DDS paragraph number that describes the design containing the implementation of the requirement, but it can also be satisfied by using diagram, figure, or table numbers if the requirement design is located in one of those. The intent is to provide a design reference for every entry in the RTM. If a requirement is deleted during this phase for whatever reason, then the requirement description entry indicates "Deleted," and the rest of the line for the deleted requirement is empty. The rationale for indicating that the requirement was deleted rather than physically removing it from the RTM is twofold. First, it is a way to indicate that the requirement was consciously removed from the project and not inadvertently deleted from the table. Second, each requirement is sequentially numbered at the conclusion of the requirements phase, and physically removing the entry from the RTM would leave a gap in the numbering sequence, necessitating renumbering all of the requirements. This, in turn, would lead to confusion, because it would not be clear whether the RTM requirement number was the original or a reassigned number. At the close of the design phases the first five columns of the RTM have been completed.

As the software development life cycle continues, the requirements are mapped into the module that implements the requirement. During the software implementation phases the RTM software component column is updated to reference the name of the software component in which the requirement is satisfied. As the VTISs are generated by the V&V group, the number of the VTIS test that verifies the requirement is entered into the RTM test number column, and the type of verification method is entered in the verification method column. Prior to beginning the software validation test phase, the RTM has been completed except for the last column, Test Results (Pass or Fail). During the software validation testing phase, the test results are recorded on the VTIS, and the corresponding result is marked on the RTM. If the test was passed, then no further action is required. If the test was failed, then appropriate changes are made to the software, and the VTIS test is repeated. If the software passes, then the RTM is so marked, and no further action is required. If the software continues to fail, then the RTM is not updated, but changes continue to be made to the software, and VTIS regression testing continues until the test is passed. By the end of the project, every requirement listed in the RTM can be traced from its high-level requirement down to the name of the module that implemented the requirement and into the validation test results, which should all be Pass.

User Interface Specification

The UIS presents the externally visible inputs and outputs of the device from the user's standpoint (Table 5-14). From the user's perspective, the user interface is the device, and the UIS is intended to specify completely the interface between the device and the external environment. The UIS describes the two-way communication between the user and the device as a system. The user usually sends information to the device by manipulating switches, depressing buttons, making selections from menus on the device's display, or performing any other action that the device can detect. The device, in turn, sends information to the user by displaying messages and digits on display panels, illuminating indicators, and emitting various audible tones.

Table 5-14   Typical Table of Contents for a User Interface Specification

Section Number	Section Title
1	Introduction
1.1	Purpose
1.2	Scope
1.3	Definition of Terms
1.4	References
1.5	Overview
2	General User Interface Considerations
2.1	Characteristics
2.2	Environment
2.3	Attributes
2.4	Rules
2.5	Critical Parameters and Functions
2.6	Capabilities
2.7	Operational Modes
3	Operational Modes
4	Front Panel Switches
5	Indicators
6	Audio
7	Displays
7.1	General Description
7.2	General Format
7.3	Character Fonts, Sets, and Styles
8	Menus and Menu Items
9	Prompts, Warnings, Alarms, and Errors
9.1	Prompts
9.2	Warnings
9.3	Alarms
9.4	Errors
10	Remote User Interface

Section 1 presents the purpose, scope, definition of terms, references, and overview required to specify the user interface. The UIS is the formal specification of all of the observable input and output behavior of the device from the user's point of view. Although one may argue that device labeling is a component of the user interface, it is not generally considered as a distinct part of the UIS document; this section should refer the reader to the appropriate labeling documents and specifications. Section 1 of the UIS includes an alphabetical list of the terms (and their definitions) related to specifying the user interface, as well as a listing of all project reference documents, by document numbers if possible, for the hardware and software, the product-level specifications, and any other specifications and documents applicable to the specification of the user interface.

Section 2 presents, for example, the user characteristics, the user environment, the attributes of the user interface, the user interface rules, the critical parameters and functions, the user interface capabilities, and the device's operational modes. Although much of this information is generic and is usually specified in a user interface guideline type of document, the specific implementation or deviation from these guidelines is presented in this section. In general, the user interface should be simple to learn, use, and operate, and it should be consistent and uniform at all levels. The functionality of the user interface should be well defined, with as few interactions between its various functions as possible. This implies that related user interface functions should be grouped together, that the different modes are clearly discernible from one another, and that errors are clearly indicated.

The user interface should observe certain rules of operation. The device should acknowledge user actions, whether the feedback is positive or negative. All input or output data that uses a common resource, such as an LCD or audio generator, should be prioritized to reduce resource contention and conflicts. The user interface design should avoid requiring the user to transpose, compute, interpolate, or mentally translate units of measure or values. The user interface should also inform the user of all changes to values that are entered manually and promptly inform the user if an attempted change to a parameter does not take place. Units entered or selected by a user should be considered the primary units of choice, and any related output quantities should be displayed in these same primary units. For example, various unit quantifiers, such as milliliters per hour and micrograms per minute, are common in a device; subsequent actions, displays, or calls to a function should default to the primary units or to units that are derived directly from the primary units. The user interface should be designed to resist casual or inadvertent changes to the device's operational mode, to attempts to turn the device off, and to parameter changes during any critical function.

User-input rules should indicate that the setting of device parameters is consistent, regardless of the parameter specified, and parameter input data should be designed for entry in the order in which the user would normally write or verbally communicate the data. Incomplete or incorrect data entry should not alter or change the current value of the parameter or device operation, and the entry should default to the previous value if the new entry is not correct. The user interface should also inform the user of incorrect or incomplete parameter entry if the user attempts to go on to another action before an entry is completed. It should be possible, however, for the user to intentionally terminate any entry sequence before the entry has been completed.

User-output rules should indicate that all displayed information is in a directly readable and usable form. The user interface should inform the user of warning conditions, and the warning should not change the operational mode of the device. For example, warnings might include conflicting units, insufficient data, low battery, or incorrect parameter entry. Information messages to the user should fit on one display, and different types of output should be distinguishable from each other. For example, warnings should be distinctly different from alarms, and alarms should be discernibly different from error indicators.

Section 3 of the UIS describes the operational modes of the device. At any given time, a device may be characterized by the major category of the task it is performing. These major tasks, the functions that the device performs, are commonly known as operational modes. From a logical standpoint, a device can be in only one operational mode at a time. For example, an infusion instrument might be in the HOLD mode or in the INFUSING mode, but not both. Operational modes serve as a convenient way of breaking the device functionality into smaller, discrete segments that can be separately described and documented. Devices that are performing in the same operational mode but displaying different messages or whose operation differs in some other subtle or less important way are considered to be in a different state. For example, two devices might be in the RUN mode, but one is operating in the AC power state while the other is in the battery state.

The user interface must be designed and implemented so that it can operate correctly and safely for each operational mode and state that the device can assume; Section 3 documents each of those modes and states. Each mode and state within the mode should be defined, and how it may be entered and exited should be described. The operational capabilities and processing logic of the mode should be presented, along with an indication of active switches, displays, indicators, and annunciators. This is laborious to document in a written format. State transition diagrams, state tables, control flow diagrams, and state matrices should be used to present this information in a compact, efficient, and convenient manner. Information in this diagrammatic form could be included in an appendix, referenced in the appropriate section. Regardless of the presentation style or format, each mode of operation must be presented in this section, along with the operational characteristics associated with the mode.

Section 4 describes the "front-panel" switches, the switches (wherever they are) the user can access to interact with the device. Section 4 indicates how the switch's action is initiated. For example, an "edge-triggered" switch activates immediately when the switch is depressed, and has no effect when the switch is released. Each switch that is to be operable by the user should be described in this section. The purpose, definition, activation, termination, and device mode(s) activation of each switch should be presented.

Section 5 describes each indicator that will be used on the device. What each indicator represents and descriptions of its icon, color and illumination, and activation mode should be included. Section 6 describes the audio components, which might, for example, emit sounds to annunciate alarms, provide switch-press feedback, and signal various other conditions to the user. This section also presents the common characteristics related to the various types of audio components, such as deviations in audio frequency percent, tone decibel minimum, and audio duration and interval deviations. It includes the specific characteristics of each audio component, such as specific frequency, tone duration and interval, initiation of tone activation, and loudness.

Section 7 presents any common characteristics of the device display(s), such as pixel resolution, backlighting, glare reduction windows, viewing angles, and contrast ratios. This section also describes in detail the display(s) to be used. For example, it might discuss color, foreground and background, border of the display, size and type of windows, alphanumeric information, and general display topology. The display topology would include the various areas of the display(s), to indicate size, principle function(s), and typical character format size. This section would also discuss backlighting and highlighting. It should include the standard character font size, character set, control characters, special characters, and style.

Section 8 describes the menus and displays to be generated for the user. In general, a menu is defined as a collection of items displayed in a window. This section should describe the collection of menus, messages, and displays that the device will generate to convey to the user its status. This section presents the generic menu rules, menu attributes, menu types, and the navigation among and between the menus. Section 8 should discuss each menu that the device will display, including the format, content, and layout of the various windows and window fields on the menu.

Section 9 describes the prompts, warnings, alarms, and errors that can be generated by the device. A prompt is a special message displayed to alert the user to a condition that requires user intervention; it may or may not be accompanied by an audio sound. A warning indicates a possible problem or condition that is of interest to the user; it may be either a continuous or a momentary message that does not change the basic operational mode of the device. Continuous warning messages are displayed until a change in the device status causes the message to be discontinued. Momentary warning messages are displayed for as long as the user continues the action that triggered the warning, or until a predefined time-out period has expired. Warning messages may also be accompanied by audio feedback for reinforcement. An alarm is a condition in which the device's operation is suspended; a message is displayed describing the problem that precipitated the alarm. The alarm message may also offer a recommended corrective action to rectify the situation. For each possible prompt, warning, alarm, and error, the format, content, display location, and display characteristics should be presented and discussed. The causes and solutions to these items should also be presented.

Section 10 describes the interface with a remote user. The communication status of the device can encompass such considerations as whether the device is under local or remote control, whether it is on-line or off-line, or whether it is in the monitor mode. Section 10 describes the various combinations of these remote interfaces and how the device will convey its status remotely to the user. This section should also present the states that the device can assume if it changes from one remote state to others.

Software Testing and Verification and Validation Documents

DTIS and the VTIS documents compose most of the structured, formalized, and documented testing process for the device software (Table 5-15). Although the content and format of the SVTPR and the SVVR documents will vary greatly on the first project or two, they will tend to become templates in which perhaps 25–30 percent of the textual descriptions remain unaltered from project to project and 70–75 percent of the documents are specific to the project.

Development Test Information Sheet

To facilitate testing of the developed software, a DTIS should be generated for each software development test performed. A typical DTIS is shown in Figure 5-1 as a form that is referenced in the SDTP.

The DTIS is the physical repository for the final results of the test that it documents. Each DTIS, therefore, should be completed in such a manner that the test is repeatable and that the objective, approach, and success criteria of the test are known. The DTIS must document the entire test setup that will be needed for regression testing, if necessary, as well as helping to ensure that the test can migrate from module-level testing into integration-level testing. The DTIS must also record the actual test results.

A DTIS should be prepared for each test defined in the SDTP. Because the SDTP, SRS, and DDS will evolve over the project life cycle, the DTIS should be kept as current as is necessary

Table 5-15   Typical Testing and Verification and Validation Documents for Software

Document Title	Acronym	Document Description
Software Development Test Information Sheet	DTIS	Test procedures, results, and verification for each test specified in the SDTP
Software Validation Test Information Sheet	VTIS	Test procedures, results, and verification for each test specified in the SVTP
Software Validation Test Procedures	SVTPR	Set of procedures for performing testing defined in the SVTP
Software Verification and Validation Report	SVVR	Final report summarizing V&V tasks and results, including status and disposition of anomalies

Notes: The SVVR serves as the "certification" that the software has passed validation testing and is acceptable for use.

until end-product acceptance. Completed DTISs are reviewed before the tests for completeness and technical adequacy of the testing to be conducted, as well as periodically audited to assess their compliance with relevant software development procedures and guidelines.

Each DTIS includes the title of the test, the requirement to be tested, the specification containing the requirement, the objective, the success criteria, and the approach to be used. In addition, the DTIS should specify the required instrumentation, the expected duration of the test, and the data collection, reduction, and analysis requirements.

Validation Test Information Sheet

Software validation tests are recorded on VTISs; one VTIS is generated for each test described in the SVTP. An example of a typical VTIS is shown in Figure 5-2 as a form that is referenced in the SVTP. Each VTIS describes the test purpose and its success criteria, the approach, and the environment; this information is used in conjunction with the SVTP to develop the SVTPR. During testing, the VTIS for each test is updated to document the test conductor, the results and associated comments, and the test completion signatures. VTISs are retained by the software V&V engineers in a central location for review by software developers, management personnel, and any quality assurance representatives.

A VTIS is prepared and maintained for each test to be conducted during the Software Validation Phase. VTISs provide an organized, accessible collection of all software validation testing and results, a means of tracking the progression and status of the validation testing, and a means of software test verification. A VTIS is prepared for each test defined in the SVTP, is generated prior to the DDR, and is maintained until the validation tests are completed. The VTISs are reviewed for completeness and for the technical adequacy of the testing that was conducted. The VTISs are periodically audited to assess their compliance with the relevant V&V procedures and guidelines. Problems detected during these audits are identified in a written summary attached to the VTIS. The VTISs are formally accepted, the results having been approved, by signature of the V&V lead engineer when the tests have been completed.

Each VTIS includes the title of the test to be conducted, the objectives, and the success criteria. It also includes the requirement(s) to be tested, the requirement's unique identifier, and the title of the specification in which the requirement was defined. The VTIS describes the test approach to the depth necessary to establish a baseline for resource requirements, the required instrumentation, and test phasing, scheduling, and duration. It also describes the data collection, reduction, and analysis requirements.

The review for approval of the VTISs occurs at the DDR and includes an assessment of the adequacy of the test methods and limits as defined in each VTIS. The VTISs are used as a basis for development of the SVTPR. The results of the testing described by the VTIS are documented on the VTIS itself, and the test conductor signs and dates the completed sheet. Completed VTISs are maintained until all of the software validation testing is completed.

Validation Test Procedures

The SVTPR are the detailed procedures to be used for performing the software validation testing on the completed software as described in the SVTP (Table 5-16). Section 1 presents the purpose, scope, overview, list of all project reference documents (by document numbers if possible) for the hardware and software, product-level specifications, and any other specifications and documents that are applicable to the specification of the validation testing procedures. It includes definitions of terms related to software validation testing.

The scope of the SVTPR is limited to the definition and description of the test procedures necessary to conduct software validation testing as defined in the SVTP. Validation testing of the software will probably be performed in an order corresponding to the phases of software development documented in the SDP. Use of this approach means that each phase of validation testing will build on the previously established software baselines and will incorporate regression testing as necessary to confirm that the newly integrated software has not adversely affected any previously validated software. Each procedure described in the SVTPR will indicate the applicable test requirements for each phase of validation testing. If no applicable test requirements exist for a specific phase of validation testing, the test procedure should reflect this fact.

For each test to be performed as a part of validation testing, a test identifier will be assigned, as well as the requirement(s) to be tested. The requirement should be identified by its unique identifier and the title of the specification in which the requirement is defined. Each test will indicate the particular phase when the validation testing will occur, the test objective and pass-fail criteria, the approach, and any required instrumentation. Each test description will include its expected duration; the data collection, reduction, and analysis requirements; and the series of individual, numbered steps that must be performed in order to conduct the test completely.

Validation testing is conducted by the software V&V engineers during the Software Validation Phase of the software development life cycle. It verifies that the fully integrated software satisfies the requirements and design specified in the SRS and the DDS, respectively. Software validation testing is conducted in accordance with the provisions of the SVVP, the SCMP, and the SVTP for the project. The SVTPR should list the specific tests to be performed and the required instrumentation for each phase of the software validation testing. The steps required to configure the required test instrumentation and to establish the instrument operation prior to the performance of each test can be generic and repetitive. Because of this, the generic test setups and procedures can be uniquely identified and described in their own test procedures, which can reduce the overall documented steps for any single individual test. These are then presented in a separate section of the SVTPR.

Table 5-16   Typical Table of Contents for Software Validation Test Procedures

Section Number	Section Title
1	Introduction
1.1	Purpose
1.2	Scope
1.3	Overview
1.4	Reference Documents
1.5	Definition of Terms
2	Generic Procedures
2.1	Test Tool Setup Procedures
2.2	Emulation Test Configuration Procedures
2.3	Mode Transition Procedures
2.4	Generic Test Setup Procedures
2.5	Test Restart Procedures
2.6	Test Wrap-up Procedures
2.7	Setup Procedures for Remote Communications Tests
2.8	Setup Procedures for Standard or Nominal Test Conditions
2.9	Setup Procedures for Worst Case Test Conditions
3	Detailed Procedures
3.1	Functional Testing Procedures
3.2	Robustness Testing Procedures
3.3	Stress Testing Procedures
3.4	Safety Testing Procedures
4	Test Reporting
4.1	Validation Test Information Sheet
4.2	Software Test Log
4.3	Software Test Report
4.4	Anomaly Report
Appendix I	Validation Test Information Sheets

The detailed requirements for test setup, measurements, and steps and the conclusion for each test to be conducted during the software validation testing are presented in a separate section of the SVTPR. The detailed test procedures are documented on a VTIS, and each is then included in the SVTPR. Each VTIS describes the test objective, approach, instrumentation, and duration; describes the data collection, reduction, and analysis requirements; and provides space for recording test results. The VTIS, with results, is delivered to the software V&V lead engineer at the completion of each test.

Prior to the start of software validation testing, the developed software's load map, its symbol file or listing, and a cross-reference file or listing should be generated from the baselined software. These files and listings are used during validation testing to identify expected test paths and memory locations. The program load map, symbol file, and cross-reference files used during software validation testing are submitted on magnetic media to the project's software configuration manager at the completion of each stage of the validation testing, for archiving in accordance with the SCMP.

Configuration files, batch files, log and trace files, and command files are generated before and during software validation testing to document test configurations, support data analysis, and ensure retestability. These files are also submitted on magnetic media to the project's software configuration manager at the completion of each stage of the validation testing, for archiving in accordance with the SCMP. Other supportive test data, such as screen dumps, that are collected during validation testing are attached to the associated VTISs at the completion of validation testing.

Section 2 of the SVTPR presents the generic software validation test procedures, the steps that are repetitive, redundant, and required for multiple validation test procedures. The steps that are required to configure the required test instrumentation and to establish and/or record the instrument operational characteristics (Section 2.1) are often generic and repetitive. These generic test tool setups are collected, grouped into categories for easy reference, and described in Section 2.1. All test tool setups referenced in this section are delivered on magnetic media to the project's software configuration manager at the conclusion of all software validation testing. The types of tools described in this section include the debugger tool(s), software performance analysis tools, automated test tools, and software complexity analysis tools.

Many of the software validation tests may require that the software and an emulation configuration be installed on a PC or workstation. The emulation system command files required to execute an emulation session with a specific emulation configuration are described in Section 2.2. All command files referenced in this section are delivered on magnetic media to the project's software configuration manager at the conclusion of all software validation testing. The types of emulation test configurations documented in this section include the emulator initialization command file, as well as the different command files used to install the required emulation configuration.

Section 2.3 presents the required steps that transfer the device from one operational mode to another. For example, it lists the procedures that would allow the device to change from the RUN mode to the HOLD mode, from the RUN mode to the ALARM mode, or from the RUN mode to the OFF mode. The remaining sections present the detailed procedural lists related to the generic test setup, the procedures necessary to restart a validation test, the wrap-up test procedures, the remote communications test setup procedures, the standard or nominal test conditions setup, and the worst case test conditions setup.

Section 3 presents the detailed software validation test procedures for functional, robustness, stress, and safety testing. Detailed procedural steps are presented for each of these categories. Where possible, the generic test setup procedures documented in the previous section are referenced in this section by name and section number.

Section 4 presents the details of software validation test reporting; the VTISs to be used for software validation testing are in Appendix I. The completed VTISs are provided to the software V&V lead engineer for review and approval, are kept in a central location, and are made available for review by the software development group and the project management group.

An SVTL (shown in Figure 5-3) is used to document all significant V&V activities that occur during the software validation testing. During and at the conclusion of the testing, the SVTL is used to evaluate the test results and to support regression testing. The Software Validation Test Report, generated at the conclusion of all testing, represents the record of software validation testing that was performed on the software. The test report may be in a format that is appropriate for technical disclosure and is governed by software V&V procedures. The report presents a summary of all of the tests that were performed, a summary of the analysis and evaluation of the test results, a summary of the anomalies and resolutions, and an assessment of the overall software quality, with any recommendations.

Anomaly Report

Reporting of software test problems uncovered through DTIS or VTIS testing is initiated by the software development and V&V engineer(s) through the use of the Software Anomaly Report (shown in Figure 5-4). The information required in the anomaly report includes how, when, and where the anomaly occurred and the impact of the problem on the system capability of the product and on continued validation testing. The Software Anomaly Report is a form in the SVVP; instructions for completing the various sections of the anomaly report can be provided in the SVVP, on the reverse side of the form, or in any other document (such as the SOPs or the guidelines). Each anomaly report contains a description and the location of the anomaly, assesses the severity of the anomaly, if it can be determined, describes the cause for and method of identifying the anomalous behavior, and includes the recommended action and the actions taken to correct the anomalous behavior. Anomaly reports are identified by a sequential serial number assigned by the project's software configuration manager. When completed, the anomaly reports are delivered to the project's software configuration manager for configuration identification, tracking, and status reporting.

Verification and Validation Report

The SVVR describes the overall status of the device software and summarizes the project's V&V tasks and results, as well as the status and disposition of anomalies. An assessment of the overall software quality and any recommendations for software and/or development process improvements are also documented in the SVVR. The report is generated after all of the V&V tasks for the project have been completed. The SVVR should include, at minimum, a summary of all V&V tasks performed, a summary of task results, a summary of anomalies and resolutions, an assessment of the overall software quality, and any recommendations for software and/or process improvements. The SVVR should include the actual results of the testing performed by the software V&V group. This document serves as the certification that the software was developed in a manner consistent with software development policies, procedures, and guidelines; that the software satisfies the documented requirements; and that the documented design was implemented.

Software Documentation Usage

Now that the software project documents have been reviewed, we can acquire a perspective of how the various documents are used. Figure 5-8 shows the typical software project documentation and how it interacts with the various software project activities. To set the perspective of

Figure 5-8   Software documentation flow and usage

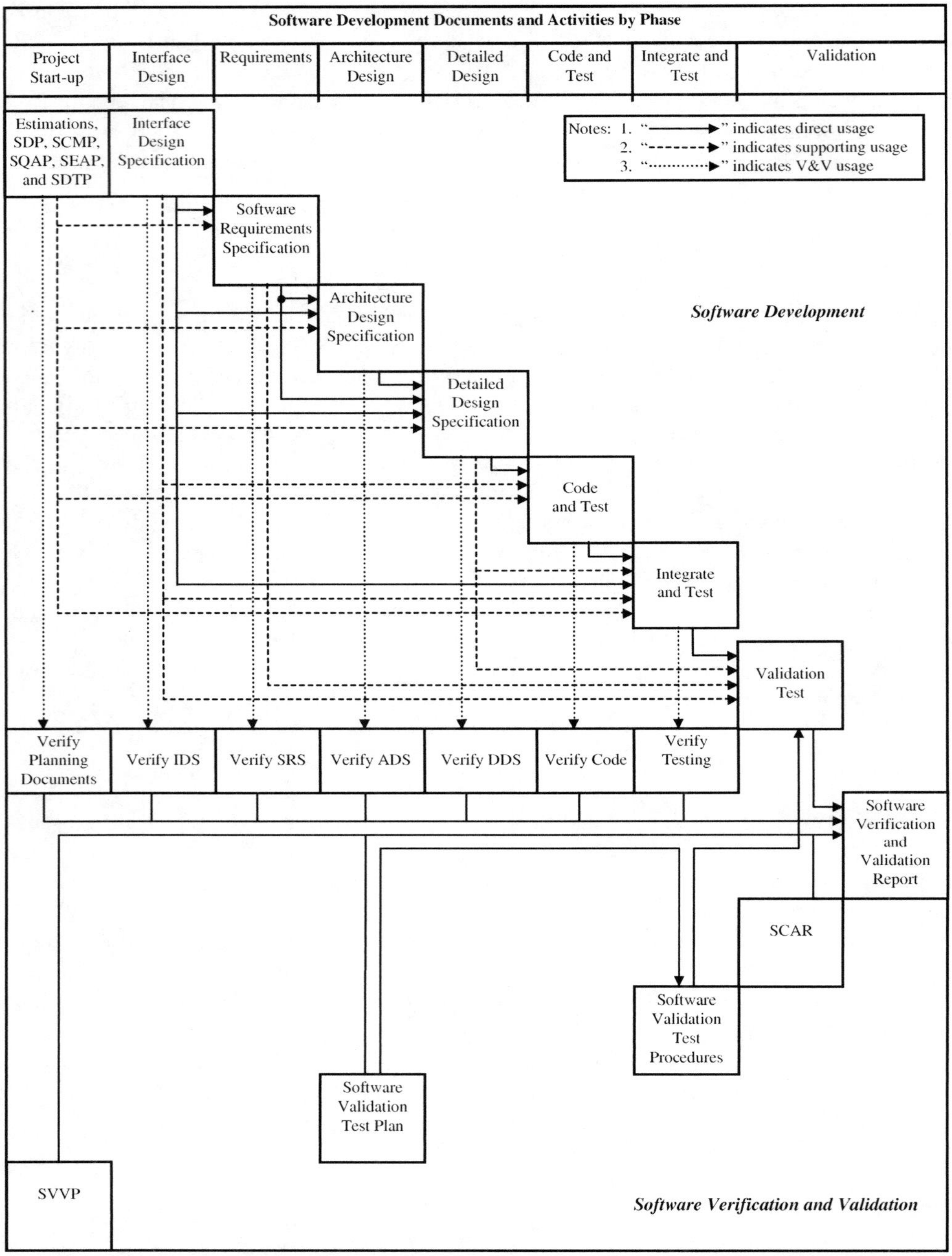

Software Development Documents and Activities by Phase

Project Start-up | Interface Design | Requirements | Architecture Design | Detailed Design | Code and Test | Integrate and Test | Validation

Estimations, SDP, SCMP, SQAP, SEAP, and SDTP

Interface Design Specification

Notes: 1. "———▶" indicates direct usage
       2. "------▶" indicates supporting usage
       3. "·········▶" indicates V&V usage

Software Requirements Specification

Architecture Design Specification

Software Development

Detailed Design Specification

Code and Test

Integrate and Test

Validation Test

Verify Planning Documents | Verify IDS | Verify SRS | Verify ADS | Verify DDS | Verify Code | Verify Testing

Software Verification and Validation Report

SCAR

Software Validation Test Procedures

Software Validation Test Plan

SVVP

Software Verification and Validation

this figure, it is assumed that the product- or system-related activities of defining product objectives, performing systems requirements analysis, and determining conceptual design have been concluded; they would be shown to the immediate left of this figure. Similarly, it is assumed that some form of challenge testing or design validation testing would normally occur after the SVVR has been generated; it would be illustrated to the right of this diagram. Across the top of Figure 5-8 are the various phases of the software project activities. Below them are the software development product documents and activities, the verification and validation (V&V) activities that transpire during the particular phase, and the associated planning documents. The lines with arrows indicate the flow of documents from several standpoints. The solid lines indicate that a preceding document or activity is used as a basis for a succeeding document, event, or activity within a particular phase. The dashed lines indicate that a preceding document or activity is required to directly support or accomplish the activities, events, or documents in a particular phase. The dotted lines indicate that documents or activities in a phase are used to perform V&V on the results of that phase.

As depicted in Figure 5-8, for example, the IDS is used to support the Requirements Phase, the Architecture and Detailed Design phases, the Integration and Test Phase, and the Software Validation Phase, because it contains part of the software design and its related requirements. The IDS must also be verified according to the policies, SOPs, and any guidelines that pertain to it. The SRS is created as a source document in the Requirements Phase; when it is completed and approved, it is then verified as part of the software V&V activities in accordance with the policies, SOPs, and any guidelines discussed in Chapter 3. The SRS is also used as a source input document, to accomplish the device's architecture design and to generate the ADS. The ADS can also be used to begin the coding of the device software's control flow, data flow, and data structures (not shown). The ADS is verified as part of the software V&V activities in accordance with the policies, SOPs, and any guidelines specified previously.

The ADS is used, in turn, as an input source document to the Detailed Design Phase and for the generation of the DDS. The DDS is then verified as part of the software V&V activities in accordance with the policies, SOPs, and any of the guidelines discussed in Chapter 3. The DDS and the IDS are subsequently used by software engineers as blueprints for coding and testing the device software. While the code is being developed and tested, the V&V group verifies that the code meets the applicable specifications. The debugged software is then used as source input information to the Integration and Test Phase. While the code is undergoing integration and further testing, the V&V group continues to verify that the code is evolving to meet the appropriate specifications. When all of the code has been integrated and a completed device software system has been achieved, the software undergoes software validation testing, followed by the generation of the SVVR.

6

The Software Quality Assurance Program: Software Development Activities

Though this be madness, yet there is method in it.

—William Shakespeare

Software engineering is a relatively new technological discipline. It is distinct from, but based on, the foundations laid by computer science, management science, economics, communication skills, and the engineering approach to problem solving. Software engineering is a pragmatic discipline that relies on computer science to provide a scientific foundation in the same way that traditional hardware engineering disciplines rely on physics and chemistry. Software engineering is a labor-intensive activity that requires both technical skill and managerial control. Consequently, management science provides the foundations for software project management. Software must be developed and maintained on time and within budget. Thus, economics builds the foundation for resource estimation and cost control. Software engineering activities occur within an organizational context; a high degree of communication is required among customers, management, software engineers, hardware engineers, and other technologists. Solid oral, written, and interpersonal communication skills are crucial for the software engineer.

Software engineering is concerned with the development and maintenance of technological products; therefore, the problem-solving techniques common to all engineering disciplines are utilized. Engineering problem-solving techniques provide the basis for project planning, project management, systematic analysis, methodical design, careful fabrication, extensive validation, and ongoing maintenance activities. Appropriate notations, tools, and techniques are applied in each of these areas by the software engineer. Engineers balance scientific principles, economic issues, and social concerns in a pragmatic manner when solving problems and developing technological products. Concepts from computer science, management science, economics, and communication skills are all combined within the framework of software engineering problem solving.

Software engineering and traditional engineering disciplines share a pragmatic approach to the development and maintenance of technological artifacts. However, there are significant differences between software engineering and traditional engineering. The fundamental sources of these differences for software are the lack of physical laws and natural or inherent interme-diate product visibility, and the obscurity of the interfaces between the software modules. Soft-ware is an intangible element that has no mass, no volume, and no physical properties. Source code is merely a static image of the software that solves a technical problem or implements a market need; while the effects produced by the software are usually observable, the source code, in and of itself, is not. Software failures are caused by design and implementation errors, not by the degradation of the software over time. Because software is intangible, extraordinary mea-sures must be taken to determine the status of a software product that is being developed. It is easy for optimistic and opportunistic individuals to state that their software product is "95 per-cent complete"; it is difficult for software engineers and their managers to assess the real progress and to spot the problem areas, except in hindsight.

Because software has no physical properties, it is not subject to the laws of gravity, ther-modynamics, or conductivity. Consequently, there are no equations to guide software develop-ment. Intangibility and a lack of physical properties for software development limit the number of fundamental guidelines and basic constraints available to shape the design and implementa-tion of the software product. Software design is comparable to the architectural design of build-ings in the absence of gravity; the excessive degrees of freedom are both a blessing and a curse to software engineering.

In a very real sense, the software engineer creates a model of a physical situation in soft-ware. The mapping between the model and the reality being modeled is the intellectual distance between the problem and the computerized solution to the problem. One fundamental principle of software engineering is to design software products to minimize the intellectual distance between the problem and its software solution. However, the variety of approaches to software development is limited only by the creativity and ingenuity of the software engineer; often, it is not clear which approach will minimize the intellectual distance, and frequently, different approaches will minimize different dimensions of this intellectual distance. This implies that use of the principles and guidelines of software engineering should always be tempered by the particular situation and the problem to be solved.

Obscurity of the interfaces among software modules also distinguishes software engineering from traditional engineering disciplines. A fundamental principle for managing complexity is to decompose a large system into smaller, more manageable subunits with well-defined inter-faces. This particular approach of divide and conquer is routinely used in engineering disciplines, in architecture, and in other disciplines that involve the analysis and synthesis of complex arti-facts. In software engineering, the units of decomposition are generally called "modules," and modules have both control interfaces and data interfaces.

Control interfaces are established by the calling or invocation relationships among the mod-ules; data interfaces are manifest in the parameters that are passed between the modules, as well as in the global data items shared among the modules. It is difficult to design a software system so that all of the control and data interfaces among the modules are explicit and the mod-ules do not interact to produce unexpected side effects when they invoke one another. These unexpected side effects severely complicate the interfaces among modules, as well as the doc-umentation, verification, testing, and modification of the software product. The data interfaces among software modules must be exact. For example, the number and types of positional para-meters passed among specific routines or modules must agree in every detail. There is no con-cept of an "almost" integer parameter or of a global data structure that is "almost" of the correct dimension(s). Constructing a stable software product is analogous to constructing a skyscraper, in which the stability of the entire structure depends on an exact fit of every door in the building, because a less than exact fit might cause the entire structure to fail.

Significant advances have been made in all areas of software engineering. For example, analysis techniques for determining software requirements and notations for expressing these requirements have been developed. Methodical approaches to the design of software products have evolved, and design notations that relate to those approaches have proliferated. Implementation techniques have been improved, and new programming languages have been developed to support these advances. Software validation techniques and quality assurance procedures have been instituted. Formal techniques for verifying the properties of the software have evolved, and software maintenance procedures have been improved. Management techniques have been tailored to software engineering. The problems of group dynamics and project communication have been explored. Quantitative models for project estimation and product reliability have evolved, and fundamental principles of analysis, design, implementation, and testing have been perfected. Automated software tools have been developed to increase the quality of the software, the productivity of the software engineer, and the management of the software project. New technical journals, as well as existing journals, devote increasing attention to software engineering topics. Domestic and international technical conferences, held on a regular basis, increasingly address software engineering.

All of this activity should not be interpreted to mean that the problems of software engineering have been solved. In fact, the level of activity is indicative of the vast number of problems remaining to be solved. Every technology evolves through the predictable phases of ad hoc invention, to the development of systematic procedures, and eventually to the culmination of a routine, handbook approach to the discipline. The technology of software engineering still involves a great deal of ad hoc invention; however, the current strategy is to document the process and get on to the handbook.

Software Requirements Engineering

In theory, requirements engineering applies proven principles, techniques, languages, and tools to help software analysts understand or describe a potential product's external behavior. In practice, product owners often wonder if anyone is really listening. The transformation of technology to a product that meets a user's requirements is difficult in every software engineering field, but the problem with requirements engineering is even more difficult. For example, customer and user needs are often impossible to realize until after the product or device has been built. Even when the requirements are stated up front, it is a given fact that they will change more than once during the software development cycle, and it is certain that they will change immediately after deployment of the device. The time between the requirements phase and product delivery is usually too long to pinpoint how specific requirements gathering techniques contributed to the device's success or failure.

It is generally accepted that a requirements document contains a description of what the product will do without describing how it will do it. In abstract form, this presents a paradox; it leaves unresolved the issue that "one person's 'how' is another person's 'what'" (Davis 1993). Furthermore, it is difficult to separate the "how" from the "what" in practice, because requirements model the device to be developed by using abstractions to produce a view of the product that is independent of the method and notation to be used. For example, the requirement "Accuracy shall be ±5 percent," is good, but you also need to understand how accurate the feature will be when implemented within the device. Measuring accuracy to within two decimal places when the overall system accuracy is good to one decimal place is meaningless. An implementation strategy that does not allow for the appropriate level of detail and precision may never meet the accuracy requirement.

Inquiry-Based Requirements Analysis

The inquiry requirements analysis model is a formal structure for describing discussions about requirements when no easily identifiable customer or customer-sanctioned requirements documentation can be identified. The model uses a conversation metaphor that follows analysis activities from eliciting requirements to documenting them to refining them. The model has three stages: documentation, discussion, and evolution. During requirements documentation, users, customers, and anyone who can provide information about the product, its implementation constraints, or the problem domain generate a list of the proposed requirements. In requirements discussion, the same individuals challenge proposed requirements by flagging and annotating them. Finally, this same group attaches change requests to the requirements on the basis of the preceding discussion and flagged requirements. The requirements are then refined when the change requests are approved.

In this model, "requirements" is a term given to all requirements-related information. This includes assumptions, scenarios, project planning commitments, implementation constraints, and the stated requirements themselves. In some projects, requirements analysis begins with some form of requirements documentation; in others, requirements may already exist as a statement of goals. However vague or well defined the starting point, the inquiry cycle model result will be a well-refined, agreed-on specification representing the requirements that describe the desired product. If there is no requirements document initially, then this model provides a systematic and incremental process for generating one.

There are several ways to analyze requirements while in the documentation stage. If a requirements document already exists, then the analysis can begin with review of that document. If such a document does not exist, then the requirements must be based on interviews, technical documentation, focus group output, or any other method used to gather fledgling requirements. One valuable technique is scenario analysis, in which a description of one or more end-to-end situations involving the required device and its environment is formulated. On the basis of these scenarios, requirements analysis is documented depending on the level of detail needed.

Although scenarios are useful in acquiring and validating the requirements, the scenarios themselves are not to be construed as a requirement. The scenario merely depicts the product's behavior only in a specific situation, whereas the specification describes what the product will do in general. An advantage of this method is that what-if questions about the product's interaction with its environment are easy to propose and analyze. Answering the what-if question by analyzing specific scenarios usually provides insights into general requirements and helps the refinement process.

The requirements discussion usually begins with questions about a requirement. This is followed by descriptive answers or solutions to the problem or question, in the form of refinements or revisions that respond to the initial question. It is likely that a question will generate many answers, and some answers may require justification if they are not immediately obvious. The intent of the answers is to evoke a clearer understanding of the requirements and help draw attention to ambiguities, missing requirements, and inconsistencies. Requirements discussions can take place gradually and informally or in formal review settings.

The ultimate result of the requirements discussion is a commitment to either freeze a requirement or to change it. A change may be traced backward to its discussion, which constitutes its rationale, and forward to the changed requirement once it has been acted on and approved. Requirements discussions can take place gradually and informally or in formal review settings.

The inquiry cycle model is not particularly rigid, and shortcuts are always possible. For example, a requirement may be changed after little or no discussion; an answer may be generated even when no question about a requirement was posed, particularly when assumptions are not articulated well or are not explicitly documented; choices may lack rationale because the reasons are viewed as obvious; and a change request may be implemented without recorded discussion. Any shortcut may be perfectly reasonable in some circumstances.

The model also embeds no assumptions about the specification language or style of the requirements expression. In addition, the model is consistent with incremental development of formal specifications, object-oriented analysis, and structured analysis models. For example, in object-oriented analysis, the requirements document evolves from a textual description of system requirements or typical use cases to a collection of object and dynamic models. The requirements discussion consists of identifying and challenging candidate objects, attributes, associations, and operations. Whatever the representation or method, the analysis progresses toward a more precise specification of the requirements through the incremental process of challenging and changing requirements.

Requirements Analysis through Scenarios

Requirements specifications are typically generated after consulting with the user or customer. There are several ways to gather and analyze requirements, and various techniques can then be applied that lead the way to a high-level or architecture design. The most popular is structured analysis, which partitions the product requirements, and object-oriented analysis, which describes the device in terms of objects, their data attributes and operations, interobject communication, object relations, and structures. In scenario analysis, hypothetical and believable situations are proposed. For these situations, possible ways to use the product to accomplish some function that the user desires are analyzed, and they can be used to describe the external product behavior directly from the user's point of view. Scenarios can also be used to support early and continued user involvement and interaction during requirements analysis and to provide guidelines to build a cost-effective prototype, help validate the requirements specification, and furnish acceptance criteria for requirements testing.

Scenario analysis is the process of understanding, analyzing, and describing product, device, or system behavior in terms of the particular ways that the product, device, or system will be used. Typically, the requirements analyst conducts scenario analysis with input from a user or customer who determines the desired functions and capabilities and the individual who operates or uses the system. The requirements analyst must understand and describe the behavior as the anticipated user perceives it. The end product of scenario analysis is a document that consists of sets of correct, complete, consistent, and validated scenarios. This document then becomes an integral part of the system or product requirements specification, and it is used as a guide for the design and testing phases.

The scenario analysis model consists of six stages; user involvement varies in each stage, but it never disappears. The model begins with scenario elicitation and the construction of a scenario tree, which describes and represents all of the scenarios for a particular user view. A user view is a set of specific scenarios as seen by a certain group of people who use the product, device, or system in a similar manner. The user view, therefore, describes the behavior of users as they interact with the product. Each user view consists of scenarios initiated by external users, stimuli, or functional components, such as modules or events. Scenarios consist of events or specific stimuli that change the system or product state, trigger another event, or both. Events are usually short and can be both an input and response that are internal and external to the system. An event type includes all of the possible events that have similar attributes. A scenario schema is a sequence of event types that accomplish a functional requirement. A scenario instance is an instantiation of a scenario schema. The scenario instance has a specific user and specific interactions between the user and the product, device, or system.

In the next stage, each scenario tree is converted into an equivalent regular grammar used to construct a conceptual state machine that models the device or system from a particular user view. In this state machine, the model nodes are system states, and the edges between the nodes are the events. The grammar and the conceptual state machine constitute the abstract formal model used to capture, represent, and display scenario system behavior.

Next, the abstract formal model is verified by manually checking the abstract model for any errors in expected behavior, to uncover inconsistencies, redundancies, and internal incompleteness in the scenario. If an error is discovered in this stage, the model returns to the first step and the formalization process is repeated. If no error is detected, the verified process is used to generate the scenarios in the verified abstract formal model by means of the conceptual state machine. In the fifth stage, rapid prototype development is used to construct the expected device on the basis of the scenarios generated previously; the result is a conceptual system. Last, the system prototype is used to validate the scenarios and demonstrate their validity to the user. If invalid scenarios are uncovered, the model returns to the first stage, and the steps are repeated until the scenarios are validated. Scenario analysis ends when both the requirements analyst and the user group are satisfied that the scenarios are valid.

This model is valid only for products, devices, or systems that have a single response to a stimulus, such as user interfaces. It is not suitable for a complex system that requires concurrent stimuli and responses. However, this limitation is not overly important because in nearly all user interface or user-machine interaction, there is generally only one event response to a stimulus. Because scenario analysis produces a set of complete and consistent scenarios, it essentially provides the input for product, device, or system acceptance testing. Whereas, in current practice, requirements must be reintroduced to drive test cases, with scenario analysis, the scenarios themselves can be used as test cases. This potentially saves the organization time because it need not create acceptance tests or form an acceptance test group. In addition, the set of scenarios can be shared among the development and test group, which ensures that the direction and goals of the project remain intact.

Prioritizing Software Requirements by Cost of Quality

System or product features, functions, and attribute requirements drive software projects, and they must be effectively and accurately managed. When the requirements have been agreed to, they can be used as a focal point for the development process and can help produce software that comes closer to meeting the expectations for the product. In real-world software development, there are usually more requirements than can be implemented with the time and resource constraints. Consequently, software lead engineers face a dilemma: Is there a way to select a subset of the requirements and still produce a system that meets the product needs? Is there a simple, effective and reproducible technique for prioritizing requirements? Beyond addressing the project scope, clear and unambiguous knowledge about requirement priorities helps to focus the development process and more effectively and efficiently manage projects. It can also help to make acceptable tradeoffs among conflicting goals such as quality, cost and time-to-market. In addition, resources can be allocated on the basis of the requirement's importance to the project as a whole. When time to market is particularly important, knowing how to rank requirements can help in planning releases by indicating which functions are critical and which can be added (and in what order) over successive releases. The cost-value approach is an analytical tool for prioritizing requirements and ranks requirements in two dimensions: according to their value to customer and users and according to their estimated cost of implementation.

A process for prioritizing software requirements must be simple and fast and yield accurate and reliable results. The prioritizing process must also satisfy quality, cost, and schedule demands; quality must be maximized, cost minimized, and time to delivery as short as possible. The cost-value approach prioritizes requirements according to their relative value and cost and, on the basis of this information, software managers can make decisions about which requirements can be excluded from the first release to keep the time to market at a minimum. In this scheme, *quality* relates to a requirement's potential contribution to customer satisfaction with the resulting system, and *cost* is the cost of successfully implementing the requirement. In practice, prioritizing based on relative rather than absolute assignments is faster, more accurate, and more reliable. The process is one of investigating project requirements by comparing requirements pairwise according to their relative value and cost. The pairwise comparison approach includes considerable redundancy and is thus less sensitive to judgment errors common to techniques using absolute assignments. An indication of inconsistencies can be determined by calculating a consistency ratio; the smaller the consistency ratio, the fewer the inconsistencies, and thus the more reliable the results.

There are five steps to prioritizing requirements by means of the cost-value approach. First, requirement engineers carefully review the requirements for completeness and to ensure that they are stated in an unambiguous way. Second, appropriate individuals apply a pairwise comparison method to assess the relative value of the candidate requirements. Third, experienced software engineers use the pairwise comparison to estimate the relative cost of implementing each requirement. Fourth, a software engineer calculates each candidate requirement's relative value and implementation cost and plots these on a cost-value diagram. Last, the appropriate individuals use the cost-value diagram as a conceptual map for analyzing and discussing the requirements. The result of the discussions is to prioritize the requirements and decide which will actually be implemented in which software release.

As an example, assume that you want to evaluate candidate requirements for a medical device to determine their relative value, and the requirements are R1, R2, R3, and R4. First, set the n requirements into the rows and columns of an $n \times n$, in this case a 4×4, matrix (see Table 6-1). Second, in all positions on the main diagonal insert the relative value 1. Third,

Table 6-1   An Example of Pairwise Comparison of Cost-Value Requirements

	Requirement			
	R1	**R2**	**R3**	**R4**
R1	1	1/3	2	4
R2	3	1	5	3
R3	1/2	1/5	1	1/3
R4	1/4	1/3	3	1

perform pairwise comparisons of all the requirements according to the criterion, using the scale shown in Table 6-2. For each pair of requirements (starting with R1 and R2) insert their relative value in the cell where the row of R1 meets the column of R2 (R1, R2) and in position (R2, R1) insert the reciprocal value (see Table 6-1). Continue to perform pairwise comparisons of R1 and R3, R1 and R4, R2 and R3, and so forth. For a matrix of order *n*, there are $n \times (n - 1)/2$ comparisons required. Table 6-3 is an example of this method in which six pairwise comparisons are required.

Fourth, estimate the criterion distribution by summing each of the *n* columns in the comparison matrix (from Table 6-1) and then dividing each element in the matrix by the sum of the column the element is a member of. For example, the sum of column R1 is 4.75 (from Table 6-1), and each element of the column has been divided by this value to produce the values 0.21, 0.63, 0.11, and 0.05, as shown in Table 6-3. The rest of the columns have been produced similarly. Fifth, the sum of the rows (Sum column of Table 6-3) has been normalized by dividing the sum of each row by the number of requirements, by 4 in this case, and the result entered into the Priority column of Table 6-3. The result of this computation is referred to as the *priority*

Table 6-2   Scale for Pairwise Comparison of Cost-Value Requirements

Relative Intensity	Definition	Notes
1	Of equal value	Two are of equal value
3	Slightly more value	Experience slightly favors one over the other
5	Essential or strong value	Experience strongly favors one over the other
7	Very strong value	Strongly favored, and its dominance is demonstrated in practice
9	Extreme value	Favoring one over another is of the highest possible order
2, 4, 6, 8	Intermediate values between two adjacent judgments	Use when compromise is needed

Note: If requirement *i* is assigned the value *v* when compared with requirement *j*, then *j* has the reciprocal $(1/v)$ value when compared with *i*.

Table 6-3   An Example of an Analysis of Pairwise Comparison of Cost-Value Requirements

	Requirement				Sum	Priority
	R1	R2	R3	R4		
Sum	4.75	1.01	0.99	1.00		
R1	0.21	0.18	0.18	0.48	1.05	0.26
R2	0.63	0.54	0.45	0.36	1.98	0.50
R3	0.11	0.11	0.09	0.04	0.34	0.09
R4	0.05	0.18	0.27	0.12	0.62	0.16

matrix, and each requirement's relative value is based on the values in the Priority column of Table 6-3. For this example, the information can be interpreted as:

- Requirement R1 contains 26 percent of the total value of all requirements
- Requirement R2 contains 50 percent,
- Requirement R3 contains 9 percent, and
- Requirement R4 contains 16 percent.

If we were able to determine precisely the relative value of all requirements, then the values would be perfectly consistent. In practice, however, we are more likely to determine that R1 is much more valuable than R2, R2 is somewhat more valuable than R3, and R3 is slightly more valuable than R1. This illustrates that an inconsistency in the comparison has occurred; consequently, the resulting accuracy is diminished. However, the redundancy of the pairwise comparisons makes this approach less sensitive to judgment errors, and it also provides a measure of the judgment errors. The *consistency index (CI)* is an indicator of the result accuracy for the pairwise comparisons and is calculated as

$$CI = (\lambda_{max} - n) / (n - 1),$$ (6.1)

where λ_{max} denotes the maximum principal value of the comparison matrix and n is the number of requirements compared. The closer the value of λ_{max} is to n, the smaller the judgment errors and consequently the more consistent the result. To estimate λ_{max}, multiply the comparison matrix (Table 6-1) by the priority vector (Priority column of Table 6-3), and then divide the first element of the resulting vector by the first element in the priority vector, the second element of the resulting vector by the second element in the priority vector, and so on. The value of λ_{max} is then calculated as the average of the elements in the resulting vector or $\lambda_{max} = [(4.66 + 4.40 + 4.29 + 4.13) / 4] = 4.37$. The consistency index can be calculated as $CI = [(4.37 - 4) / (4 - 1)] = 0.12$. The final step is to determine if the resulting consistency index ($CI = 0.12$) is acceptable; that is determined by calculating the *consistency ratio.*

The *CI* of randomly generated reciprocal matrices from the scale 1 to 9 is called the *random index (RI)*. The ratio of *CI* to *RI* for the same-order matrix, called the *consistency ratio (CR)*, defines the accuracy of the pairwise comparisons

$$CR = CI / RI.$$ (6.2)

According to Table 6-4, the *RI* for matrices of order 4 is 0.90, and the consistency ratio for our example is $CR = (0.12) / (0.90) = 0.14$. As a general rule, a consistency ratio of 0.10 or less

Table 6-4 Consistency Indices of Randomly Generated Reciprocal Matrices

Matrix Order	Random Indices	Matrix Order	Random Indices	Matrix Order	Random Indices
1	0.00	6	1.24	11	1.51
2	0.00	7	1.32	12	1.48
3	0.58	8	1.41	13	1.56
4	0.90	9	1.45	14	1.57
5	1.12	10	1.49	15	1.59

is considered acceptable. For the example, the result is less than ideal, although in practice consistency ratios exceeding 0.10 are common.

Although the cost-value approach is intuitive and more useful than traditional approaches, making all of the required pairwise comparisons is not only tedious but sometimes requires backtracking to check the consistency of earlier pairwise comparisons. Moreover, the method does not account for interdependencies between requirements. For example, the implementation of a low-cost, high-value requirement requires the implementation of a high-cost, low-value requirement as well. This situation probably will not be a factor in cases in which the requirement sets are small, but with a larger number of requirements, it could be a major impediment. A case of more requirements also raises the issue of complexity, since the number of pairwise comparisons is of order n^2 where n is number of total requirements considered. This is offset by the fact that the cost-value method is based on a well-established analytical technique and, with reasonable effort, provides a clear indication of the relative costs and values of all candidate requirements.

Quality Function Deployment in Software

In response to the need for software quality, manifested by intense and global competition, Quality Function Deployment (QFD), as the implementation of Total Quality Management (TQM), has become prevalent. Specifically, QFD has been proposed as an effective approach for implementing quality improvement programs in a variety of product and service environments and has been adapted for the development of software (Haag, Raja, and Schkade 1996). This adaptation, termed Software Quality Function Deployment (SQFD), represents the transfer of QFD technology from its traditional environment to the software development environment. SQFD focuses on improving the quality of the software development process by implementing quality improvement techniques during the requirements solicitation stages of the product development life cycle. These quality improvement techniques lead to increased analyst and programmer productivity, fewer design changes, a reduction in the number of errors passed from one phase to the next, and quality software systems that satisfy customer and user requirements. The new software developed with SQFD also requires less maintenance and, consequently, allows organizations to shift resources and funds to new product development.

SQFD, adaptable to any software engineering methodology, quantifiably solicits and defines critical customer and user requirements. SQFD precedes the system development life cycle process and allows it to remain intact. Specifically, SQFD is an adaptation of the A-1 matrix, the House of Quality, which is the most commonly used matrix in the traditional QFD methodology. In this adaptation, SQFD consists of five distinct steps.

In the first step, customer or user requirements are solicited and recorded on the left y-axis of the A-1 matrix. The customers or users would include end users, managers, system development personnel, and any individual who would benefit from the use of the proposed software system. The requirements are recorded as short statements, specifically in the terminology of the user, and are accompanied by a detailed definition that forms the data dictionary of SQFD.

In step two, the requirements are converted to technical and measurable statements of the software and are recorded along the top x-axis of the A-1 matrix in cooperation with the customer. For example, "easy to use" may be converted to "time to complete the tutorial," "number of icons," or "number of on-line help facilities" and "user friendly" might be converted to "number of menus," "number of menu levels," or "number of input fields." It is important to understand that some user requirements may convert or translate into multiple, technical product specifications, which require crucial and extensive user involvement. In addition, the technical product specifications must be measurable in some form, because they will be used to generate the metrics that will help to guide subsequent implementation. For example, the user requirement "provides multiple print formats" may be converted to "number of print formats," and "provides strip chart output" translates to "yes" or "no," a Boolean value.

In step three, users are asked to complete the A-1 correlation matrix by identifying the strength of the relationships between the various requirements on the left and the technical specification at the top. For example, "easy to learn" is highly correlated with "time to complete tutorial," moderately correlated with "number of input fields" and has no correlation with "number of print formats." In the SQFD scheme of things, high correlation is given a score of 9, and no correlation would receive a score of 0. Because all of the identified customers and users participate in this activity, it is important that a consensus be reached about the strengths entered in the correlation matrix.

On the basis of customer survey data about the proposed product, the requirements priorities for the stated customer requirements are developed and listed on the right y-axis (step four). At this point, additional information may be gathered from customers and users concerning assessments of competitor products. Data on sales and improvement indices may be gathered from the development team.

Step five involves developing priorities of the technical product specifications and entering them on the bottom x-axis. This is done by summing the results of the multiplication of user requirement priorities by the correlation values between the customer requirements and the technical product specifications. These raw priority weights for the technical product specifications are then converted to a percentage of the total raw priority weights. Additional data may be solicited from the development team concerning targeted measures of the technical product specifications, along with estimates of cost, difficulty, and schedule feasibility. The end result of the SQFD process will contain measurable technical product specifications, their priority, and targeted measures. All of this information is then carried into the software development life cycle.

Heuristics, Rigor, and Cost in Software Design

The fundamental basis for maintaining the conceptual integrity of software development is a rigorous design. As described in Chapter 1, it was originally imagined that heuristic design methods were sufficient to ensure the integrity of the developed software. After all, it seemed a simple, although tedious, task for clever individuals to think up all of the pieces that had to be built, implement them, and make sure that nothing was left out. As we have seen, there is still a legacy of heuristic thinking in software development.

The principal difference between heuristics and rigor in the design of software systems is in the integrity and stability of the design and that a heuristic design almost always works. When it does not work, however, it must be fixed and patched. After a series of such failures and subsequent fixes, the design becomes highly idiosyncratic, as a function of its failure history. In reality, this dependence on failure histories begins before the start of software design. The software designers practice a mental heuristic design process in which they mentally test and fix a heuristic design by thinking up situations and cases and flexing the design to discover deficiencies. The design thus becomes idiosyncratic as a function of the imaginary history of the perceived failures. A rigorous design will take more creativity and thought than its heuristic counterpart but, once created, the rigorous design is more stable. A rigorous design should survive its implementation, not be overcome by it, and provide a framework for the intelligent control of changes to the implementation as the requirements change.

The difference between heuristics and rigor in design can be illustrated in the construction of a tic-tac-toe program that commences play from any point within any game. Anyone with a pad and pencil can readily figure out what to do next in any situation, but writing down all such possibilities may be impractical. A heuristic approach could be based initially on the analysis process performed with pad and pencil, and it will account for some reasonable moves. However, it will fail in many situations, and subsequent analysis of these failures will suggest additional criteria of play for the program. As each addition is made, a less obvious situation may still lead to a failure, but after many additions, the program may be capable of perfect play. However, it will be difficult to prove perfect play outside of an exhaustive analysis, which will in turn be hard to prove complete. As noted, a heuristically developed design, even though possibly correct, will be highly idiosyncratic, on the basis of the history of the imagined and real failures encountered in play.

Getting a program to work is a by-product of getting it right, and a well-designed program can be expected to run correctly from the start. It is well known that no foolproof methods exist for determining that the last error in a program has been found; confidence is stronger when the first error in a program is never found. Program correctness is key to good program design because a discipline of rigor has been imposed on the software in place of heuristics. Any structured design process produces a stepwise refinement of the software that is derived and validated as successive functional expansions into simpler, more primitive functions. When the design moves from heuristic invention to rigorous deviation, the design structure survives the coding and becomes available for use in maintenance and modification, as well as implementation. Each refinement in effect marks the top of a hierarchy that later serves as an intermediate starting point for verification of the software correctness, or for adding capability to the program.

One of the most vexing problems of a software project is meeting cost and schedule commitments. One way to circumvent this problem is to reinterpret cost estimates as a design-to-cost methodology. If cost is to be fixed, then a new and fresh examination of the software specifications is required. For nearly any function needed within the device, software can be defined over a wide variety of costs; the basic functions of a software module are usually a small fraction of the total software that is ultimately built. The rest of the software deals with being friendly to the user, handling errors automatically, reaching fail-safe states, shutting down the system gracefully, and so on. All of these are important, but they can be prioritized in terms of the funds and time available for the project. For example, the typical split of basic to exception code in software is that 20 percent of the code handles 80 percent of the functions required. If the basic code is underestimated even by 100 percent, then the 20 percent is actually 40 percent and the split now becomes one of 40 percent of the code handling 60 percent of the function. This is most likely tolerable because it still allows 75 percent (60/80) of the exceptions to be handled, but the critical software management job is to make sure that the original basic 20 percent or new 40 percent is up and running within schedule and cost, at the expense, if necessary, of the original 80 percent or new 60 percent.

Design-to-cost is not a new idea, although it seems that way, given the historical track record of software projects. The basic design-to-cost methodology comes from simple, multilevel budgeting, in which a certain amount is withheld for a function and the rest is then available for other functions. In a software project, this can be applied at very nearly its full effect. For example, given a budget for an item of software, an appropriate fraction can be allocated to its overall design, starting at the top and working down the software structure. A critical part of this overall design is the allocation of the remaining funds to the construction of the software at the lower levels. The design-to-cost methodology forces the actual costs of starting construction at the top of the software to be taken out of the funds before the remainder is allocated to the rest of the software. The WBS structure is a good mechanism for arraying the funds of the software project.

Software Requirements versus Software Design

As medical products encompass more features and technology, they will grow in complexity and sophistication, and the hardware and software will be driven by necessity to become highly synergistic and intricate, which will, in turn, dictate tightly coupled designs. The dilemma is whether to tolerate longer development schedules to achieve the features and technology or to pursue shorter development schedules, but there really is no choice, given the competitive situation of the marketplace. One solution that achieves shorter software development schedules is a reduction of the number of requirements that represent the desired feature set to be implemented. By documenting requirements in a simpler way, the software effort can be reduced. When the complexity is reduced, the overall hardware and software requirements are reduced. In turn, the overall software test and V&V times are reduced. Limiting the requirements set helps because the number of requirements is directly proportional to the number of lines of code required to implement a feature; the number of lines of code is directly proportional to the development effort and schedule; and the development effort is directly proportional to the amount of time consumed in software testing and V&V.

One issue is how to reduce the number of documented requirements without sacrificing feature descriptions. This reduction can be achieved by limiting the number of documented requirements, being more judicious about how the specified requirements are defined, or recognizing that some requirements are really design requirements. A large part of requirements definition should be geared toward providing a means to delay making decisions about product feature requirements that are not understood until they are better understood.

V&V must test the product software to assure that the requirements have been met and that the specified design has been implemented. At worst, every software requirement will necessitate at least one test to demonstrate that it has been satisfied. At best, several requirements might be grouped such that at least one test will be required to demonstrate that they all have been satisfied. The goal for the software engineer is to specify the smallest number of requirements that still allow the desired feature set to be implemented. To understand these points, a few examples should be examined.

Refinement of Software Requirements

Suppose a mythical device has the requirement, "The output of the analog to digital converter (ADC) must be accurate to within plus or minus 5 percent" (see Figure 6-1). Although conceptually this appears to be a straightforward requirement, to the software engineer assigned the task of performing the testing to demonstrate satisfaction of this requirement, it is not as simple as it looks. As stated, this requirement will necessitate at least three independent tests, and most likely five or more tests. One test will have to establish that the ADC is generating the specified nominal value. The second and third tests will be needed to confirm that the output is within the plus or minus 5 percent range. To a good software engineer, the 5 percent limit is not as arbitrary as it may seem, because of the round-off errors associated with the percent calculation with the ADC output units. Consequently, the fourth and fifth tests will be done to ascertain the sensitivity of the round-off calculation.

Figure 6-1   Software requirements refinement, example 1

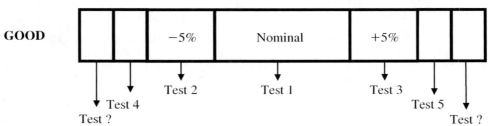

"The output of the ADC must be accurate to within plus or minus 5%."

GOOD

−5%   Nominal   +5%

Test 2   Test 1   Test 3

Test 4   Test 5

Test ?   Test ?

"The output of the ADC must be between X and Y."

BETTER

X   Y

Test 1   Test 2

Test ?   Test ?

A better way to specify this requirement is to state, "The output of the analog to digital converter (ADC) must be between X and Y," where the X and Y values correspond to the original requirement of plus or minus 5 percent. This is a better requirement statement because it simplifies the testing. In this case, only two tests are required to demonstrate satisfaction of this requirement. Test one is for the X value, and test two is for the Y value. The requirement statements are equivalent, but the latter is better because it has reduced the test set size, resulting in less testing time. Consequently, the product may reach the market earlier.

As another example (see Figure 6-2), suppose the marketing people want the next product to be user friendly and that they already know the basic content, layout, and navigation among the menus and features of this user-friendly product. There are several ways to document the user interface requirements of this new product. The question now becomes, Which one supports the corporate requirement of getting new products into the marketplace fastest? Let us examine the situation before analyzing how to document the user-friendliness requirements of the product. First, the marketing people already know that they want menus, and they have definite requirements on how the menus should function. Second, the menu particulars will need to be documented at some point so that the software engineers can implement what is needed. Third, the question to be asked is whether this user interface is requirements or design.

One option is to specify, "The user interface shall be user friendly." This is an adequate requirement statement but lacks credibility because it does not lend itself to testability and V&V. The phrase *user friendly* is not quantifiable and is not testable in its current form. Furthermore, the "user-friendly" interface is too generic, because a menu system is what marketing wants. Furthermore, the term *user friendly* is ambiguous, and additional information is needed to

Figure 6-2   Software requirements refinement, example 2

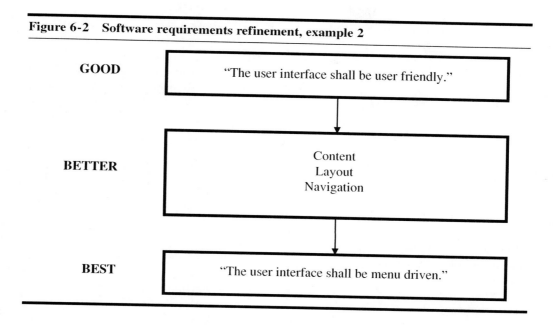

GOOD — "The user interface shall be user friendly."

BETTER — Content / Layout / Navigation

BEST — "The user interface shall be menu driven."

transform it as a requirement into the detailed content, layout, and navigation that are already known by the marketing group as the desired implementation.

A second option is to specify in the requirements document, "The user interface shall be menu driven." This is a well-defined requirement because it conveys what the user interface is without specifying how it will work. In this approach, the software verification is easy and straightforward to accomplish. The product either has a menu-driven interface or it does not, and demonstration of this requirement takes minutes, not hours. The details of how the menu-driven feature is implemented are already known and can be placed within the software design specification.

Another option is to specify in the software requirements document the known content, layout, and navigation of the menus. This option is viable but not as attractive as option two. In this instance, software verification must examine each menu for content and layout and then validate the navigation among the menus. This can be extremely time-consuming and laborious. Furthermore, the marketing people will alter the menus as they continue to refine their understanding of what they really want, and the requirements document must then be updated, approved, and re-released. Another drawback to this approach is that it might even be too early in the project to understand completely the interplay among the menu items, which means that changes are inevitable. Additionally, this option may complicate the design process, because the menu system may have been designed and documented prior to the rest of the system, which means that the design is now contained in two separate documents. As the overall product design matures over time, more changes and document updates are inevitable.

Assimilation of Software Requirements

Consider the situation in which several requirements can be condensed into a single, equivalent requirement. In this instance, the total test set can be reduced through careful analysis and insightful design. As an example, suppose that the user interface of a product is required to display several fields of information that indicate various parameters, states, and values; that it is a requirement for the user to be able to edit the fields interactively; and that it is required that key system critical fields must flash or blink so that the user knows that a system critical field is being edited. Further, assume that the software requirements document captures this by specifying: "All displayed fields can be edited. The rate field shall flash while being edited. The exposure time shall flash while being edited. The volume delivered field shall flash while being edited."

These statements are viable and suitable for the requirements specification, but they may not be optimum from an implementation and test point of view. For example, there are three possible implementation strategies for these requirements (see Figure 6-3). First, a monolithic editor routine can be designed and implemented that handles all aspects of the field editing, including the flash function. Second, a generic field editor can be designed that is given a parameter that indicates whether the field should flash during field editing. Third, an executive editor could be designed that selects either a nonflashing or flashing field editor routine, depending on whether the field was critical. Conceptually, on the basis of the documented requirements statements above, the validation tests would ensure that (1) only the correct fields can be displayed; (2) the displayed fields can be edited; (3) critical fields blink when edited; and (4) each explicitly named field blinks.

The first monolithic design option potentially presents the severest test case load and should be avoided. Because the design is monolithic in structure and performs all editing functions internally, all validation tests must be performed within a single routine to determine whether the requirements are met. The validation testing would consist of the four test scenarios presented above. Furthermore, inclusion of in-line code tests into a single routine might alter the execution environment and provide misleading results.

The second design option represents an improvement over the first. Because the flash/no flash flag is passed as a parameter into the routine, the testing internally to the routine is reduced because part of the testing burden has been shifted to the interface between the calling and called routines. This is easier to test because the flash/no flash discrimination is made at a higher level; it is an inherent part of the calling sequence of the routine and, therefore, it can be visually verified without formal tests. The validation testing would consist of test situations 1, 2, and 4 presented above. The third design option represents the optimum from a test standpoint, because the majority of the validation testing can be accomplished with visual inspections. This is possible

Figure 6-3   Software requirements assimilation, example 1

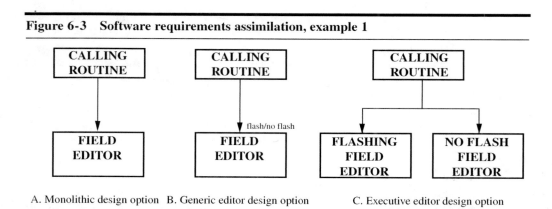

A. Monolithic design option   B. Generic editor design option   C. Executive editor design option

because the flash/no flash discrimination is also implemented at a higher level, and the result of the differentiation is a visibly flashing field or a nonflashing field. The validation testing would consist of test situations 2 and 4 presented above.

As presented here, these requirements and their design implementation options are well defined and can be used for the released code. However, on the basis of the design options, the requirements could be rewritten to simplify testing even further. Assume that the third design option requires less testing time and is easier to test. The requirement statements can then be written to facilitate this situation even more. The following requirement statements are equivalent to those above and tend to drive the design in the direction of the third design option: "All displayed fields can be edited. All critical items being edited shall flash to inform the user that editing is in progress." In this instance, the third design can be augmented by creating a list or lookup table of the fields required to be edited. A flag can be associated with each, indicating whether the field should flash. This approach allows a completely visual inspection to replace the testing, because the field is either in the edit list or it is not. If it is, then it either flashes or it does not. Testing within the routine is still required, but it now is associated with debug testing during development and not with formal validation testing after implementation.

As another example of collapsing several requirements into a single equivalent requirement (see Figure 6-4), consider the following case, which is a derivation of the previous example. Suppose that an instrument has several modes of operation and that its requirements are: "Audio feedback is required to indicate the status of the instrument. Audio signals are required to indicate errors, alarms, warnings, and when the instrument is in the HOLD state." An obvious requirement question to be addressed is, What audio signal(s) should be generated if two or more of these conditions exist simultaneously? One solution would be to expand the requirements definition and enumerate in the requirements specification each and every permutation and combination of errors, alarms, warnings, and operational audio signals. For each entry, the requirements specification would explicitly state which signal takes precedence over the other(s).

The disadvantage to this approach is that a specific validation test must be generated for each specified requirement, as well as the potential combinations, even if they might not be realistic. The alternative to this is to generate the requirement statements: "Audio feedback is required to indicate errors, alarms, warnings, and when the instrument is in the HOLD state. Whenever more than one audible sound is enabled at the same time, only the highest priority sound shall be audible." The advantage to this is that it, too, can be validated by visual inspection rather than by formal validation testing. For example, during software design, the list of audio signal conditions could be created along with an indication of their priority. A simple inspection of the implemented list would indicate whether the condition requires an audible sound, and what the priority of that sound is relative to the other sounds. Validation testing can then be relegated to whether the sound can be generated and the proper frequency and volume.

Requirements versus Design

It is tacitly agreed that there is a lot of overlap between requirements and design, and, in fact, design itself can be considered a requirement. The division between these two is not a hard line. However, many individuals do not appreciate that the distinction between them can be used to simplify testing and consequently shorten overall software development times. Requirements and their specification concentrate on the functions needed by the system or product and the users. Requirements must be discussed in terms of what must be done and not how it is to be done. For example, "Hardcopy strip chart analysis shall be available" is a functional requirement, and "Hardcopy strip chart analysis shall be from a pull-down menu" has design requirements

Figure 6-4   Software requirements assimilation, example 2

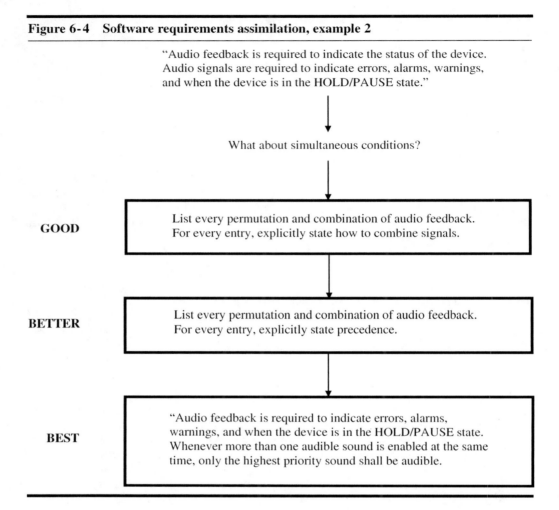

"Audio feedback is required to indicate the status of the device. Audio signals are required to indicate errors, alarms, warnings, and when the device is in the HOLD/PAUSE state."

What about simultaneous conditions?

GOOD

List every permutation and combination of audio feedback. For every entry, explicitly state how to combine signals.

BETTER

List every permutation and combination of audio feedback. For every entry, explicitly state precedence.

BEST

"Audio feedback is required to indicate errors, alarms, warnings, and when the device is in the HOLD/PAUSE state. Whenever more than one audible sound is enabled at the same time, only the highest priority sound shall be audible."

mixed with the functional requirements. Consequently, there are times when requirements specifications will contain information that can be construed as design. However, resist placing the "how" design requirements in the software requirements specification and concentrate on the underlying "what" requirements.

As more "how" requirements creep into the software requirements specification, more testing must occur, principally on two levels. First, there is more detail to test for, and second, but strategically more important, more validation than verification needs to be done. Because verification is qualitative and ascertains that the process and design were met, low-key activities have been transferred from the visual and inspection methods into validation testing, which is more rigorous and requires formal proof of requirements fulfillment. The distinction of design versus requirements is difficult, but a careful discrimination of what goes where is of profound benefit. As a rule of thumb, if it looks like a description of "what" needs to be implemented, then it belongs in the software requirements specification. If it looks like a description of "how," or if a feature can be implemented in two or more ways and one of those ways is preferred over another, or if it is indeterminate whether it is requirements or design, then it should rightfully belong in the software design specification.

There is another distinct advantage to moving as many "how" requirements to design as possible. The use of computer-aided software engineering (CASE) tools has greatly automated the generation of code from design. If a feature or function can be delayed until the design phase, it can then be implemented in an automated fashion. This simplifies the verification of the design, because the automation tool has been previously verified and validated, so the demonstration that the design was implemented is almost a fait accompli.

The Software Life Cycle in Practice

This section presents, in detail, how the pieces of the software life cycle fit together in practice, from project start-up through analysis, requirements, design, code and test, integrate and test, and validation testing to configuration change control, as shown in Figures 6-5 through 6-11 and Table 6-5.

A few explanatory notes are in order relative to these figures and their description. First, most of the acronyms presented here have been discussed in detail in previous sections. Second, the criteria column of the figures represents decision points in the project at which the software lead engineer has either met obligations in the software planning documents or decides that enough information and data have been gathered for the current software phase and continued work will not yield significant additional information. Satisfaction of the criteria is a joint agreement by the software development team and the V&V team; both participate in defining the criteria during project planning, and both are required to agree when ad hoc decisions are to be made. Satisfaction of the criteria allows the project to move on to the next phase. Third, the baseline column of the figures represents a stable increment in the capabilities of the software and serves as an intermediate release to the V&V team, as well as a fallback position in case something goes wrong during testing. Satisfaction of the baseline criteria was defined in the planning documents and can be augmented at the discretion of the software lead engineer whenever an additional, logical configuration or capability of the software has been reached that was not envisioned when the planning documents were generated.

Fourth, the build column in the figures represents a completed intermediate release of the software, and formal V&V testing can commence on the configuration released to the V&V team. This version of the software represents the "golden" copy of the software that has already passed V&V testing, and it is used to help form the basis of the next software baseline version to be developed by the software development team. Fifth, as each phase begins, some of the phase inputs are the outputs from the previous phase's activities. Consequently, a phase will always produce new information, data, and work products, and it will most likely output some modified version of previous work products. Last, within any given phase, an arbitrary but finite number of builds can be accomplished. These builds can encompass both code and documentation. The intent of these incremental builds is to provide stable platforms or releases that are well defined and well controlled, to facilitate testing, development, V&V, configuration control, and audit activities.

At the time of the project start-up (Figure 6-6), a software lead engineer is appointed to lead and manage the software activities, and at some time after that the software V&V lead engineer is selected. The V&V lead engineer reports to the software lead engineer for technical direction, to understand the plans, strategy, and general direction to which the software team is committed. The V&V lead engineer, however, is also reporting to the software engineering manager who

Figure 6-5 Overview of the software engineering life cycle process

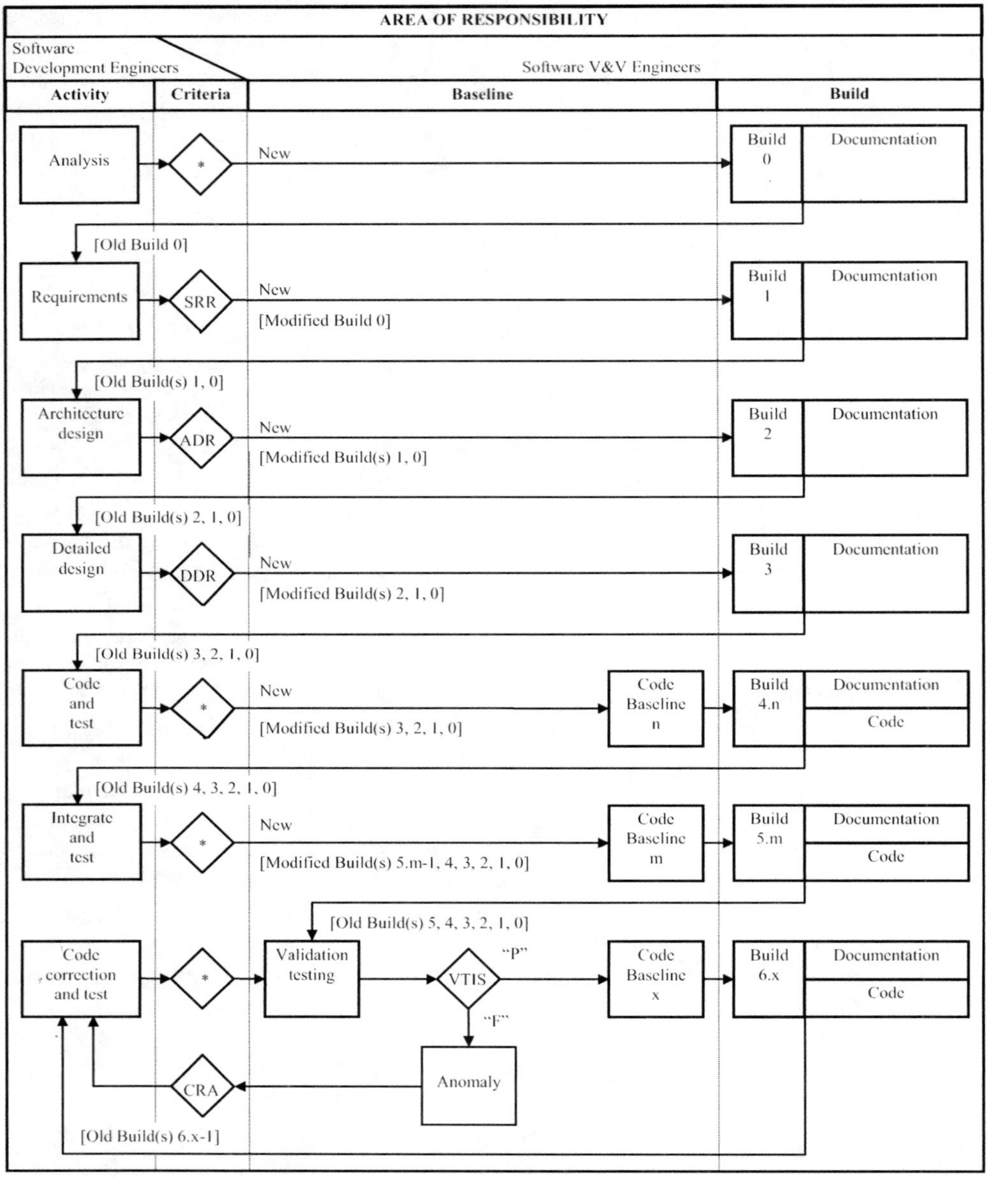
AREA OF RESPONSIBILITY
Software Development Engineers
Software V&V Engineers
Activity
Criteria
Baseline
Build
Analysis
*
New
Build 0
Documentation
[Old Build 0]
Requirements
SRR
New
[Modified Build 0]
Build 1
Documentation
[Old Build(s) 1, 0]
Architecture design
ADR
New
[Modified Build(s) 1, 0]
Build 2
Documentation
[Old Build(s) 2, 1, 0]
Detailed design
DDR
New
[Modified Build(s) 2, 1, 0]
Build 3
Documentation
[Old Build(s) 3, 2, 1, 0]
Code and test
*
New
[Modified Build(s) 3, 2, 1, 0]
Code Baseline n
Build 4.n
Documentation
Code
[Old Build(s) 4, 3, 2, 1, 0]
Integrate and test
*
New
[Modified Build(s) 5.m-1, 4, 3, 2, 1, 0]
Code Baseline m
Build 5.m
Documentation
Code
[Old Build(s) 5, 4, 3, 2, 1, 0]
Code correction and test
*
Validation testing
VTIS
"P"
"F"
Code Baseline x
Build 6.x
Documentation
Code
Anomaly
CRA
[Old Build(s) 6.x-1]

* Indicates software lead engineer has either met obligations in software planning documents or decided that enough information and data have been gathered for the current phase, and continued work will not yield significant additional information.

is ultimately responsible for the quality assurance of the software. The intent of this reporting structure is twofold:

1. It gives the software lead engineer the capability to govern, manage, and control both the development and V&V aspects of the project.

Table 6-5   Reporting and Resolution of Configuration Changes

ACTIVITY	CONFIGURATION CHANGE REPORTING—DOCUMENT AND RESOLUTION						PRECIPITATES
	Reporting Document				Resolution		
	Type	Classification		Defintion	Who	Result	
New capability, function, or feature development, test, and debug	None				None		Baseline items
Testing of any type	Anomaly	High		Change is required to correct: a condition that prevents or seriously degrades a system objective and no alternative exists; a safety-related problem	Software Lead Engineer	Misunderstanding or misinterpretation	No action
						Future baseline	No action
						Correction required	CRA generated
		Medium		Change is required to: correct a condition that degrades a system objective; provide for performance improvement; confirm that the user and/or system requirements can be met		Misunderstanding or misinterpretation	No action
						Future baseline	No action
						Correction required	CRA generated
		Low		Change is desirable to: maintain the system, correct operator inconvenience, or other		Misunderstanding or misinterpretation	No action
						Future baseline	No action
						Correction required	CRA generated
Testing of any type; CRA generated	CRA	Baseline items	Class I	Changes that affect performance, function, technical requirements	SCRB	Authorized changes	Baseline item change
			Class II	Changes that are not Class I			
		Class III		Changes to nonbaselined items	Software Lead Engineer	Authorized changes	Configuration control item change
Update, modify, or alter an item	CRA	Baseline items	Class I	Code and documents	Software Engineer	Altered items	New baseline
			Class II	Documents			
		Class III		Configuration-controlled items			

2. The V&V results are ultimately the responsibility of management and are out of the control of the software lead engineer.

When these two individuals are in place, the rest of the team begins to form, and the project takes on more formality. At this time, project estimates and some preliminary analysis are performed and documents are generated. The preliminary analysis deals with technical issues such as the user interface, hardware analysis and trade-offs, hardware and software interface definition, and conceptual design approaches. At some point, the software lead engineer decides that enough analysis has been performed, and the information is formally saved as new software documentation. In the next stage of the project (Figure 6-7), requirements analysis begins, new documents are generated, and several data items are revised. This phase is concluded when the SRR is held.

In the Architecture Design Phase (Figure 6-8), the requirements from the previous phase are converted into a software architecture design that specifies the upper levels of the software design; several new data items are created, and others are modified. Some of the data items that are germane to this phase are used in the next phase, while others are not needed until later in the project. The Architecture Design Phase concludes with the ADR. The next phase (Figure 6-9) expands the architecture of the previous phase and begins the detailed specification of the software design, which concludes with the DDR. In the next two phases (Figure 6-10), construction on the code begins, and it is released to the V&V group for testing as incremental builds. As the lower software modules are created, they are also integrated and assimilated into larger aggregates as the product software evolves into its final configuration.

In the last phase (Figure 6-11), validation testing begins on the completed software; while this is in progress, the software development team updates the documentation to ensure that the

Figure 6-6 Phase 0 of the software life cycle in practice

SCHEDULED MILESTONE	AREA OF RESPONSIBILITY					
	Software Development Engineers		Software V&V Engineers			
	ACTIVITY	CRITERIA	BUILD			
				created	SQAP	SDE
				created	SVVP	V&V
	Project start-up and preliminary analysis	*		created	Project estimations	SDE
				created	Analysis information	SDE
Phase 0						
Build 0.*n*				created	Phase Report	V&V
				created	SCSR	SCM
	Interface analysis and design	*		created	IDS	SDE
				updated	Analysis information	SDE
Next phase	Phase 1 Phase 2					

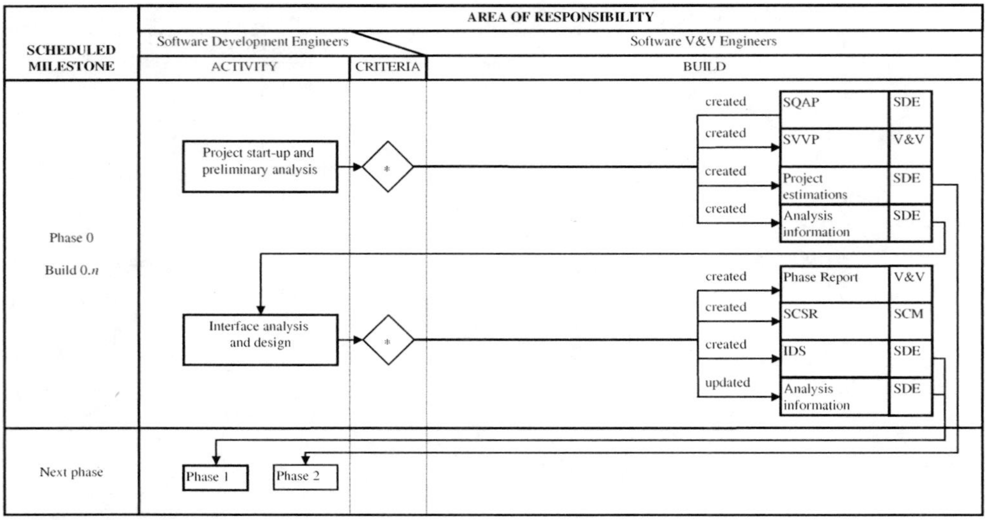

Note: SDE is software development engineer(s), and SCM is software configuration manager.

Figure 6-7 Phase 1 of the software life cycle in practice

SCHEDULED MILESTONE	AREA OF RESPONSIBILITY					
	Software Development Engineers		Software V&V Engineers			
	ACTIVITY	CRITERIA	BUILD			
Previous phase	Phase 0					
				created	Phase Report	V&V
				created	SCMP	SCM
				created	SCSR	SCM
				created	RTM	V&V
Phase 1				created	SDP	SDE
Build 1.*n*	Requirements analysis	SRR		created	SEAP	SDE
				created	SRS	SDE
				updated	IDS	SDE
				updated	Analysis information	SDE
Next phase	Phase 2					

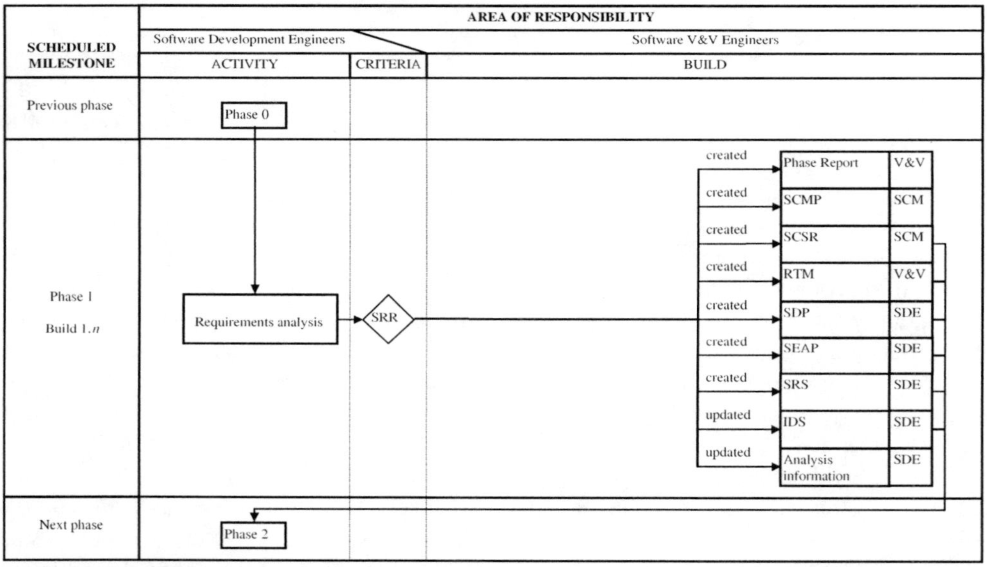

as-built code is correctly reflected in the documentation. If the code does not pass the validation tests, an anomaly is generated and its disposition determined. If changes need to be made, a CRA is generated, authorizing a specific change to the baselined code. The software is corrected, documentation is updated, if necessary, and the fixed code is submitted for validation regression testing. The code stays in validation testing until all outstanding anomalies have been closed.

Figure 6-8   Phase 2 of the software life cycle in practice

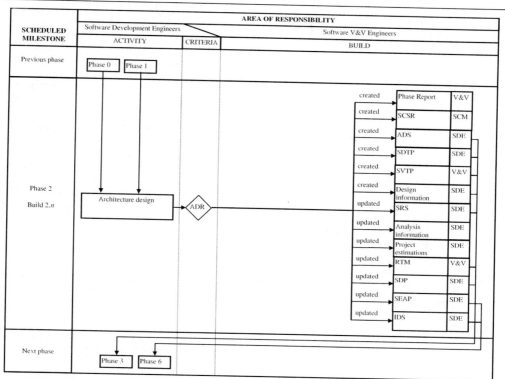

When all anomalies have been closed, the software is certified for use and formally released into the documentation system.

Because of the significance of this last phase, Table 6-5 describes the processing of configuration changes. It is important to understand the implications and relationship among all project documents, Software Anomaly Reports, baselines, and CRAs. In Table 6-5, the first row indicates the configuration change activities that occur during the development of new capabilities, functions, or features not included in the software prior to the start of the project. The second row indicates the configuration change activities that occur when a Software Anomaly Report is generated during V&V testing or any formal testing. The third row indicates the activities accomplished when a CRA is generated that affects a baseline that has already been released or has passed V&V testing and is considered a "golden" copy. The last row indicates the responsibilities to complete the authorized CRA.

As V&V or any formal testing continues, it exposes errors or anomalies in the code. This means that either the code is correct and the documentation does not adequately reflect the code operation, or the documentation is correct and the code did not implement the specification. A Software Anomaly Report is generated and given to the software lead engineer, who analyzes and evaluates the reported problem. If the problem disclosed by the Software Anomaly Report is within the code currently under construction or within the corresponding documentation, the anomaly can be closed, because the existing project documentation represents the authorization to change the baseline code (see first row of Table 6-5).

Figure 6-9   Phase 3 of the software life cycle in practice

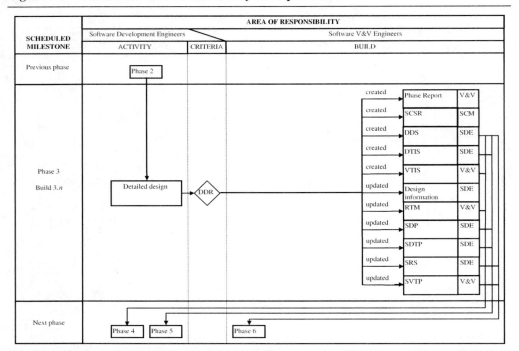

However, if the anomaly is against a previously baselined, validated code that is under configuration control, then its disposition is determined differently (see second row of Table 6-5). The software lead engineer can decide on one of three dispositions of the anomaly:

1. If the anomaly was a misunderstanding or misinterpretation of the specifications or code by the tester, then no action need be taken, and the anomaly can be closed.

2. If the perceived anomaly is a defect that must be corrected, it will, in fact, be corrected because of a future baseline that is already an integral part of the project's development activities. No action need be taken to correct this defect, and the anomaly can be closed.

3. If the anomaly is a condition that needs to be corrected, then a CRA is generated, and the CRA serves as the authorization to modify a previously baselined item that is not currently in a change state.

In addition to a CRA being generated from an anomaly, it can be known a priori by the tester that the discovered error affects a baselined item, and a CRA can be generated directly. In either event, a disposition of the CRA is necessary (see third row of Table 6-5). Class I and II CRAs are issued against prior baselined items; a Class III CRA is issued against nonbaselined items. For example, a Class I or II CRA would be issued to alter or modify code, requirements documents, or design specifications; a Class III CRA would be issued to change any of the software planning documents or test specifications or the acceptance plan. For Class I and Class II items, the SCRB reviews the configuration management implications of the change, assures that proper configuration practices have been observed, and determines disposition of the CRA; for Class

Figure 6-10   Phases 4 and 5 of the software life cycle in practice

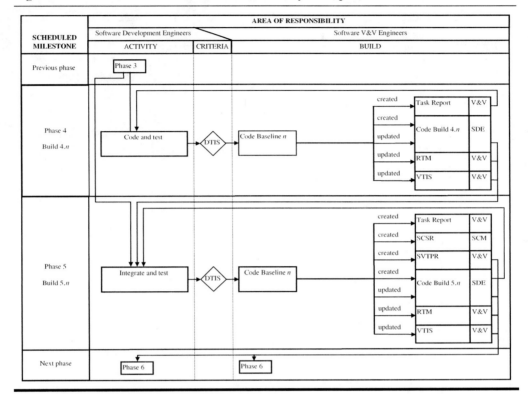

III items, the software lead engineer determines dispositions of the CRA. Assuming that disposition of the CRA has been approved, the specified items must be changed (see last row of Table 6-5). A project software engineer then alters the specified items, thus creating a new baseline version for those specific items. The altered items are then submitted to the V&V group along with the CRA and Software Anomaly Report, so that they may also be validated as correct. The items that were changed can then be put back as soon as practicable, or may wait for the next baseline to be released by the software development team to the V&V team.

Prototypes

The difficulty of defining just what the user wants the software to do has been a frequent source of inadequate requirements specifications. There is no doubt that the form and content assumed by the SRS has much to do with the quality of the software being developed. Software engineers who have had to work with incomplete, inconsistent, or misleading specifications have experienced the frustration and confusion that invariably result from these types of specifications. The quality, timeliness, and completeness of the software, and ultimately of the product, suffer as a consequence. Often a product will be defined in terms of a set of general objectives that do not identify the detailed inputs, processing, or output requirements. In other cases, the development

Figure 6-11   Phases 6 of the software life cycle in practice

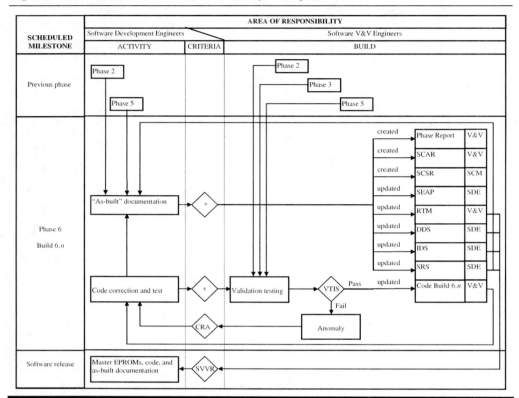

team may be unsure of the efficiency of an algorithm, the adaptability of software from a previous product, or the form and function that the user interface should take. In these and several other situations, a prototype approach to software engineering is a valuable means of reducing the uncertainties and enhancing overall communications.

Prototypes are models of the software to be built. They can assume one of three forms:

1. A paper prototype that depicts or describes in text the user interactions in a form and enables the user to understand how the interactions will occur. This form assumes that the user can grasp and mentally picture the operations described.

2. The working prototype that implements some subset or limited functionality of the final product's features and allows the user to get a "hands-on" feel for the ultimate features as they will be implemented in the product. This is an improvement on the paper prototype, because it allows the user to interact with a physical realization and react to the tactile feedback.

3. An operational prototype, consisting of an existing program that performs all or some of the functions the user desires. It also has other features that need to be improved upon in the new development effort. This form of the prototype provides all of the advantages of the second form and has an additional advantage.

Although to the user there is little or no difference between prototype forms two and three, there is a world of difference to software developers. Form three is usually a software product developed by the software group that will ultimately construct the new software; therefore, developers are intimately familiar with the software—its features and the product it represents.

The form that the prototype assumes can be grouped into two generic classes. The evolutionary prototype evolves into the final product, and the prototype code is used as a part or subset of the delivered software. A simulation prototype provides for user feedback, feasibility studies and analysis, and human factor evaluation. In this instance, the prototype code is not necessarily used in the final product. Simulation prototypes can also be used to explore and evaluate various candidate designs for software control that could be used in the final product.

All software projects require some degree of analysis, and software prototypes are no different. As previously discussed, software analysis is performed regardless of the software engineering methodology to be applied on the project; in software prototype production, the form that the analysis takes will vary. In some instances, it is possible to apply fundamental principles of analysis and derive a paper specification of the software, from which a design can be developed. In other situations, requirements are gathered, the analysis principles are applied, and a model or prototype of the software is constructed for assessment. In still other instances, circumstances require the construction of a prototype at the beginning of the analysis, because the model is the only means through which the requirements can be effectively derived, and the model then evolves into the production software. In many, but not all cases, the construction of a prototype, coupled with systematic analysis methods, is an effective approach to software engineering.

Paradigm of Prototypes

As in all approaches to software development, a prototype (Figure 6-12) begins with requirements gathering and analysis. The software engineer and the customer or user meet and define the overall objectives, define the known requirements, and outline the areas where further definition is required. From this, a quick design focuses on a representation of those aspects of the software that are visible to the user, such as input alternatives and approaches, output formats, and display topology and content. The design then leads to the construction of a little code that is tested to assure that it will not break during the user's evaluation of the resulting prototype. The generated prototype is evaluated by the user or customer and used to refine and focus the requirements for the next version of the software.

In a series of iterations, the prototype is then refined to satisfy the needs of the customer and user, while at the same time enabling the software engineer to better understand what needs to be done. At a minimum, the prototype serves as a mechanism for identifying and solidifying product requirements; if a working prototype is constructed, however, the software developer attempts to make use of parts of the existing prototype software for inclusion in the new prototype version or of tools that directly enable working programs to be generated. When the prototype has matured into the final product, the appropriate software documents are created, and the software is verified and validated just as in the more traditional software development methodologies. This paradigm stresses the incremental enhancement of the software as it grows from the prototype into the final product software. This is not a license to circumvent the established software development methodology. In fact, most of the structured software engineering techniques are still needed.

The prototype serves as the first system in effect and tests the viability of the new concepts and technology. When it has satisfied its intended goals, the prototype is usually thrown away,

Figure 6-12   Software prototype paradigm

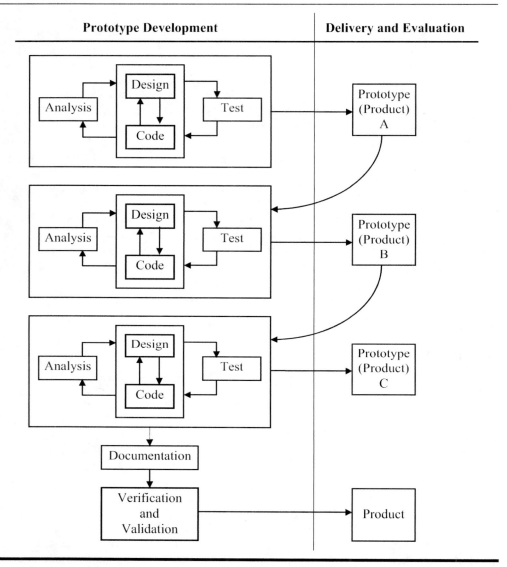

because it probably does not fully comply with or meet its specified requirements in all areas. However, the management question is not whether to build a prototype product and then throw it away, because that will happen to some degree anyway. The real question is whether to plan in advance to build a throwaway prototype, or promise to deliver what would have been the throw-away to the customer as the final product. This is not easy to decide.

Throwing away the prototype may be too idealized. Prototype production as a paradigm for software engineering is problematic. For example, the customer sees and experiences what appears to be a working version of the "product software" and is unaware that the prototype does not meet software quality standards, that it is not particularly efficient, and that long-term software maintainability has not been considered. Furthermore, if the prototype software has been developed with the use of a fourth-generation language that, usually, cannot be used in the final product, then the prototype software must be converted into the programming language of choice for the product. When informed that the prototype "product" must be rebuilt, the customer usually applies pressure and demands that a few fixes be made to the prototype to get a working product sooner.

However, in making the prototype operational, the software engineer has made implementation compromises to get the prototype working quickly. Inappropriate code may have been used simply because it was available and familiar to the software engineer; inefficient algorithms may have been implemented simply to demonstrate the capability. After a while, even the software engineer may become used to the prototype's feature implementation and forgets the reasons why the features were important. In both of these instances, the less-than-ideal choice has become, by definition, an integral part of the product.

If a software prototype is constructed in parallel with product development, it is possible that feedback from the prototype software effort can result in significant product redevelopment and rework. Since a prototype is an early development engineering step, the likelihood of redevelopment, and its consequent impact on the product's schedule, requires that senior management supports the goals of the prototype and that the development team be prepared for potential additional work. Furthermore, the users and customers who will be testing and evaluating the prototype must understand that the "product" they will test and examine is unfinished and that they can play a formative role in its development.

If an operational prototype is implemented for a subset of the product's full features, then it should accomplish several goals:

- Demonstrate whether the specific product features are feasible and viable in the combination presented;

- Help to gather data on the usability and performance issues associated with the product;

- Confirm that the design and the implementation concepts for the product can be communicated and expressed explicitly;

- Solicit and focus user feedback about the product and its feature set, which may include statistics that measure the prototype against product requirements.

Prototypes and Evolutionary Design

Prototype software as an evolutionary design approach was started by Donald McCracken in the late 1970s; it was refined by Boar, Martin, and several others in the mid-1980s. Regardless of the specific approach used for prototype production, it begins with a request from a customer, just as the more traditional software development processes do. The request can be verbal or written and can have the informal tone of a memorandum or the formal context of a specification. Whatever the media, the prototype software begins a life cycle of its own that starts with the user's or customer's request.

McCracken's approach to prototype software is composed of four distinct steps:

1. Use of an application generator, such as a fourth generation language, to develop a prototype with key parts of the desired capability;

2. User exercise and evaluation of the prototype to determine where it needs improvement;

3. Refinement of the prototype through the use of the application generator that iterates and evolves the prototype until the user is satisfied with the results;

4. If the performance of the resulting prototype is adequate, establishment of it as the user's product, continually updated and maintained via the application generator. If higher performance is required, then either the prototype can be refined further, or the prototype itself can be used as a de facto specification for the development of a high-performance product.

The McCracken prototype software model assumes that the prototype developers and the customer work closely with one another and that the user is fully capable of determining when the prototype is complete and ready to be viewed as a full-fledged product.

The Boar prototype software model comprises six steps. The first step is analysis of the software request and determination of whether the software to be developed is a good candidate for a prototype. Any application that creates dynamic visual displays, interacts heavily with the user, or demands algorithms or combinatorial processing that must be developed in an evolutionary fashion is a strong candidate for a prototype. In this model, it is essential that the customer be committed to the evaluation and refinement of the prototype and be capable of making requirements decisions in a timely fashion.

The second step begins with an acceptable candidate project and a software analyst who then develops an abbreviated representation of the user requirements. This representation conveys both the information and functional domains of the application as well as a reasonable approach to partitioning requirements easily into prototype pieces. This representation and the resulting partition are then reviewed with the customer, and approval of the results is reached.

In the third step, a set of abbreviated design specifications is created for the prototype. The design must be completed before prototype construction can commence, but the design typically focuses on top-level architecture and data design issues rather than on the detailed procedural design.

In the fourth step, the prototype software is created, tested, and refined in an iterative process. Ideally, preexisting software is adapted to create the prototype rapidly. However, rapid is a relative term, because the prototype software will most likely be a conglomeration of modified existing code, new code, and code generated from fourth-generation application languages. This means that at times the code will come together quite quickly and at other times very slowly. Specialized prototype construction tools, languages, and fourth-generation coding techniques can be used to help with the development of the prototype software.

When the prototype has been carefully and fully tested, the fifth step is presentation of the prototype to the customer or user. The customer or user must be willing and committed to evaluation of the prototype. The user will be expected to exercise, test, and evaluate the prototype to provide modification suggestions, but the customer or user must also be prepared to be extremely patient. Crashes and failures may be frequent, and the trick will be to differentiate between failures of the prototype and failures of how the prototype was assembled. The sixth step is the repeated iteration of steps four and five until all of the requirements are formalized, or until the prototype has evolved into a production system.

Prototypes and Structured Design

Regardless of whether the goal of the prototype is gathering user requirements or evolution of the prototype into a production system, both of these life cycles conclude by entering the design phase of the traditional structured software development life cycle. This means that the prototype is not intended to be an operational system per se, but rather a means of modeling the user requirements, as well as providing an early version of the final production software. Philosophically, the top-down structured software development methodology is another form of prototype construction. Instead of using written analysis methods, the various prototype versions provide a working model with which the software analyst and the user can interact to obtain a more realistic feeling of the product's functions.

The prototype life cycle involves development of a working model that is, in effect, thrown away and replaced by a production system that is more efficient and better structured and that has been optimized for system requirements. There is significant danger that either the user or the software development team may try to turn the prototype itself directly into the production software and system. This usually leads to disaster because the prototype lacks operational detail, is not full featured, and does not have the necessary support documentation required for verification, validation, and maintenance. On the other hand, if the prototype is literally thrown away and replaced by the production system, there is a danger that the project may finish without having a permanent record of the final user requirements. This is likely to make the maintenance of the software increasingly difficult over the product's life cycle.

The prototype approach does provide an alternative to the generation and validation of written requirements specifications and draft user's manuals. It ensures that the software will be responsive to the user's needs. The prototype approach provides a much more realistic validation of the user requirements than does the review of a set of textual specifications and manuals. The prototype approach can also raise second-order issues and problems that the product will have in the user's mode of operation. Rapid development of the prototype minimizes the problems of accommodating the inevitable requirements changes during long development periods. The rapid prototype capability also makes it possible to generate several alternatives for comparative trials and feasibility studies and provides quick-response, how-about-this? solutions to user difficulties.

Probably the most common claim in support of the prototype approach is that written requirements specifications and design documents are no longer needed. This claim is usually espoused by individuals who are eager to please and provide quantity results, not necessarily quality results. To market most medical devices, some degree of regulatory approval is required; regulatory approval is predicated in most instances on the V&V of the software. In order to verify and validate the software, the requirements and design of the software must be in writing. When they are, there is tangible evidence of what and how the software is to perform. Therefore, since written documentation is required in the end, it is counterproductive to begin work on a prototype with the expressed goal of not producing any written documentation.

Although fairly good, rapid prototype capabilities exist for some applications, they are not universally applicable to real-time distributed processing applications; command and control system applications; and large, integrated, corporate information system applications. Furthermore, the flexibility of the prototype is often negated by the organizational inertia and environment of company. For example, existing standards and the "traditional way of doing business" often do not lend themselves to the prototype approach. In addition, the functional groups of an organization may not be structured to be mutually supportive, a fundamental requirement of prototype development projects. As an illustration, suppose a prototype development team, consisting of a mechanical engineer, an electrical engineer, and a software engineer, develops a new type of lead-screw drive for a device. As the lead-screw drive evolves and matures, the final prototype of the mechanism becomes the physical representation that will be incorporated into the device itself. From the mechanical engineering standpoint, the final prototype is, in fact, the production design. The drive motor and its prototype circuitry will probably also be in their final form and ready for use in the device. From the electrical engineering standpoint, the final prototype is also, in fact, the production design. However, the software is probably a long way from inclusion into any device, because it must be repackaged for efficiency, safety, and optimization; retrofitted with the existing software design and architecture standards; documented; and then tested and finally validated. Whereas hardware functions perform most of their work up front with design and during the actual prototype generation and their efforts conclude with a de facto production design, software activities are generally concentrated at the end of a project; much of the effort continues after the hardware disciplines have completed theirs.

If the initial prototype deviates radically from the user's needs, desires, and requirements, then it may lead to disastrous results. For example, the product may be perceived as unresponsive; consequently, the users are turned off by it. However, this is usually a more palatable result than waiting until the product has reached the marketplace and then finding it unacceptable. The prototype approach also concentrates on near-term user needs and frequently neglects the foreseeable longer term needs, often until it is too late to recover and make amends for the deficiency. Furthermore, the development of a suboptimal product through the prototype approach requires substantial rework to correct the negative effects that the prototype has associated with the overall, integrated product.

Prototype development allows early and focused feedback on a product before the full-scale product is released by allowing early, hands-on evaluations with selected and knowledgeable customers while the product is being developed. Through judicious selection and screening, only a subset of the product's full features is implemented. The development team can gain valuable information about whether the product has the right features and is meeting its requirements.

Throwaway Prototypes

Throwaway software prototypes are software programs created in a quick and dirty manner and discarded once they have fulfilled their purpose. They are frequently used to validate presumed requirements, to gain experience necessary to uncover new requirements, or to validate possible design options (see Figure 6-13). Throwaway software prototypes greatly reduce the

Figure 6-13   Throwaway prototype model of the software development life cycle

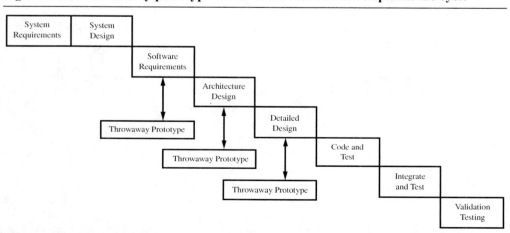

risk of building a product that does not satisfy the needs of the user; reduce development costs, because fewer changes need to be made during the software life cycle; and increase the probability of project success, as a result of enhanced communication between the software developer and the user.

Comparatively, there are few software engineering difficulties with the use of throwaway software prototypes as long as the throwaway prototype does not end up as the product itself. There are also numerous approaches to constructing throwaway prototypes. Among them are using languages that facilitate very rapid product development, although the resultant prototype is relatively difficult to maintain; reusing software components from a repository; reusing previously released software in some degree of totality; and using tools that are available to assist in the rapid creation of user interfaces.

Difficulties with throwaway prototypes include those related primarily to the management of throwaway software relative to costs and conversion of the throwaway into a production system. Software developers involved in throwaway prototypes occasionally find it difficult to declare that the throwaway product is ready for customer inspection; they want to continue to play with and evolve the prototype into something more elegant (Bersoff and Davis 1993; Gordon and Bieman 1994). This practice adds to nonrecoverable engineering costs. When this happens, management should remove the prototype as soon as possible from the software engineer and present it to its evaluator. The problem with converting the throwaway into a production system is that quality, robustness, and reliability cannot be retrofitted into software.

There are few software configuration management issues associated with throwaway prototypes. The appropriate level of configuration management is about the same as for small development efforts; an automated code management system that tracks all changes to code by date, time, and programmer is adequate. Of course, if code from a reusable software component repository or from a prior validated product or system is being used, the configuration management practices related to that repository or system should be applied. Software configuration management problems arise primarily when throwaway prototypes are combined with evolutionary prototypes to create an operational prototype.

Evolutionary Prototypes

Evolutionary prototypes are high-quality programs used to validate presumed requirements, to gain the experience required to uncover new or additional requirements, or to validate a possible software or product design. The difference between the evolutionary prototype and the throwaway prototype is that the evolutionary prototype is repeatedly and deliberately modified and redeployed whenever new information is learned or new data are gathered (see Figure 6-14). The net effects of this type of prototype generation are a greatly reduced risk of constructing a product that does not satisfy user needs, and an increased probability of project success that results from the enhanced communication between the software developers and the user.

Throwaway prototype production is quite different from evolutionary prototype production. In a throwaway prototype, only those parts of the system that are not well understood are built, whereas in an evolutionary prototype those parts of the product that are well understood are built first, to continue development from a solid foundation. Each increment of the evolutionary prototype is slightly more risky than the preceding one, but experience with the preceding version(s) provides enough insight into the problems to make a step much less risky. Another major difference between these two prototype approaches is in quality. Throwaway prototypes are built with little or no concern for quality, robustness, or reliability, whereas the quality of evolutionary prototypes must be built in up front or they will not be able to withstand the necessary

Figure 6-14   Evolutionary prototype model of the software development life cycle

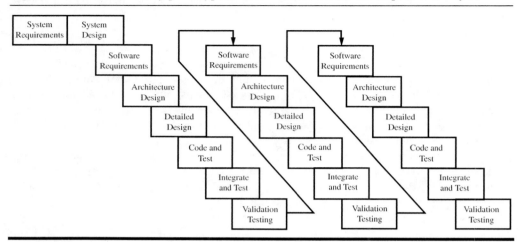

levels of use and modification. The names of the two approaches indicate the most profound and fundamental philosophical differences between them: you cannot build a prototype and then later decide whether it is to be discarded. The decision to discard must be made initially or resources may be wasted, by building quality into something to be discarded, verifying the wrong features, trying to retrofit quality, or trying to maintain a schedule of planned enhancements on top of a shoddy foundation.

There are both engineering and management problems associated with evolutionary pro-totyping (Bersoff and Davis 1993). First, appropriate levels of quality and documentation for an evolutionary prototype are usually unknown. If it is treated as a full-scale development effort, there will be sufficient but probably unnecessarily high levels of effort. If a new increment results in a dead end and must be reverse engineered out of the prototype, resources will have been wasted in building in a quality level. A middle-of-the-road position is needed to reduce the risks yet achieve sufficient quality. One possible solution to this issue is a set of evolutionary prototype standards and guidelines similar to those defined for normal software quality assur-ance, only less stringent and tailored for prototyping. Another solution is the operational proto-type approach discussed below.

A second problem is, How is feedback from the users of the evolutionary prototype obtained, and how will it be obtained in a timely manner so that it can be incorporated into the next iter-ation? This problem may also be solved through the operational prototype approach. A third difficulty is that as experience is gained, as the evolutionary prototype incorporates more require-ments, each new feature becomes incrementally more risky. This, too, can be controlled by the operational prototype approach. Last, building software to accommodate large numbers of major changes can be controlled by any number of documented software processes, such as informa-tion hiding, low intermodule coupling, high module cohesion, object-oriented development, and sound documentation practices.

There are also configuration management problems associated with the production of evo-lutionary prototypes. By definition, it forces software configuration management into the very heart of the development process. Then all of the configuration management challenges of the standard life cycle development become magnified. Configuration identification is challenged because there will inherently be many viable, in-use variants of all components that require identification by purpose, feature mix, and baseline. Configuration control itself is probably most challenged because it is almost guaranteed that there will be multiple versions of all viable baselines deployed at the same time, multiple new versions will be under development simultaneously, and there will be multiple teams of developers endeavoring to make all of these evolving prototypes. The issue becomes how to plan, orchestrate, and control the changes and how to coordinate those changes with all interested parties, all of whom probably have disparate goals. Configuration status accounting is challenged simply by the need to adequately inform all of the participants in an evolutionary prototype project of the status of a multivariate product in several simultaneous stages of development and deployment. Configuration auditing is challenged by rapidly changing baselines and by the need to ensure timely promulgation of audit results, which may dramatically impact any of several in-use and developmental baselines.

The solution to these problems lies in judicious and strict use of proven software configuration management practices, not in the creation of new ones. Evolutionary prototyping is not so much a brand-new life cycle model as it is a lower risk acceleration of the conventional waterfall model. Consequently, any configuration control boards that are formed for this type of life cycle model should have at least one member who is intimately familiar with and has a clear understanding of the full family of evolutionary prototypes underway. This will help to ensure sensible decision making concerning simultaneous changes being proposed on a single component being readied for multiple future releases.

Operational Prototypes

Operational prototypes probably combine the best of throwaway prototypes with the best of evolutionary prototypes. In this form (see Figure 6-15), a stable base is constructed using sound software engineering principles, while the prototype incorporates only those features that are well known, understood, and agreed on. When completed, the resultant stable software base is officially baselined by conventional methods of software configuration management; this version is deployed at operational field sites so that users may review and critique the product as it is currently configured. In addition, an expert prototype developer is commissioned to observe the system in operation.

As the users flex the system, they will uncover problems, but they will also think of new features that would be helpful in fulfilling their duties when using the product. Instead of having to make telephone calls or write their comments, the users express their views and ideas directly to the prototype developer present. When the users stop using the system, the prototype developer constructs a quick and dirty implementation of the desired changes on top of the working baseline. When implementation of the new feature is complete, users experiment with the modified system to ensure that the prototype developer understood the need correctly and that the requested feature really is what is needed. Over time, a collection of these temporary, quick and dirty changes are made to the operational baseline. Eventually the prototype developer returns to the office with those changes.

As the features that were incorporated by the quick and dirty changes are merged with others from other sites, they are analyzed as a whole. The site-generated code is discarded, but the features it implemented are properly engineered into a new, single baseline that follows well-defined and accepted software engineering and software configuration management practices. Finally, as these features are bundled into new versions of the software, new releases are baselined and redeployed with on-site prototypes, just as before, and the procedure repeats.

Figure 6-15   Operational prototype model of the software development life cycle

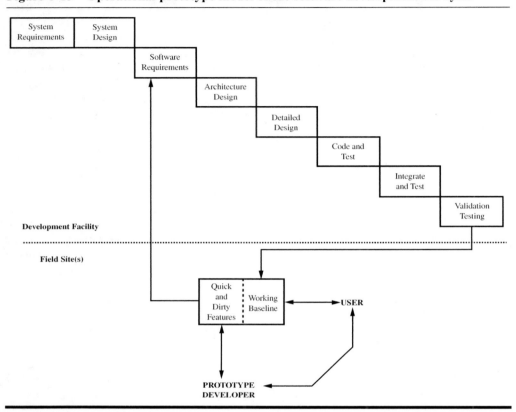

Operational prototype production solves most of the problems associated with the two ear-lier prototype techniques. In particular, it ensures a stable, quality-controlled product, the ability to gain immediate user feedback without unnecessary effort by the user, and the ability to provide users with rapid incorporation of their expressed desires into the presumed product for immediate validation. There are, however, also some problems with operational prototypes. First, the on-site prototype developers must work well with customers and users, understand the application, be extremely effective, and be willing to travel, possibly for extended periods. Second, if the quick and dirty changes are left at the site, along with the prototype product, they may prove to be unreliable and may even adversely affect the rest of the system; this is particularly problematic if the product is deployed in a truly operational mode. Removing the prototype is not necessarily good either, however. If it is taken away, users may become irate because the feature is being removed and they have come to rely on it.

The third area of operational prototype problems is in software configuration management, which must accommodate additional inputs not dealt with before (Bersoff and Davis 1993). The operational prototype is developed with conventional techniques; the functional baseline is created and placed under configuration control when the initial system-level requirements are approved. On approval, the software requirements specification is placed under configuration control as part of the allocated baseline. On completion of system-level testing, the product baseline is created to help control changes to the design, code, test, and user products and their associated documentation. The software is then fielded, with the knowledge that the baseline is under control. As problems are reported from the field, the software undergoes the normal and familiar process of configuration control. Change requests are written, reviewed, approved, categorized as requirements change or error fixes, and prioritized, and their fixes are scheduled for subsequent releases. The prototype developers in the field, however, are making their changes using a tool that maintains a trace of what changes to the code are being made by whom and when. After returning home, the prototype developers have electronic media containing code changes and a mental record of modified requirements that correspond to the new or modified features realized by those electronic patches. Both sets of enhancements must be channeled into the software configuration management process of the developing prototype. The easiest way to do this is to initiate change requests for each field change and indicate that this is a proposed change to the software functionality that has already been field tested as a prototype at a specific site. The normal configuration control process can then merge these changes with the error fixes and the functionality enhancements requests that have not been put into the prototype. All of these change requests are then evaluated by a change control board composed of developers and customers, or their qualified representatives, on the basis of benefit to the customer and cost and schedule impacts. The changes are then prioritized and scheduled into built releases. High priority must be given to those changes originating from the field prototypes, because the customer has already justified these enhancements.

Prototype Documentation

When prototype generation techniques are to be used on a software development project, documentation is a concern. If the prototype is intended to address some unknown aspect of the product, timely documentation could help to ensure that little or no time is lost waiting for the prototype's information. Several possible approaches might be utilized.

First (see Figure 6-16), the product software documents could be generated in the conventional manner. However, for those areas for which the prototype is to provide information, the documents could be left blank. The prototype would then be developed and the necessary information or data collected. On the basis of results of the prototype effort and activities, the

Figure 6-16   Prototype place holder in product software documentation

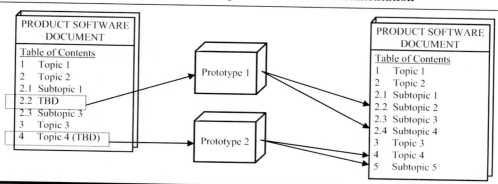

documents could then be updated in the appropriate locations to replace the blank sections with the data gathered from the prototype. Second (see Figure 6-17), a complete set of conventional project software documents could be generated for the prototype project. The prototype would then be developed and deployed to the users, and the information and data gathered. The prototype documents would be updated to reflect the results of the prototype reviews, and these would then serve as the formal documentation of the software work products. Last (see Figure 6-18), a complete set of conventional project software documents could be generated for the prototype project(s), as in the second option. The prototype(s) would then be developed and deployed to the users. The information and data gathered would then be used to update the initial prototype documents, reflecting the results of the prototype activities. The various prototype documents, however, would then be merged to create the conventional product software documents. The prototype documents would serve as a formal baseline configuration item that would provide operational and requirements references for the product, as well as establish an audit trail for formal verification of the presumed requirements and design.

Figure 6-17   Prototype as documentation of stand-alone product software

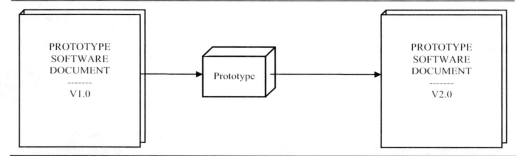

Figure 6-18   Prototype as a generator of product software documentation

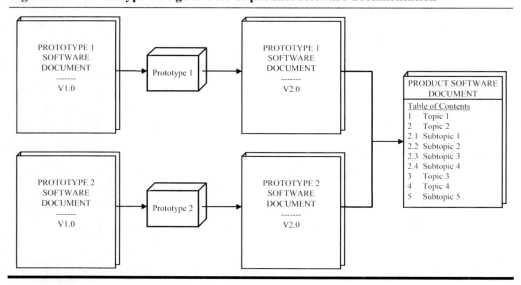

Software Reviews

Software development reviews are organized around and follow the Software Development Plan (SDP). Until the code development phase begins, the software development group's reviews end each of the software development life cycle phases, and the material to be reviewed is the end product for the particular phase. For example, the Requirements Phase produces the Software Requirements Specification (SRS) as an end product, and the phase terminates with the Software Requirements Review (SRR). The end product of the Architecture Design Phase is the Architecture Design Specification (ADS), and the phase concludes with the Architecture Design Review (ADR).

The software life cycle phase activity is gated by the successful conclusion of each phase review, implying that the software project cannot begin the next phase until the current phase is successfully closed out. However, assuming that no show-stopper issues arise at the review, it is more expedient for the project to keep track of the deficiencies that come up at these phase reviews through the use of an action-item list. The project is then allowed to begin the next software life cycle phase, with the stipulation that these action items will be explicitly and individually addressed as the first order of business at the review of the next phase, and they must be closed out at that time. Although this sounds very ominous, threatening, and risky, it should be remembered that the software quality assurance program is deliberately defined and set up to avoid this type of situation by detecting major catastrophes and issues early enough to react and correct them. Thus, these situations are prevented from happening in the first place. If they were to occur, the entire software quality assurance program would have failed, and there would be more serious problems to address.

Starting with the software Detailed Design Phase, the software review process begins a transformation. In addition to the formal and structured Detailed Design Review (DDR) that concludes the Detailed Design Phase, the in-progress design is scrutinized through the design review mechanism. This review is a much less formal meeting, at which the current software design results are presented by one or more members of the software design team to other peer-level software engineers. When the software project has achieved the code implementation phase, the formal review process is abandoned, and the reviews take on a work-in-progress characteristic. In both of these cases, it should be expected that software memorandums, listings, simulations, prototypes, and any other readable and suitable outputs from the analysis and implementation activities can be used to frame the form of the review.

The teams should understand that these design and code inspections and reviews are mandatory and extremely productive, because they are inextricably tied to quality control for two reasons:

1. Any design errors detected at these reviews are corrected immediately and are not propagated any further into the software life cycle.

2. The errors produced and detected during coding activities have no opportunity to be propagated as further sources of error, because they contribute immediate points of failure when directly tested.

Consequently, these types of reviews contribute immensely to the overall quality and reliability of the software.

Software and System-level Reviews

The relationship of software reviews to software development and the V&V activity phases as shown in Figure 6-19 does not include any product-level or system-level reviews, because

Figure 6-19   Relationship of reviews to the software development life cycle

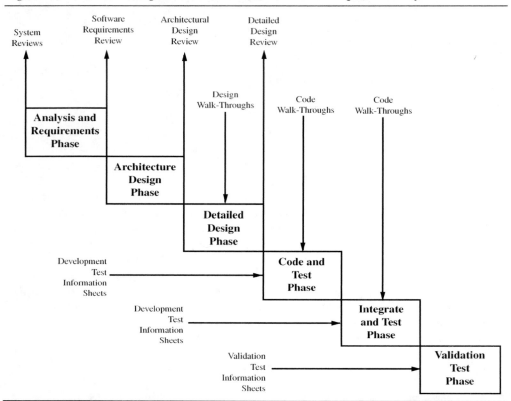

it is assumed for the sake of clarity and focus that these types of reviews have already been conducted. However, some discussion of system reviews is necessary because they do affect software quality assurance. Although a system concept or architecture review can seldom be structured on the basis of formal software documents, software quality assurance should consider the following types of questions at those reviews:

- What was used as the basis for the understanding of the user needs—specifications, reports, surveys, discussions, focus groups, or any other form?

- If a system architecture has been selected, have various alternative configurations, such as distributed, monolithic, or networked processors, been considered?

- If a specific processor has been selected, has consideration been given to both hardware and available support software?

- Will the specific processor selected require capital acquisitions of additional hardware and software?

- Has an alarming schema for system failures been considered?

- Have the critical elements of the system concept or architecture been identified?

- Has the handling of these critical elements been validated by simulation or analysis, or at all?

- Does the system concept embody software maintenance that is consistent with the corporate philosophy as well as with the capabilities of the individuals who will perform the maintenance?

- Can the effort to create the SDP, the Software Quality Assurance Plan (SQAP), and the Software Configuration Management Plan (SCMP) documents be started on the basis of the information from these system-level reviews?

Software Requirements Review

The SRR is based on the product requirements document(s) and the SRS. The software quality assurance group must be satisfied that several items have been properly addressed by the software analysis activities. First, the hardware resources and the available memory should have been defined relative to the known processing needs, growth margins, and future product improvements. This should also include response times, processing bandwidths, and the minimum reserves for memory and processor load. In addition, the input/output (I/O) channels should have been stipulated such that no new configurations will be needed or added. Second, the interfaces to the software should have been adequately defined, including the external hardware interfaces, interfaces to any other software, and user interactions with the product. The interface specifics of the data that relate to format, range, scale, sources, and rates, as well as the software linkages and relationships to the data, should also have been adequately identified and defined. In addition, global data and constants should be agreed to and defined.

Third, all functions that are required by the user and by the system design must be accounted for. These include the definition of key algorithms, the stipulation of the frequency of computations associated with each function, agreement on and definition of accuracy, and standard units used in any of the calculations to be performed.

Fourth, the initial device state must be provided. This should include any initialization operations that are required of the user as well as of the software to satisfy any external, internal, safety, or regulatory requirements. In addition, it should include any self-test, diagnostics, fault-tolerant, or predictor-corrector processing requirements for the external or internal hardware.

These types of items frame the substance of the SRR. The central question to be answered at the conclusion of the review is whether the requirements for the software and the environment in which it will operate have been specified in a manner consistent with the use to which the software will be put.

Software Architecture Design Review

The ADR is the first review related to the physical implementation of the code. As such, it is usually centered on the ADS that presents the architecture of the software. This is a crucial and nontrivial review because it marks the point in the software development schedule at which development of the product code can begin. The ways the various elements of the design may be apportioned among the mechanisms for capturing the design include textual descriptions, flow diagrams, state diagrams and matrices, event tables, and logic tables. These design-capturing mechanisms may be bound, set down on loose-leaf paper in a single document, or spread over several documents.

Whatever means are used, design documentation should be reviewed with several questions in mind. First, software quality assurance should assure that the development environment has been adequately specified. For example, has the programming language been specified along with its required support software? Are any unique programming conventions, tools, or techniques anticipated that are not covered by the SDP? Will it be necessary to acquire any additional software or hardware resources to carry out further software development that is consistent with the SDP? Second, software quality assurance should ensure that the data have been fully identified, structured, and allocated appropriately. For example, will the proposed design force global constants to be expressed in terms of hard-coded values or parameters? Are the data specified in terms of size or dimensions, format, range, scale, rates, accuracies, and response times?

Third, software quality assurance should ensure that the software architectural structure has been adequately described. For example, is the scope of each identified module narrowed to a specific set of operations? Does the modular decomposition reflect intermodular independence? Have the requirements of each module been specified to a level of detail sufficient to permit detailed design to begin? Have all of the requirements of the software specification been addressed? If an execution processing budget has been specified, does the design support the processing timeline? Does it provide adequate reserve? Does the design predicate any constraints or limitations beyond those found in the specifications, and, if so, are they compatible with the end use of the product?

Fourth, software quality assurance should ensure that the software design adequately conveys the safety aspects of the device. For example, is the software control system clearly defined? Does the software avoid potential problems that could be caused by defective external components? Does the software control trap infinite loops, deadly embraces, or runaway conditions? Have validity checks been defined, and can corrective action be taken within any critical processing windows? In summary, the software quality assurance concern with the architecture design is to verify that the software specifications will be met, that the course of further design and development is well defined, that the software architecture reflects an approach that will help reduce software complexity, and that the design conforms to the intended application.

Software Detailed Design Review

The DDR is intended primarily to review most of the module designs, but it should also include review of any updates to the overall software architecture and design. Design changes come to the attention of the software quality assurance group through its representation on the change control board, which will be discussed later. Such updates, other than outright alterations to the design, are generally in the form of the addition of more detail to the overall software architecture and design. These may be reviewed informally for their responsiveness to the software specifications through the use of design walk-throughs.

The bulk of the DDR, however, is concerned with reviewing the design of the tasks and the high-order modules first identified in the ADS and described in the low-level modules of the Detailed Design Specification (DDS). Software quality assurance must address several areas. First, it should assure that the software architectural structure of the modules and submodules has been adequately defined. For example, are the function and interface of a module with other modules specified? Do the various design-capturing mechanisms clearly indicate the scope of the code that will implement it? Have numerical techniques or algorithms been analyzed for accuracy and range? Are they consistent with module specifications and with the end purpose of the software? Are the timing estimates consistent with module specifications? Have the memory requirements been estimated? Has each of the functions defined in the module specifications been addressed? Does the module design imply any limitations or constraints not previously known?

Second, software quality assurance should ensure that the software detailed design conforms to programming standards. For example, assuming that the software development policies and the programming standards refer explicitly to the use of structured design techniques, does the detailed design conform to the precepts of structure?

Third, quality assurance should ensure that the software detailed design adequately reflects safety-related processing. For example, has critical timing been analyzed? Can all processing occur within the critical window and within adequate margins? Are corrective actions for potentially invalid conditions reasonable in regard to minimizing their effect on the system or on user inputs? In summary, a successful DDR ensures that the planned construction of the software will permit the software end product to fulfill its assigned requirements within the system as a whole, and that the software is ready to be developed completely.

Code Walk-throughs

Code inspections can be viewed as an extension to the software test function. In fact, code reviews are formally structured activities, and software quality assurance personnel should be prepared to examine code and look for specific logic or processing errors, as well as general adherence to good software engineering practices. First, software quality assurance should ensure that the code supports the programming standards and conventions. For example, are there any violations of the accepted programming standards? Are the entry and exit interfaces consistent with other modules and the overall design? Are the standards and conventions related to internal comments and documentation supported? Second, quality assurance should ensure that the code reflects the detailed design. For example, does the code deviate from the detailed design document? Are there any unreachable code sections? Are there any unidentified variables? Are pointers and index variables checked for validity prior to use and, if not, is the rationale for ignoring the test acceptable? Do module descriptions and names match those in the design documentation? If the code is written in or uses assembly language, is the use of registers consistent with the overall design? In summary, a software quality assurance program should not be implemented without code inspections; the practice and its subsequent positive results are well regarded within the software industry, as will be discussed in more detail later.

Software Test Plan and Procedure Review

Software development test plans are prepared early in the software development phase, and they are reviewed several times during the software development life cycle to permit the test procedures to be prepared and additional test resources to be procured or developed. The final review and approval of the development test plans occurs at the time of the DDR. Regardless of the particular type of software development test being planned, certain aspects of the test plan documents should command software quality assurance personnel's attention. First, software quality assurance should ensure that the test environment is clearly identified. For example, are all of the hardware and support software that are implicit in the plan clearly identified? Are any to be acquired; if so, are any specifications required? Have additional support personnel beyond software engineers been identified; if so, has their availability been established? Second, software quality assurance personnel should examine and critique the test philosophy and strategy.

For example, will simulation, emulation, or both be used for any of the testing? Should the further use of automated test tools be considered as a viable alternative and cost-effective approach to defect removal? Will end-product hardware be required prior to software integration; if so, when will it be available? Have the sequences of software integration events been identified? Are the test procedures defined well enough to support the demonstration of software adequacy and completeness?

In summary, test plans are derived by software developers and generated to test the development of the software. The primary software quality assurance concern for these tests is that each test should be planned to make effective use of that part of the software allocated to the test and that all necessary hardware, software, and resources will be available when needed.

The test procedures are initially identified in the software test plans, and they govern the conduct of software tests. The test procedures assume the availability of all resources, as well as the personnel identified in the test plans, and indicate how they will be used. The sequence of the tests and the testing itself represent a gradual progression from the level of the code to the level of the completely integrated software as an end product. Although it may prove difficult to state all of the test conditions to be satisfied, the test procedures must provide specifics for those tests that demonstrate the compliance of each module with the module specifications and of the integrated code with the software requirements. Each validation test should be sufficiently explicit in the definition of input stimuli to assure the repeatability of the test, as well as in the definition of the expected results to permit auditing of the testing later. The test procedures should name or describe any data reduction procedures that will be followed. Because software quality assurance personnel are privy to the preparation of these test procedures, it is probably not necessary for the procedures to be formally reviewed. Instead, the software quality assurance team merely reviews them as a qualitative measure of how well they will validate and qualify the implemented software relative to design and requirements.

Software Audits

As stated above, the software quality assurance group reviews the SCMP to ensure two conditions:

1. To make certain that there will be no ambiguity concerning the software developed on the project—that the actual code was tested and executes within the device.

2. To answer any questions related to the currency of the software documents that serve as the references for software validation.

Beyond the establishment of a reasonable plan, the software quality assurance group must assure itself that the plan is being followed. This implies that the configuration management procedures and version control methods must be audited at periodic or frequent intervals, depending on the items audited.

The process of following a change order to the product or system requirements into the software requirement document(s) and into the design documents is a fairly simple matter of inspection. However, software library and code changes initiated during the testing of software and then worked backward to the design and possibly into the software requirements present a more difficult problem. Library control becomes an inherent feature of the library package for version control and should be spot checked at periodic intervals. During the early coding efforts, the checking could occur biweekly or weekly, depending on the level of coding activity. During software integration, library and code audits should be made at least weekly, possibly even daily during the final testing activities.

Test-derived code modifications to baselined items are generally documented through the use of a change request form. The change request form assures that the code and, if necessary, the documents will be changed. From the software quality assurance perspective though, this entails examination of the source code and the document files. Realistically, it is impractical to do this for all changes, so periodic audits are relied on to verify that the configuration management procedures are being followed and that the requested changes are being made.

Discrepancies in the version of any baselined item can create mischief very quickly. Although it may be practicable to permit substantial delays in the implementation of corrective action for defects found in any of the other reviews, problems encountered or exposed by configuration management audits must be rectified immediately. The software quality assurance group must have the authority to freeze all code, if such action is deemed necessary, to straighten out the discrepancies found; this freezing period might even include suspending or halting any test activity. The rationale for this is readily apparent to those who have known software development projects in which the software has gotten out of control. Taking such a drastic action implies, usually, one of two conditions. First, the frequency of the audits was inadequate and should be increased. Increasing the frequency of the audits is a relatively minor irritant, but any discrepancies can be readily remedied. The second condition is that software engineers who are charged with implementing the corrective action in the defective software are performing irresponsibly; this is not a minor irritant, but a major catastrophe in the making.

Another area for the software quality assurance group is the auditing of conducted tests. This is performed by verifying that the test procedures are being followed and that the recorded output is accurately logged or attached to the test procedure, if it is an automated output. Verification of test execution as planned and authentication of the results apply only to those tests for which procedures actually exist. This means that the validation of tests occurs only to the formally reviewed and approved testing and not to testing that is performed to get the software to execute successfully. The software quality assurance group need not be present during the actual test conducted; the issue is not the honesty of the software developers or of the software testers but, rather, the extent to which the test discipline adheres meticulously to procedures and data recording practices. As in most areas of human behavior, it is all too easy to find shortcuts that appear harmless, but some individual must be able to verify that testing is not permitting the gradual erosion of the standards of precision and that testing was performed in the way that both project management and the customer expected it would be. Occasional visits by the software quality assurance group during the testing operations will help to provide this reassurance, even if the group does nothing more than draw the testers' attention to the extent of their departure from the standards. The frequency of the visits will depend on the individuals involved; the appropriate average interval between the visits can be derived only through experience.

Software Reuse

Although there has been debate on the merits of software reuse, the mere fact that debates occur indicates that the concept provides its own set of problems as well as an insight into the software development process. In fact, software reuse is becoming so widespread that medical software development organizations need not pick just one reuse technology for their software development, but may select two or more reuse technologies that provide the best and most economical coverage for their applications. The reason for this is risk management.

Adoption

Software reuse is a viable strategy for dealing with the marketplace when demand is growing but budgets are shrinking, competition is increasing, and organizations are streamlining. However, instituting reuse effectively in product and software development is a challenge; a variety of technical, managerial, economic, social, and legal factors must be recognized, addressed, and resolved.

Reuse adoption refers to the process of transforming an organization's way of conducting business from one-of-a-kind product development to a reuse-driven approach, where the goal is to reorganize resources to meet the customer's needs with greater efficiency. Intuitively, software engineers grasp what the technologies are designed to accomplish because they use reuse daily; when presented with a new task, they often draw on related experiences of their own or of others. On occasion, and anticipating similar tasks in the future, they design their work for reuse, although they generally think of this as a good engineering practice rather than reuse. Many organizations now want to institutionalize the practice.

The essence of adopting reuse is implementing a program to institutionalize reuse. It begins with the identification of reuse opportunities, showing how reuse would contribute to the organization's objectives and developing a plan for managing the reuse program. Next the organization's current reuse situation is assessed, goals are established, and alternative strategies for adopting reuse are formulated. Each strategy must be analyzed so that risk and economic factors are taken into account. Next, the organization develops a plan that implements the strategy of choice, begins the plan, and reviews its progress.

Under reusability, software construction will add two additional activities to its process model (see Figure 6-20); component development and component retrieval. During software development, the construction process will be modified by inclusion of a component policy that addresses those modules to be reused. Specifically, the component policy must cover the development and implementation standards for data management and interfaces, encouraging the adoption of standard software architectures and inhibiting insular activities that encourage software development from scratch. V&V policies will also need modification to support reuse. Specifically, the policy must address the implementation of systematic evaluation techniques that go beyond the traditional testing techniques. It must also include a more careful and detailed

Figure 6-20   Software development life cycle with reuse

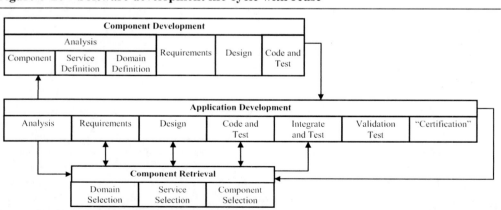

visual inspection of the software components for reuse to ensure that they comply explicitly with the programming standards and conventions.

An added stage to the conventional software construction activities must be integrated into the software life cycle. Component development may occur independently of the software application. For example, a particular software requirement might be identified that requires a specific data structure and access interface that could be developed as a stand-alone and independent task from the mainline software development effort. Another aspect of this independent stage is the conversion or generalization of a specific function that has already been developed. For example, an editing function used in the user interface task might require alteration from its current configuration to make it compatible with the current requirements. Another example might be the encapsulation of a units conversion routine that was once embedded within a module and is now a reusable library function.

Component retrieval must also be added to the software development life cycle to retrieve those reuse modules that were archived by prior projects. The retrieval function or service should be based on an archiving system that uses keywords and documentation techniques to select and extract the reusable components. The archiving also requires configuration management to handle the existing component base and modifications and updates, and classification techniques for storing and retrieving components.

Three distinct activities must be accommodated in reuse: production, technology, and certification. These activities may be assigned to a group other than the normal software construction group or team, or they can be additional activities for the standard development team. The production activity, the central one, creates software applications from reusable components. Production utilizes analysis and design techniques similar to those used in the traditional software engineering activities. The technology activity supplies, maintains, and manages the reuse components and provides general support for the production activity. The certification activity applies strict quality control procedures to the reuse components to ensure that all components satisfy the quality requirements and that the resultant applications meet the user or customer requirements.

Strategies

The beginning point for software reuse is the recognition that both reuse and development represent the construction of an entirely new product by combining two forms of functionality. Invariant functionality is the reuse of components or modules without change. For example, mathematical routines, unit conversion routines, real-time executives, and CRC calculations can be reused without modifications. By definition, unchanged code alone cannot create a new system, because it lacks the customization needed to meet the new set of requirements. Variant functionality is the set of new software that must be added to customize the invariant modules. Variant functionality can be as simple as a few parameters passed to an invariant functionality package, or as complex as fully developed new software modules or systems. Regardless of how simple or complex the software, it will always contain some mix of these two functional types. Invariant functionality provides the kernel around which the new software can be constructed; variant functionality lets the software address the new set of requirements.

The intent of reuse development is not to do away with the variant components, since that would, in effect, prevent addressing of any new needs. The objective of effective reuse development is the creation of invariant components that help focus the development of variant functionality into very precise, succinct statements of the differences between the old and new software usage. Reuse intensive development is, paradoxically, best accomplished by focusing more on how to change the software effectively than on how to keep it from changing at all; well-focused mechanisms for expressing variant functionality will do far more to keep large sections of code invariant than will arbitrary attempts to build around existing code components.

The concept of variant and invariant functions can be readily extended to activities outside code development by analyzing how they can be built. This can be done by combining baseline components of various sizes and types. Just as with executable code, the objective in building a reusable system specification is to develop a set of baseline components that support concise and succinct descriptions of how the new reuse specifications differ from the existing specifications.

Because reusable systems are constructed from some mix of invariant and variant functionality, the manner in which they are combined is an important criterion for evaluating a code's reuse characteristics. In general, this has led to two broad, complementary reuse strategies. Adaptive reuse uses large code segments as invariants and restricts variability to lower level and isolated locations within the overall code structure. Examples of this include changing arguments to parameterized modules, replacing input and output modules, and altering individual lines of code within a module. Adaptive reuse can be thought of as the equivalent of software maintenance; both try to isolate changes to minimize their global impact. Compositional reuse uses small code parts as invariants and variant functionality as the structure that links those parts. Examples of this strategy are the reuse of code from a reuse library and programming in a high-level language. Compositional reuse is similar to conventional programming, in which individual functions of moderate complexity are composed according to a grammar and assembled to create new and more powerful functions.

Adaptive and compositional reuse are very different. Adaptive reuse endeavors to maintain the overall structure invariant; it tends to be application specific and comparatively inflexible. However, it does help keep reuse costs under control. Compositional reuse is very flexible if the original set of reusable components is sufficiently rich and generalized. However, the initial cost of constructing such a generalized component set can be very expensive for reuse. In fact, if compositional reuse is extended to the extreme, it begins to take on the look of conventional programming. Compositional reuse also has a coverage level characteristic that refers to the ability of a set of reuse parts to address an application area without forcing the use of a lower level language. Full coverage sets are sufficiently rich and complete to solve new problems within a well-defined application area by using only those reusable parts. Partial coverage sets provide representative parts that act as examples of the component types needed to solve problems in an application area. Partial coverage sets are not sufficiently generalized to solve a problem in the application area without resorting to the use of lower level languages.

Economics

Software reuse usually focuses on reusing source code, but other areas of the software development cycle can also qualify for reuse; architecture and design, user interface, project planning, and testing are the most readily apparent artifacts. However, some very serious barriers must be overcome before software reuse can approach its economic potential. First, successful reuse demands that the reusable materials be certified to levels of quality that seriously approach or actually achieve zero defects. Poor quality, poor quality control, and careless software practices are common, and they preclude producing reusable software artifacts. Not only is there the added cost to clean up a quality-deficient artifact, but also, to make it ready for reuse it must undergo additional V&V scrutiny, which contributes to longer delivery times. The concept is to produce only quality and validated software that sits on the shelf waiting for the next project;

anything else is an added burden that goes beyond the fundamental scope and costs of the software development project.

Second, a reuse artifact must be constructed so that reuse is straightforward and efficient. This means that the initial construction of the reusable materials is more expensive and time-consuming than building ordinary software, but the succeeding projects benefit greatly. In fact, such construction is about 50 percent more expensive than normal construction and requires about 30 percent longer schedules (Jones 1994c), but subsequent projects can take advantage of the reuse project artifacts. The reason for the additional cost is the effort required to generalize and validate the reusable components. However, reusing a component costs 25 percent of the development cost of an equivalent function (Troy 1994), because of the effort needed to locate the required component, gain an understanding of how it works, and then integrate it into the reuse application. The cost of maintaining reuse components represents 10 percent of their development cost (Troy 1994).

Third, assuming that a library is created and stocked with useful, reusable artifacts, incentives must be offered to project management and technical personnel for using the materials. The ordinary time and materials accounting approach to most software projects is a severe disincentive to reuse; a change in practice must be forced at both the cultural and financial levels. To overcome these barriers and convert to software business practices that encourage reuse is a switch in the focus of measurements from what is developed to what is delivered. Another helpful shift is the use of modern functional metrics as the basis of software development. For example, suppose a device company decides to deliver an application containing 500 function points (about 60,000 C statements) for a development cost that is not to exceed $250 per function point, or $125,000. Assume that the average industry cost is $1,000 per function point. It is obvious that to be successful, the development team would need extensive reuse capabilities for many of the project deliverables.

Fourth, software is a key to competitiveness and therefore represents a valuable company resource. Ten years ago, software represented 30 percent of the functionality of an average information system. Currently, that figure is about 70 percent; five years from now, software will represent 90 percent (Troy 1994). As efforts concentrate on those factors that set a company apart from the competition, reuse performance will become a critical part of software processes.

Last, any given software project that envisions the usage of reusable artifacts or materials must be planned and designed initially with reuse in mind. This means that software life cycles, estimating tools, planning tools, standards, and design methods must include specific capabilities for dealing with reusable materials. Currently, most software management tools and practices have no provisions for reuse.

The Software Postmortem

Software postmortems are meetings in which continuous improvements in software processes are made. From these meetings, the effective, efficient, and productive software activities and procedures are formalized, institutionalized, and fostered. The software activities and products that did not work or produced poor results are scrutinized to determine their root causes. Then they are either eliminated or modified, to achieve a more robust software engineering process. Although the postmortem can be expected to last a full day, it is not uncommon for this meeting to last for more than one day, particularly for large, multiyear, multiperson projects. To achieve full effectiveness, the meetings should be held off-site from the company facility.

The attendees can be varied, but if the combined software development, V&V, and software quality assurance staffs are small, say 20 or fewer, then it is usually beneficial for the entire staff to attend. If the size of the staff is large or not everyone can attend because of other project schedules and commitments, then software lead engineers from all current projects, along with all of the software engineering staff who participated on the project just concluded, should attend. It is probably also appropriate to have the project's lead electrical engineer attend, to provide a valuable perspective of the software effort from a different point of view.

A typical software postmortem (Table 6-6) begins with the setting of ground rules (Table 6-7) for the meeting and a review of the agenda. Although setting meeting ground rules is not too common for technical meetings, the intent of the postmortem is to be nonconfrontational, to

Table 6-6   Typical Agenda for a Software Postmortem Meeting

Agenda Item	Description
1	Introduction
1.1	Ground Rules
1.2	Agenda
2	Surveys—Part I
2.1	Report Card
2.2	Process Maturity
3	Historical Perspective
3.1	Project
3.2	Software Team
3.3	Results—Actuals
3.4	Results—Prediction
3.5	Process, Methodology, and Practice
4	The Postmortem
4.1	Process
4.2	Methodology
4.3	Practices
4.4	Documents
4.5	Metrics
4.6	Management
5	Surveys—Part II
5.1	Report Card
5.2	Process Maturity
5.3	Result Comparison

Table 6-7   Typical Ground Rules for a Software Postmortem Meeting

Rule Number	Description
1	Attack ideas, not the person
2	Any subject is fair discussion
3	There are no right answers
4	Nonvolatile, unemotional discussions only
5	Respect for the dignity, position, and rights of others
6	Privileged and private discussions
7	All decisions, rulings, judgments, close calls, conclusions, determinations, resolutions, decrees, edicts, pronouncements, sentences, and so on, are the reserved rights of the referee and/or management

elicit honest and frank observations and comments about the project and its results. Because of the nature of the meeting, it is important that a strong facilitator, knowledgeable about software, be present to guide and monitor the progress of the discussions and, most important, to ensure that meaningful dialogues take place.

As shown in Table 6-6, the first item on the agenda is two surveys. The intent of the surveys is to ascertain the perceived effectiveness of the project as a whole, and of the software process that was used on the project. The first survey is a report card (Figure 6-21), to be completed by both software developers and the software V&V members who participated on the project; each group circles a grade for each subject under the respective column head. The second survey is used to assess the effectiveness of the software process itself. An effective survey to use is a modified and shortened version of the Software Engineering Institute's software process maturity self-assessment. The results of both of these surveys will help to calibrate the software group's understanding of how well the process works from the development as well as the V&V perspectives. The results of this survey should be tabulated but withheld from presentation to the group at this time.

The third item on the agenda is the historical perspective of the project. This should be presented by the software lead engineer, but it is not uncommon for other individuals to make parts of this presentation. The intent is to review the project software activities, starting with the first day of the project and concluding with the last day. The software lead engineer should review all of the project software planning documents generated during the project start-up, to become refreshed and familiarized with the original intent and direction of the project. The primary documents to be reviewed are the SDP, the SDTP, the Software Verification and Validation Plan (SVVP), and the SVTP, and of secondary importance are the SCMP, the Software End-Product Acceptance Plan (SEAP), and the SQAP. The SDP, SDTP, SVVP, and SVTP are of particular importance because they represent the presumed and predicted course of events for the project. Within those documents, the sections describing schedule, techniques, methodologies, strategies, testing, and activities should be reviewed for comparison with the actual events in the project.

The software lead engineer should then gather the actual, final development metrics on the project relative to the total time spent on the project, the total number of software engineers

Figure 6-21   A typical software team report card

PROGRAM/PROJECT SOFTWARE TEAM

REPORT CARD

Please grade how well the software team performed the following software aspects of the project from your perspective as either a software DEVELOPER or as a software V&V individual.

The grades run from the highest (1) to the lowest (5).

SUBJECT	DEVELOPER	V&V
Analysis	1 2 3 4 5	1 2 3 4 5
Requirements	1 2 3 4 5	1 2 3 4 5
Design	1 2 3 4 5	1 2 3 4 5
Code	1 2 3 4 5	1 2 3 4 5
Test	1 2 3 4 5	1 2 3 4 5
Integration	1 2 3 4 5	1 2 3 4 5
Verification and validation	1 2 3 4 5	1 2 3 4 5
Configuration management	1 2 3 4 5	1 2 3 4 5
Hardware interaction (*)	1 2 3 4 5	1 2 3 4 5

* How well, overall, did the software aspects interact with the hardware teams?

who worked on the project, and the software metric counts. The project software lead engineer then presents this information to the attendees and contrasts the values that were estimated at the outset of the project with the actuals at the end of the project. Last, the software lead engineer reviews the process, methodology, and practices employed in the project, especially any that differed from the documented policies, SOPs, or guidelines. The rationale for this historical perspective is to remind everyone of the project and to refresh their memories, to help stimulate and facilitate the following discussions.

The fourth agenda item is the discussion of the project itself. This part may be structured or informal, but it is essential that several key areas of the project be discussed. These areas are the process, methodology, and practices that were used; the documents that were generated; the metrics that were captured; and project management. From the discussions related to the software process, methodology, and practices will come suggested changes and modifications to the existing policies, SOPs, and guidelines. The software project documents should be examined from the standpoint of their information content, usefulness, and format. The metrics should be examined from several directions. First, they should be compared to past projects as well as to current, ongoing projects to determine if improvements have been made. Second, they should be examined for their relevancy, usefulness, and timeliness. Last, they should be examined for their relative merit as meaningful predictors of the software process in general and of a project specifically.

The results of these discussions are twofold. First, these results are reflected, as appropriate, into the policies, SOPs, and guidelines as updates and revisions after the meeting concludes. The updated and revised documents then compose the set of software engineering documents for any new projects that are about to begin. Second, because the software lead engineers from current projects are present, they can install some of these suggestions immediately into their projects at their discretion.

The last agenda item is to repeat the same two surveys taken earlier. It is not unusual for the results of these same surveys to be different, for two fundamental reasons. First, because the project just recently ended, there can be negative feelings and perceptions about the project that can influence an individual's evaluative thought process. Second, at the end of the postmortem, the individuals who participated in the project will generally tend to feel better about it and its results as a whole. Therefore, the results should be generally more positive than the previous results. The results of the first and second surveys should then be compared and contrasted with the group. The "truth" about process maturity, and how software engineers perceive their overall effort, will usually lie somewhere between the two results.

7

The Software Quality Assurance Program: Software Testing Activities

To test the products produced or captured by analysis, design, and coding, testers must not only understand the components themselves, they must also understand the interrelationships among these products and the processes that captured or produced them. In short, they must have a good understanding of development methods and tools.

—Edward V. Berard

Assume that you are a software engineer. You know that as soon as you have finished the coding of a particular assignment, you will want to prove that it works right. However, there is a hidden fallacy in this mind-set. This is the right approach in the sense that this is a fairly factual representation of real life, but it is wrong if you expect testing to be a productive means of making the code more correct. The primary goal of testing is not the demonstration of the correctness of the software but, rather, the uncovering of as many defects within the software as possible. Just like death and taxes, there are defects in software.

The design of a test case is not the only ingredient that contributes to the productivity of a test. The type of software being tested can also influence the quality of the test. For example, assume that the test cases are based on the operational environment for which the software to be tested has been developed. It is reasonable to expect that the responses of the software to the test stimuli will be partitioned in a manner that reflects the structure of the software. Therefore, the testing of software that is related to keypad inputs should be processed in that part of the software concerned with user inputs, and it should be ignored in all other areas of the software, such as motor control or sensor monitoring. This illustrates that testing need not check the response of the software at all key test points, but only at certain predetermined points; because of this the software has an attribute of functional modularity.

Functional modularity is one of the four characteristics of testable software found in the IEEE Computer Society's definition of "testable." The other characteristics refer to the facility with which diagnostics may be invoked; the inclusion of additional code for evaluation of invariants; and the annotation of evaluation criteria that is placed in the source code at the points at which measurements are made. Fundamentally, a software end product is testable to the extent that it facilitates the establishment of verification criteria and supports evaluation of its performance. It would be difficult to argue with the intent of this definition since it promotes those software features and attributes that improve the productivity of the test process. However, once the code has been written, this definition is not particularly useful to the development of test methodologies. The design of a test by the software engineer, who is knowledgeable in the design of the software, leads to the verification of the code with respect to the design, without regard to design faults.

Software Nodes and Paths

Software cannot be said to have been properly tested until all of the code has been executed. However, a single, successful execution of a code segment does not prove that the segment is free of defects. The segment may, in fact, execute correctly with certain combinations of some segments, but not at all with other code segments. Consequently, software testing should focus on the paths between the segments, not merely the segments themselves, since they were tested during the construction of the segment. This means that, at the very least, the path between each pair of code segments or nodes is executed before testing can be completed. Because code construction tests the segments through the activity of debugging, and if all paths between these segments are executed, then the software can be certified as fully tested because all of the segments will have been executed during the execution of the software control path mechanisms.

In an unstructured program, this approach is impossible, and testing should probably not even begin. In a structured program, however, testing can take advantage of several good coding practices that should be documented in the software development SOPs and guidelines. For example, the single-entry and single-exit construct produces a valuable test environment, because it forces many obvious terminal node pairs that sufficiently bind the software to finite ranges to permit the testing as discussed above.

Among other things, a directed graph of a software segment (Figure 7-1) is a way of illustrating the accessibility of any given node as the iterative function of the accessibility of the nodes separating it from the root of the graph. An additional feature of the directed graph is that it can portray either an individual module and its internal logic structure or a conglomeration of modules and the logic path between the modules. As shown in Figure 7-1, the directed graph consists of five unique paths from N_{11} to N_{51}. They are easy to identify and can be exercised by suitable test data that will cause the switching between the various conditional branches at N_{11}, N_{21}, N_{22}, and N_{33}.

In addition, there is a loop in this specific example from N_{51} to N_{11} that, if it is executed n times, increases the number of paths that can be executed from five to 5^n. The original five paths have, in effect, become concatenated in n different ways. It is not the intent of this discussion to present the exhaustive theory of software directed graphs and testing, since there are numerous sources that are devoted to this topic, but rather to set the context in which software testing must become practical rather than impossible, random, or hit-and-miss.

This illustration of a simple software segment and its directed graph provides the intuitive understanding that within even a modest software module of five code segments, a 100 percent

Figure 7-1　Example of a directed graph representation of software

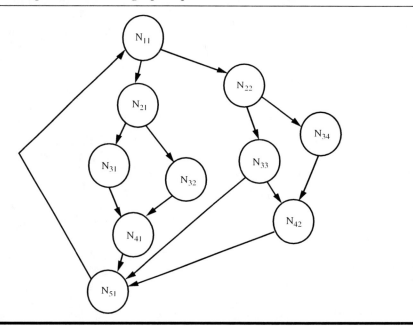

path testing is possible, but that a simple loop condition creates virtual paths that cannot reasonably be tested. The expectations and limitations of path testing can be summarized, in general, by using three categories of implementation defects: missing control flow paths, inappropriate path selection, and inappropriate or missing actions.

Missing control flow paths cannot be tested because, by definition, they are not present, yet their absence can cause software failures. For example, if the path around a division operation should be taken when the test for a divide by zero is not present, then the software will most likely fail, because the path does not exist and division by zero will be attempted. An example of an inappropriate path selection is the incorrect or inadequate branch condition specification in which each individual path may, in fact, have been exercised and tested, but some of the paths will be taken under the wrong conditions. Inappropriate or missing actions are the real, value-added aspects of path testing. This type of testing would uncover, for example, the addition, rather than multiplication, of two numbers; passing of the wrong data from one module to another; and failure to initialize data properly. As a fundamental test method, the deliberate execution of sequences of paths is a productive technique at the code construction phase, because it relies on the software engineer's knowledge of the software. It is also viable when the software module size is modest and when structured programming approaches have been applied.

However, there does exist a diabolical aspect of software path testing. It is possible, and not uncommon, to include software paths that are impossible to reach. For example, suppose module *A* checks to determine if some error condition exists before it passes control to module *B*. If the error condition exists, then module *A* passes control to an error routine rather than to module *B*. Suppose that module *B* also checks for the same error, because its software engineer wanted assurance that module *B* would not cause a catastrophic failure if it were to execute under the error condition. During the integration testing of both modules, it should be apparent that the path in module *B* to avert a software failure will never be taken and, therefore, will never be tested. Although this may be a harmless coding error that will never be caught by testing, a subsequent change to the software could expose this untested path to execution. It is not unusual to have paths in the software that, to be completely tested, require assessment of an impossible set of conditions.

Stress and Boundary Tests

Tests that apply to the operational or functional capabilities of the product are straightforward and fundamentally demonstrate the satisfaction of specified requirements. Tests that attempt to assess the operational limits of the software are independent of the path tests. Boundary tests determine the operational limits of the software in predictable environments. For example, a syringe pump is usually designed to infuse fluid into a patient at some maximum rate. Because of computations within the instrument and subsequent round-off error, boundary testing should be conducted at the prescribed maximum rate, plus a small increment beyond that value. Boundary tests are usually used to calibrate the performance envelope of the software. The tests of the individual modules within the software may also include boundary tests. For example, if the device contains a keypad for user inputs to command the device, then the modules performing the processing related to the keypad inputs should be exposed to data at minimum and maximum magnitudes and rates, as well as several sensitive points in between. These boundary tests are conducted primarily to expose inadequate software design or faulty code, rather than to explore the performance of the software.

The distinction between stress and boundary tests is often not great, but the subtle differences can be distinguished. Stress tests are analogous to the destructive physical tests to which hardware parts are frequently exposed. For example, to stress test the rate of the serial communications lines in a medical device before the device software can no longer keep up, the rate of meaningful data packets is increased until the device stops. Commonly, stress and boundary tests result in "breaking points" being reached that are below the expected, designed, or required thresholds. This condition may indicate a software defect in the code, the design, or even the specified device requirements. In any of these cases, it usually reflects the condition in which a combination of software logic paths is being executed for the first time. The tests have achieved the effect of testing against the postulated operational environment.

Stress and boundary tests have several similarities to the environmental testing performed on the hardware. Although failures are expected, these tests are not specifically directed toward exposing outright defects. Instead, they are designed to define the software performance in given environmental conditions. Consequently, only if the performance falls below the accepted limits when confronted with a quantified environment, as specified in the requirements definition, does the software really become a failure. Because definition of the device's environment is usually difficult, two situations arise. First, software engineers who are searching for either defects or proof of performance easily overlook these tests. The difficulty with this is that it will be the user or customer who will discover the device's software deficiencies and inadequacies. Second, the failure of a boundary or stress test is, at best, a judgment call decided by the best engineering judgment used to analyze the environmental conditions. Consequently, what the software quality assurance engineer may raise as a software anomaly, relative to the quantified environment, may be adjudicated by the software and system architects. In summary, although stress and boundary tests do not apply to all software within a device, they will apply to a part of it; when they do, it is the responsibility of the software quality assurance engineer to ensure that the tests are performed.

Software Testing Strategy

The primary purpose of software testing is to find interior defects so that they can be corrected. The secondary purpose of the testing is to determine the operational limits of the software. Path testing provides good test coverage during code construction, and stress and boundary testing flexes the software from an environmental standpoint. The testing that occurs between these two test approaches requires a strategy that is as deliberate in its methodology as was the systematic development of the analysis, design, and implementation of the code. Just as code development evolved from the general, at the product level, to the specific, at the code level, the software testing strategy proceeds in the opposite manner. It starts with specific module testing and progresses up to validation testing of the software end product. The process from system specification to code implementation is mirrored by the progression of tests that validate the results and accomplishments of each stage. Examples of functional tests, robustness or boundary tests, and stress tests are shown in Tables 7-1 through 7-3.

At each stage of software construction, it is obvious that the exposure of as many defects as possible is desirable and that the total number of defects found is the sum of the number of

Table 7-1　Typical Examples of Software Functional Testing

Functional Area	Types of Testing
Functional mode tests	Transitions between operational modes Correct inputs generate correct outputs Inputs and outputs include switches, tones, messages, and alarms
Remote communications tests	Connect and disconnect Valid commands inquiry Handling of invalid commands and inquiries For all baud rates supported Corrupted frames Error handling in general and the interface to the error handler Control mode, with emphasis on safety aspects Monitor mode, with emphasis on fidelity of values reported
Timing tests	Active failure tests are completed within system critical time(s) Passive failure tests are completed within the operational window
Battery tests	Ramp up and ramp down of voltages Various levels of warnings, alarms, and errors

Table 7-2   Typical Examples of Software Robustness Testing

Robustness Area	Types of Testing
Boundary testing	Over and under specified limits Numerical values that determine logic flow based on minimum or maximum value Negative numerical values
Overflow and underflow values	Too large for all algorithms Too small for all algorithms
User interface	Enter unexpected values Enter unexpected sequences
Execution time-line processing	Routines that have execution time limits are altered to introduce delays Tasks that have execution time limits are altered to introduce delays Routines with execution constraints due to parametric calculations are altered
Data transmissions	Unexpected commands are transmitted to the remote communications handler Unexpected data are transmitted to the remote communications handler

Table 7-3   Typical Examples of Software Stress Testing

Stress Area	Types of Testing
Duration tests	Overnight runs Weekend runs Other types of software burn-in tests
Buffer overload tests	Global buffers under loaded and overflow conditions Global data structures under loaded and overflow conditions
Remote communications load tests	Verify the transfer at the maximum transfer rate Verify the transfer at the maximum rate under maximum load conditions
Worst case scenario tests	Verify the product and equipment operating capability under projected worst case Highest execution rate Event overload for event-driven systems

defects found at each stage. A less obvious reason for exposing as many defects as possible in each test suite is that the longer a defect remains in the software, the more expensive it is to remove it. For example, a defect detected during the construction of a module is known to be in the module under test, by definition. If the defect is initially discovered during software integration, then before it can be removed it must first be isolated to one of the modules that compose the current software integration being tested, because the defect may not, in fact, reside in the current module being integrated. If the defect is found during validation testing, it must be isolated to a module in a software system of even larger scope. In addition, as the software becomes integrated, the access to individual low-level nodes becomes more restrictive, and this limits the effectiveness of any diagnostic procedures. Furthermore, as the software gets closer to its release date, if the defects have not been isolated nor their cause found, work might have to be suspended on the remaining, unfinished parts of code. This suspension permits additional resources to be applied to locate the defect, as well as to prevent the software from becoming even larger, further complicating the search for the root cause of the defect.

Software test tactics should be formulated not necessarily on the number of defects found per unit of time nor per unit of work hours, but on a measure of the effectiveness that incorporates both the success in exposing the defects and the failure of leaving some defects still uncovered. Let us consider a hypothetical case. Mathematically, the efficacy of testing can be measured as follows:

$$E = [D_f/(D_f + D_r)] \times 100, \qquad (7.1)$$

where D_f is the number of defects found and D_r is the number of defects remaining after the test. For example, Table 7-4 shows a comparison of two mythical software products that underwent four types of testing. Assume that program *A* initially harbored 400 defects and that at the time of system release only 375 of those defects had been found. The overall efficacy is $(375/400) \times 100 = 93.75$. Assume that program *B* also had 400 initial defects, but the emphasis of the testing methods was changed to improve the efficacy of earlier testing at the expense of later testing. This might be accomplished, for example, by deliberately spending more in time and tools for module and integration testing than for validation and system or product testing. This approach found 383 defects out of 400 for an overall efficacy of $(383/400) \times 100 = 95.75$. The net number of defects remaining in the program has been reduced from 25 to 17, representing a total improvement of 32 percent.

Although this example is purely hypothetical and has little, if any, practical value, it does allow three valid conclusions to be drawn:

1. The efficacy of the test techniques must be measured and used as a basis for quality improvement.

Table 7-4   Example of Testing Efficacy for Two Software Programs

	Program A[1]			Program B[1]		
Testing Type	**Efficacy**[2]	**Defects Found**	**Defects Remaining**	**Efficacy**[2]	**Defects Found**	**Defects Remaining**
Module	50	200	200	70	280	120
Integration	50	100	100	70	84	36
Validation	50	50	50	30	11	25
System	50	25	25	30	8	17

Notes: 1. Programs are known to have 400 total defects.
    2. Efficacy = [(Defects found)/(Defects found + Defects remaining)] × 100.

2. The emphasis of the early tests should be entirely on the exposure of defects, while the later tests should focus on performance.

3. It is unconscionable to cut short module and integration testing to meet a previously established schedule.

Selection of Orthogonal Array Testing

Depending on the survey and the industry, testing consumes 30 to 70 percent of software development life cycle resources, and yet many faults escape the testing phase and are discovered in the field. This often causes customer dissatisfaction, high field maintenance cost, and a perception of poor product quality. This should motivate the software test group to find and plan more efficient software tests. Testing effectiveness can be improved in many ways, but, fundamentally, testing should wisely determine which tests must be executed. One way is to use the mathematical tool of orthogonal arrays to select the test cases intelligently. Test cases selected in this manner efficiently cover the test domain and, therefore, greatly improve the test engineers productivity. The success of the orthogonal arrays method can be attributed to two important factors. First, it encourages focused attention on the usage of the software being tested, and, second, it provides a mathematically sound way to span the entire operating domain with a minimum number of test cases.

Mandl (1985) suggested the use of orthogonal arrays for testing software. Although a review of the most commonly used test methods would clarify the advantages and differences of the orthogonal arrays testing method, an example using the orthogonal arrays software testing method is more illustrative. Consider a function to be tested that contains the four parameters A, B, C and D. These parameters could be the arguments of a command line entered from a PC, the state of an interface, input from a connecting device, or the initial states of internal parameters. Suppose each parameter has three possible levels, values, or conditions as shown in Table 7-5. The level could be a priority scheme in which level 1 is higher priority than level 2 and level 2 is higher than 3; or initial, intermediate, and final values; or state values. The test domain consists of 81 possible combinations of the test parameter levels, and it is assumed that the software must perform correctly for all possible values of these parameters. A thorough analysis of the software requirements document and understanding of the usage of the software are needed to prepare the parameter-level table, but knowledge of how the software is written is usually not necessary to generate the level table.

Table 7-5   Example Parameters and Levels of Orthogonal Array Testing

Test Parameter	Level		
	1	2	3
A	A_1	A_2	A_3
B	B_1	B_2	B_3
C	C_1	C_2	C_3

   In the orthogonal array–based testing method, the effort to generate the test plan can be small, and the test cases generated by this method have the highest effectiveness as measured in terms of the number of faults detected per test. Table 7-6 shows the orthogonal array–based test cases. The nine rows correspond to test cases, and the four columns correspond to the test parameters. As shown, the first test case comprises Level 1 for each parameter, and it represents the combination A_1, B_1, C_1, and D_1. The second test case comprises the combination A_1, B_2, C_2, and D_2, and so forth. Orthogonal array–based testing has the property that for each pair of columns, all parameter-level combinations occur an equal number of times. In the orthogonal array testing matrix shown, there are nine parameter-level combinations for each pair of columns, and each combination occurs once.

   By conducting the nine tests indicated by Table 7-6, the following faults can be detected. First, orthogonal array testing can detect and isolate all single-mode faults. A single-mode fault is a consistent problem with any level of any single parameter. For example, if all cases of parameter A at Level 1 cause an error condition, it is a single-mode failure, and test cases 1, 2, and 3 will show errors. By analysis of the information about which tests show the error, the identity of the factor level causing the fault can be determined. Second, orthogonal array testing can detect all double-mode faults, the condition of a consistent error existing when specific levels of two parameters occur together. A double-mode fault is an indication of pairwise incompatibility or harmful interactions between two test parameters. Third, orthogonal array testing can detect multimode faults. Although orthogonal array testing of strength 2 can assure the detection of only the single- and double-mode faults, it may also detect multimode faults. This can be determined by studying the interaction tables of the test cases.

   Software faults can be divided into two categories: region faults and isolated faults. Faults that occur for only one specific combination of test parameter levels, such as by data-entry errors, are called *isolated faults;* assurance against them is not possible without testing all combinations. However, when the underlying logic is faulty, there is a tendency for a region of the test domain to exhibit a malfunction; such faults are called *region faults.* Single- and double-mode faults are special cases of region faults. Orthogonal array testing is highly effective for

Table 7-6   Matrix for Example of Orthogonal Array–based Testing

Test Case	Test Parameter			
	A	B	C	D
1	1	1	1	1
2	1	2	2	2
3	1	3	3	3
4	2	1	2	3
5	2	2	3	1
6	2	3	1	2
7	3	1	3	2
8	3	2	1	3
9	3	3	2	1

the detection of region faults with a relatively small number of tests. Consider a geometric visualization example of software with only three test parameters A, B, and C. The test domain is cube-shaped because each parameter is represented by one axis and consists of 27 lattice points. Test cases based on one factor at a time cover only the cases on each of the three axes, which is a small region of the test domain. The orthogonal array–based test cases are dispersed uniformly throughout the test domain and greatly increase the possibility of detecting region faults, compared to any other test plan with the same number of test points not uniformly distributed in the test domain.

Unit and Module Testing

Testing at the unit level is directed toward the discovery of faults within each routine. These faults can either be a failure of the code to reflect the design or a failure of the code and design to satisfy the module's specified requirements. If the module has other modules subordinate to it, then the unit test of the topmost module of the set will, by definition, include the testing of the entire set. Unit testing is, therefore, a subset of module development and provides a more cohesive test strategy. Unit testing is mostly an informal process and activity per se; the formality attached to it is the proof that the module has been properly exercised. It can be concluded that the greater part of unit testing is based on the software engineer's informal test runs and that the module test procedure really only demonstrates compliance with the module's requirements specification.

Unit testing should include test cases for the execution of specific control paths and for the correlation of these test cases with the code or with design documentation. Unit testing is more likely to profit from contrived input rather than operational input, whereas module testing would use operational inputs adapted to the specific module's processing specification and design. For example, the input to unit tests encompasses all of the limit conditions applicable to the module, even if some of the conditions are considered to have no probability of occurrence in the operational environment. Although this sounds like overdesign, rigorous testing of this type provides a degree of tolerance to any errors made during design activities that would normally manifest themselves as interface failures at a later date. In addition, this type of testing also produces error calibration data in the boundary conditions, a place where exploratory boundary testing is appropriate at the module level.

Diagnostic input is also a better way to test path branching rather than data related to system requirements. It is not nearly as important *why* a path was taken as it is that it *was* taken. Error handling paths within software are the most likely of all software paths to be unexercised. Although software engineers are fairly good at including error traps, they are not particularly diligent about testing them, for three reasons:

1.   The absence of error traps and handlers is usually easy to spot in design reviews.

2.   The fact that an error is trapped is no assurance that corrective action can be taken.

3.   Some error traps are extremely difficult to test, even with contrived or diagnostic input.

Static Testing

Another technique used to augment the exposure of faults by testing is static analysis, which attempts to single out structural and semantic defects in the software. The target for this analysis is both design data and code, which can be implemented via software tools.

Compilers and linkers have for years been performing static testing and analysis, although they are traditionally not considered as such. Other types of static analysis output include the count of each type of code source statement used in the software, cross-references for the operands used, and cross-references of called and calling module entry points. Other static analysis outputs include lists of unused variables, mismatched module interfaces, inconsistent use of common data areas, and uninitialized variables. Some of these static analysis outputs are global and can be used to help with unit testing as well as module testing.

The use of static analysis prior to actual testing can reduce the time it takes to track down the cause of a particular test failure. In fact, it is reasonable to expect that static analysis will expose some defects that would slip past execution tests, because it exposes latent faults from a different test perspective. In a published experiment, static analysis was responsible for the detection of 16 percent of the errors seeded in a large program, while path testing found 25 percent (Gannon 1979).

One of the more attractive techniques for finding defects at the module level is a detailed inspection of the code itself. Software can be inspected, just as the requirements definitions and the various design documents can be inspected, by the software quality assurance group for consistency and accuracy. Code inspection is not a substitute for the actual exercise of the code, but rather a means of exposing faults that might otherwise go undetected. A more important subtlety of the code defects found by inspection is that they are more easily removed. For example, Russell (1993) found that approximately one defect was found for every person-hour invested in the inspection process; this was two to four times faster than detecting code errors by execution testing. When compared to defects found after release to the customer, Russell determined that each problem reported by the customer required an average of 4.5 person-days to repair and that one hour spent on inspection thus avoided 33 hours of subsequent maintenance effort, assuming a 7.5 hour workday.

The inspection effectiveness is also directly related to the speed at which source code statements are examined; slower paces yielded the best results. For example, inspections that proceed at the rate of 150 lines of code per hour detect the most errors—about 37 defects per 1000 lines of code, excluding comments. Inspections carried out at 750 lines of code per hour detect the fewest errors and average fewer than eight defects per 1000 lines, excluding comments. C. Jones (1986a) indicated that the defect density of software ranged between 49.5 and 94.6 defects per 1000 lines of code, and, therefore, Russell's 37 per 1000 may represent up to 80 percent of all defects in the code.

It is important to distinguish between code inspection, code walk-throughs, and code audits. Code audits are conducted to determine the fidelity with which the coding standards have been followed. They are concerned with matters such as comments and header documentation, labeling of instructions and operands, and location of declaration statements. These audits are usually conducted periodically and at random by the software quality assurance group.

Code walk-throughs are rather like show-and-tell meetings. Normally, the software engineer explains the code to a group of peers, and all participate in the attempt to find flaws. The subtle advantage to this strategy is that the group will then naturally begin to solve the flaws they find. The walk-throughs are usually informal, to keep the presenting software engineer from becoming defensive about the code being reviewed. The presence or absence of management is usually a function of the comfort level of the presenter and the assembled group. However, it is always a good idea to include someone from the software quality assurance group to verify that the code walk-through was held in accordance with software development policies and SOPs.

Although code inspections are more formal than code walk-throughs and audits, they should not be conducted as adversarial proceedings. Defects found in the code should be logged for subsequent corrective action. Whereas the code walk-through would usually occur with other software engineers, the code inspection group is probably not so homogeneous. The membership should comprise software engineers who have different roles on the project, such as design and test as well as coding. Checklists should be used to make certain all branches and interfaces have been examined and that no potential source of defects has been overlooked. For example, did the team check for remedial action and error logging for stack overflow? Did it check for inadvertent extensions of global data beyond what was allocated? Although the routine seems cumbersome, after a few of these inspections, it will become familiar, and the team will proceed more quickly.

The result of this organized approach is that code inspections may find more errors than actual code executions. For example, Gannon's (1979) experiment with path testing and inspection showed that in seven error categories, path testing found the greater number of computational and logic errors, while inspection uncovered the greater number of errors in I/O, data handling, interface, and data definition, and with the database. More important, the average time to find and correct an error was less for inspection than it was for path testing in all seven categories. Net increases of productivity that show a savings of 94 hours per 1000 lines of code have also been reported (Fagan 1976). As attractive as code inspection appears, it does not replace module execution testing. It does, however, augment it tremendously. Of course, the members of the inspection team must be fluent in the programming language under inspection. On the downside, the advantage of code inspections will be negated if the design documentation is not thorough, explicit, or current.

The contribution of the software quality assurance team is less involved with unit testing than with the other test phases, but less is still quite a lot. Software quality assurance personnel must review the test plans and procedures to make certain that they yield a good harvest of defects and are not contrived to prove correctness of the software. Static analysis is compellingly analogous to inspection activities, in which quality has traditionally provided cost-effectiveness. A software quality assurance person as an objective auditor should be present on every code inspection team, but need not be present during most of the actual testing. However, software quality assurance personnel should witness the execution of those test cases cited in the formal test procedures, to affirm operation in accordance with the procedures and to authenticate the data and results.

Integration Testing

Integration testing is primarily the test of the interfaces between the modules. The speed with which it can be accomplished is directly related to the care and detail with which the design and unit tests have been planned and performed. Integration testing is the location where the first cost savings that can be realized from the verification process show up. Under ideal circumstances, integration testing will take about as long as all of the unit testing. Under the worst of circumstances, it will require multiples of the work hours consumed by unit testing.

That the objective of integration testing is to expose interface defects suggests that only the linkages between the modules need be examined for failure sources. However, the source of the faults is usually not within the explicit module interface; rather, it tends to be in the internal logic of the module itself. Therefore, integration tests should be directed toward the manner in which the modules operate with each other. The order in which the modules are joined to the evolving software end product must be planned with the thought that the new paths created through the software, with the addition and integration of a new module with the existing set, will be sufficiently well defined to facilitate the design and application of the appropriate test cases. On the surface, this seems straightforward, until software logical iterations become a consideration; then the ability to exercise a few paths with a given test case is often impaired by the missing modules. To simplify the implementation of integration test cases and get the software functioning in an operational mode as quickly as possible, the modules that interface with the device's external world should be integrated as early as possible.

Although the density of path testing is not nearly as exhaustive in integration testing as in unit testing, certain multimodule paths will most likely be executed if the interfaces are to be properly exercised. There are several issues to be considered in determining the order in which the modules should join the system. If the integration order is not settled by careful planning, then productivity or thoroughness, or even both, will suffer. If the order strategy is not documented in the test plans, then careful planning will have been wasted. In addition to presenting the integration paths that will be taken, the test plans should state the environment needed, particularly with emphasis on any special hardware or software resources needed. Often, this requires the development or procurement of new equipment, and new or additional software tools. Because these items may require long lead times, it is important that the test plans be prepared early in the software development planning cycle.

The test plans should also outline the procedures that must be developed for each stage of the integration testing. The procedures must start by identifying the purpose of the test so that it can be tracked back to the testing plans. Input stimuli, and their point of application, must also be specified, as well as the expected results and their point of observation. Other information required to assure the productivity and repeatability of the testing should be included as appropriate. What should not be in the procedures are the type and qualifications of the test personnel, the order of the switches that must be energized, or any other information more appropriate to factory inspection.

The procedures and the test plans should be reviewed in terms of the verification of the software end product design. The review should focus on the capability of the test designs to flush out the defects. Software quality assurance personnel should be on hand during integration testing to certify the authenticity of the data collected, the adherence to library control practices, and the fidelity with which the procedures are being followed. It is not feasible to turn the conduct of integration testing over to an independent test team, because although the tests must demonstrate that the design of the software has been satisfied, the primary purpose of the integration tests is to expose faults. A good set of test designs will find the faults and tell the development team to further isolate and repair the faults found. In fact, it is not uncommon to spend a large part of the integration time in devising and executing diagnostic tests beyond those for which the original procedures were prepared. Integration testing is an integral part of software development; the role of software quality engineering is restricted to monitoring and auditing.

The sum of the testing used during integration will cover much of the software. Module-to-module path testing will have been performed, and there will have been software execution testing, in which representative operational input data require the modules to work together in various logical configurations. Some of these tests might even reflect stress and boundary testing. Software quality assurance personnel will have reviewed the integration plans and the integration test plans and procedures, monitored the integration testing to confirm conformance to the procedures and to library control standards, and certified the results. At the conclusion of the integration tests, ownership of the software is logically transferred from the software development team to the software quality assurance team. The testing of the software will no longer be controlled by the software developers, but by the independent software V&V group.

Validation Testing

Validation testing is the validation of the software end product by the V&V team or by the software quality assurance group. The successful conclusion of this phase means that the software is ready for integration with the associated hardware. It also indicates that the software is certified as being ready for manufacturing and for use within the device. In addition, the validation testing of any independent software end products developed under contract may also serve as tests for product acceptance. Although this is not of great importance, the contractor's testing plans and procedures should be reviewed by the software quality assurance group, which should also monitor the actual testing. Validation testing results in a demonstration under a formal regimen that the software end product meets its stipulated requirements.

By the time validation testing has been reached in the software development life cycle, the testing emphasis has shifted from the search for defects toward proof of performance. However, the design of validation tests should ensure that the opportunity to uncover defects that might not have been accessible previously is not wasted. Defects found during validation testing are those related to the software's nonconformity with requirements specifications. Even though the design was verified against the requirements specifications and integration testing demonstrated the software's compliance with the design, there are differences of specification interpretation to contend with, as well as human errors by developers and verifiers. The testing procedures are reviewed in relation to the requirements specification only, not to the design documentation.

During validation testing, the inner workings of the software are generally of little interest. Validation testing must include a sufficient variety of discrete combinations of representative operational inputs over the entire operational range of the device to provide confidence in the structural integrity of the software. The input must include invalid data or combinations of data to defeat the error-handling mechanisms of the software. Usually, however, the number of input combinations is so great that it is impossible to determine the inputs that are representative of the software's full capability. The only feasible solution is to include the use of random inputs during expected operational data inputs. However, this set of test input conditions should be used only after the validation tests have been performed with the predetermined conditions, to measure the salient performance characteristics.

Because it is expected that some defects will be found during validation testing, a mechanism is required to repeat previous tests after a defect has surfaced and been repaired. The efficiency of these regression tests (Table 7-7) can be improved greatly if the input for each test case can be captured and reused at the time of the regression test. No matter how achieved, it is absolutely essential that the procedures used for validation testing can be repeated and that regression testing can be performed. If at all possible, regression testing should be automated.

Validation testing can be viewed as the stress test of the integrated software. In reality, stress tests are directed toward measurable performance and not specifically toward the manner in which the earlier interface problems were resolved. If defects are discovered as a result of stress tests, there is a good likelihood that they will be traceable to the places in the overall software design where the interfaces were initially defined, or to the modifications of that design that were made during integration testing. In diagnosing causes of defects during validation testing, it is helpful to regress to the original integration tests, as well as to earlier validation tests. Careful comparisons of the software's behavior during the tests may provide a clue about the hidden defect.

One of the toughest problems that software quality assurance must deal with is the establishment of the basis for accepting the software end product. It is not sufficient to state simply that the software must be proven to conform to its specification, because it is impossible to

Table 7-7   Typical Sequence of Software Regression Testing

Step	Test Activity
1	Compare the new software to the existing baseline
2	Generate a cross-reference listing to assess changes and to ensure no unintended side effects
3	Assess the number of changes and the criticality
4	Determine the level of effort required and assess the risk
5	Test the new functions and the debug fixes
6	Execute a predetermined set of core tests to confirm that no new unintended changes have been introduced

qualify explicitly the software for all operational conditions. Acceptance must be based not only on the capability of performing the nominal functions within some predefined error limits at a few fixed points, but under as wide a diversity of circumstances as can be imagined. This brings us back to random inputs as the vehicle that will ensure that defects occur. Validation testing works toward including in its acceptance criteria a requirement for evidence, from which an inference can be drawn that the number of defects remaining at the conclusion of the testing does not exceed a specified limit. This does not suggest that any defects found should be ignored but, rather, that those defects should be repaired immediately. It indicates that the number of defects found during validation testing with random stimuli should be an indication of the number that remain.

Given random input, there is a typical decay in the rate of defect discoveries. This suggests that the rate at which the time between defects increases is a more valid criterion than merely specifying a maximum number of defects or the maximum number of defects within a given time period. If the data exhibit an adequate fit to a predetermined reliability model, then the software equivalent of mean time to failure, or other statistical inferences, can be calculated, and software acceptance can be based on that value. Criteria based on the rate of defects rather than the number of defects will avoid nonacceptance of a potentially usable program in favor of delaying acceptance until reliability has been demonstrated. This solution serves the best interests of development, quality, management, and the customer or user.

Validation supports the usability of the software. At most, it establishes the software usability as a system; at the least, it affirms the usability of the software to the same level of success that the specifications anticipated the operational use of the software in the device. Even in the best of all worlds, specifications are not detailed enough to cover every operating circumstance to which the software will be exposed, which was why the previously discussed testing required random inputs. The specifications are never prescient, and the actual environment in which the software operates may differ from that visualized at the time the requirements were defined. Many software programs have lacked the flexibility to handle all of the problems that the user would expect. The full measure of usability cannot be taken during validation testing; evaluation must be used to help augment the usability determination. Basically, validation testing will only determine whether the software satisfies its specified requirements; system or device evaluation determines whether the specification accurately reflects the physical world.

Device System Testing

The software end product that has emerged from software validation testing has been deemed acceptable. However, it must now work in concert with other electrical and mechanical subsystems and components. To do so, it will need to be exercised in another series of tests geared to validate the device as an integrated, working, fully functional system. This does not imply that the software end product has not already communicated or interfaced with one or more parts of the operational hardware. The software testing discussed so far will, in fact, require some degree of hardware operability to test software functionality properly. Table 7-8 lists the testing sequence at the system level.

The testing of the software in this configuration was not mentioned earlier because it is important to have confidence in the software end product prior to the testing of its execution in the more complex system environment. This is analogous to performing unit tests on modules prior to incorporating them into the evolving software end product. Attempting to test the coordinated operation of newly minted software with old or even new hardware configurations can be demoralizingly slow, tedious, and irritating. For example, if a test fails, then the difficulty

Table 7-8   Typical Sequence of Software System Level Testing

Step	Test Activity
1	Complete the RTM, except for the test results
2	Validate the process used to generate and build the system
3	V&V testing proceeds from a known and controlled test bed
4	Perform software fault insertion
5	For embedded software: Utilize an in-circuit emulator with the latest configured software and hardware to test function, robustness, stress, and safety Remove the in-circuit emulator and perform functional and robustness testing of the user interface and stress testing of the communications interface
6	Execute the appropriate test suite to: Locate software design errors Locate suspicious coding practices Locate unused and improperly scoped variables Reverse engineer the software in generating test cases
7	For embedded software: Validate the EPROM burn-in procedure
8	Complete and review the RTM to verify that all requirements have been tested and satisfied
9	Complete any reports, to provide closure
10	Complete the SVVR and submit it to a controlled environment: Include the CRC identifier List all baselined items that were verified with this version of the software

is to determine whether the failure was because of the old software configuration, the newly installed software module, the old hardware configuration, or the new hardware configuration. Even when the failure location has been determined, more testing may be required to further amplify the cause of the failure and, once this has been done, correct the failure. This is followed by a delay, to rectify and correct the deficiency, rebuild the system, and perform the tests again. This can consume an enormous amount of time, particularly if hardware changes must be made on items or components needing long lead times.

However, as much as it is ideal to merge only validated software end products with other validated software products or hardware, this may not always be possible. Not infrequently, the software is so inextricably bound to some aspects of the hardware that the capability of simulating that hardware with software or with simpler, less sophisticated hardware is too limited to be of any real use. From a software standpoint, this situation can be improved by a certain amount of simulation from other elements of the system as system-level stubs and drivers. Real-time input can then be synthesized with adequate realism; some hardware responses can be creditably dubbed, but real interaction is difficult to achieve. The extent to which it is difficult to test the software is an inverse measure of the success with which the system design was the product of a functional, modular decomposition. The more independence among the elements of the system or device, the simpler the functional interfaces will be and, therefore, the simpler it will be to test the software.

In spite of these factors, even in a well-designed system there may be circumstances that warrant some early multiconfiguration hardware-software testing. This means that part of the device testing, which is really system integration testing, may be less a distinct test phase than an ongoing operation that threads its way through the previously defined software integration and validation phases. System-level integration testing, or whatever remains of it after multiconfiguration validation testing, is conducted within the same managerial disciplines as overall program development and integration planning. System integration requires the early formulation of plans and procedures that must be approved before testing begins; test cases are directed at exposing the defects in the system design just as software integration was directed at the top-level software design. The pretest documentation is reviewed in terms of the verification of the overall design; software is only a black box of the system.

The role of the software quality assurance group during system testing is to audit the system and provide information relative to software performance as based on the software tests discussed earlier. The respective system architects, designers, or engineers are the owners of the system elements or components; their function is to actually operate the system and track down the source of each problem encountered. A separate system integration team is usually the most productive way of welding the various elements of the system into a unified whole, although in most companies this may not be feasible.

System validation, or acceptance testing, is the final, formally defined test phase in the preoperational software life cycle. The management aspects of software validation apply equally to system acceptance. Independent testers validate the system or device against approved specifications and procedures; regression testing may be necessary if software or hardware changes are made during these tests. After all specific performance tests of the system have been satisfied, then testing with abundant random stimuli should be conducted as a basis for acceptance or rejection criteria.

Embedded software follows this same type of testing, except that it does require a few unique considerations. First, embedded software commonly must intermittently test the operation of its associated hardware. This is not inherently different from any ordinary diagnostic procedures, except that the tests are interleaved with the primary operational functions of the system rather than being performed off-line; the specifics of these integrity tests are not usually given in the system specifications. The validation of software capability through fault insertion or hardware degradation will usually be performed with respect to the software requirements definition. Second, for embedded software, the stimuli and the observed results of the hardware-software tests are not all easily converted to machine readability or machine generation; therefore, automated regression testing and analysis are not always practicable.

Third, embedded software resides in semiconductor ROM or PROM devices. Thus, the software intended to be resident in these devices should be acceptance tested using this operational memory. Until now, the easily modifiable memory was no particular problem, because the uncovering of multiple defects was anticipated, along with their alterations. However, the execution of real-time embedded software with anything other than the actual operational configuration is not a totally valid test. For example, the software storage that is substituting for ROM or PROM may operate with different fetch time characteristics, which will affect the rate at which the operational software can process data. Unless the semiconductor devices are erasable, the devices that begin any of the software-related testing must be considered expendable, because at least one software repairable error will occur. Even if a rigorous certification of the ability of a substitute memory to emulate accurately the final storage medium can be found and used, some software testing with the operational memory will still be required to validate the mapping into ROM or PROM.

Automated regression tests are especially useful for the operation and maintenance phases of the software life cycle. After the repair of a defect during the operation and maintenance period, it is necessary to repeat the tests that were used to establish the original operability of the software. Of course, these tests are performed after the execution of the tests to confirm the success of removing the particular defect. A peculiarity of software is that after a repair, its state is not restored to the original factory conditions, but rather to a state that has not existed before. Before the new software version can be claimed to be ready for use, software quality assurance personnel must make certain that new defects have not been introduced into the software because of the changes. The same problem exists when modifications are made to enhance the operation or to adapt the software to a new environment. In this case, however, the original validation test cases may no longer fully apply, and planning is required to define the new set of tests. When that occurs, they will preserve the appropriate parts of the original tests and prove the operability of the new software.

The embedded software in this case also presents the concern about whether it can simulate the outside world environment and capture the test results. The earlier test bed must either be maintained during operation and maintenance or must be capable of assimilating the new tests. This is an expensive proposition, and it must be reckoned with early in the determination of the software support cost of the software life cycle.

Software Safety Testing

A key element of software safety testing (see Table 7-9 for examples) is the production of a hazards analysis and a software failure modes and effects criticality analysis (SFMECA). This analysis starts at the system level and decomposes the product into its mechanical, electrical, and software components. It then attempts to mitigate single point failures or justify a single error trap by calculating a low probability of its occurrence. Consequently, the hazard analysis and SFMECA generated earlier in the project must be updated to reflect the as-built software. Software safety testing of the product requires the use of the updated documents as part of the

Table 7-9   Typical Software Safety Testing Examples

Safety Area	Types of Testing
Fail-safe tests	Verify the fail-safe provisions of the software design Error conditions and handling Limited, non-destructive fault insertion Data corruption
Active failure tests	Completion within system critical time ROM via CRC computation and comparison to stored value RAM for stuck bits in data and address paths RAM for address decoding problems Cyclic program execution checked with a timer and a watchdog circuit Motor speed check by monitoring lead screw rotation flag Backward calculations for motor speed and pressure Relative execution rates between tasks LED indicator(s) voltage LCD display(s) comparison Processor and controller Digital to analog converter Pressure transducer and pre-amp
Passive failure tests	Watchdog timer Watchdog disable Hardware RAM CRC generator Battery Audio generators and speakers EEPROM
Safety tests	Critical parameters and their duplicates Events that lead to a loss of audio and/or visual indicators Events that lead to tactile errors such as key presses Error handling for corrupted vectors, structures, and sanity checks Sufficiency of periodic versus aperiodic
Safety testing from the hazards analysis	Single point failures Normal power-up, run-time, and power-down safety

software validation effort. When applied to test and manufacturing equipment, safety testing takes on another meaning. Safety in this context requires surveying the environment and the role that the equipment plays in supporting the production of a safe product. For example, if the equipment is used to make a pass or fail determination of a product on a production line, then the safety issue is elevated appropriately to the proper level. If the equipment is the sole check for a particular function of the product before it leaves the production line and is boxed for shipment, then the safety issue is elevated to the level of the product it supports. In contrast, if the equipment consists of a label generator, then safety testing merely ensures control of the software. For test and manufacturing equipment, validating that the process is in place minimizes the chances of an error occurring, possibly by using human intervention.

The preferred software test approach to all products or equipment is white-box testing rather than black-box testing. This may not be warranted for all functions, such as user interface testing. Furthermore, code inspection, as the sole technique for safety validation testing, should be avoided unless the software changes are hard-coded data alterations such as strings or constants, rather than logical changes that alter the program's instruction order.

Software testing of a product or equipment is normally performed at the software component level and the software system level. Component-level testing concentrates on individual components or a grouping of components; system-level testing focuses on the performance of the software as an entity. Software component-level testing is performed during the code and test phase of the life cycle and during the integrate and test activities of code construction. This type of testing is best performed by the software development engineers themselves; Development Test Information Sheets (DTISs) should be generated to support and document this testing. Software system-level testing is performed during the software system testing activity and should be performed by the software V&V engineers; Validation Test Information Sheets (VTISs) should be generated to support and document this testing.

Event-driven systems are time dependent, and it is essential to understand the software execution architecture. To accomplish this, four basic testing activities must be done to capture the software's execution architecture. First, produce a timing event diagram that identifies all interrupts, their priority, and their type. The interrupt type can be classified as synchronous, driven by a timer, or asynchronous, driven by external events. The interrupts should also be classified as software interrupts, hardware external interrupts, or hardware internal interrupts. Examples of hardware external interrupts are sequential input and output, motor control, and keyboard inputs; internal hardware interrupts can include divide-by-zero and over- or underflow calculations. All software not directly related to an interrupt should be identified. This background software should be documented with a structure chart that indicates the control execution logic and execution duration. After all of this information has been gathered, the timing event diagram should be plotted. For this plot, the operational time window should be shown, along with the synchronous interrupts and their interval and priority and the asynchronous interrupts and their priority; noninterrupt software should be shown as a block of time.

The second test activity is to gather information about the power-on tests or power-on self-tests (POSTs). These tests are not really time dependent, because whether the POST requires three seconds or five seconds to complete is not important. The POSTs are referred to as tests for passive failures because they must execute once in each operational window, or at least once between power-up and power-down. In addition to self-tests, this mode also encompasses the initialization of software variables and the hardware itself. For the POST, outline the self-tests performed. If a test is perceived to be missing, then the software and product fail this safety test, unless the software developer can prove that it is not a single point failure condition, or that there is a low probability of occurrence. Assuming that the product passes this test, functional testing of the self-tests themselves can then be performed.

The third test activity is to gather information about the run-time tests that begin after the POST has successfully finished and the product begins operation. These tests are concerned only with the activity that occurs when the product is in a normal working cycle, and they are time dependent. This means that the safety tests are being performed on a cyclic basis in the background, checking for active failures, and must be complete within the product's time-critical window. In this operational mode, the self-tests being performed should be outlined and compared to a template that is representative of other products. If a test is perceived to be missing, then the software and product should fail this safety test, unless the software developer can prove that it is not a single point failure condition or that there is a low probability of occurrence. Assuming that the product passes this test, functional testing of the run-time tests themselves can be performed. The run-time tests must be timed to prove that they start and complete execution during the time-critical window under both nominal and worst-case conditions.

The last test activity is to gather information about the power-down tests. To accomplish this, identify all of the conditions under which the product can shut down, including loss of power, error trap or halt instruction, and normal power-off by the user. All conditions must be tested to ensure that critical parameters are saved or, at least, not corrupted. In addition, if a RAM failure occurs, then an error flag should be set and checked on the next power-up so that default run-time values may be loaded from protected storage. Analysis and test of all error traps that test for error conditions should be performed, along with the subsequent branch error handler, and the results should be compared against the SFMECA. Any other power-down tests being performed should be outlined and compared to a pro forma template representative of other products. If a test is perceived to be missing, then the software and product should fail this safety test, unless the software developer can prove that it is not a single point failure condition, or that there is a low probability of occurrence. Assuming that the product passes this test, functional testing of the power-down tests themselves can be performed.

Allocation of Software Testing

To achieve uniform, consistent, and sufficient software test coverage, it is of benefit to allocate the various aspects of software testing to corresponding software life cycle activities (Figure 7-2). During the design process and activities, software designers accomplish their design activities and store the resultant design. While the design evolves, designers should generate test information sheets to specify the testing to be conducted to validate the implemented design. The test information sheets should be used and reviewed as a part of the design walk-throughs. Since these tests are done at the discretion of the designer, they should be prioritized by safety, reliability, effectiveness, performance, and any other appropriate criteria. These tests should target the integrated software components, the interfaces among the integrated tasks or functions, and paths among the various tasks and functions.

When the design has been completed, it is given to the programmers who will create the source code. As the programmers generate the code, they should also create test information sheets to specify the testing to be conducted to validate the implemented design and requirements. The test information sheets should be used and reviewed as a part of the code walk-throughs. Since these tests are at the discretion of the programmer, they should be prioritized by safety, reliability, effectiveness, performance, and any other appropriate criteria. These tests should target the individually completed components for functionality, robustness, and stress. The code constructed by the programmer will also undergo debug testing. This level of testing is at the function, routine, or component level and satisfies path testing, interface testing, and logic or branch testing.

After the code has been implemented and integrated, formal testing commences. This type of testing is performed by both software development engineers and software V&V engineers. Software developers will do their testing on the basis of test information sheets generated as the design and code evolved. Software V&V engineers will have produced a second set of test information sheets based on the design and the code that was documented in the software requirements and software design document. At the conclusion of this formal testing, both types of

Figure 7-2   Typical allocation of software testing

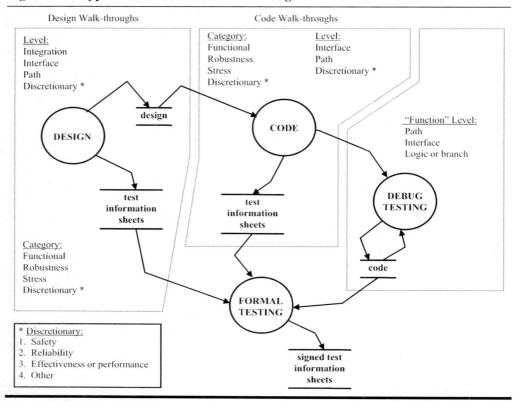

test information sheets are reviewed for adequacy, completeness, and coverage and are signed off and archived.

Software Reliability Engineered Testing

The testing of software is subject to strong conflicting forces. A product must function sufficiently reliably for its application or use, but it must also reach the market at least at the same time, if not before, its competitors and at a competitive cost. Some products may be less market-driven than others may, but balancing reliability, time of delivery and cost is critical. One of the most effective ways to perform this balancing is to engineer the test process through quantitative planning and tracking. Software reliability engineered testing combines the use of quantitative reliability objectives and operational profiles of system or product use. Loosely, the standard definition for *software reliability* is the probability of execution without failure for some specified interval. This definition is compatible with that used for hardware reliability, although the failure mechanisms may differ, and software reliability engineered testing is generally compatible with hardware reliability technology and practice. This is important because no product is purely software; all systems encompass a mixture of software and hardware components. In fact, a "software system" is really a "software-based system."

Software reliability engineered testing can be applied to any product containing software and for most kinds of testing. The only requirement is that testing be spread broadly across the system or product functions. For example, it can be applied to product feature, load, performance, regression, and certification or acceptance testing, but it is not appropriate for testing an isolated set of functions, such as product error recovery capabilities. Software reliability engineered testing should be applied over the entire software life cycle, including all releases, with particular focus on testing the phases from subsystem to delivery or release. Software test engineers are the prime movers in implementing software reliability engineered testing, but software engineers, architects, and designers and users are also involved. There are two types of software reliability engineered testing; development testing, in which you find and remove faults, and certification testing, in which you either accept or reject the software. In many cases, the two types of testing are applied sequentially.

Development testing precedes certification testing, which in turn precedes product acceptance testing. During development testing, failure intensity, the failures per unit execution time, are estimated and tracked; execution time is the actual time used by a processor in executing a program's instructions. Failure intensity is an alternative way of expressing software reliability. Software test engineers use failure intensity information to determine corrective actions that might need to be taken and to guide and gauge the software release. The release decisions could include release from software test to system test, system test to beta test, and beta test to manufacturing or to the field. Development testing typically comprises feature, loading, and regression testing and is generally used for software developed within the organization. Certification testing, on the other hand, does not involve debugging, and there is no attempt to resolve or fix the failures that are identified. Certification testing typically includes only load testing and is generally used for software that is acquired, including commercial-off-the-shelf or packaged software, reusable software, and software developed by an organization outside of the company.

The software reliability engineered testing process follows a spiral model, in a manner analogous to the software development process, and iteration occurs frequently. Figure 7-3 represents an unwound coil of this model, in which Execute Tests and Interpret Failure Data occur simultaneously, or at least in parallel, and are closely linked, the relative emphasis being

Figure 7-3   Core application steps in software reliability engineered testing

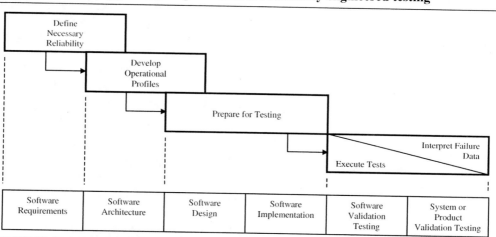

on interpretation increasing with time. Software test engineers define necessary reliability and develop operational profiles in partnership with the software development engineers and architects. There are several advantages to this. First, the software test engineers depend on these activities and are thus more strongly motivated to ensure their successful completion than if the development group alone generated them. Second, the software test group can get more contact with users, which is valuable in determining what product behavior would be unacceptable and how unacceptable it would be and in understanding how users would employ the product. Third, the software development engineers and architects obtain a greater appreciation of testing and of where requirements and design need to be made less ambiguous and more precise, so that test-case and test-procedure design can proceed. Last, software test engineers can make valuable contributions to reviews by pointing out important capabilities that are missing.

Software reliability engineered testing has seven major steps. The first two steps, consisting of decision making, form the basis for the following five steps and generally take only a few hours. The core steps (Figure 7-3) take considerably longer. The core steps are virtually identical for development and certification testing, except for the first and last ones. The first step is to determine which associated systems require separate testing. In addition to testing the entire system, software test engineers may need to test major system variations. For example, the medical device may have different hardware configurations, or it may work with different communication protocols in different countries. Software test engineers should test any major components of unknown reliability and any smaller components that are expected to be reused extensively. If the product interacts strongly with other software systems or products, then testing should include a strategy that represents these systems functioning together as an integrated whole. The second step is to decide which type(s) of software reliability engineered testing are needed for each system to be tested. Using the example above, development testing might be assigned to product configurations but certification testing to communication protocols. Development testing is appropriate only for systems that are coded at least in part by the organization.

The third software reliability engineered test step is to define the required or necessary reliability. The first activity is to determine operational modes, the distinct patterns of system or product use and/or environment that need separate testing because they are likely to stimulate different failures. A separate operational mode may also be established to provide for accelerated testing of rarely occurring but critical operations; "Critical" in this context means that an operation adds considerable extra value when it executes successfully and results in an extreme impact when it fails. The terms "value" and "impact" refer to safety with respect to human life, cost, or service. Division into operational modes is based on engineering judgment; however, more operational modes can increase the realism of the test, but they can also increase the effort and cost of selecting test cases and performing system tests.

The second activity is to define failure in terms of severity classes. A failure is the departure of software behavior during execution from defined requirements; it is a user-oriented concept. A fault is the defect in the software that causes the failure when executed; it is a developer-oriented concept. Consequently, failures implicitly express the users' negative requirements for software behavior. The reliability definition process itself consists of outlining these negative requirements in a system-specific way for each severity class. A severity class is a set of failures that affect users to the same degree; it is often related to the criticality of the operation that fails. Common classification criteria include impacts on human life, cost, and service. In general, classes are widely separated in impact, because their impact cannot be estimated with high accuracy.

The third activity is to set the failure intensity objectives for the developed software. The objectives can be defined for the product as a whole or separately for each operational mode and severity class; there may be different objectives for the end of system testing and the end of beta testing, for example. Setting failure intensity objectives for the developed software is accomplished by:

- Establishing the system or product failure intensity objectives from an analysis of specific user needs, existing system reliability and the degree to which users are satisfied with it, and the capabilities of competing systems.

- Determining and summing the failure intensities of the acquired hardware and software components.

- Subtracting the total acquired failure intensities from the system failure intensity objectives in wall-clock hours, which yields the failure intensity objectives for the developed software.

- Converting the results into failure intensity objectives for the developed software per unit of execution time.

The last activity is to engineer the reliability strategies. The three principal reliability strategies are (1) fault prevention, which uses requirements, design, and coding technologies and processes, as well as requirements and design reviews, to reduce the number of faults introduced in the first place; (2) fault removal, which uses techniques such as inspection and development testing to remove faults in the code once it is written; and (3) fault tolerance, which reduces the number of failures that occur by detecting and countering deviations in program execution that may lead to failures. Engineering these reliability strategies means finding the right balance among them to achieve the failure intensity objective in the required time and at minimum cost.

The fourth step of software reliability engineered testing is to develop operational profiles for the product. An operation is a major task that the system or product performs. An operational profile is simply the set of operations and their probabilities of occurrence. Activities in this step include developing two types of operational profiles, overall (across all operational modes) and operational mode. The overall profile is used to select the test cases to prepare for; the operational profile for each operational mode is used to select operations for execution when that mode is tested. An operational profile is obtained from the occurrence rates of individual operations; it can be presented in tabular form or graphically as a network of nodes and branches. The tabular representation is generally better for systems whose operations have few attributes; the graphical representation is generally better for systems whose operations have multiple attributes. For example, an operational profile for an infrared (IR) thermometer could be captured in tabular form, an infusion device as either tabular or graphical, and a heart lung machine as graphical. In a graphical representation of a system or product, the nodes represent attributes of an operation, and the branches represent the attribute value or occurrence probability. A path through the network represents an operation; the occurrence probability could be conditional on the previous path to that point in the network. Regardless of which representation is used, the procedure to develop an operational profile is similar. The procedure for generating the representation is:

- Identify the initiators of operations. System or product users are most commonly the initiators of operations, but initiators can also be external or other systems and the system controller.

- List the operations that each initiator produces for the tabular representation or the operation attributes and attribute values for the graphical representation. The system requirements are the most useful source of information for this task, but other sources include work-process flow diagrams for various job roles, draft user manuals, prototypes, and previous versions of the product.

- Determine the occurrence rate per wall-clock hour of the operations for the tabular representation or of the attribute values for the graphical representation.

- Determine the occurrence probabilities by dividing the occurrence rates for each operation by total operation occurrence rates for the tabular representation or the occurrence rates for each attribute value by total attribute occurrence rates for the graphical representation.

The fifth step of software reliability engineered testing is to prepare for testing by generating test cases, test procedures, and scripts for any automated tools to be used. Particularly defined terms figure in these activities. A *run,* a specific instance of an operation, is characterized by that operation and a complete set of values of its input variables. *Input variables,* which exist external to the run and influence it, are *direct* because they control processing in a known, designed way, or they are *indirect* because although they influence processing, it is not in any predictable way. A run differs from a *test case,* in which values of only direct input variables are provided. A test case becomes a run when the values of indirect input variables are specified. This impacts testing productivity because by changing the indirect input variables, software test engineers can use a moderate number of test cases to generate a very large number of different runs.

The first activity of test preparation is to estimate the number of test cases that can be prepared cost effectively, on the basis of the effort needed for each. The test cases can be selected in two steps. First, select the operations in accordance with their occurrence probabilities, using the overall operational profile modified appropriately for any critical operations. For example, if the occurrence probability of an operation is 0.71, then 71 percent of the test cases should be from the operation. Second, complete the selection of the test cases by choosing levels for all direct input variables where a *level* is a value or a range of values for an input variable for which failure behavior is expected to be the same because of processing similarities. For example, in an infusion device, a value of the input variable "volume to be infused" would be a volume number, but the value "100 ml" would be a level of that input variable because the product would probably behave in the same way for all volumes input. Only one value within a level for a test case is needed and, in some cases, a level has only one value. Second, list the levels for each direct input variable and then randomly choose a level for each direct variable. The choice should be made with equal probability from the set of levels. The operation and the set of direct input variables selected specify a test case. The last activity is to write the test script if automatic testing is to be used to implement the test case selected.

The next step of test preparations is to define the *test procedure,* the specification of the set of runs and environment associated with an operational mode. In general, providing values of operation occurrence rates statistically specifies the set of runs, so that when executed, the test procedure will select test cases at random times from the prepared set, following the occurrence rates. In feature testing, test runs are executed essentially independently of each other, and data are frequently reinitialized to reduce interactions between runs. In load testing, large numbers of test runs are executed in the context of an operational mode and are driven by the test procedure. Load testing stimulates failures that can occur as a result of interactions among runs, both directly and through interactions and corruption. In regression testing, feature test runs are repeated after each baseline to determine if changes made to the software have spawned faults that cause failures. The last step of test preparation is to prepare the automated tools. Software reliability engineered testing can be performed without test automation, but test management and failure identification tools usually make the process faster and more efficient. Recording the operations executed provides a way for comparing the test operational profile with the profile expected in the field. Actually, operation recording should be more than a feature of the test platform; it should be an integral part of the system or product itself that can facilitate the collection of extensive field data, both to evaluate the current product and to provide a base for engineering future systems.

The sixth step of software reliability engineered testing is to execute the tests, by conducting the test and identifying failures, determining when they occurred, and establishing the severity of their impact. During this step, the sequence is to begin with feature testing and follow that with load testing. Regression testing is typically done after each baseline that involves significant change. In load testing, each operational mode is executed separately. It is wise to allocate execution time among the operational modes for testing in the same proportions that they are expected to have in the field, adjusting for critical operational modes. Test execution involves identifying failures, determining when they occurred, and establishing the severity of their impact. Failures can be identified by deviations of program behavior; determine which deviations affect the user, because only those that do are failures. Generic tools can detect many types of deviations, including interprocess communication failures, illegal memory references, and deviant return code values. Manual insertions in the code can be used to detect programmer-defined deviations. Some manual inspection of test results will be required to identify failures not amenable to automatic detection and to sort out deviations that are true failures. If it can be demonstrated that the ratio of failures to deviations is essentially constant, then deviation data can be used in place of failure data by adjusting by the known ratio. Of special interest are circumstances such as cascaded failures, repeated failures, and failures that will not be resolved. Testing should determine the time of failure or number of failures per time period during the execution time; if execution time is not readily available, use an approximation. A special approach will be needed to handle failure data if testing is done on multiple platforms, systems, products or machines.

The last step of software reliability engineered testing is to interpret the failure data with the understanding that this interpretation is different for development testing and certification testing. In development testing, the goal is to track progress and compare present failure intensities with their objectives. In certification testing, the goal is to determine if a software component, product, or system should be accepted or rejected, with limits on the risks taken in making that decision. For development testing, failure data are generally interpreted at fixed intervals. For certification testing, interpretation is performed after each failure.

The first development testing activity is to consider trends in feature, load, and regression testing by estimating the failure intensity over all severity classes and across all operational modes and plotting it against time. The failure intensity trend plot should present the most likely estimate along with the upper and lower 95 percent confidence bounds. Comparison with the overall failure intensity objective helps to identify at-risk schedules or reliabilities and allows for appropriate and timely corrective actions. Long, large upswings in failure intensity commonly indicate that either the system or product has evolved or the test operational profile has changed. System evolution can be an indication of poor configuration control and a change in the test operational profile may indicate poorly planned test execution. In either case, corrective action is necessary to achieve a dependable test. The next activity is to guide release decisions. If the failure intensity objectives were defined as severity class by operational mode, then the failure intensities should be estimated that way and compared with the failure intensity objectives chosen for the system or product. If only an overall failure intensity objective was defined, then the estimate is only for the overall failure intensity and compared to the objective. Release decisions should include component test to system test, system test to beta test, or beta test to manufacturing and field release. Failure intensity can be estimated on the basis of software reliability models and statistical inference, from failure times or the number of failures per time period.

The first certification testing activity is to generate a reliability demonstration chart (Figure 7-4) that plots the normalized failure times. Multiplying each failure time by the appropriate failure intensity objective produces a normalized value. Each failure is plotted on the chart and labeled with its severity class. Depending on the region in which the failure falls, it may indicate accept and or rejection of the software being tested, or that testing should continue. Values falling in the Accept region indicate that sufficient data have been collected to demonstrate that the software can be accepted at the risk levels for which the chart was constructed. Other reliability demonstration charts can be constructed for different levels of consumer risk (the risk of accepting a bad program) and supplier risks (the risk of rejecting a good program).

Software Statistical-Based Testing

Engineering is traditionally defined as the application of science to produce useful artifacts. Software engineering, then, could be characterized as the application of science to the development and testing of software. Most software engineers, however, would be at a loss to cite the scientific basis for their methods of work. The scientific approaches to product testing and certification that are used in mature engineering disciplines are applicable in software production as well. In other industries, products are typically certified under protocols in which random

Figure 7-4   Typical reliability demonstration chart

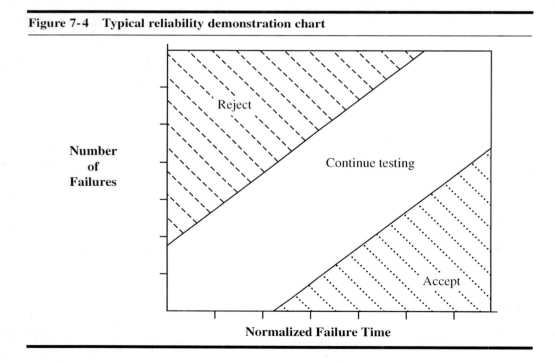

samples of the product are drawn, tests characteristic of operational use are applied, analytical or statistical inferences are made, and products meeting a standard are certified as fit for use. Statistical testing based on a software usage model is the application of such a protocol to software. In statistical testing, an operational usage model of the software is developed, test cases are randomly generated from the usage model, and test results yield statistically valid measures of software quality and test sufficiency.

Scientific Software Testing Foundation

A principle of fundamental importance to this approach is that when a population is too large for exhaustive study, as is the case for all possible uses of software, a statistically correct sample must be drawn as a basis for inferences about the population. In the case of software testing, the population is the set of all possible scenarios of use, the frequency of occurrence of each use being accurately represented. The premise that must be accepted as a starting point in this analogy is that it is not possible to test all ways in which the software may be used.

As a different and simple example to demonstrate the impossibility of testing all possible scenarios of use, assume that a medical product uses software designed with an unbounded input sequence length. Although the design intends to use a finite number of input sequences, it has a theoretically infinite number of possible usage scenarios. For software with only two user inputs, A and B, the possible scenarios of use are A, B, AA, AB, BB, BA, AAA, AAB, ABA, BAA, BBB, and so on. There is really no question about whether all possible scenarios of use will be tested, because they will not be. The only questions are how the population of uses will be characterized and how a subset of test cases will be drawn. A random sample of test cases from a properly characterized population, if applied to the software under proper test control, will allow valid generalization of conclusions from testing to operational use. Any other set of test cases, no matter how thoughtfully constructed, will not.

The challenge is first to characterize the population (all uses) from which a sample (test cases) will be drawn. The representation of the population must include all possible uses, including the infrequent and exceptional as well as the common and typical. Software use can be viewed as a stochastic process that is a series of events that unfold over time in a probabilistic way. Software use can be modeled as a stochastic process known as a Markov chain, and the standard analytical results for Markov chains can be interpreted to yield insights about operational use. The engineering formalism, a Markov-chain usage model of software, provides the basis for an approach to software testing that is grounded in well-understood science and supported by widely used engineering practices. For this discussion, the term *usage model* refers to an operational model of a software system that represents the population from which a sample of test cases will be drawn. The model may be designed to represent normal usage conditions, stress conditions; hazardous conditions, maintenance conditions, or any other conditions about which operational performance information is desired.

Statistical testing involves the six steps depicted in Figure 7-5. As shown, a usage model is developed for each usage environment or user class that is important for the application. Quantitative analysis of the model yields data that may be used to refine the model and to guide both development and testing. Test cases are generated from the model. Some combination of model coverage testing, importance testing based on probability mass, and random testing is used, and it may be supplemented by crafted testing as needed. Random testing allows statistical estimates of the operational reliability of the product. The software has been "certified" to be of known quality when a well-defined, statistically valid, repeatable process has been used, and the resulting measures of the product meet pre-established quality requirements.

Figure 7-5   Typical statistical testing process

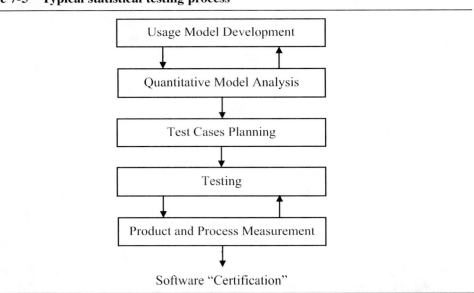

Usage Model Development, Testing, and Measurement

The first step in usage model development is to characterize general operational conditions and stratify the classes of usage. For example, software is "used" by a "user" in some "environment." The definitions of user, use, and environment define the operational environment to which inferences about the software apply. The basic task in model building is to identify the states of use of the system and the possible transitions among the states of use. Every possible scenario of use is represented by the model and is potentially generated from the model as a test case. A usage model may be represented as a graph, in which the nodes represent states and the arcs represent inputs that cause transitions between states. Figure 7-6 portrays a simple usage model as a directed graph with transition probabilities on the arcs.

The structure of the usage model represents the possible use of the software. A probability distribution is next imposed on the structure to represent expected use of the software under specified conditions. Transition probabilities between states in the usage model may be based on field data, on engineering judgment, or on estimates from customer inputs. The probabilities associated with states and state transitions in a usage model may be set to reflect either routine or nonroutine conditions. As the system progresses through the product life cycle, the probability set may change several times, because of maturation of system use and availability of more information.

Although usage models may be represented in other forms, Markov-chain usage models are prominent in statistical testing practice because of the insights that may be gained from calculations on a Markov chain. Standard calculations on a Markov chain provide expected values for measures that are highly useful in test planning.

Once the usage model has been developed, test cases can be automatically generated, and they constitute a "script" for use in testing. The test cases may be annotated during test planning to include instructions for conducting and evaluating tests and during test execution to record

Figure 7-6   Typical Markov-chain usage model

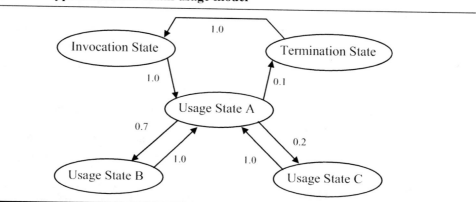

results and observations. The test cases may be executed by human testers or used as input to an automated test tool; test sufficiency and software reliability metrics are calculated throughout the testing process.

Benefits of Statistical Testing Based on a Usage Model

Software usage modeling produces benefits throughout the software life cycle. Since a usage model is based on specifications rather than code, the insights that result from model building can influence product decisions in the early stages of a project, when the opportunity to prevent problems is greatest. The usage model and statistical testing can help with requirements validation because the usage model is an external view of the system specification that is readily understandable by system engineers, developers, customers, and end-users. Interfaces and requirements are often simplified or clarified when these parties review the usage model.

The usage model can also help with resource and schedule estimation. Standard calculations on a usage model provide data for effort, schedule, and cost projections such as the minimum number of tests to cover all states and transitions in the model. Furthermore, "what if" analyses can be conducted to bound the best- and worst-case outcomes of testing based on failure data. In terms of automated test case generation, the usage model can help define the test scripts.

In addition, usage models help to develop effective, efficient testing. Faults are not equally likely to cause failures because faults that lie on frequently traversed logic paths have a higher probability of causing failures than faults that are on infrequently traversed paths. This simple fact is the primary motivation for statistical testing; faults are discovered in roughly the order in which they would cause failures in the field. The test budget is therefore spent in a way that maximizes the increase in operational reliability resulting from testing.

Usage models also facilitate quantitative test management. Statistical testing based on a usage model provides quantitative criteria for management decisions about completion of testing and system release. The sufficiency of testing can be measured as the statistical difference between expected usage as represented in the usage model and tested usage as recorded in testing. Last, the usage model will help to validate the estimate of the software reliability. Under a statistical testing protocol, a valid estimate of expected operational performance can be derived from the performance of the software during testing. The test results, through correct or incorrect software performance for each input, are recorded on the model, and reliability is calculated as the probability of correct performance on every input in a random use.

Designing an Integrated Corporate Test Strategy

In practice, it is not unusual to find that several groups within an organization are performing tests on a product and, in fact, that certain aspects of the testing are duplicated. This is particularly true of products that require complex testing. Stand-alone test development by engineering, quality, manufacturing, and field support personnel needs to reflect an integrated approach to test design and execution. An integrated approach tends to overcome the inefficient, time-consuming practice of developing tests in isolation and transform what is often an inefficient and ad-hoc approach to designing tests into a structured and methodical one that views the entire test process as a composite and seamless entity. Medical device manufacturers often make product-test decisions that result in piecemeal solutions. For example, engineering test approaches are developed for specific products with a narrow focus on a particular process technology, feature set, or operational characteristics, or giving a product limited test capabilities. The same holds true for field service in which installation and fault diagnostics are addressed on a product-by-product basis. All this makes planning for high quality difficult, because six-sigma processes require close and seamless coupling with flexible test procedures. Integrated test processes, methods, and standards hold the promise of structured guidelines for designing an enterprise-wide test approach that can provide high-quality products and services at low cost.

There are as many paths to an integrated approach to test design as there are different organizational structures and methods within a given company; carefully integrating the various inputs and other parameters can hold subjectivity to a minimum. A close examination of how the various groups influence the creation of the test strategy is important (Figure 7-7). The test-user community comprises such functions as product development, quality, reliability, manufacturing and service, and their inputs are essential in setting up a test strategy because they are in an ideal position to assess current test deficiencies and the range of defects involved.

The driving force behind an effective test strategy is, of course, test technology itself, and the current status and future trends in the different test fields must be investigated thoroughly.

Figure 7-7   How various company groups influence creation of test strategy

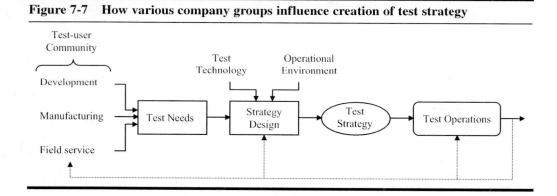

Diagnostic self-test capability becomes extremely important as the complexity and inter-functionality of products increases and when the use of external test equipment becomes too costly. Self-testing implies an intelligent product that can detect and diagnose its own defects, and with the advent and widespread usage of the Internet, remote and on-line diagnostics features are a necessity as products are characterized more and more for their cross-functional features and networking capabilities. Final testing fails if good test-process planning is overlooked at the front end of the manufacturing process.

In most companies, there are many separate integration and test setups within each product group that are limited in scope. This frequently results in black-box software testing that lacks comprehensiveness; the product evaluation performed by these setups is not thorough, because the test facilities are unable to simulate real or worst-case situations. Furthermore, the distributed setups lend a narrow focus to the product evaluation and fail to gauge interproduct functionality. Lack of automation in software testing, which is common, limits test coverage. Enhancing these test setups with longer and more thorough testing can improve the situation, but the distributed nature of the setups continues to provide a narrow focus and overlooks functionality at the inter-product level.

All tests must work in harmony with company goals related to concurrent engineering, higher quality, and shorter cycle times and still be cost-effective. Concurrent engineering requires that tests are created early in the design cycle, and high-quality operations need tests that are thorough, robust, and flexible. The careful, logical unification of the test-user community input with an assessment of the testing environment and current test technology constitutes most of the work in creating a sound test strategy; participative working meetings are the key to stream-lining the synthesis effort.

Formulating a company-wide strategy is difficult when a varied product test mix is con-sidered all at once; it is best to segment the products into classifications based on their tech-nical complexity. Classifying products in this way usually will have the greatest impact on the selection of test approaches. The criteria used for the classification are based on the degrees of complexity in the product's hardware, software, and applications elements; for example, the clas-sification can be from low to high complexity, in three to five levels. Examining the test-user community's needs, the present test processes, and emerging test trends will reveal areas for improvement. Suitable test technologies can be selected and carefully matched to satisfy needs while maintaining harmony with operational criteria and goals. Capturing the results yields new test approaches for the future with specific recommendations. Each product classification and phase segment would go through this procedure.

A convenient form can be used to capture the test strategy for a specific product classifi-cation (see Table 7-10). The first row of the table would contain the test users' needs and issues specific to the particular product classification for each area that provides or requires testing of the product. In the second row of the table the current test process for each area is repre-sented by a flow diagram and below that the product life-cycle steps would be illustrated in flow-diagram form. From the needs and issues list and pictorial descriptions, the fourth row would be generated; it contains the lists of recommended solutions to the needs and issues of the first row. These solutions are then translated pictorially to create a recommended test process and should include the transfer of test data or results and the flow of the test process across the var-ious test groups. It is important that the recommended test process is shown relative to the appro-priate product life-cycle steps and to the present test process, because the portrayals show how and why the recommended test approaches differ from the present one. Major risks and impacts presented by this change are also listed in the last row of the table. The finished charts can serve as a guide for mapping a test strategy for a new product.

Table 7-10   Typical Form for Test Strategy Development Analysis

	Development Phase	System Design Validation Testing Phase	Reliability Phase	Manufacturing Phase	Service Phase
Needs and Issues	1. 2. 3.	1. 2. 3.	1. 2. 3.	1. 2. 3.	1. 2. 3.
Present Test Process Flowchart					
Product Life-cycle Steps Flowchart					
Recommended Solutions	1. 2. 3.	1. 2. 3.	1. 2. 3.	1. 2. 3.	1. 2. 3.
Recommended Test Processes Flowchart					
Major Impact and Risk	1. 2. 3. 4.	1. 2. 3. 4.	1. 2. 3. 4.	1. 2. 3. 4.	1. 2. 3. 4.

When similarly constructed and proposed test approaches for all of the different product classifications are viewed together, a picture of an integrated test strategy begins to take shape. When taken as a whole, the multifunctional test elements and the new test approaches form the company's integrated test strategy. This approach is not flawless; certain key success factors should be present. One critical success factor is the willingness to adopt proper test technologies and the selection of correct test processes at the earliest possible point in a product life cycle. Other key factors include the use and acceptance of test tools for automating test generation and the migration capability of current tests to other phases of the life cycle. However, it should be remembered that, overall, the test efforts will diminish as quality improves.

To estimate the financial impact of the new test strategy, a chart can be created for a given product model that compares the costs for both the old approach and the new strategy. The cost comparisons would, it is hoped, show that the new strategy would save money. Intuitively, the estimates will point to some key financial implications. First, even though the extra test effort has added to design-phase costs, better quality and superior tests have reduced the quantity of testing, resulting in a shorter development cycle and less costly manufacturing. Second, the greatest cost savings are realized during the service phase, which is usually the worst time to detect and solve problems and deficiencies that were easily correctable during design, because of its manually intensive nature.

When Is "Good Enough" Good Enough Testing?

Nearly everyone agrees with the engineering maxim that engineers will continue to improve their design until forced to cease activities. From the engineer's perspective, there are always changes to be made that improve the product. The test group is usually better about this than the design engineer, but even the testers have this mentality. Unfortunately, many companies opt for the opposite end of the spectrum: do as little testing as possible and, if more time is needed for development, steal the necessary time from testing and reduce the allocated test time. Regardless of whether the engineer is a developer or a tester, at every point in the software development life cycle, the present quality of the product must be weighed against the cost and value of further improvement. The challenge is to be able to articulate and quantify why demanding test techniques might make sense for a medical product project, and, if so, how much testing is really needed. It is a given that exhaustive testing is impossible in both principle and practice, but sufficient testing is possible, depending on the circumstances. The concept of a good enough test approach must be distinguished from the approach that advocates exhaustive testing. There has been criticism of the good enough approach from the exhaustive testing perspective, particularly by quality and reliability groups not intimately familiar with software and software testing. However, the exhaustive approach not only is fiscally irresponsible, but the test manager who refuses to face the fact that exhaustive testing is impossible chooses instead to seek an impossible level of testing. When management ships the product over the inevitable objections, the test manager can blame management for every bug found in the field because the testing wasn't completed.

Within the testing community, there is no clear-cut consensus of how to know when to say when. In any situation, the good enough testing approach poses the question, "How do I know if I'm doing, or have done, enough of the right type of testing?" There is no objective or rigorous calculus for answering this question, but the identification of what to consider in attempting to answer it can be. Good enough testing is the process of developing a sufficient assessment of quality, at a reasonable cost, to enable wise and timely decisions to be made concerning the product. This means that, at a high level, it is useful to think about the value of testing as having four parts:

1. Assessment of the product quality. How accurate and complete is it?

2. Assessment of the cost of testing. How reasonable is it? Is it within project constraints? Is there a good return on investment, such as the extent of information gained per test?

3. Decision-making. How well do the assessments serve the project and the business?

4. The timing associated with all the above. Is it soon enough to be useful?

In practice, testing is better if the assessment of quality is more accurate, the cost of testing is lower, the basis for making decisions is better, and the time frames are shorter. In theory, perfect testing would instantly and effortlessly give the right information to allow any part of the company to make any necessary decision concerning the product.

The important point is that if the testing is not coupled with a decision to be made and it is not providing data for future use, then that testing has no purpose. The good enough testing approach is about conscious and purposeful testing and not about "have to" testing, in which test plans are written because some person or organization said that such a test was required. Testing should be striving to contribute more value and less clutter to projects. A good enough testing approach involves, first, assessing the four dynamics above and, second, deciding if they are good enough as a whole. Table 7-11 lists the testing valuation area and the types of questions to be considered. When every aspect of the first part of the assessment has been completed, the individual answers must be considered in total relative to the questions, "How good is our testing?" and "Is it worth improving?" However, it is often easier to answer these questions with hindsight by comparing the testing information to information revealed by other means or test results from other groups within the organization. In addition, most software goes through many iterations of development and release, so that the iterations of the same code provide a means to assess, contrast, and improve the test process. The challenge, however, is to use this knowledge to know that testing is good enough while doing it the first time.

The Last Test

The last software test is a rather philosophical question, and it fits into the same category as trying to determine when the last snowfall of the season will occur. The software end product at release has survived the unit tests of its parts, the integration and testing of those parts, the validation testing of the integrated parts and perhaps some degree of system integration testing, and, finally, product validation testing. However, this is not tantamount to a statement that the software has been delivered free of errors. The proof of error-free software lies in the tests that are conducted during the operation and maintenance phases of the software. All of these tests are a fraction of the total number of tests that will be run against the software in its life cycle. Given the astronomical number of discrete states that are potentially inherent in the structure of the software, each and every execution of the software is potentially a unique one and, therefore, requires a new test. The last test performed is the last execution of the software prior to the retirement of the device, and therefore its software, from the market. Only then does software quality assurance collect its records, update its metrics for the last time, and send them off to the archives.

Table 7-11   Good Enough Testing Evaluation Questions

Testing Valuation Area		
Step	**Testing Valuation Area**	**Questions to be Considered**
1.1	Assess product quality	How are we assessing and reporting the quality of the product? Are we sure our assessment of quality is justified by our observations? Are we aware of the stated and implied requirements of the product when we need to know them? How quickly are we finding out about important problems in the product after they are created? Are our tests covering the aspects of the product we need to cover?

Continued on next page.

Continued from previous page.

	Testing Valuation Area	
Step	**Testing Valuation Area**	**Questions to be Considered**
		Are we using a sufficient variety of test techniques or sources of information about quality to eliminate gaps in our test coverage? What is the likelihood that the product could have important problems we do not know about? What problems are reported through means other than our test process and that our testing should have found first?
1.2	Evaluate the cost of testing	How much does the testing cost and how much can we afford? How can we eliminate unnecessary redundancy in our test coverage? What makes it difficult and thus costly to perform testing? How might the product be made more testable? Are there tools or techniques that might make the process more efficient or productive? Would testing be less expensive overall if we had started sooner or waited until later?
1.3	Check how well testing supports decision-making	Is the test process aware of the kinds of decisions that that management, developers, or other groups need to make? Is the test process focused on potential product and project risks? Is the test process tied to processes of change control and project management? Are test reports delivered in a timely manner? Are test reports communicated in a comprehensible format? Are the test process and test results communicated and are we reporting the basis for our assessment and our confidence in it? Is the test process serving the needs of technical support, publications, marketing or any other business process that should use the quality assessment?
1.4	Timing of the above	Is the above information generated soon enough to be useful?
2.1	How good is the testing?	With respect to the preceding questions, are there any pressing problems with the test process? Is our test process sufficient to alert management if the product quality is less than they want to achieve?

Continued on next page.

Continued from previous page.

Testing Valuation Area		
Step	**Testing Valuation Area**	**Questions to be Considered**
		Are any classes of potential problems intolerable and, if so, are we confident that our test process will locate all such problems?
2.2	Is it worth improving?	What strategies can we use to improve testing? How able are we to implement those strategies? Do we know how? How much cost or trouble will it be to improve testing? Is that the best use of resources? Can we get along for now and improve later? Can we achieve improvement in an acceptable time frame? How might improvement backfire and introduce bugs or impact other projects, for example? What specifically should be improved? Are there any side benefits to improving it? Will improvement make a noticeable difference?

8

The Software Quality Assurance Program: Software Verification and Validation Activities

Unlike the fairy tale Rumpelstiltskin [sic], do not think that by having named the devil that you have destroyed him. Positive verification of his demise is required.

—System Safety Handbook for the Acquisition Manager,
U.S. Air Force

The words software verification and validation (V&V) embody philosophic, methodological, and process aspects of software engineering without actually encompassing a tangible item. Consequently, it is very difficult to discuss V&V in a manner that allows the non-software engineer to come to grips with the physical activities of V&V. Most of the discussion up until now has been primarily related to software development as a systematic approach to the software life cycle. Verification and validation are activities that shadow and parallel the software development activities in such a way that they are sometimes assumed to consist of a single, additional software testing phase that follows the final software integration phase. In practice, this step does exist, but software V&V is so ubiquitous that it is usually misunderstood and misaligned. Contributing to the illusion that software V&V are inherent software characteristics and activities is the fact that nearly all of the preceding discussions related to software development methodology, process, documentation, analysis, and design and testing are equally applicable to the software V&V activities.

The goals of software V&V activities are to assess and improve the quality of the work products generated during development and modification of software. The software quality attributes of interest include correctness, completeness, consistency, reliability, usefulness, usability, efficiency, conformance to standards, and overall cost-effectiveness. To be an efficient checker, software V&V should be performed throughout the software life cycle, and it should be disassociated from software development or modification team members.

Software development is an exercise in problem solving, in which the solution is embodied in the various software end products. These end products consist of the software code, the documents describing the software, and the manuals that describe the use of the software; the execution of the software with its inputs provides the solution. During software development, several intermediate products produced by the software development group are passed through the various V&V functions and activities, to enhance the overall correctness and quality of the final product. In problem solving, a key activity is to determine that the solution is correct; the V&V process is composed of the set of procedures, activities, techniques, and tools that are used to ensure that the software end product does, in fact, solve the intended problem.

Conceptually, two types of activities achieve software quality independently from software development: life cycle verification and formal validation. Life cycle verification is the process of determining the degree to which the software development work products of any given phase in the development cycle fulfill the specifications that were established during previous phases. It also verifies whether those work products adhere to documented policies, SOPs, and guidelines. Formal validation is a rigorous demonstration that the source code conforms to its documented specifications for requirements and design. It is the process of evaluating the software at the end of the software development process to determine its compliance with its specified requirements. In addition to this final testing phase, validation will also include the random regression testing of some of the previously completed software development tests.

High-quality software cannot be achieved through testing of the source code alone. Although the software should be totally free of errors, this is seldom the case, except in very small programs. Even if source code errors were the only measure of software quality, testing alone cannot guarantee the absence of errors in the software; it can only guarantee that all of the known errors have been found. In fact, it is a well-known maxim of software engineering that the number of errors remaining in a program is proportional to the number already discovered. This is so because from a software engineering perspective, the most confidence is placed in software found to have no detected errors after thorough testing, and the least confidence is placed in a program with a long history of fixes.

The best way to minimize the number of errors in software is to catch and remove them during analysis and design so that fewer errors are introduced and propagated into the source code. Although the testing of the code is an important technique for assessing software quality, it is only one of several techniques available. (See Chapter 7 for a discussion of those testing techniques. In summary, V&V is a pervasive concept that permeates all phases of the software development life cycle. It is not just a set of activities that follow the implementation of the software.

V&V involves the assessment of the software work products to determine their conformance to specifications. These specifications include requirements, design documentation, various guidelines, software language implementation standards, project standards, organizational standards, and user expectations. The requirements must be examined for conformance to user needs, environmental constraints, and notational standards. Design documentation must be verified with respect to the requirements and notational conventions, and the source code must be examined for conformance to the requirements, the design documentation, user expectations, and various implementation and documentation standards. In addition, supporting documents, such as the user's manual, test plans, and operation procedures, must be examined for correctness, completeness, consistency, and adherence to standards.

Errors occur when any aspect of a software end product is incomplete, inconsistent, or incorrect. There are three major categories of software errors: requirements, design, and implementation errors. Requirements errors are caused by an incorrect statement of the user's needs at the product level, by the failure to specify the functional and device performance requirements completely, by inconsistencies among the requirements, and by translating the product-level requirements into infeasible software requirements. Design errors are introduced by the failure to translate product-level and software requirements into correct and complete software solution structures, by inconsistencies within design documents, and by inconsistencies between the design specifications and the product-level and software requirements. A requirements error or a design error that is not detected until source code testing can be very costly to correct; therefore, it is important that the quality of the requirements and design documents be assessed early and often. Implementation errors are those made in translating the design specifications into the final source code. They can occur in data declarations, data referencing, control flow logic, computational expressions, functional routine interfaces, and I/O operations.

The quality of software work products that are generated during analysis and design can be assessed and improved by using systematic quality assurance procedures, walk-throughs and inspections, and automated checks for consistency and completeness. Techniques for assessing and improving the quality of the source code include systematic quality assurance procedures, walk-throughs and inspections, static analysis, symbolic execution, software unit and module testing, and systematic software integration testing. Formal validation techniques can be used to show, in a rigorous manner, that the software end product conforms to its requirements.

Verification and Validation in the Software Life Cycle

The V&V activities occur throughout the software life cycle; typical V&V tasks during the development phases as required by the Standard for Software Verification and Validation Plans (ANSI/IEEE Std 1012-1986) are shown in Table 8-1. The tasks shown in Table 8-1 are the minimum required for the development phases required by the standard. The standard also specifies the minimum input and output requirements for each task. A V&V task cannot begin without specific inputs, and it is not completed until the task-specific outputs are completed. The V&V activities can be tailored by adding or deleting tasks from the minimum set. Table 8-2 lists some of the optional V&V tasks and considerations that might be assigned to the V&V group. Fundamentally, the V&V group is responsible for verifying that the software product at each life cycle phase satisfies quality attributes and that at each phase the software product also satisfies the requirements of the previous phase. It is also responsible for validating that the software satisfies the system requirements and objectives.

Although its activities are directed at the software, the V&V group must also consider how the software interacts with the system as a whole, and this includes the hardware, users, other software, and other external systems. The V&V group maintains its own configuration management and data management functions on code, data, and documentation received from the development team, to ensure that V&V discrepancy reports are made against controlled documents and to perform regression testing against controlled software releases.

The V&V group's documentation evaluation and testing are different from those conducted by other groups. The V&V quality assurance team reviews documents for compliance to standards and performs a logical check on the technical correctness of the document contents. The V&V group may perform in-depth evaluations through activities such as rederiving the algorithms from basic principles, computing timing data to verify response time requirements, and

Table 8-1   Typical Minimum Set of Recommended V&V Tasks

Phase	Tasks	Key Issues
Concept	Concept documentation evaluation	Satisfy user needs; constraints of interfacing systems
Requirements definition	Traceability analysis	Trace of requirements to concept
	Requirements validation	Correctness, consistency, completeness, accuracy, readability, and testability; satisfaction of system requirements
	Interface analysis	Hardware, software, and operator interfaces
	Begin planning for V&V system testing	Compliance with functional requirements; performance at interfaces; adequacy of user documentation; performance at boundaries
Design	Traceability analysis	Trace of design to requirements
	Design evaluation	Correctness, consistency, completeness, accuracy, readability, and testability; design quality
	Interface analysis	Correctness, consistency, completeness, accuracy, readability, and testability; data items across interface
	Begin planning for V&V component testing	Compliance to design; timing and accuracy; performance at boundaries
	Begin planning for V&V integration testing	Compliance with functional requirements; timing and accuracy; performance at stress limits
Implementation	Traceability analysis	Trace of source code to design
	Code evaluation	Correctness, consistency, completeness, accuracy, readability, and testability; code quality
	Interface analysis	Correctness, consistency, completeness, accuracy, readability, and testability; data and control across interfaces
	Component test execution	Component integrity
Test execution	V&V integration test	Correctness of subsystem elements; subsystem interface requirements
	V&V system test execution	Entire system and at limits; user stress conditions
	V&V acceptance test execution	Performance with operational scenarios
Installation and checkout	Installation configuration audit	Operations with site dependencies; adequacy of installation procedure
	V&V final report generation	Disposition of all errors; summary of V&V results

Table 8-2 Typical Optional V&V Tasks and Suggested Applications

Tasks	M	C	R	D	I	T	X	O	Considerations
Algorithm analysis			×	×	×	×		×	Numerical and scientific software using critical equations or models
Audit performance									When the V&V group is part of the quality assurance or user group; for large developments to help quality assurance; or for user group staff audits
Configuration control					×	×	×	×	
Functional					×	×	×	×	
In process			×	×	×	×	×	×	
Physical						×	×	×	
Audit support									When the V&V group is part of a systems engineering group or is independent; for large software developments
Configuration control					×	×	×	×	
Functional					×	×	×	×	
In process			×	×	×	×	×	×	
Physical						×	×	×	
Configuration management		×	×	×	×	×	×	×	When the V&V group is part of the user group
Control flow analysis			×	×	×				Complex, real-time software
Database analysis			×	×	×	×		×	Large database applications; if logic is stored as parameters
Data flow analysis			×	×	×			×	Data-driven real-time systems
Feasibility study evaluation		×						×	High-risk software using new technology or concepts
Installation and checkout			×	×	×	×	×	×	When the V&V group is part of the systems engineering or user group
Performance monitoring								×	Software with changeable user-machine interfaces
Qualification testing			×	×	×	×	×	×	When the V&V group is part of the systems engineering or user group
Regression analysis and testing			×	×	×	×	×	×	Large, complex systems

Continued on next page.

Continued from previous page.

Tasks	Phases (*)								Considerations
	M	C	R	D	I	T	X	O	

Reviews support
  Operational
   readiness
  Test readiness
					
					×
						
						×
							
							×
							×
								
								×
								×
									When the V&V group is part of the systems engineering or user group

Simulation analysis			×	×	×		×		No system test capability or the need to preview the concept for feasibility or the requirements for accuracy
Test certification					×	×	×		For critical software
Test evaluation			×	×	×	×	×	×	When the V&V group is part of the quality assurance or user group
Test witnessing					×	×	×		When the V&V group is part of the quality assurance, user, or systems engineering group
User documentation evaluation		×	×	×	×	×	×		Interactive software requiring user inputs
V&V tool plan generation	×						×		When acquiring or building V&V analysis and test tools

Walk-throughs
  Requirements
  Design
  Source code
  Test
			
			×
			
				×
				
					×
					×
						
						×
							
							×
								
								×
								×
								×
								×
									When the V&V group is part of the quality assurance or systems engineering group; for large software developments to staff walk-throughs

* Phases: M = management; C = concept; R = requirements; D = design; I = implementation; T = test;
  X = installation, integration checkout; and O = operations, maintenance

developing control flow diagrams to identify missing and erroneous requirements. The V&V group may also suggest more optimal approaches to what they find. The V&V group's testing is usually separate from the development team's testing; in some cases, the V&V group may use development test plans and results and augment them with additional tests.

A major influence on the responsibilities of a V&V group and its relationship to other groups is to whom the V&V group technically reports on the software project. There are fundamentally four ways to organize the V&V effort. First is the traditional approach, where the

V&V group is independent of the development team and is usually referred to as independent V&V or "IV&V." In this relationship, the V&V group establishes formal procedures for receiving software releases and documentation from the development group. The V&V group sends all of its evaluation reports and discrepancy reports to the development, user, and management groups. To maintain an unbiased technical viewpoint, the V&V group does not use any results or procedures from the quality assurance or systems engineering groups. The independent V&V group's tasks are oriented toward engineering analysis and comprehensive testing. The objective is to develop an independent assessment of the software's quality and determine whether the software satisfies critical system requirements. The advantages of this approach are detailed analysis and test of the software requirements, independent determination of how well the software performs, and early detection of high-risk software and system errors. The disadvantages are higher costs and additional software development interfaces.

In the second organization example, the V&V group could be embedded within the system engineering group. In this case, the V&V tasks are to review the group's engineering analysis and testing. In some instances, the V&V group may be the independent test team for the systems engineering group and share its data. The V&V group's results are reviewed and monitored by the systems engineering and quality assurance groups. An independent V&V group reporting to the systems engineering group is another form of this organizational approach. Advantages of using systems engineering personnel in the V&V tasks are minimum cost to the project, no system learning for the staff, and no additional software development interfaces. A disadvantage to this approach is the loss of objective engineering analysis.

In the third organization example, the V&V group could be embedded within the quality assurance group, in which case the V&V tasks are monitoring, auditing, and reviewing the content of the software development end products. In these tasks, the V&V group works as part of the quality assurance group and maintains its relationship to the systems engineering and other development groups in the same way that the quality assurance group does. The advantages of embedding V&V within the quality assurance group are low cost to the project and entry of V&V analysis capabilities into reviews, audits, and inspections. A disadvantage of this approach is the loss of independent systems analysis and testing.

Last, the V&V group could be embedded within the user group, in which case the V&V tasks are an extension of the user group's responsibilities. Its tasks are configuration management support of products under development, support of formal reviews, user documentation evaluation, test witnessing, test evaluation of the development test planning documents, and user testing support. As an extension of the user group, the V&V group would receive formal software deliverables and provide comments and data to the development's project management team, who distributes the information to its own development team. An advantage of this approach is the strong systems engineering and user perspectives that can be brought to bear on the software during its development. The disadvantages are loss of detailed analysis and testing of incremental software, because the incremental builds are not formal deliverables, and loss of error detection and feedback to the development group. If the user group has an independent V&V group reporting to it, these disadvantages can be overcome, but an additional software development interface is created.

Quality Assurance

The purpose of the software quality assurance group is to provide assurance that the procedures, tools, and techniques used during the product software development and modification phases are adequate to provide confidence in the work products. Often, software quality assurance personnel are organizationally distinct from the software development group. However, this is not a prerequisite if the individuals performing the software quality assurance tasks on a project are different from the individuals performing the software development activities. This implies that an individual can fulfill a software quality assurance role on one software project and a software development role on another project, if they are not the same two projects. Frequently, both software quality assurance engineers and software engineers report to the same management person. The reporting structure is not as important as the two groups and their activities being separate and distinct on any project. This adds a degree of impartiality to quality assurance activities and allows the quality assurance personnel to become specialists in their discipline. In some organizations, the software quality assurance personnel function is advisory; in others, the software quality assurance group actively develops the standards, tools, and techniques and examines all software work products for conformance to the specifications.

Software quality assurance personnel are sometimes in charge of the arrangements for design and code walk-throughs, code inspections, and phase reviews. In addition, they are often responsible for the software project postmortem; they write the software project legacy documents and provide long-term retention of the software project records. The software quality assurance organization can also serve as a focal point for the collection, analysis, and dissemination of the quantitative data that relate to cost distribution, schedule slippage, error rates, and any other factors that influence software quality and productivity.

Typically, the software quality assurance group will work with the software development group in an advisory capacity to derive the Software Development Test Plan (SDTP). This allows the software quality assurance group to provide guidance to the software development group concerning the testability and repeatability of the proposed tests, for example. The SDTP specifies the objectives of the testing, the test completion criteria, the system integration plan, the methods to be used on particular modules, and the particular test inputs and expected outcomes. This collaboration also helps the software quality assurance group formulate their own validation testing plan and strategy to maximize the test effectiveness and document that strategy in the Software Validation Test Plan (SVTP). The insight gained by the software quality assurance group about the type of testing to be performed by the software development group will allow the software quality assurance testing to yield a more thorough and orthogonal testing strategy, for example. Although software quality assurance tests are of the same type as development tests, they usually take on a slightly different aspect. The function tests and the performance tests of the V&V group are based on the requirements specifications. They are designed to demonstrate that the software satisfies both the software requirements and the product-level requirements. Therefore, the SVTP can only be as good as the specified requirements, which must be phrased in quantified, testable terms.

For validation testing, functional test cases specify the typical operating conditions, input values, and expected results. Functional test cases also test the software behavior just inside, on, and just beyond the software's functional boundaries. The performance tests are designed to verify the software response times under varying loads, the percentage of execution time spent in various segments of the software, the throughput, the primary and secondary memory utilization, and the traffic rates on the data channels and communication links. The stress tests are designed to overload the software in various ways. For example, stress tests would include overloading the device's keypad and button inputs while operating remotely at the maximum baud rate or physically disconnecting the communications link while operating remotely.

Validation structure tests examine the internal processing logic of the software and the particular routines called; the logical paths traversed through the software routines are the objects of interest. The goal of structure testing is to traverse a specified number of paths through each routine to establish the thoroughness of the testing. A typical approach to structure testing is to augment the functional, performance, and stress tests with additional test cases to achieve the desired level of test coverage. Frequently, some of the structure tests cannot be designed until the software has been implemented and subjected to the predefined tests.

In some cases, software quality assurance personnel will work with development personnel to derive the software test plan. In other cases, the software quality assurance group will merely verify the adequacy of the test plan for the source code. In either case, the test plan is an important work product of the design process; it should be developed in a systematic manner and evaluated by the software quality assurance group.

Attributes of Quality Software

Studies related to the determination of the appropriate factors for software quality in terms of software code and specifications include those by C. Jones (1976), McCall, Richards, and Walters (1977), and Boehm et al. (1978). The attributes shown in Figure 8-1 are representative of those proposed; most of these attributes are qualitative rather than quantitative. As shown, the top-level characteristics of quality software are reliability, testability, usability, efficiency, transportability, and maintainability. In practice, efficiency will often turn out to be in conflict with transportability, maintainability, and testability; however, as hardware costs continue to decrease, the efficiency of machine code usage will become much less an issue and, consequently, a less important attribute of software quality. At present, all reasonable software development methodologies support the creation of software with all of these quality characteristics. While a specific segment of code may not be as efficient locally as a skilled software engineer can write it, disregarding all other factors, it must be designed to be as efficient as possible while still exhibiting the other desired qualities.

For the purposes of this discussion, reliability and testability stand out. Although the other characteristics are equally important, they are less related to testing and validation issues and more related to qualitative rather than quantitative issues. Reliable software must be correct, complete, consistent, and feasible at each stage of the software development life cycle. An infeasible set of requirements will lead to an inadequate design and probably to incorrect implementation. Assuming that the software meets these adequacy requirements at each stage of the software development process, then to be reliable, it must also be robust. Robustness is the ability of the software to survive a hostile environment, because all possible events cannot be anticipated.

At all stages of the software life cycle, the software must be testable; to accomplish this, the software must be understandable. Although the desired products are the requirements and design, the actual product is the code, which should be represented in a structured, concise, and self-descriptive manner so that the desired and actual products may be compared easily and unambiguously. In addition, the software must be measurable. This will allow the means for actually instrumenting the software or inserting probes to test and evaluate the software end product at each stage.

The emphasis on particular quality factors will usually vary from project to project, although not by much, as a function of the application, environment, and other considerations. The specific definition of quality and the importance of the given attributes should be specified during the requirements phase of the project. Even if good quality is difficult to define and measure, poor quality is glaringly apparent. Software that is error prone or does not function correctly is

Figure 8-1   Taxonomy of software quality

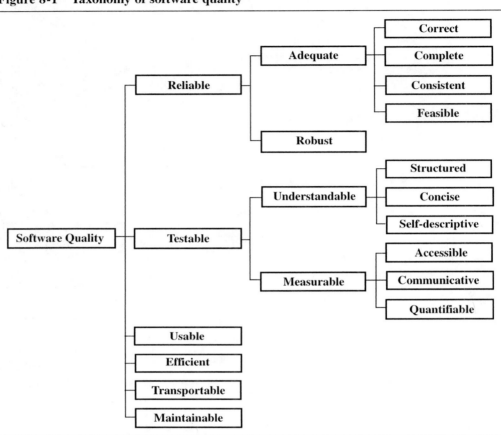

Reprinted with permission from *Microprocessor Software Project Management,* E. T. Fathi and C. V. W. Armstrong, p. 143, courtesy of Marcel Dekker, Inc., New York, 1985.

obviously of poor quality; discovering the errors in the software is the first step toward software quality assurance. Execution of the software with representative data samples and comparison of actual results with expected results have been the fundamental techniques used to uncover and determine software errors. However, testing is difficult, time-consuming, and not fully adequate; consequently, increased emphasis has been placed on insuring software quality through the development process.

Attributes of Quality Software Specifications

The four basic V&V criteria for software requirements and design specifications are completeness, consistency, feasibility, and testability (Figure 8-2).

A specification is complete to the extent that all of its parts or sections are present and each part is fully developed. In software engineering, a "complete" specification is probably not

Figure 8-2   Taxonomy of a satisfactory software requirements and design specification

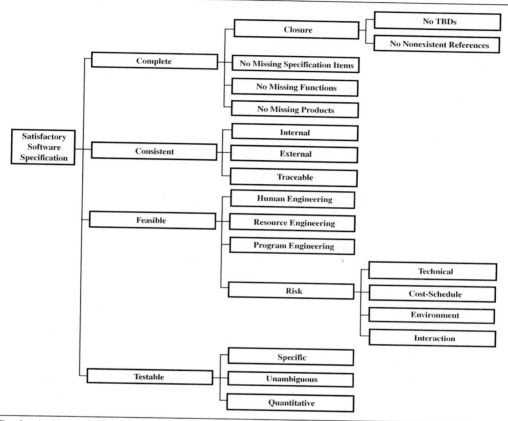

Reprinted with permission from "Verifying and Validating Software Requirements and Design Specifications,"
B. Boehm, in *Milestones in Software Engineering*, P. W. Oman and T. G. Lewis (eds.), p. 128, © 1990 IEEE.

possible. The aim must be to have as nearly a complete specification as is feasible given the aggregate understanding of the product. Completeness will actually stem from the concept that whatever is documented should be entirely whole, rather than that the documentation should contain the totality of information.

A software specification must several properties to assure its completeness. The specification cannot have any to-be-determined (TBD) entries within it. TBD entries are items for which decisions have been postponed and a placeholder has been entered in their stead. For example, "The device shall deliver fluid at a maximum rate of TBD ml per hour." There can be no nonexistent references in the specification to functions, inputs, or outputs that are not defined elsewhere within the specification. For example, "A record of all errors shall be logged in the Error Log Table," where the "Error Log Table" is undefined in the specification. There can be no missing specification items—items that should be (but are not) present as a part of the standard format of the specification. There should be no missing functions—functions that should be part of the software product but are not called for in the specification. For example, no recovery capability is specified that would ordinarily be associated with the device's functional recovery following alerts or warnings. There should be no missing products within the specification—products that should be a part of the delivered software but are not called for in the specification. For example, test tools or device error output postprocessors are needed to facilitate testing, field service, or maintenance, but they were not specified in the documentation.

The first two properties, "no TBDs" and "no nonexistent references," form a subset of the completeness properties that are called closure properties. Closure properties are those that can be verified by mechanical means. The last three specification properties generally require some human intuition to verify and validate them.

A specification is consistent to the extent that its provisions do not conflict with each other or with any governing specifications or objectives. Internal consistency implies that the specification does not conflict with itself. As a counterexample of internal consistency, one section of the specification states that real-time control interrupts shall have top priority at all times, and another section of the same document states that the safety subsystem shall take precedence over all other processes and interrupts. External consistency means that the specification items do not conflict with information items in another specification or entity. Traceability is the property that items in the specification have clear antecedents in earlier specifications or in statements of system objectives. In large specifications, each specified item should indicate the item or items in the earlier or higher level specification from which it is derived. This will prevent misinterpretations and "creeping elegance" embellishments, such as adding adaptive control features to a device when best engineering judgment had determined that they were not needed for the job and that they may not even work as reliably as simpler approaches.

A specification is feasible to the extent that the life cycle benefits of the specified system exceed the software life cycle costs. Feasibility involves more than verifying that the software satisfies its functional and performance requirements. It also implies validating that the specified system will be sufficiently maintainable, reliable, and human engineered to keep a positive life cycle balance sheet. In addition, feasibility implies identifying and resolving any high-risk issues before committing a large group of software engineers to any detailed development. Verifying and validating from a human-engineering standpoint involves ascertaining that the specified system provides a satisfactory way for users to perform their operational functions, that the system will satisfy human needs at various levels, and that the system will help the user to fulfill his or her human potential.

Resource engineering feasibility involves the V&V that a system can be developed to satisfy the specified requirements at an acceptable cost in resources and that the specified system will cost-effectively accommodate the expected growth in its operational requirements over the product life cycle. Software engineering feasibility addresses V&V by endeavoring to determine whether the software will be cost-effective to maintain and will be portable, and whether it has sufficient accuracy, reliability, and availability to satisfy cost-effectively the operational needs over its life cycle.

If the life cycle cost-effectiveness of a specified software end product is extremely sensitive to some device aspect that is not well known or understood, then there is high risk associated with the device or system. If such issues are not identified and resolved in advance, then there is a strong likelihood of disaster if and when this aspect of the system is not realized as expected. The four major sources of risk in software requirements and design specifications are technical, cost and schedule, environmental, and interaction effects.

Technical risks cover a broad spectrum of uncertainties, primarily associated with the ability to resolve the specified high-risk issue. Examples of technical risks involve achievable levels of overhead in the processor budget and processing timeline, achievable levels of device safety and protection, achievable speed and accuracy of new algorithms, and achievable overall software performance as well as hardware performance. The cost and schedule risks relate to the sensitivity of cost goals and schedule constraints. Examples of cost and schedule risks include the availability, stability, and reliability of the underlying hardware and operating system; and the support tools, such as compilers, linkers and loaders, and debuggers, that the software will be developed with and eventually run on. In addition, cost and schedule risks involve the availability of key personnel and the processing strain on available memory and execution time.

Some of the environmental risk issues are the expected volume and quality of the data to be used for input and testing; the availability and performance of the interfaces among the various hardware and software components; and the expected sophistication, flexibility, and degree of cooperation between system developers and users. Another concern related to interaction effects is the second-order effects caused by the introduction of the new device. For example, the system may experience overloads because the new capabilities stimulated additional and unexpected customer requests, high input data volumes, and system network transactions. This sort of reaction cannot be predicted precisely; the important thing is to determine where the system performance is highly sensitive and to concentrate risk-avoidance efforts in those areas. If software development is high risk in several areas, then the risks tend to interact exponentially. Unless the high-risk issues are resolved in advance and independently of the project, software development will eventually fail to provide any significant operational capability in a reasonable and timely manner.

A specification is testable to the extent that it can identify an economically feasible technique for determining whether the developed software will satisfy the specification. To be testable, the specification must be specific, unambiguous, and quantitative wherever possible. As counterexamples, the statements, "The device must be easy to clean," "The software shall provide accuracy sufficient to support effective fluid delivery," or "The software shall provide real-time response to user inputs" are not testable. These are good for product goals or objectives, but they are not precise enough to serve as the basis of a pass-fail acceptance test. These can be converted into testable requirements by the addition of quantifiable criteria or with the addition of clarifying conditions or definitions.

For example, the above requirements could be rewritten as, "The device shall be easy to clean with a sponge or paper cloth," "The software shall provide ± 2 percent accuracy in the control of fluid delivery," and "The software shall respond to user inputs within 0.5 seconds." In many cases, even these revisions will not be sufficiently testable without further definition. It will often take considerable effort to eliminate vagueness and ambiguity in a specification, to make it testable, but such an effort is well worthwhile because it will have to be done for the test phase anyway; doing it early eliminates expense, controversy, and possible bitterness in later software phases.

Verification and Validation of Off-the-Shelf Software

Off-the-shelf software is being used increasingly in medical device software systems. When integrated with the device's custom software, it sometimes becomes the critical piece that must function safely, accurately, and in accordance with the system requirements. Current software-related standards and FDA regulations recommend that manufacturers perform V&V of safety-critical off-the-shelf software. Rather than rely on the original software manufacturer's guarantee of safety, and to allay process-management concerns regarding the software vendor, V&V can be accomplished by performing process audits. A typical audit would entail a visit to the vendor's facility to review process documentation and perform spot checks to verify process compliance.

The visit to the vendor would provide the opportunity to acquire documentation, meet key technical personnel, and interview management.

The V&V personnel should begin the vendor audit by reviewing the software coding standards, software development plans, configuration management plans, quality assurance plans, and software management plans. The V&V personnel should also review any subcontractor documents and verify that the subcontractor's design and development staff also complied with the standards. Spot checks should be conducted of the vendor's software development library, development folders, and schedules, and a few quick discussions with key engineers should be conducted. The intent of this audit is to uncover undocumented or unexpected operational characteristics of the vendor's software. For example, certain combinations of conditions may not have been verified, parts of the software may not have been tested, and appropriate stress tests may not have been performed.

Requirements levied on off-the-shelf software must be traceable, testable, and compatible with the intended operation of the device. Commercial software releases and even availability of the software on the market for several years also help to validate that the software met the vendor's expectations, but it does not necessarily ensure that the device requirements will be met. To verify that the proposed software will meet the device requirements, V&V must correlate the device, interface, and software requirements with the off-the-shelf software requirements. Compliance with some requirements can be ascertained by an examination of the testing performed by the vendor. This includes a review of the vendor's available requirements, test plans, procedures, and results. When done early in the system development phase, the device manufacturer's test documentation can be reviewed and upgraded to both assist in off-the-shelf software compliance and incorporate vendor testing.

Characteristics of off-the-shelf software design and operation are potentially critical for software safety. Functions that perform I/O, task management, processor interface, and support libraries must operate securely, reliably, deterministically, and within the device's system specifications. The I/O management functions can be checked through available documentation, test results, and inductive test techniques. I/O functions will include data communications among hardware, software, and users, device addressing, data vectoring, and service calls. Task management encompasses the operational sequence of the software, the starting and stopping of processes, and management of the various process states. These functions should be analyzed for scheduling, timing, task communications, and memory management performance. V&V must ensure that processor interfaces, such as processor interrupts, memory access, and run-time precision, are consistent with device requirements. Libraries must be inspected to ensure that all of the proposed utilities meet the precision requirements of the system, perform properly over the entire range of possible device environments, and handle all errors in a manner consistent with system requirements.

Verification and Validation of Software Safety

A proof of software safety involves showing that the software cannot get into an unsafe state and that it cannot direct the device into an unsafe state, or showing that a software fault that does occur is not dangerous. Although verification can prove the correspondence of the source code to software requirements and specifications, it commonly does not capture the semantics of the hardware. What is needed is a proof of software safety; several analytical methods exist.

In one such procedure, instead of attempting to prove the correctness of the software relative to its original specification, a weaker criterion of acceptable behavior is selected (Anderson and Witty 1978). If the original specification is denoted by P, then a specification Q is chosen such that any software that conforms to P will also conform to Q. Q then prescribes an acceptable behavior of the software. The program is then designed and constructed in an attempt to conform to P, but so as to facilitate the provision of a much simpler proof of correctness with respect to Q than would be possible by using P. Such a proof is called a proof of adequacy; a special case of adequacy is termed safeness. This weaker specification interprets Q to be "P or error." This means that the program should either behave as originally intended, or it should terminate, giving an explicit indication of the reason for the failure. In these terms, a proof of safeness can rely on assertion statements that hold when the software is executed; otherwise, a failure indication would be generated. A complete proof of adequacy for safety would also require that the recovery procedures involved when the assertion statement failed be verified to ensure safe recovery.

Another verification method for safety involves the use of software fault-tree analysis (Leveson and Harvey 1983). When the detailed design or code has been completed, software fault-tree analysis procedures can be used to work backward from the critical control faults that were determined by the top levels of the fault tree through the program to verify whether the program can cause the top-level event or mishap. The basic goal of this safety assertion is that, by definition, the designers did not intend for the system to have mishaps. The incorrect software states can be divided into those that are considered safe and those considered unsafe. Software fault-tree analysis attempts to verify that the program will never allow an unsafe state to be reached. This is essentially a proof by contradiction; it is assumed that the software has produced an unsafe control action, and it is shown that this could not happen, because it leads to a logical contradiction. Although a proof of correctness should theoretically be able to show that the software is safe, it is often impractical to accomplish because of the magnitude of the proof effort involved and because of the difficulty in completely specifying the correct behavior of the software.

Fault trees have also been applied at the assembly-language level to identify the hardware fault modes that cause the software to act in an undesired manner. Such hardware fault modes could be erroneous bits in the program counter, in the registers, or in memory. Software fault trees can also be applied to the software design before the code construction actually begins. This enhances the safety design of the software while reducing the amount of formal safety verification needed later in the project.

Software common mode analysis is derived from techniques of hardware common mode analysis (Noble 1984). Redundant and independent hardware components are often used to provide fault tolerance; a hardware failure that affects multiple redundant components is called a common mode failure. In analysis of hardware common mode failure, each connection between the redundant hardware components is examined to determine whether the connection provides a path for failure propagation. If there are shared critical components, or if the connection is not suitably buffered, then the design must be changed to satisfy the independence requirement.

There is a potential for a hardware failure to affect more than one redundant component through a software path, as well as through a hardware path. For example, a processor could fail in such a way that it sends out illegal results that cause a supposedly independent processor to fail. Software common mode analysis examines the potential for a single failure to propagate across hardware boundaries via a software path, such as through serial or parallel data links or shared memory, through the use of structured walk-throughs. All of the hardware interconnections identified in hardware common mode analysis are examined to identify those with connections to software. All software processes that receive input from the connection are then examined to determine whether any data items or combinations of data items can come through this interface and cause the process to fail. It is not unusual to have to trace a path through several modules before it can be ascertained that there is an undesired effect.

Management Interface

There is a delicate balance between data used by engineers and data used by project managers. Unless the same data are used and interpreted under the same rules by both, the idea of data as a helper is likely to be distorted into data as a weapon. In the project manager's job description are the tasks to measure the progress of the project, provide visibility for management reviews, and ensure the success of the project in a non-threatening way. To accomplish this, the project manager's activities include estimating, planning, scheduling, and tracking.

Data that are too difficult and time consuming to obtain are usually crucial for the decision-making process. Delivery of metrics to the various individuals concerned with the data is varied. For example, software engineers often need metrics within seconds to minutes to understand and alter their work products. Managers typically need metrics within hours to identify trends and potential problem areas, within weeks to adjust the schedule, and within months to adjust plans and revise project estimates. Project data represent a continuum that varies from real-time feedback for engineers to much longer sampling periods that are more appropriate to tracking and managing the activities of teams. Consequently, the use of tools, such as PERT (Program Evaluation Report Technique) programs, provides little direct, real-time support for managers; project trend indicators are much more effective in alerting managers that events and activities on the PERT chart need attention.

Metrics are an invaluable supplement to these other tools for project management. Integration of project milestone data and the data from various work-product analysis tools into a convenient, accessible summary for project managers provides a powerful capability for managing more effectively. The difficulty is that the data displayed in such a project status table need to be available for updating by the engineers, but still be relatively private for the project manager, to prevent incorrect interpretations by various individuals. For example, suppose that the actual count of noncomment source statements for a particular module exceeded the original estimate by a predefined boundary condition or threshold. This condition alerts the project manager that a potential problem is developing, when in reality it is a normal indication of growth for that particular type of module.

Several types of graphical and tabular data can be used to convey and derive trends meaningfully. A simple plot of engineering effort against project deliverables is probably the easiest to generate. For example, a plot of source code statement generation versus time or defects identified versus defects remaining open provides both engineers and management with feedback about the progress of the project, as well as an indication of whether the software effort is being expended according to the original estimates. Other measures can be used to plot effective engineering effort, such as percentage of weighted functionality completed, design weight completed, and function points implemented. Of course, their success depends heavily, if not entirely, on the accuracy of the up-front estimated values and the projected end point.

The graphs of effort versus time are generally by-products of work product analysis tools. A necessary complement to these types of graphs comes from a defect-tracking system, even though defects are all too often accurately tracked only after software release, not before. The most natural time to require accurate reporting of defect data is before release and after formal testing begins. Nevertheless, defect reporting is labor intensive, and timely recording of defect information requires considerable energy. This is particularly necessary when the development team members are performing their own formal testing in support of their design. However, highly useful to both software engineers and project management are graphs of defects versus time. These graphs show both the trend of defects discovered and the trend of defects that remain unfixed or open. In the later stages of the project, these are just as important as the trends of effort versus estimates were during the beginning stages of the project.

One of the most difficult times for a project manager is the period early in the project when no code or modules exist, a time when it is very difficult to quantify progress because design metrics are a function of the creative period of the project. An alternative way of looking at this period is to calculate the number of design defects that are expected to be found during inspections and to plan and plot the inspections or design reviews that will be necessary to discover these defects. The estimated number of design defects and the time to find them during inspections are, by definition, based on historical data for past projects and the accuracy of that data by phase.

9

The Software Quality Assurance Program: Software Configuration Management Activities

The level of thinking that got us into this mess is not the level of thinking that will get us out.

—Albert Einstein

Configuration control is one of the software disciplines of the 1980s that grew in response to the many failures of the software industry throughout the 1970s. Over the years, the computer has been applied to solve many complex problems; the ability of software to manage these applications in the "traditional" way has all too frequently failed. In the 1970s, software engineering managers learned the hard way that the tasks involved in managing a software project were not linearly dependent on the number of lines of code produced but rather were exponentially dependent. As the 1970s ended, software engineers examined their failures in an effort to understand what went wrong and how it could be corrected. The software development process was dissected, and techniques were defined by which the development process could be effectively managed. Consequently, the most talented and experienced members of the software community began to develop a series of new disciplines intended to help control the software process. One of those disciplines became known as software configuration management.

To understand properly the role that software configuration management plays in the software development process, a review of the goal of that process is valuable. Software engineers are individuals who respond to the needs of another set of people by creating software that is designed to satisfy those needs. The software is a tangible output of the software engineer's thought process of converting someone else's idea into a product. The goal of the software engineer is to construct a software product that closely matches the real needs of the people for whom the software will be developed. Ideally, the perfect achievement of this goal would be a product having an intrinsic set of attributes that characterize product integrity. Product integrity would

315

then fulfill the user's functional needs, could be easily and completely traced through the product life cycle, would meet the specified performance criteria, and would ensure that cost and delivery expectations could be met.

This rather pragmatic view of the product demands that product integrity be a measure of the satisfaction of the real needs and expectations of the software user. It places the burden for achieving the software goal squarely on the shoulders of the software engineer, because that is who is in control of the development process. While the user can establish safeguards and checkpoints to gain visibility into the software development process, the primary responsibility for the success of the software is with the software engineer. Therefore, the goal of software engineering is to build software that exhibits the characteristics of product integrity. However, software is not simply a set of programs, but includes the documentation required to define, develop, and maintain these programs. Although this notion is not new, it still frequently escapes product development and maintenance management groups who assume that controlling a software product is the same as controlling the computer code.

Software engineering involves a complex set of interacting organizational entities. When a software project is undertaken, software engineering activities are in three basic discipline sets: project management, development, and product assurance. The various activities of software project management are directed both inward and outward. They support general management's need to see what is going on in the software project and to ensure that the company consistently develops products with integrity. At the same time, these activities look inside the software project in support of the assignment, allocation, and control of all project resources. In that capacity, software project management determines the allocation of resources to the software development and software product assurance disciplines. It is management's prerogative to specify the extent to which a given discipline will be applied to a given project. Historically, management has been handicapped when it comes to deciding how much of the product assurance disciplines are required, because of both inexperience and organizational immaturity.

The software development discipline represents those activities traditionally applied to and associated with a software project. This includes analysis, design, engineering, code development, testing, installation, documentation, training, and maintenance. In the broadest sense, these activities are needed to transfer a system concept from its beginning through the development life cycle. It takes a well-structured, disciplined, and rigorous technical approach to system development, along with the right mix of development disciplines to attain software product integrity. The concept of an ordered, procedurally disciplined approach to software development is fundamental to product integrity. This type of development approach provides development baselines, each of which provides an identifiable measure of progress and forms a part of the total foundation that supports the final product. Moving sequentially from one baseline to another with a high probability of success necessitates the use of the right development disciplines at precisely the right time.

The software product assurance activities used by software project management to gain insight into the software development process include configuration management, quality assurance, V&V, and test and evaluation. The proper use of these activities by software project management is basic to the success of the project, because they provide the technical checks and balances over the software product being produced.

Generically, configuration management is the discipline of identifying the configuration of a system at discrete points in time for the purposes of systematically controlling changes to the configuration and maintaining the integrity and traceability of the configuration throughout the system life cycle. Software configuration management does not differ substantially from the configuration management of hardware components, which is generally well understood and effectively practiced. However, many attempts to implement software configuration management have failed because the particulars of software configuration management are not directly analogous to the particulars of hardware configuration management, and because software configuration management is a less mature discipline than is hardware configuration management.

Generically, quality assurance as a discipline is commonly invoked throughout government and industry organizations with reasonable standardization when applied to systems composed only of hardware. However, there is enormous variation both in thinking and in practice when the quality assurance discipline is invoked for software or for a system containing software. Quality assurance has long been practiced on hardware projects. It is, therefore, mature in that arena, but it is relatively immature when applied to software development. Quality assurance consists of the procedures, techniques, and tools that are applied by quality assurance professionals to ensure that a product meets or exceeds pre-specified standards during a product's development cycle. Without specific prescribed standards, quality assurance entails ensuring that a product meets or exceeds a minimum industry standard or commercially acceptable level of excellence.

The quality assurance discipline has not been uniformly treated, practiced, or invoked relative to software development for several reasons.

- Very few organizations have software design and development standards that compare in any way with the hardware standards for detail and completeness.

- It takes a high level of software expertise to assess whether a software product meets prescribed standards.

- Few software buyer organizations have provided for or developed the capability to impose and monitor software quality assurance endeavors in the software seller organizations.

- Few organizations have tried to define the difference between quality assurance and other product development disciplines.

However, software, as a form of information, cannot be standardized; only the structures or framework for defining and documenting the software can be standardized. Thus, software development techniques can be meaningfully standardized only in relation to information structures, not to the content of the information.

V&V came into being expressly for the purpose of coping with software and its development, unlike configuration management and quality assurance. The V&V process deals with how well software fulfills its functional and performance requirements, as well as whether the specified requirements are indeed stated correctly and properly interpreted. Verification assumes more of the traditional quality assurance duties and activities; it is concerned with ascertaining that the software was implemented in accordance with prescribed and standardized processes. Validation ensures that the software end product is what it was intended to be relative to the previous baseline, that it meets its predefined design, and that it satisfies system-level requirements. Validation is invoked to ensure that the user receives the right product. To enhance objectivity in software quality assurance, an organization other than the software development organization must perform the V&V function.

Testing and evaluation are probably the best understood of the software disciplines, but they are practiced with the least uniformity. Testing and evaluation are imposed outside the software organization to independently assess whether a product fulfills its objectives. Testing and evaluation do this through the execution of a set of test plans and procedures. Specifically, in support of the end user, testing and evaluation entail evaluating the product performance in a live, or as close as possible, environment. Testing and evaluation are usually major undertakings involving one or more systems that are to operate together but that have been developed and accepted as stand-alone entities. Some organizations formally turn over test and evaluation responsibility to a group outside the development project organization after the product reaches a certain stage of development. This philosophy espouses the feeling that developers cannot be objective to the point of fully testing and evaluating what they have produced.

Configuration management, quality assurance, V&V, and testing and evaluation overlap in the required skills, functions, duties, responsibilities, and activities. All must be performed to assure software end-product performance. Depending on many factors, the actual overlap may be significant or slight. Some people in the software industry contend that V&V and test and evaluation are subfunctions of quality assurance. The contrasting argument is that V&V and test and evaluation have come into being as separate disciplines because conventional quality assurance methods and techniques have failed to do an adequate job of providing software end-product quality. In fact, software quality assurance is not really a discipline as much as it is a concept reflected in configuration management and V&V, just as testing and evaluation are probably reflected in all phases and types of testing. What is important is that all of the functions that have been defined are performed, not what they are called or who is responsible for their execution.

Baselines

The term *baseline* was originally used as an engineering survey term for an established line with a fixed direction and end points that allowed further extensions into unmapped areas. In the configuration management sense, a baseline is a document, a set of documents, or a particular version of code that is formally designated and fixed at a specific time during that configuration item's life cycle. However, the original concept still applies; the establishment of software configuration item baselines allows the orderly extension or development of the software or system, from specifications into design and then into the hardware and software items themselves. In practice, series of different baselines are established in order to permit an ordered flow of development work.

Software baselines establish a sequence of unambiguous references to the known properties of the software at any given time during software development or its operational life. This includes the period before any code physically exists. Even from the point at which the need for a software solution is determined, something about the software is actually known. From that point on, the software gradually emerges; in a controlled development process, it incrementally takes on more concrete definition through a sequence of documentation and code releases. Certain sets of releases constitute the baselines, and all of the baselines are subject to change at any time. The changes to the baselines reflect both necessary and desired revisions of the external characteristics of the software, such as the addition of a new feature or capability, or of the internal characteristics of the software, such as defect removal. Configuration control is the control of changes to the software baselines.

Baselines are planned milestones in the evolution of the software end product. They represent a discrete stage of the software evolution in which the features, capabilities, and functions of the software are well defined and known. There are several types of formal baselines, some of which may not be appropriate to all software development projects and some that are tied to software development phase-ending deliverables. Software development baselines can consist of documents, code, or both.

The software functional baseline contains the definition of the problem and represents the description of the software end product to be developed. The allocated baseline is the apportionment of the functions to be performed by the software to the specific hardware and software elements. Depending on the type of application, the allocated baseline and the functional baselines may be the same. The software top-level design baseline represents the overall architecture of the software for meeting its requirements. The detailed design baseline, the scheme of how the software will be built, includes the description of what will be built. The software end-product baseline, a hybrid baseline, contains the code as well as the documentation describing the code; the description is usually relative to an as-built version of the detailed design baseline. The software operational baseline is the product baseline that is updated as necessary during the life of the device.

The above are the formal software development baselines. Additional informal baselines are also necessary for the code and data during development of the software. The scheme of informal baselines will be derived from the SDP development method(s) to be used. For example, during the Integration and Test Phase, a group of procedures, functions, or capabilities are added as a single, logically functional module to the evolving software end product. The descriptive documentation and source code of this incremental addition to the software end product will be under some form of control from the time the set of tests directed at the module were completed.

Just as the informal baselines provide additional control points, there may also have to be several top-level and detailed design baselines for a single software end product. This would allow and account for the decomposition of the software into several subsystems and the assignment of those subsystems to different software development teams. This would facilitate and account for the delivery of a succession of software "builds" that can be used to demonstrate the evolving software's capabilities. The criterion for determining whether to establish a baseline has to do with the fundamental concept of a baseline. A baseline must define the descriptions of the properties of the software to be controlled if it is to provide accurate knowledge of the software in its current state. From an implementation standpoint, this means that at discrete points in the development or operational life of the software, existing documentation and code must be frozen, placed in a master library, and modified only through some established change procedure with signature authority.

Each software baseline includes the materials of its preceding baseline. For example, once the software requirements specification is placed under configuration control, it remains under control throughout all successive baselines. This does not necessarily mean that a code change inconsistent with the requirements specification cannot be made without formal authority. If the discovery were made, for example, during hardware and software integration that the value of an external flag was reversed in the specification, then the code would be changed to conform to the hardware reality. At that time, a change request would be filed to indicate the correction. In this way, the change request becomes the documentation of a fait accompli. The software baseline may or may not contain software planning documents. The decision to control these plans depends on how the planning documents will be used in the future and whether any changes made to the plans need to be, or will be, disseminated to the individuals who should be aware of the changes.

There are three fundamental reasons for defining baselines when only documentation of the software and not the code exists:

1. The documents define the current state of the software and are useful to software engineers who are about to continue software development in the next development phase.

2. The documents define the software in a manner that will permit the results of one development phase to be verified with respect to the results of the preceding phases.

3. The documents ensure the accuracy of the documentation for the benefit of those software engineers who will be responsible for the software during its operational life.

Code Control

Special problems surface with baselines that contain code. The most obvious problem is the fact that it is impossible to look at a physical code file and immediately judge its currency; physical code files are not marked-up pages with red lines that indicate the interim changes. Not until the header of the file is displayed and the revision or version status of the file becomes apparent do its interim changes become known, assuming that the file header has been filled out or is even present at all. Another major problem with code baselines is that permanent changes to the code may be made relatively effortlessly through the invocation of the source file editor. This may be done several times a day during the test and debug periods and, therefore, the revision or version status of the file may not be kept up to date.

Special problems require special solutions, and several solutions have been developed for controlling the changes in software code files. Common to nearly all of them is the concept that control should be avoided until the subject code begins to stabilize. Although this probably sounds antithetical to these discussions concerning software quality assurance, it is a rather sensible approach as long as the period of avoidance is not excessive. There is no need to control the code if the code remains entirely in the hands of its author. While a software engineer is testing or debugging the function or module, the only control necessary is the one required for the software engineer's own purposes; in this context, almost any mechanism will work. In reality, control may not be appropriate even at the time the code is released to the integration team, because the first attempts at its integration may evoke too many changes in the code for any external control to be effective. However, when the time comes for the next set of functions or modules to be added to the evolving software end product, it is necessary to place the integrated code under configuration control.

The basic problem of code control is making certain that only the latest validated edition of the code is linked with the other authorized editions to form the tested software end product. The most straightforward way to ensure this is to make sure that each code edition has a unique identifier that would be generated by the source code editor. The most recent version is then given to the compiler that automatically passes the edition information intact to the header record of the output object file. The link editor examines the edition information before linking begins, to confirm that it agrees with the edition currently in the link output file. Although not all software development systems are configured to perform this task in the manner specified, most systems do provide various aspects of it.

In a variant of this method, the operating system adds a flag to the last edited version of the software, deletes the flag from previous versions, and allows the compiler to operate only on source files containing flags. Software engineers can still compile earlier versions of the software by defining additional compile time parameters, but they cannot do so inadvertently. Regardless of how the software development environment is set up, the objective is to avoid software testing with obsolete editions of the software.

When mechanized controls for the source code, the constituency of the load modules, and the executable composite software to be used for testing are in place, the subject of software librarians comes up. A software librarian is an essential part of the software development environment, because no matter how diligent the software engineers are at recording the changes to the various software editions, invariably something will slip through, and the software is no longer under control. Although a human librarian will be helpful in keeping track of the myriad software changes and may even be the funnel through which all source code changes are made, the likelihood of perfect performance even over a few days is small at best.

It is better to have a powerful library control tool and system, and to use the human librarian mostly as an auditor of the use of the tools, to make certain that the affected documentation has also been revised. The more elegant automated software librarians allow for the re-creation of a module as it had existed in any previous edition, as well as permitting the concurrent editions of a module to be controlled. In this way, during debugging, several temporary variants of a module may be used for diagnostic purposes. Once the bug has been found and eliminated, the capability of recalling the authorized version for repair makes it easy to strip any diagnostic code from the debugged module.

In summary, code control is the domain of automated librarians but is augmented by human librarians or configuration managers. Through the use of the automated librarian, the time for code control to pass from the software engineer to the configuration manager can be delayed until the initial set of software errors has been removed from the software end product. At that time, the source code files are placed under configuration control and become a part of either an interim or formal baseline.

Firmware

Configuration control of code must be carried one step further when the operational memory for the software is a set of ROMs, PROMs or electronically erasable PROMs (EEPROMs). Consider the operational situation in which it becomes necessary to replace one of these firmware devices because of some failure. This is possible only if the partition or mapping of the load module is unambiguously known; alternatively, ambiguity can be avoided only if the mapping of the software is repeatable.

For example, suppose a load module of 3000 sixteen-bit binary addresses is transferred to a set of twelve identical ROMs of 1000 four-bit memory locations. The way in which the address space of the load module is mapped into that of the ROM array is through the use of a partitioning program. In order to replace any one of the 12 ROMs, the load module is reprocessed through the partitioning program, but only the 1000 bits unique to the failed ROM are delivered to the ROM fabrication facility. This means that the partitioning program itself must be under configuration control, because any change in it may affect the final partitioning result. If the partitioning program is deliberately modified, then the original version of the program must be saved as part of the product software support library, which is peculiar to the programming product for which the ROMs were made.

Another difficulty with firmware that complicates the manufacturing engineer's world, but is pedestrian to the software engineer, is the certainty that the correct firmware device is inserted into its allocated place on the printed circuit board—and on the correct board. This problem is usually alleviated by one of several number-labeling schemes that can be affixed to some part of the firmware device's anatomy. For example, most firmware devices can allow an 18-character label to be printed on the device. If 10 to 12 of these characters are used to identify the hardware, then there remain enough characters to record the software edition as well as some ancillary information peculiar to the manufacturing system. The software edition identification is particularly useful if several concurrent versions of the software are maintained. With proper labeling, the semiconductor devices can be stockpiled in parts bins in the hardware assembly area without creating the hazard that an insertion error will escape the notice of inspection personnel.

Configuration Management

Configuration management is a discipline that applies technical and administrative direction and surveillance to:

- identify and document the functional and physical characteristics of the configuration items;

- audit the configuration items to verify conformance to specifications, interface control documents, and other requirements;

- control changes to configuration items and their related documentation;

- record and report information needed to manage configuration items effectively, including the status of proposed changes and the implementation status of approved changes.

Thus, a configuration item is a collection of hardware, software, firmware, or documents that satisfy an end-use function and are designated for configuration management. As shown in Figure 9-1, configuration management consists of four major divisions: identification, change control, status accounting, and audits.

The various elements of configuration control must be organized into a system with appropriate paperwork to record certain control activities and ensure distribution of change information. Responsibility for compliance with the configuration control plan must be fixed and a system of audits installed to ensure that compliance must be worked out. These types of matters, and others already mentioned, are also the components of configuration management. Although software control boards, through release and change notices, consume much of configuration management, the most basic concern of configuration management is creating a sensible labeling scheme.

Labeling Practices

Consistent labeling practices are of inestimable help in relating documents to code as well as to each other. A labeling scheme that encompasses all controlled material must have three major

Figure 9-1   Major divisions of configuration management

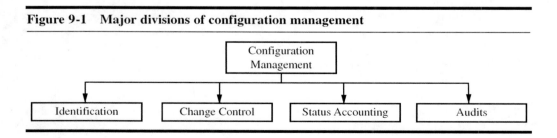

parts: an identifier, a subject, and an edition. Although these parts can be in any order, the edition information is rarely first. The identifier carries the description of the type of configuration item that is labeled. The subject field refers to the final product or some part of it, and it is usually assigned a numeric value, although alphanumerics can be used. The edition information is usually divided into two parts, one for the version level and one for the revision index. The version level is updated when a new logical function is added, when the software is reconfigured for a new operating circumstance, or even to indicate the addition of new modules during software integration. The revision index is incremented when a defect has been removed or a minor improvement in the performance of the software has been made. By definition, all new versions start with the revision index set to zero.

For example, the software configuration identification section of the Software Configuration Management Plan (SCMP) governs the explicit assignment of software version and document numbers. In general, and during development, a generic version and document identification numbering scheme is employed, so that the number easily conveys the name of the project, or product model number, the initials or abbreviation of the document type, and the release identification number. If the project is a general medical product, then the detailed design specification might be numbered GMP-DDS-001; the Device Model 123 improvement project software requirements specification might be numbered 123-SRS-002. It is helpful to label documents with numbers beginning with the digit 0 (zero) for the version level until the final version of the software is released. For example, the initial, first-time-ever draft would be labeled 0.0; review version one of that draft would be 0.1, review version two would be 0.2, and so on until the document was approved and released in final form as 1.0. This scheme will also work well for documents that have already been released but are undergoing updates, to reflect the current code version.

The software version or release numbers conceptually function in the same manner; they are release numbers with "fix numbers" appended. As the software evolves through its life cycle, each baseline is assigned an incrementing release number that is a whole number. As fixes are made to repair errors and remove bugs, the fix number is appended to the release number. The first release of software could be 1.0, followed by release 2.0, then 3.0, and so on. As intermediate releases are made, the software number might be 1.01, 1.1, or 1.2, depending on the granularity required to track fixes and upgrades. When software is ported to a new platform or host, a new release number should be assigned, as if the software were being released as a major update. This should be done even if a major upgrade was made. The reason is that the new number provides a baseline for validation testing since the version from the old platform became operational; the new platform can be validated as equivalent to the old platform version, and then the new upgrades, enhancements, or capabilities can be installed. If this sequence is not performed, it will be difficult, but not impossible, to determine if the software does not work because of the new platform or because of the implemented changes.

Precisely how the labeling scheme is set up and how it formulates rules concerning the correspondence of editions among material of different identifiers depend on the type and size of the systems being developed and the number of characters used. In addition, and most important, the software labeling scheme should satisfy any labeling conventions that are already predicted by the elements of the software development environment. Whatever method is used, the key should be consistency among the code, code files, and corresponding documents. For example, Routine A Version 1 Revision 3 should be found in a file that has the same version index number, 1 in this case, and the software specifications should also be at version level 1. It should be understood that the revision levels may be inconsistent, because the defects may be removed from either the code or the documentation without affecting the other.

Software Change Practices

Three types of events can affect a controlled document or file: release to the control system, formal requests for a change, and formal notification that a change request has been complied with. Much of configuration management has to do with avoiding nonproductive, improvised measures of handling and marking these types of events, while at the same time ensuring that unauthorized alterations are not encouraged by cumbersome bookkeeping. Accordingly, it is customary to initiate or record each type of event by using a unique instrument, which is usually a printed form, that reduces the likelihood of incomplete information and incomplete dissemination.

The software release notice is the vehicle for placing a document or code file into a baseline. The form to be used as the software release notice should request: the document or file identification number; the name of the system; the name of the subsystem, component, or applicable project description; the date; the authorized person releasing the item; and a list of the individuals to whom the notification will be sent. Obviously, a software release notice applies to any new documentation or code, but it should also be used to mark new versions of software products that are already in operation, normally at the conclusion of validation testing on the new version. This will act as a trigger to alert the appropriate individuals in charge of the distribution of code and manuals to take appropriate action.

Documents and code require alteration for external or internal reasons. The external reasons are generally viewed as changes in the functional or allocated baselines that affect the software design or architecture, such as the addition of a new requirement or the alteration of the user interface. Internal changes are those required to improve efficiency, improve maintainability, remove code no longer used, and remove defects. Whether the change is internal or external, the first step in altering controlled material is the generation of a software change request.

Related to defect removal, a software change request is generated when controlled software produces a failure, debugging found the defect, and a fix has been found. The debugging process is often preceded by a software trouble or problem report that lists the symptom and the part of the software responsible for the problem, if it is known. The software problem report is commonly used as the basis for the decision that an attempt should be made to solve the problem. This occurs during any formal testing or operational period, when a confrontation with a defect is often avoided in favor of some sort of work-around. If the decision is made to fix the problem, then a software change report or Change Request/Approval (CRA) is generated.

The information contained in the CRA (see Figure 3-8) includes: the identification numbers or names of all code files and documents that are affected by the change; the names of the system, subsystem, or components; a description of the change; an estimate of the severity or impact of the change; and other versions of the system to which the change should also be made. If the CRA is the result of a software problem report, the report is referenced, and the CRA includes the date and identity of the requestor. The CRA may attach additional information that explains, amplifies, or further supports the requested change. For example, the CRA may have a listing showing the differences of the source code files or VDIFFs, listings of the files themselves, and even red-lined document pages. The CRA should be a complete review package, and any information that helps to facilitate its approval should be attached.

The software change request then goes to the Software Change Review Board (SCRB), where the decision is made to proceed with the completion of the requested change. This is usually a perfunctory decision for CRAs that are related to bug fixes, in contrast to the other types of changes mentioned. The purpose of the SCRB is principally to ensure that all relevant personnel know the status of the baseline. While waiting for the board's decision, the CRA assumes the status of an interim software change notice and is used to justify further testing with the altered program. Usually, the SCRB is convened quickly and reaches its decision and approves the change in a matter of hours or less; the procedure need not be laborious, formal, or restrictive.

The notification that a software change has been made is implemented through the use of the software change notice, which is, in effect, an abbreviated software request notice. The librarian or configuration manager issues a software change notice when the change has been satisfactorily tested and the correctness of the documentation updates have been verified. The software change notice contains the name of the issuer, the date of issue, and the system name, identification number, or description. In addition, the notice includes a reference to the software change request that was its progenitor, the identification number or description of all controlled items that were affected, and a brief description of the change and its effect, if any, on the baseline performance definition. For operational systems, a single software change notice may affect several different software versions that are distributed at diverse installations. Inclusion of the version identification numbers for each of these indicates that the change was tested on each version. One of the functions of the SCRB is to look for the documentation indicating that those tests were indeed done. The software change notice is sent to the SCRB and presented by the author of the software trouble report, the appropriate software management personnel, and quite possibly a separate function responsible for the distribution of software updates.

The SCRB's constituency is a function of the type of software system that gets reviewed, although some generalizations are possible. If the system involves elements other than software, such as embedded software, or a product or device composed of related software systems, then the configuration control board may have greater scope. A software management person is certainly on the board, as well as a representative of the software quality assurance function from the project whose software is under review. A member of either marketing or program management may be present, although usually not unless the agenda includes consideration of changes in the functional or allocated software baselines. The board should include the software librarian or configuration manager from the project whose software is under review.

At the project level, decisions to authorize work on an enhancement or on the repair of a noncritical problem would normally be made elsewhere, although the individuals who make those decisions might also be people who attend SCRB meetings. The real decisions faced by the board are those pertaining to procedural matters; the board's role in configuration management is to make certain that control is maintained. In fact, its composition reflects the purpose of ensuring awareness, not deliberation.

The questions that would normally arise have to do with making certain that estimates of cost or impact were made or that the documentation associated with the code change was correspondingly altered. Thus, it is not necessary for the SCRB to meet immediately each time a software change request or change notice has been prepared. It is generally adequate to meet weekly, or as necessary, during software development, possibly monthly during the first year of operational life, and less frequently thereafter if few changes are being made. For the majority of the changes presented to the SCRB, the board approves work that has already been performed, either the actual changes or their associated paperwork.

Externally caused software modifications, such as enlarging the scope of the project or adding new features or functions, are usually driven by the project and concern cost and schedule. For these cases, the SCRB may be charged with advising project management that the software estimations are in accordance with established procedures, or it may even be given the authority to make the final decision. A board meeting dealing with such matters may be called at any time for the specific business at hand. Moreover, the board's composition may differ from that required to sanctify the changes already made.

This type of change often tends to blur the distinction between configuration control practiced during development and the control practiced during the operational period. It is probably more often the rule than the exception that major alterations of the requirements specification start to crop up well before the first release of the finished software. The reasons for this are numerous, but they begin as early as the software design phase and continue to wreak havoc in their own special way, even up through validation testing. Without a diligently pursued system of control, software engineers may soon find it difficult to be certain of the external specifications they are supposed to be working toward.

Control of Installed Variants

Although nearly every device manufacturer has the best of intentions and initially intends to release only one product version, additional versions will begin showing up during the development effort, as well as during the operational period. Each version must be treated and maintained as a concurrent operational baseline. In the sense that afterthoughts occur with less frequency as the time since the conceptual phase of the project increases, control is somewhat less difficult during the operational period. On the other hand, more of these external changes will result in permanent diversity of the baseline content, creating a new set of problems. At any given moment, several versions of the software may be extant, needing to be maintained. Commonly, the versions are at different revision levels.

The situation only gets worse with time, with the maturation or evolution of the software, and with the operating environments under which it is installed. For example, suppose that a defect is found in Version 4, Revision 19 of operational software, and a decision is made to fix the problem. Even before the repair is made, an investigation is undertaken to determine which of the other versions have the same problem. This may not be as simple as ascertaining if the others have the same version-revision level as the faulty module found in Version 4, Revision 19. The same defect may, in fact, exist in other editions of the module, and in some variants of the software, or the module may have been removed or logically bypassed. As an illustration, an input error-checking routine may be blocked off for systems that connect to hardware devices that contain their own error checking. It is also possible that other parts of other variants have code that compensates for the bug or that simply cannot be affected by it. For example, in Version 4, Revision 19, the module at fault may, under certain circumstances, fail to provide an adequate timeout before accepting a user command. However, Version 4 is the only interactive version, while all of the others are off-line processors. In addition to determining which versions of the system are affected and how they should be properly tested, the costs associated with regression testing of an operational system should be considered. Although the practice has very obvious disadvantages, it can be a viable exercise to determine if it is more prudent to leave any of the variants alone.

All of this points out the fact that it is necessary to know unambiguously the exact composition of each installed system—its modules, any databases, and their editions. Only with this type of control can a proper investigation be made to determine the effect of a change on each software version, as well as the manner in which the change must be verified. Rigidly controlled configuration records are nowhere more important than for the distribution of the correct updates to the right installations. This is a problem faced by firms whose business is selling products that have different but interrelated software systems within them, those that sell volumes of instruments, and any others who have a large, geographically widely distributed user base. To support this, a database information system is required, and even that requires an extension of a quality control system to include the update distribution, because the shipment records in the mailroom must be compared to those in the database. If the updates can be downloaded through a network controlled by the user database and can be coupled to the master librarian, then some of the quality assurance functions can be reduced.

10

The Software Quality Assurance Program: Software Hazards and Safety Activities

We build systems like the Wright brothers built airplanes—
build the whole thing, push it off a cliff, let it crash, and start
over again.

—R. M. Graham

In recent years, software and microprocessors have replaced many of the electromechanical components traditionally used in medical devices and control systems. Software has been substituted for the hard-wired relay logic and keyboards, and video displays have been substituted for switches and dials. Device manufacturers have the potential to improve their products without making changes to the hardware by simply distributing a new copy of the control software. But this advantage does not come without a price. Not only is the production of high-quality software very difficult and time consuming, it introduces the possibility for new kinds of hazards. For example, the linear accelerators that are used for cancer radiation therapy treatments pose risks to the patient and to the device user from electrical shock, radiation exposure, and mechanical collisions caused by runaway software.

Software, in and of itself, is not unsafe, but the physical systems that it may control can do damage. Software safety considerations do not arise for software applications that perform the more traditional data processing or scientific computations. Only when the software is coupled to control systems that are themselves potentially unsafe do software safety issues arise. The results of software control computations and decisions are usually not subjected to human review prior to their implementation and, therefore, humans cannot intercede as a safety check. After the software control function has been implemented, the software controlled system can rarely be returned to its prior state.

Safety engineering, a recognized engineering discipline, emerged when it became clear that complex modern technologies demanded a systematic approach to the control of hazards. Safety requirements may, in fact, conflict with other system requirements in such a way that a radically different design might be achieved if cost and performance were the only considerations for the device design. The resolution of these conflicts in a consistent and intelligent manner demands that safety requirements be explicitly separated from other device requirements and that the responsibility for fulfilling them is assigned to someone with authority.

Software designers must assume that during the operational life of the product, the control software will fail spectacularly and unexpectedly. This does not mean that a computer-controlled device is necessarily unsafe; it means that software designers must anticipate software failures and protect against them. In systems having a serious potential hazard, regulations have traditionally directed that no failure of a single component should be able to cause a serious accident. For the purpose of these directives, any combination of computers, microprocessors, and control software that share common memory should be considered a single component. Thus, no safety-critical function can be allowed to depend solely on a single computer system that does not have an independent backup; systems should be designed to fail into a safe and harmless state. Only a few simple functions should be required to enter or preserve the safe states by terminating or preventing potentially hazardous conditions. These functions are usually called interlocks, lock-outs, or shutdown systems, and they should be designed to work properly despite the failure of the other systems. Many regulations and guidelines specify that these safety functions should not be performed by the same computer system that provides normal operating functions.

Risk Management

The FDA's quality system regulation is intended to give medical device manufacturers the flexibility to determine the controls necessary to be commensurate with the risks for the device being developed. Although the FDA sees risk analysis as an essential requirement of the regulation, it gives little guidance on specific risk analysis approaches and procedures, such as fault-tree analysis (FTA) or failure modes and effects analysis (FMEA). Medical device companies can manage and reduce risk more effectively by including risk consideration as early as possible in device or process development and revisiting those issues systematically throughout the development process. Fundamentally, the risk management process involves the steps shown in Figure 10-1. To manage risk, hazards must first be identified; by evaluating the potential consequences of those hazards and their likelihood, a measure of risk can be estimated. The likelihood value is then compared to the company's risk-acceptability criteria; if it is too high, the risk must be mitigated. Because risk cannot be completely eliminated, the risk that remains must be managed. The following steps can be used in an overall risk management program:

- Develop written definitions of what needs to be done and how to do it.

- Define responsibilities and accountability.

- Define what needs authorization and who is responsible for handling it.

- Define the skills and knowledge necessary to implement the system and a provision for training those who do not have these skills.

- Develop and maintain written documentation to demonstrate conformance to the risk management policies and procedures.

Figure 10-1   Typical flowchart for risk management of identified hazards

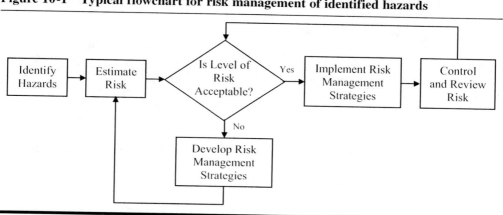

- Incorporate measures that cross-check and verify that risk management procedures are followed.

- Verify that risk management systems are in place and functioning properly.

Whereas many companies have good hazard and risk assessment programs, effective risk management is not always in place.

Early in the design stage, a preliminary hazard analysis can be conducted to establish the baseline hazards associated with a device. In essence, the analysis consists of listing the major components and operating requirements of the device and evaluating their potential hazards. The components and operating requirements should include raw materials and wastes, hardware monitoring and control systems, human device interfaces, services, and the operating environment. Potential hazards that should be evaluated include toxicity, flammability, and reactivity of raw material and wastes; sensitivity to environmental factors such as temperature and humidity; mechanical or electronic hazards; and human factors associated with the operator-device interface. The patient-to-device interface can also be hazardous because of unsafe or ineffective delivery of energy, administration of drugs, or control of life-sustaining functions. In addition, incorrect information could lead to a misdiagnosis or to wrong treatment or therapy being ordered. When conducting a preliminary hazard analysis, a what-if or brainstorming approach to identify possible failures can be used to evaluate potential consequences and develop risk management strategies. In general these strategies will lead to an improved, lower cost design.

Failure scenarios developed as part of the failure approach can be prioritized by the severity of each hazard. At this stage there is often insufficient detail to evaluate hazard likelihood accurately, but comparisons may be made with similar devices and their histories from medical device reports as well as from the company's experience with a similar product. The goal is to eliminate all high-severity hazards and to reduce as many medium- and low-severity hazards as possible. Because of the considerable flexibility in this early design stage, major changes can made in the device to make it inherently safer at minimal cost. For example, if use of a chemical was determined to be a significant hazard, then other, less toxic chemicals or a diluted form of the original chemical might be a reasonable mitigating measure.

During prototype development, a more detailed hazard and risk analysis can be performed. Usually at this stage of the design process, block diagrams, preliminary software, and mechanical drawings are available, and the basic operations of the device have been defined. The device and its operation can be reviewed by analysis techniques that include top-down and bottom-up approaches. A hazard and operability (HAZOP) study is a bottom-up approach that can be used for new or complex designs that involve HAZOP studies conducted on individual steps, each of which has a design intent. For example, the loading of a solution bag into a large-volume IV pump could be one step of the process for delivery of intravenous solutions to the patient. When this method is used, deviations from the design intent are explored by applying a series of guide words, such as flow: more, less; temperature: less, more; and pressure: none, high, to applicable design parameters. If the deviation defined by the combination of a design parameter and guide word (for example, more flow or less flow) can result in a hazard, then potential causes and any existing controls are identified. The risk level can be evaluated using a risk matrix in which consequence and frequency ranges have been established according to the company's internal risk-acceptability criteria (see Figure 10-2). Deviations that have category A or B risks should be reduced to level C or D risks, for example.

When a device contains many mechanical components, an FMEA should be considered. However, an FMEA is time-consuming and is generally applied only to Class III devices, the safety-critical parts of any device, and devices that contain many electrical components. The FMEA is another bottom-up approach that focuses on a particular component of a medical device and explores the possible failure modes. For each failure mode that results in an undesirable consequence, the potential causes and existing controls are evaluated, and the level of risk can be determined by using a risk matrix.

An FTA is a top-down approach in which the design team starts with the undesired consequence or top event and identifies the initiating and contributing events that must occur to produce it. The identified events are combined, using logic gates, at the point where two or more independent events join to produce a higher-level event. The logic gate determines whether the subevent probabilities or frequencies should be multiplied or added. If all events under a gate

---

Figure 10-2   Typical matrix of risk acceptability

FREQUENCY		CONSEQUENCE			
		1 (low)	2	3	4 (high)
high	4	C	B	A	A
	3	C	B	B	A
	2	D	C	B	B
low	1	D	D	C	C

are necessary for the higher event to occur, an *and* gate is used. If each of the events is sufficient to produce the higher event on its own, an *or* gate is used. Both physical failures and human errors can readily be included in a fault tree. An example of an FTA is presented later in this chapter. If failure rates for each event on a fault tree are available or can be estimated from generic data, then the top-event frequency could be calculated and compared to a company's internal risk-acceptability criteria. Although the fault tree is a powerful risk-analysis tool, its greatest limitation is the availability of relevant failure data; consequently, it is generally best used to compare risks of various alternatives. The greatest benefit of a fault tree is that the events that contribute most frequently to the top event can readily be identified, and mitigating measures can be focused on reducing the frequency of these events.

The risk analysis should include any risks associated with the manufacture and delivery of the device to its intended location. For devices that involve solutions or components that can be degraded by environmental factors such as heat, humidity, cold, or light, storage and transportation methods must be reviewed. Identified problems could lead to changes in packaging or warnings on storage or packaging containers. It is important that any changes made during the design process be reviewed to ensure that new or additional safety hazards are not being introduced into the design. Small changes are generally reviewed using a what-if approach, whereas larger changes may require a HAZOP or FMEA.

Hazard Analysis

A hazard analysis is a disciplined analytical approach used to identify the hazardous elements within a device and to help assess their safety implications. The hazard analysis is a global or system-level look at the device as a whole from the viewpoint of safety to the patient and user; more detailed analyses can be performed subsequently on specific components, functions, or subsystems. The findings and recommendations from the hazard analysis are usually transmitted to the design team, if the design team did not actually perform the analysis, and appropriate changes are made in the device design to reduce the identified accidents and minimize their consequences. Table 10-1 presents a partial list of the standards that govern hazard analysis.

The hazard analysis procedure consists of three basic steps: collection of data, identification of the hazardous source(s), and preparation of a hazards and effects table. The team performing the hazard analysis should examine all available information that relates to the hardware, software, materials, processes, test, and operation of the device. Any of these items that could, under certain conditions, cause loss of life, personal injury, or property damage is considered a hazardous source or element. Under normal circumstances these hazardous elements are harmless, but certain abnormal conditions can trigger them, causing an accident.

For example, consider a hypothetical medical device that monitors eye dilation in conjunction with a therapeutic bath that follows eye surgery. The system consists of a sensor unit that observes the dilation of the eye and a monitoring and control unit that displays the percentage of eye dilation. The sensor also measures the background illumination that the monitor uses in its algorithm to determine the percentage of eye dilation; the threshold values used by this device are set by a clinician. The device also accepts a tubing set and automatically clamps the tubing closed at below threshold dilation values. If the pupil size drops below its preset threshold value, an audible alarm is triggered and the system automatically shuts off delivery of the therapeutic drug. Under normal operation, the sensor unit, the monitoring unit (consisting of the threshold values and the alarm mechanism), and the control unit (consisting of the clamping mechanism and the device shutoff) do not pose a threat to the patient. However, an incorrect threshold value,

Table 10-1   A Partial List of Hazard Analysis Standards

Standard Number	Standard Title
ANSI/ASQC-1.15-1979	Generic Guidelines for Quality Systems
ANSI/IEEE STD 730-1984	IEEE Standards for Software Quality Assurance
ANSI/IEEE STD 830-1981	Guide to Software Requirements Specifications
ASQC C1-1968	Specification of General Requirements for a Quality Program
MIL-STD-109B	Quality Assurance Terms and Definitions
MIL-STD-217B	Reliability Prediction of Electronic Equipment
MIL-STD-472	Maintainability Predictions
MIL-STD-483	Configuration Management
MIL-STD-781C	Reliability Design Qualification and Production Acceptance Tests: Exponential Distribution
MIL-STD-785B	Reliability Program for Systems and Equipment Development and Production
MIL-STD-1521A	Technical Reviews and Audits for Systems, Equipment, and Computer Programs
MIL-STD-1629A	Procedures for Performing Failure Modes, Effects and Criticality Analysis
NASA SP-6502	Elements of Design Review for Space Systems
NASA SP-6504	Failure Reporting and Management Techniques in the Surveyor Program
NHB 5300.4(A)	Reliability Program Provisions for Aeronautical and Space Systems Contractors
N68-10120	Parts and Materials Application Review for Space Systems
N68-20357	An Introduction to the Assurance of Human Performance in Space Systems

a sensor malfunction, an alarm malfunction, or a clamping mechanism error are triggering events that could lead to an accident.

For the hazard analysis, all hazardous sources associated with the device should be listed and identified. These sources should include hardware, software, materials, processes, operation, labeling, and any directions for device use. Hazard identification should extend beyond the operation of the system and should include the installation, testing, maintenance, and retirement of the device from the market. Secondary device events should also be considered as a hazard source because they could lead to a secondary accident. These types of events occur when a seemingly harmless triggering event interacts with a hazardous source. In the example given above, a triggering event could be that the commands from the monitoring and control unit to the infusion pump become garbled on the communications bus, because of EMC problems, thus causing the infusion pump to begin over-washing the eye, possibly depleting the supply of natural tears from the tear ducts.

If the preliminary hazard analysis has determined that there are no hazardous sources associated with the device, the hazard analysis may be terminated at this point. However, if hazardous sources are found, they should be documented in a hazards and effects table (see Figure 10-3). The format of the table can vary, and some table items may be omitted or left blank depending on the scope of the hazard analysis. The first item(s) listed in the table should be the hazardous source(s) that were identified as the second step of the analysis. The next item to list in the table is the location and identification of the hazardous source. The identifying name or number could be a part number or component name referred to in other documents or drawings. The location of the hazard could be identified by part number, component number, subassembly number, or even grid numbers. If the device is a relatively simple one that involves only a few components, the location information could be omitted if the identifying name or number is a unique descriptor.

Figure 10-3   Typical example of a hazards and effects table

HAZARDS AND EFFECTS TABLE		
Device or system description: Hazards and effects investigator(s):		Date:
Item Description	**Hazards and Effects**	
	(1)	**(2)**
1. Hazardous source		
2. Location and identification of hazardous source		
3. Trigger mechanism		
4. Accident		
5. Effect of the accident		
6. Warnings		
7. Accident prevention safeguards		
8. Effects mitigation safeguards		
9. Accident frequency		
10. Criticality of the accident		
11. Remarks		

The next item to document in the table is the trigger mechanism. This mechanism can be identified by name or number; in some instances, environmental conditions or operating procedures might be entered to augment the description of the trigger mechanism. In addition, cautionary notes might add useful information to the table. The next item to be entered into the table should be the accident that occurs when the hazard element interacts with the trigger mechanism. In addition to the accident that results, the effect of the accident as perceived by the user or patient should be documented (for example, death, sickness, injury, and/or property damage). Some accidents are not of a sudden or catastrophic nature, and the effects may be mitigated if there is an early-warning system or capability. If such a warning system is present or used, it should also be noted as a warning in the table, although it is commonly omitted in some hazards and effects tables.

Accident prevention measures may not completely eliminate an accident, but they could significantly reduce accident probability. Safeguards are typically thought of as a piece of hardware, but they could just as easily be a procedure. If an accident prevention safeguard is built into the device or system, it should be noted under this item in the table, although accident prevention types of safeguards are commonly omitted in some hazards and effects tables. The adverse effects of the accident could be mitigated by the installation of appropriate hardware or software as well as through appropriate operating procedures. If a mitigation of effects safeguard is built into the device or system, it should be noted in the table under this item, although these types of safeguards are commonly omitted in some hazards and effects tables.

Expected accident frequency or probability is most likely not known when the preliminary hazards analysis is performed. However, if rough estimates can be made, then the estimate is entered into the table. Warning systems and preventive safeguards could reduce the accident probability and should be entered individually into the table and be considered as a part of the overall estimate for the system or device. Frequently, instead of a numerical estimate of the accident probability being entered into the table, a frequency classification is used for the preliminary hazard analysis. For example, a sample accident frequency classification could be defined as "extremely remote" for accident probabilities that are less than 10^{-6} per hour; "remote" for accident probabilities between 10^{-5} and 10^{-6} per hour; "possible" for accident probabilities between 10^{-4} and 10^{-5} per hour; and "probable" for accident probabilities greater than 10^{-4} per hour. This is not the only possible classification scheme for accident frequency; a classification should be used that directly reflects the specific device and its operating environment. This table item might also be left blank if an estimate of the accident frequency is not available nor easily derived, and other hazards and effects tables may omit this item altogether.

The next table item presents the effect of the accident ranked as a function of its criticality. Warning systems and mitigation safeguards could reduce the criticality of an accident and should be entered into the table and be considered as a part of the overall criticality assessment. Commonly, a ranking classification rather than a complete description of the criticality is used for the preliminary hazard analysis. For example, a sample criticality ranking could be defined as "insignificant" for accidents that cause very limited damage; "minor" for accidents that can cause damage to the device or system and require repair, but death, sickness, or injury are not possible; "critical" for accidents that may cause death, sickness, or injury, but a response time to the accident is available; and "catastrophic" for accidents that will cause death, sickness, or injury immediately. This is not the only possible criticality ranking scheme; a ranking should be used that directly reflects the specific device and its operating environment. This table item may be left blank if insufficient information is available to estimate the ranking; other hazards and effects tables may omit this item altogether.

Last, any general remarks should be entered into the table, and any comments that are relevant to the safety of the device. Recommendations for warning systems, safeguards, and alterations in the hardware, software, or operating procedures may also be entered. This item may be left blank if there is nothing to remark or comment about or to recommend.

The preliminary hazard analysis examines the device from the perspective of safety. All hazardous sources are identified, and all hardware, software, materials, and operations that can interact with the hazardous source and trigger an accident are identified and documented. The results of this analysis and the table can be used to improve the device safety. The preliminary hazard analysis can also identify those areas that require further study through the use of more rigorous reliability analysis techniques. The findings of the preliminary hazard analysis are also useful in developing training procedures, test and maintenance schedules, and emergency plans.

The preliminary hazard analysis results can also be used to decide an optimal allocation of engineering resources to achieve maximum safety by making it possible to decide which potential accidents require priority consideration. For example, an accident with both a high criticality ranking and a high frequency classification is more serious and should therefore receive more attention. If appropriate, the accident priority decision can be made after quantitative information about the accident frequency and criticality is obtained through detailed reliability and risk assessment.

The preliminary hazard analysis is best suited to identification of accidents that involve only one or two hazard sources and one or two triggering mechanisms. More complex situations involving two or more hazard sources and several triggering mechanisms are difficult to analyze through a preliminary hazard analysis. Deductive and more detailed techniques, such as fault-tree analysis and FMEA, are better suited for these situations. Another limitation of the preliminary hazard analysis is that its findings are primarily qualitative, even though some rough estimates of the frequency of accidents may be included. Fault-tree analysis can be used to compute accident frequencies in a more rigorous and disciplined manner. In spite of these limitations, the preliminary hazard analysis is a valuable aid in identifying potential safety problems during the early design stages, when sufficient information may not be available for a more rigorous analysis. The results of the preliminary hazard analysis enable the device designers to avoid many potential safety problems at an early stage of the device design process.

Hazard Analysis Models and Techniques

Many different types of hazard analysis are in use. Some differ primarily in their names, whereas others truly have unique characteristics. One of the greatest problems in performing hazard analysis is selecting appropriate models and techniques that match the product and project goals, tasks, and skills. Because the methods have different coverage and validity, several may be required during the life of the project. No one method is superior to all others for every objective or even applicable to all types of systems. Very little validation of any of these techniques has been performed, so all results should be scrutinized carefully. This does not mean, however, that the techniques are not useful, only that they must be used carefully and combined with engineering judgment and expertise.

The resources and time for any analysis are limited. Not all resources should be put into one single method or into one single phase of the analysis process. In planning the analysis and selecting appropriate procedures, consideration should be given to its purpose, who will use the results and what kind of information is expected, the seriousness of the potential hazards, the complexity of the system or product, the nature of the project and the uniqueness of its design and technology, the degree of automation, the types of hazards to be considered, and the role of humans and processors in the system.

Failure Modes and Effects Analysis

The FMEA is a qualitative procedure that identifies potential component failures in a medical device and assesses their effects on the device. During this procedure, the device is scrutinized to determine which components can fail, what the effects of that failure are, how critical the consequence of that failure is, whether the failure can be detected, and what possible safeguards exist. All significant failure modes of the different components are identified, their detection and safeguards are documented, and the effects of their failure on the device are determined.

The FMEA is used to ensure that all conceivable device failure modes and their effects are understood. It can also assist in identifying design flaws and providing a basis for selecting design alternatives during the design stage of device development. The FMEA can provide a basis for recommending design improvements, for assessing priorities of corrective action, and for recommending test programs. It can also be used to assist in the troubleshooting of an existing system or device that is encountering operational problems. A well-organized FMEA can benefit the design team by examining the entire device from the standpoint of failures, which will help to highlight potential design flaws. This analysis can help facilitate communication about the effects of potential failures that must be passed among the various component design teams, as well as the system or device design team.

The preliminary hazard analysis is not a prerequisite for the FMEA. The FMEA may be conducted at any point in the development of the medical device design. In fact, it is often an advantage to conduct progressively more detailed FMEAs at different stages of the design process. For example, an initial FMEA can be conducted at the conceptual design stage. The findings may then be used in improving the conceptual design, as well as providing insight for the preliminary design stage. One or more FMEA activities may then be conducted during the preliminary design phase, which could improve the current design phase effort and impart new understanding for the detailed design phase.

Some reliability analysis projects may end with the completion of the FMEA, whereas other projects may proceed to conduct more rigorous analyses, such as the fault-tree analysis. The decision of whether to progress with more or even more detailed FMEAs depends on the purpose and scope of the device. In existing devices with operating problems, the FMEA can also be used for identifying failure causes. If an FMEA was previously conducted during the design phase of the device, the information from that analysis can be used to troubleshoot the current operational problem(s). If necessary, the analysis sheets from the previous analysis may be updated by using any new information.

The FMEA consists of four basic steps:

1. Establish the scope of the analysis.
2. Collect data for the analysis.
3. Prepare a components list for the device.
4. Prepare the failure modes and effects sheets.

The scope of the FMEA should clearly identify the system or device boundaries such that no device component is left out of consideration. This is relatively simple for small medical devices, but careful consideration and scrutiny may be required for larger devices or systems. The scope should also delineate the extent of the analysis. For example, all FMEAs include information relative to the underlying causes and possible effects of the failure. Additional information that might be useful to capture concerns failure detection, safeguards, frequency of the failure, and the criticality of the effects of the failure. The extent of the information to be included should be specified in the scope of the FMEA. The extent of the FMEA may depend on when it is to be performed. For example, if two analyses are performed for the same device, one at the conceptual design stage and one at the detailed design phase, the extent of the latter analysis may in fact be broader than that of the former analysis. The extent of the scope of the FMEA should be decided on a case-by-case basis.

The team that performs the FMEA should have access to all pertinent documents that relate to the device's configurations, design, specifications, schematics, drawings, and operating procedures. Not all of these documents may be available at the time of the analysis, but the team should use whatever documentation is available. It is also recommended that the analysis team interview the design, operations, testing, and maintenance personnel. If necessary and prudent, the interviews should be extended to include component vendors and any outside experts. The intent of the FMEA team is to gather as much information as is possible and necessary; any interviews that may be conducted in support of this can be in person, by telephone, or even by questionnaires. In some instances the analysis team may also be the design team members.

A list of all components in the device is prepared before examining the potential failure modes of each of the components. The components list may include device functions; operating conditions, such as temperature, pressure, and loads; and the environmental conditions for each component. All of this information will usually prove to be very useful in preparation of the analysis sheets of failure modes and effects.

The FMEA findings are recorded in a tabular format on the analysis sheet shown in Figure 10-4. The format of the analysis sheet can take many different forms. Some of the items listed on the sheet may be omitted if the scope or the information available at the time of the analysis precludes them. The first item entered on the analysis sheet is the component description, which should be a unique and well-defined identifying name or code for the specific component. It is best if this name corresponds to the names or codes used in the device's drawings, schematics, specifications, or other salient documents. It may also be necessary to refer to any subsystem or component names in order to completely and uniquely convey the component description.

A brief statement of the intended function of the component should be entered for each mode of operation that the component is intended to perform in, although some FMEAs may omit this item. The next item to be entered is the failure mode. The possible ways in which the component can fail to function as intended are listed. Also contributing to these device failures are the failures attributable to degradation with age; all operating modes of interest, operation, or shutdown under all environmental conditions as applicable; and failure to shut down properly when necessary. Other considerations should include premature operation, failure to operate at prescribed times, failures during operation, excessive deformation of components, and structural failures. All possible causes of the failure are entered on the sheet, followed by specifying all of the possible effects of the failure.

The next item to be entered is failure detection, which relates how the failure will first become apparent to operating personnel or users. Some FMEAs may omit this item. Failures may initially be detected by auditory alarms, meter reading, or cessation of operation. Some failures may not be detected until maintenance or even testing of the device. Any provisions built into the device that will help to reduce the failure probability or mitigate the effects of the failure are listed next, although some analysis sheets may omit this item. If the failure probability or

Figure 10-4   Typical example of an analysis sheet of failure modes and effects

FAILURE MODES AND EFFECTS ANALYSIS SHEET

Device or system description: Date:

FMEA investigator(s):

Item Description	Failure Modes and Effects		
	(1)	(2)	(3)
1. Component			
2. Function			
3. Failure mode			
4. Causes of failure			
5. Effects of the failure			
6. Failure detection			
7. Safety features			
8. Failure frequency			
9. Criticality of the effects			
10. Remarks			

failure frequency is known, it is the next item entered on the analysis sheet. Instead of the numerical estimate of the failure probability, a frequency classification may be used that is similar to the scheme discussed above for the preliminary hazard analysis. This item may be omitted in some FMEAs, or left blank if sufficient information is not available to estimate the failure frequency at the time the analysis is conducted.

Criticality of the effects is the next item entered on the analysis sheet. The effect of the failure is ranked according to its criticality; commonly, a ranking classification is used for the FMEA rather than a complete description of the criticality. For example, a sample criticality ranking could be defined as "insignificant" for failure effects that are not a safety hazard and have very little effect on the device's reliability and availability; "minor" for failure effects that are not a safety hazard but will affect the device's reliability and availability; "major" for failure effects that are not a safety hazard but will affect the device's reliability and availability significantly; and "critical" for failure effects that are potential safety hazards. This is not the only possible criticality ranking scheme that can be used; a ranking should be used that directly reflects the specific device and its operating environment. Whatever scheme is used, however, should be used consistently throughout the FMEA. This table item may be left blank if insufficient information is available to estimate the ranking. Other analysis sheets may omit this item altogether.

Last, general remarks should be included on the analysis sheet. Any comments that are relevant to the failure modes and effects of the device may be entered. Recommendations for warning systems, safeguards, and alterations in the hardware, software, or operating procedures may also be entered as a part of this item. This item may be left blank if there is nothing to comment about or to recommend.

The FMEA concentrates on identifying possible component failures and their effects on the device. In addition, design deficiencies are frequently identified that lead to improvements to correct the deficiency. If potential failures of the device are identified, effective test programs and procedures can be derived or recommended. Failure modes may be prioritized according to their frequency and criticality, so that more engineering time can be spent fixing the higher-priority failure modes; this is similar to the preliminary hazard analysis strategy discussed previously.

A limitation of the FMEA is that each failure mode is considered individually. If a failure mode, all by itself, affects the device performance, this is identified by the FMEA. In more complex medical devices, a single failure may not adversely affect the device, but two or more failures in combination may. The FMEA is not particularly well suited for assessing the combined effects of two or more failures. Deductive methods, such as fault-tree analysis, are better suited for this type of analysis.

Analysis of Software Failure Modes and Effects

The FMEA forms shown previously are sometimes not convenient for documenting the software FMEA (SFMEA). The FMEA produces, in general, two items: an analysis that shows each failure mode—its cause, corresponding effects, and a statement of the severity of the potential risk; and a report that identifies the high-risk failures and the design activities that will be implemented to minimize them. As an alternative for capturing the SFMEA, the data may be set up in a tabular format (see Figure 10-5) or as a series of records in a database that can be utilized in summary reports in a tabular format. The latter approach is attractive because it supports overall analysis with the options of sorting and searching by element and risk.

The elements necessary to begin the SFMEA are the device FMEA results, the system architecture, the design documentation, fault trees if available, and any relevant failure probability

Figure 10-5   **Typical example of a table of software failure modes and effects analysis**

Software Function	Failure Mode	Cause	Effect on System	Possible Hazard(s)	Risk Index	Applicable Control

lists. Each failure mode is entered into a row of the SFMEA, starting with the software function column. The software function can be a generic operation such as set alarm, clear alarm, battery level, or reset clock, or the name of a specific module, routine, or function. The failure mode and cause are entered in the next two columns. The failure mode indicates the way in which the system device component or element fails; the cause is the combination of the defect and the triggering event that can produce the failure. For example, the failure mode could be stated as CPU failure, speaker failure, or LCD failure; the failure cause could be electrical breakdown, analog conversion error, or corrupted program. The system effect column indicates the consequences of the failure on other system elements and could be, for example, loss of control, alarm change, or rate value incorrect. The possible hazards column indicates the potential hazard that the failure might cause, and the risk index could be an arbitrary value or a frequency classification as described for the hazard analysis and FMEA. The applicable control column represents the implemented mitigation method. This may be with electronics or mechanisms, but if other software safeguards are to be used, then the names of variables, routines, or code location should be entered. For example, if a single function is to be used to detect variable corruption, then the name of the routine would be entered. On the other hand, if the error checking is embedded within assembly language code, then the statement labels immediately preceding and following the code logic would be entered.

Although not shown, additional data might be entered into the SFMEA. These entries might include the effects of the failure at various levels within the software as well as up to and including the impact on the safe operation of the device. For example, failure of the watchdog timer and its code detection logic might be traced from lowest level logic up through each operational module and finally into the system itself. Another piece of information might be a statement of how the device will detect a specific failure and notify the user. For example, corrupted flow rates might be indicated by an audible warning or an LCD row being out might be indicated with a visual alarm, such as an entirely highlighted LCD display.

Fault-Tree Analysis

Fault-tree analysis is probably the most widely used method for analysis of system or device reliability and safety. It is a formal deductive procedure for determining the various combinations of component-level failures that could result in the occurrence of specified undesirable events at the system or device level. This analysis encompasses not only hardware component failures, but also human errors and software errors. Within the context of fault-tree analysis, the term *failure* refers to both failures and faults. Fault trees can also be used to compute the probability of the undesired event as a function of the probabilities of the various component failures; each undesired event will have its own fault tree.

Fault trees can be generated at any point during the device design. If a fault tree is constructed early in the design process, it may be updated as more precise information becomes available or as design changes are implemented. Fault trees may also be used for operational devices, to identify the root causes of system-level failures that are encountered during device operation. A fault-tree analysis may follow a preliminary hazard analysis or an FMEA, but neither activity is a prerequisite.

A fault-tree analysis consists of the following three steps:

1. The fault tree is constructed.
2. The fault tree is analyzed qualitatively.
3. A quantitative fault-tree analysis is performed.

Depending on the scope of the reliability and safety effort and the nature of the device, the fault-tree analysis will actually consist of steps 1 and 2, or 1 and 3, or 1, 2, and 3 because of the nature of the analysis.

If two engineers develop a fault tree for the same device, it is possible that the two fault trees may not be identical. In fact, depending on the complexity of the device, the two fault trees may seem vastly different at the very outset of fault-tree construction. This difference in construction reflects the difference in how the engineers logically modeled the device for analysis. The two fault trees must provide the same results, however, when the end of the analysis is reached.

A fault tree is a diagrammatic representation of the relationships between component-level failures and an undesired event associated with the device. The fault-tree diagram depicts how component-level failures propagate through the device to cause a system-level failure or an undesired event. Component-level failures are called the terminal events, primary events, or end events of the fault tree. The undesired event at the system or device level is called the top event of the fault tree.

The best vehicle for understanding a fault tree is to examine one that has been generated for a simple device. In the example shown in Figure 10-6, a fault tree of a mythical medical device, the undesired event is termed *patient hazard*. This example presents only a few of the many events that could affect the patient with a real-world device. The undesired event (the patient hazard) is placed at the top of the tree.

Figure 10-6   An example of a fault tree for a mythical device

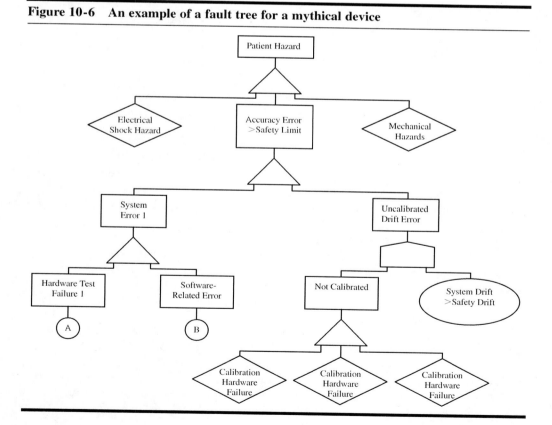

The next step is to consider all of the possible ways, means, and conditions that could possibly pose a hazard to the patient with the device being considered. Probably the most effective way to phrase this consideration is, "What is necessary and sufficient to cause a patient hazard?" As presented here with the mythical device, there exists the possibility of electrical shock, mechanical hazards, and an accuracy error that exceeds the predefined safety limit. These three events are then placed below the top or undesired event. Because the top event can be precipitated by any one of these three events, an OR gate is used to convey this condition symbolically. At this juncture, the analysis could continue with any of the three events just identified.

However, the electrical shock hazard and the mechanical hazards were deemed terminal events by the engineering analysts, on the basis of their best engineering judgment. Terminal events, those that will not be resolved any further into their respective causes, are represented by circles, ellipses, or diamonds. Whether an event should be further resolved into its causes is a decision made by the engineering analysts. The decision depends on the availability of quantitative data related to the event and the level of resolution that the analyst wants to incorporate into the fault tree. In this case, these two events are placed within the diamond terminal symbol, which represents causes that are terminal because they are undeveloped events. Undeveloped terminal events are those that, with further resolution, will not improve the understanding of the problem, or they are events that are outside the scope of the analysis, or they are placeholders in the early analysis versions that will be resolved at a later date.

We continue arbitrarily with the *accuracy error* intermediate event. This event is placed in a rectangle and the question is asked, "What is necessary and sufficient to cause the accuracy error to exceed the safety limit?" In the example given, the accuracy error can be caused by a *System Error 1* OR an *uncalibrated drift error.* Continuing down the uncalibrated drift error branch, the question is, "What is necessary and sufficient to cause the uncalibrated drift error?" There are two causes shown for this error, a *not calibrated* event and a *system drift that exceeds the safety limit* event. In this case, both conditions must occur for the uncalibrated drift error to happen, so an AND gate is depicted leading from these two causes to the uncalibrated drift error rectangle. Best engineering judgment was used to determine that the *system drift exceeding the safety limit* event is an intermediate event that will not be resolved further, so it is placed into the circle or ellipse terminal event symbol. The circle terminal event symbol represents a basic event, one that is either a component-level (and thus not resolved any further) or an external event. Examples of component-level events are component failures, system failures, or human errors. Component failures and system failures represent a condition in which the component or system either does not perform its intended function correctly or performs an unintended function. External events are those that are exogenous to the device under analysis, such as earthquakes, tornadoes, and fires.

The *not calibrated* intermediate event is examined next. The question is, "What is necessary and sufficient for the drift error to be uncalibrated?" As shown, three causes can contribute to this event, the *Software Calibration Error 1* event, a *hardware calibration failure* event, and a *procedural error* event. For each of these causes it was decided by best engineering judgment not to pursue them any further; consequently, they were placed within a diamond terminal symbol as defined above.

Returning to the *System Error 1* event branch, it was determined that *Hardware Test Failure 1* OR a *software-related error* were necessary and sufficient to cause the system error event. Consequently, they were placed in rectangles following an OR gate. The circle symbol represents a transfer-out connector to another diagram. The analysis of the hardware failure branch is continued in Figure 10-7. Here, the circle depicts a transfer-in symbol and represents the point at which the analysis is to begin in this diagram. It is connected to a rectangle symbol that repeats

Figure 10-7   An example of a fault tree for a mythical medical device—branch A

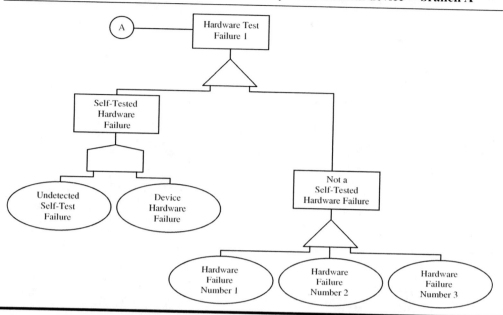

the intermediate event that the corresponding transfer-out symbol was connected to, in this case the Hardware Test Failure 1 event. Either a *self-tested hardware failure* OR a *hardware failure that is not self-tested* can cause the hardware failure.

The necessary and sufficient causes that can produce the self-tested hardware failure are an *undetected self-test failure* AND a *device hardware failure*. In our best engineering judgment, these two are basic terminal events, and so they were placed in the ellipse symbol. The hardware failure event that is not self-tested can be caused by three necessary and sufficient events, appropriately called *Hardware Failure Number 1, Hardware Failure Number 2,* and *Hardware Failure Number 3*. In this device, these failures are well known and defined in the design schematics or drawings as developed by the hardware engineers, and they are all deemed to be basic terminal events. They may represent, for example, voltage drops, pin shorts, or a lead screw bottoming out at a specific location.

The analysis of the *software-related error* branch is continued in Figure 10-8. The software-related error can be caused by one of four events, a *design specification error* event, the *Program Execution Error 1* event, a *coding error* event, and the *corruption of a critical variable* event. The design specification error is a basic terminating event, by engineering judgment, and no further resolution is to be undertaken for this event. The *Program Execution Error 1* can be caused by a *transient noise* AND if the *execution error is not software detected*. Both of these events are deemed to be basic terminating events and are placed in the ellipse symbol. The coding error can be caused by an *algorithm error* AND *incomplete verification* of the coded software. These were decided by engineering judgment to be basic terminating events.

As shown in Figure 10-9, the necessary and sufficient conditions for a critical variable corruption can be a *stuck RAM bit*, a *Software Error 1*, OR a *transient noise*. The RAM stuck bit and the transient noise were deemed to be basic terminal events by engineering judgment. The

Figure 10-8   An example of a fault tree for a mythical medical device—branch B

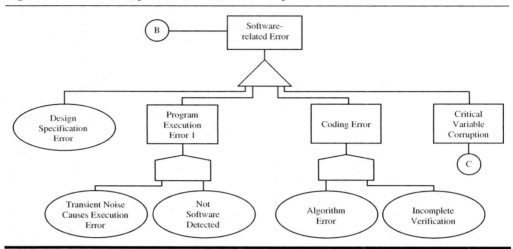

software error event can be caused by a *data path error* OR a *critical module error.* The data path error is determined to be an undetermined terminal event that will contribute little to the understanding of the current analysis.

The *critical module error* event has been analyzed further. The necessary and sufficient conditions causing the critical module error are *insufficient verification* of the developed software AND an *algorithm error.* The insufficient verification is deemed to be a basic terminating event. The algorithm error event, however, can be caused by a *source information error* AND an *implementation error.* Both the source information error and the implementation error were considered the terminating events by best engineering judgment.

This example illustrates the basic concepts and procedures associated with the construction of a fault tree and introduces some of the symbols used in the fault tree. It also serves as the vehicle to define some of the terms used in fault-tree analysis, such as top event, intermediate event, basic and undeveloped terminal events; and the symbols, such as OR gate, AND gate, transfer, and rectangle. Other symbols and terms can be used, but these represent the minimal set that will adequately convey the device design for a hazard analysis and fault-tree construction.

As discussed previously, a terminal event is one that is not further resolved into its causes. The decision not to resolve an event into its causes depends on the availability of quantitative data for the event and the level of resolution to be included in the fault tree. However, if the probability of the undesired event is to be computed, then the probabilities of the terminal events are necessary. Just because the probability of an event is known, however, it need not be treated as a terminal event. It can be dealt with as an intermediate event and then further resolved.

The level of resolution needed, desired, or required to adequately complete the fault tree and any analysis depends on several factors. Usually, the terminal event is a component-level event, an event caused by another system, or an external event. Component-level terminal events include component failures, human errors, and software errors. Examples of terminal events that are caused by other systems are a high operating temperature due to an air-conditioning failure or a power failure due to a power outage. External terminal events might be events such as earthquakes, floods, tornadoes, and fires.

Figure 10-9   An example of a fault tree for a mythical medical device—branch C

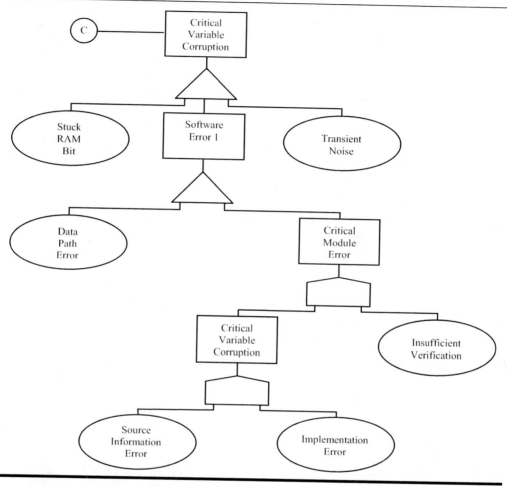

The probabilities of the terminal events should be available if the computation of the probability of occurrence of the undesired event is the objective of the analysis. This would extend, of course, to the probability of occurrence for any of the intermediate events in the fault tree. If the quantification of the fault tree cannot be readily determined at any given level, it would be prudent to continue the fault tree down to those levels at which the information is available or where it can be determined easily. If the probability of a component-level event is not known, it may also be treated as an intermediate event that would then be further resolved into failures at the constituent parts level for which failure probabilities are known. A component may have more than one failure mode, and each failure mode may constitute an event. Some of these failure modes may be treated as terminal events, whereas others may be treated as intermediate events.

In some situations, subsystem-level events are treated as terminal events if further resolution of the event will not improve the understanding of the problem. This is acceptable if the probability of the subsystem-level event is available, the components of the subsystem-level event do not enter the fault tree as terminal or intermediate events elsewhere in the fault tree, and there is no statistical dependence between components of the subsystem and other events in the tree. This discussion does not discuss fault-tree analysis exhaustively, provide detailed guidelines on how to progress, nor provide definitive information related to fault tree analysis methodology. The intent here is to present enough of the methodology and process to adequately cover fault-tree analysis for the vast majority of medical device software projects. More complicated devices will require a more thorough analysis than that presented here.

Although a manual fault-tree construction was assumed for the sake of this presentation, fault-tree construction algorithms suitable for implementation as software tools are available. Several commercial tools execute on a wide variety of platforms. However, do not expect any of these tools to accept a brief description of the system and then produce the required fault tree. The user of these automated tools must still specify as inputs the effects of each failure mode for each component and subsystem, as well as the functions of the system, subsystems, and components. This means that the user must have a good understanding of the device logic and functional operation, whether a manual or automated version of fault-tree analysis is used. In addition, data preparation and collection can be as time consuming in the automated environment as in the manual one. If the decision is made to automate the fault-tree construction process, a method or program should be selected that has the capability to support all of the features of the fault trees that must be constructed.

Fault-Tree Analysis Probabilities

Quantitative probabilities for any undesired event may be determined from the fault-tree analysis. Which quantities are computed from the analysis depends on the purpose for which the fault tree is to be used. For example, if the top event of the fault tree represents an accident, then the probability that no accident occurred anytime between time zero and time t would represent the reliability of the top event at time t. If the top event were *device failure,* then the probability that the device is in an operational state at time t could be determined. In addition, device parameters, such as failure rate, mean time to failure, mean time to repair, and expected number of failures, may also be determined. Reliability, availability, and other such related parameters may also be calculated for the intermediate events of the fault tree. In this case, instead of the complete tree, only that part of the tree below the intermediate event of interest would be used in determining the intermediate event probability. Although constant failure rates and constant repair rates are assumed for the components in most fault-tree analyses, other types of failure rates and repair rates may be considered. Even if all of the components of the device have constant failure rates, it does not necessarily mean that the device as a whole will also have a constant failure rate.

The estimation of the probability of a hazard using the fault tree begins with knowing or being able to determine the probability of the occurrence of the basic fault conditions. Then, for any intermediate or top event, the appropriate hazard probability may be estimated using basic statistics and probability mathematics. The probability that both event a and event b will occur is the product of the probability that a will occur times the probability that b will occur. The probability that a or b will occur is 1 minus the probability that a will not occur times the probability that b will not occur. Mathematically, these probability formulas are given by the following.

$$p(\text{AND}) \; = \; p(a) \times p(b), \tag{10.1}$$

$$p(\text{OR}) \; = \; 1 - \{[1 - p(a)] \times [1 - p(b)]\}. \tag{10.2}$$

Equations 10.1 and 10.2 are used in the following example. Figure 10-10 gives an example of a fault tree associated with another mythical medical device, and assumes that the terminal events illustrated have the probabilities shown. The probability that a "device failure" will occur is the probability that *Subsystem 1 fails* times the probability that *Circuit 1 fails.* Mathematically,

$$p(\text{device failure}) = p(\text{Subsystem 1 fails}) \times p(\text{Circuit 1 fails})$$
$$= (0.6) \times (0.2) = 0.12.$$

The probability that the *pressure limit will exceed the device threshold* is given by the following:

$$p(\text{pressure} > \text{limit}) = 1 - \{[1 - p(\text{Sensor 1 drifts})] \times [1 - p(\text{reference drifts})]\}$$
$$= 1 - [(1 - 0.75) \times (1 - 0.25)]$$
$$= 1 - (0.25 \times 0.75)$$
$$= 1 - 0.19$$
$$= 0.81.$$

Figure 10-10   Example of a fault-tree probability calculation

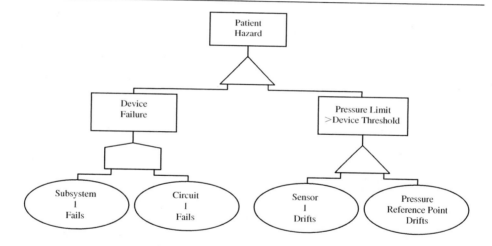

Fault Description	Probability of Failure
Subsystem 1 Fails	0.6
Circuit 1 Fails	0.2
Sensor 1 Drifts	0.75
Pressure Reference Point Drifts	0.25
Device Failure	0.12
Pressure Limit > Device Threshold	0.81
Patient Hazard	0.85

Notes: $p(\text{AND}) = p(a) \times p(b),$
$p(\text{OR}) = 1 - \{[1 - p(a)] \times [1 - p(b)]\}.$

The probability of a *patient hazard* for this mythical device is determined from the probabilities of the causing events. Namely,

$$
\begin{aligned}
p(\text{patient hazard}) &= 1 - \{[1 - p(\text{device failure})] \times [1 - p(\text{accuracy} > \text{limit})]\} \\
&= 1 - [(1 - 0.12) \times (1 - 0.81)] \\
&= 1 - (0.88 \times 0.19) \\
&= 1 - 0.15 \\
&= 0.85.
\end{aligned}
$$

Another useful calculation using the fault-tree analysis is the criticality of the device. This technique establishes the relative weighting of the issues identified as a result of the fault tree analysis. To calculate the criticality, assume that a particular failure occurs and compute the top event probability. Next, multiply that result by the actual probability of the assumed failure. The criticality is then established by the numerical ranking of the relative weights. Figure 10-11 presents a criticality example that is based on the fault-tree analysis and probabilities that were used in the previous example.

Figure 10-11   Example of a fault-tree criticality calculation

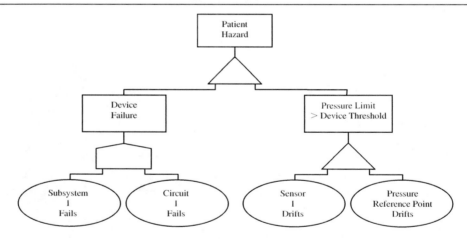

	Probability of Failure					
Fault Description	**Actual**	**Assumed**	**Device Failure**	**Pressure Limit**	**Patient Hazard**	**Criticality**
Subsystem 1 Fails	0.6	1.0	0.2	0.81	0.848	0.509
Circuit 1 Fails	0.2	1.0	0.6	0.81	0.924	0.185
Sensor 1 Drifts	0.75	1.0	0.12	1.0	1.0	0.75
Pressure Reference Point Drifts	0.75	1.0	0.12	1.0	1.0	0.25

Notes: $p(\text{AND}) = p(a) \times p(b)$
$p(\text{OR}) = 1 - \{[1 - p(a)] \times [1 - p(b)]\}$
Criticality $= p(\text{actual fault}) \times p(\text{top event})$.

This example illustrates that the failure of Circuit 1 is not critical to the probability of a patient hazard relative to the occurrence of the three other events. Of those three other events, the failure of Subsystem 1 is twice as critical as the drifting of the pressure reference point, and the failure of Sensor 1 is three times as critical as the reference point drift. In absolute terms, the drift of Sensor 1 is most critical to the probability of a patient hazard, followed by the failure of Subsystem 1 and then the drift of the pressure reference point. This approach can be used to give guidance on which events, components, or subsystems might need additional design considerations to bolster their safety and reliability.

Hazard Analysis Difficulties

Hazard analysis is not without its own difficulties and traps. Because the process and procedure depend heavily on human involvement and engineering judgment, the team generating the hazard analysis must consider several factors when applying the procedures (Charette 1991). The amount of time spent in generating any of the hazard analysis information is not uniform. In general, conducting an FMEA requires more time, effort, and expense than a hazard analysis or fault tree and a fault tree more than a hazard analysis. The extent of the effort required is a function of how familiar the analysts are with the device, their familiarity with the analysis procedures, and the level of detail and rigor chosen to document the analysis. Care should be exercised so that the time required to complete the analysis is not so extensive and burdensome that the development team becomes reluctant to make further design changes.

Inexperienced analysis teams usually fail to consider fully the spreading impact of the failure modes. Development team designers and engineers participating on the analysis team can become so focused and single-minded about a failures consequence in one part of the system that they forget about its interaction and consequences with other system components. For example, they may focus on the electrical component consequences to the degree that they forget to consider its failure impact on the software or mechanical components. The degree to which user or operator errors can trigger system errors and defects is also commonly underestimated.

If the analysis team overestimates the number or severity of potential hazards in a device, then an excessive amount of engineering time might be spent in mitigating them. This can quickly deplete the assets of a product development program, which usually has limited resources. Further, extra engineering eats away at the time to market for the product, and that can be extremely costly for any company. Conversely, the analysis team initially underestimating the number or severity of the hazards can lead to a false sense of security, which could in turn lead to a faulty or risky device being introduced into the marketplace, thereby placing lives in jeopardy and causing large liability losses for the company. It may also lead management to underfund the required device maintenance phases and discovered-risk response. Underestimating hazards initially may also produce a reactionary response from management as more hazards are discovered; resources are wasted and personnel frustrated by creating explanations for potential failures related to the device design. The discovery of failures after underestimation, particularly after what is believed to have been a thorough hazards analysis, also prejudices management against hazard analyses on future projects in general. The request for subsequent hazards analyses are often met with skepticism by management, and the recommendations may not be seriously considered.

As juxtaposition, the hazard analysis can be overly accurate and lead to a false sense of security. The purpose of using a hazard analysis is to produce an operationally safe and efficacious medical device. If this result is accomplished, then some individuals may question whether it was the hazard analysis or another process that actually helped produce the correctly functioning device. This kind of skepticism is frequently driven by a feeling that the development team is so solid and competent that subsequent device versions do not need a hazard analysis.

During the 1970s and 1980s, device manufacturers attempted to shift identification with product design from individual ownership to team ownership, but the approach failed because the engineering staff took great pride in the products they designed. It is now tacitly agreed that ownership is crucial in team dynamics, but that ownership complicates the situation with respect to the defects of hazard analysis. Some engineers interpret hazard analysis as "finger pointing," "blame analysis," or a demonstration by management of their lack of talent and skills. Development management may see the hazard analysis as an unnecessary delay to the production of a device because it may require several years to determine with any degree of certainty that a device is safe and effective.

The argument that the direct added value of a hazard analysis cannot be determined is valid, but it is important to at least consider its impact from a generic economic standpoint. The effectiveness of a hazard analysis can be determined by counting the number of failures that could have resulted in recalls had the hazard analysis not detected them, by determining the cost of making the necessary changes, and by calculating the total amount of effort spent performing the analysis. The effectiveness of the hazard analysis in dollars saved is the number of potential recalls times the individual recall cost per unit times the number of units recalled minus the cost of the design engineering change to mitigate the hazard minus the cost of the engineering time to generate the hazard analysis. Although hazard analysis is relatively new and has not been fully applied to medical device development, its use will improve and its results will become more trustworthy, so that the costs incurred will be seen as an investment and not an expense.

Safety

All medical devices must be safe, effective, and reliable for their intended use. This is true for both the hardware and the software of the device. Safety is always the most important design consideration for medical devices. A medical device must never function or malfunction in a way that will place the patient or user in jeopardy or cause harm to either one. Safety is not an option, and it cannot be attained solely through compliance with appropriate standards. Although the definitions of safety vary, the standard judicial test of safety relates to negligence. Under the theories of strict liability and warranty, the safety test for a device is whether the device itself is free of defects and not unreasonably dangerous for its intended and foreseeable use. Another way of examining the safety definition is determining whether the device is one that the ordinary, prudent manufacturer would design, manufacture, and sell.

The device's compliance with applicable safety standards is not enough to assure a safe and effective device in and of itself, primarily for two reasons: (1) Standards tend to trail the best engineering practices within any given industry by several years. (2) Proof of compliance with applicable standards does not necessarily enhance a medical device manufacturer's judicial defense. However, proof of noncompliance usually serves as the basis for punitive damages. A perverse but good measure of a medical device manufacturer's quest for safe, effective, and reliable medical devices is success in both the marketplace and the courtroom.

In relation to safety, two aspects should be considered during the design of the device. First, failures must be analyzed relative to risk assessment. Failures and misuse that could cause harm to the user or patient must be assessed and designed out of the device. Good assessment techniques are the fault-tree analysis and the FMEA. Second, device liabilities must be analyzed and addressed. All possible failure modes must be explored and designed out of the device. All possible misuse situations must also be removed from the device, or at least a design-around must be provided. Courts may assess special punitive judgments to device manufacturers who have knowledge about unsafe device conditions but do nothing to neutralize them.

One line of argument says that there is really no such thing as software safety, because software, in and of itself, cannot be unsafe. However, this is a rather parochial view of software's role in the medical device, since the state of the device is composed of the states of the various components within the device, and one of those components is software. Software can have various unexpected and undesired effects when used in a complex device. Software safety entails the assurance that the software executes correctly within the context of the device as a whole without resulting in any unacceptable risk. What constitutes an acceptable or unacceptable risk is difficult to determine and must be defined for each device, but the definition will often include economic, political, and moral decisions.

Similar to hardware safety, software safety is achieved through the identification of potential hazards early in the development process. This allows for the establishment of software requirements and design features that are intended to eliminate or control those hazards. The other potential hazards to be considered relative to software lie outside of the normal operating mode of the device. They include maintenance modes, device failure modes, failures or unusual incidents in the device's environment, and errors in human performance. The fault-tree analysis and the FMEA are effective techniques to help define the device hazards relative to software. Device component failure is always one of the most logical and natural hazards to control.

Active and Standby Redundancy

One method used to address the high failure rate of certain components is the use of redundancy. Redundancy is the practice of using more than one component for the same circuit in hardware or of having duplicate code in software. The philosophy behind the concept of redundancy is that if one component fails, there is a second component that will function in its place and allow the device operation to continue safely. An example of this would be a primary and secondary alarm speaker in a medical device that would allow the device's alarm subsystem to continue to function even if the primary alarm speaker failed.

Redundancy is usually thought of as active or standby. Active redundancy is a design strategy in which two or more components are placed in parallel and all components are operational. In this case, the device operates satisfactorily when at least one of the two components functions. If one of the parallel components fails, then the remaining part continues to function, and device operation is sustained. Active redundancy is important in improving the reliability of a device because the mean time between failures (MTBF) for the circuit, and therefore the device, is increased and reliability greatly improved.

Although originally a hardware concept, active redundancy is also applied to software. Critical parameters or variables can be stored in nonvolatile memory so that redundant checks can be made to compare the current "working" value with the preserved value. Code and data corruption can likewise be guarded against via a CRC (cyclic redundancy check) calculation, in which a value is generated from the individual characters within the code and data. Watchdog circuits can be used to nullify software instances of deadly embraces, stuck keys, or race conditions.

Active redundancy, whether in hardware, software, or both, does have a price. It is expensive to implement in relation to actual parts count and additional design time. The implementation of active redundancy in hardware has as a downside the additional cost of purchasing two components instead of one. The designing and implementation of watchdog circuits and timers are also additional hardware burdens for the device. Active redundancy in software causes some difficulties also. All safety checks must be completed within a regular cycle that steals processor time and bandwidth resources. Timing among the software tasks that must execute within the device in normal operations must be scrutinized to avoid any time-out situations. The design for the active redundancy aspects of the device from both a hardware and software standpoint becomes much more complicated and sophisticated.

In standby redundancy, two or more components are placed in parallel, but only one component is active, and the other components remain in a standby mode until activated. This method of redundancy is usually a hardware option that can also be achieved in software. The concept for software implementation of standby redundancy is to have two copies or versions of the device software that execute in parallel. One copy is deemed the master copy and the second the slave, backup, or ghost copy. At predefined checkpoints, the results of the executions are compared; if the master copy disagrees with the secondary copy, then the master is shut down, and processing continues with the secondary. The price for this parallelism is often two sets of hardware for the software to execute on. There is also the added burden of coordination and synchronization between the two programs. More elaborate schemes must be developed for the device software to determine accurately when, if, and how the master is deemed unfit for continuing operations.

Device Misuse

An area of design concern of paramount importance to software is device misuse. When the user fails to read the user manual properly, misunderstands device labeling, or is inadequately (or not at all) trained, medical devices will be misused and even abused. Every medical device manufacturer has stories about the ingenuity of users in misusing and abusing its products. From a practical standpoint, it is impossible to make a medical device completely misuse and abuse proof. However, it is incumbent on the design team to design around as much misuse and abuse as can be reasonably anticipated.

The categories of misuse and abuse are varied. They include excessive application of cleaning solutions; physical abuse; spills; excessive weight applied to certain parts or areas of the device; excessive torque applied to controls or screws; excessive pressure applied to contact buttons or switches; improper voltages, frequencies, and pressures; and improper or interchangeable electrical or pneumatic connections. Historically, most of these misuses and abuses were relegated to the hardware areas. However, as user interfaces have become more prevalent and sophisticated and software has become more common, misuse and abuse has become manifest in the software area also.

As an example, key presses and software key debounce time must be considered. The processing timeline of software tasks now must be considered so that the inputs from the device keypads have had the time to be registered and acted upon correctly by the software. As users become more familiar with the user interface, the sequences of button pushes, and the device's menu navigation, they will become more adept at anticipating the next response required by the device. This, in turn, can cause inputs to the device to become garbled, leading to frustrating nuisance alarms and processing delays. At worst, this can happen when the state of the instrument becomes fatal to the user or the patient, because the software designers failed to consider all possible conditions and states the instrument may be in during these types of inputs.

Software developers should discuss the types of device misuse with marketing representatives to define as many possible misuse situations as can be anticipated. Software designers must then design around these situations to increase the reliability and safety of the device. Software designers should also allow for safety margins that will ensure proper processing time-line budgets. Where design restrictions limit the degree of protection that can be offered against misuse and abuse, the device should give an alarm or malfunction in a manner that is harmless to the user and also makes it obvious that the device is not operating in its intended manner.

Reliability versus Safety

Software safety and reliability are often equated, but these concepts are in the process of being separated. Software reliability is generally thought to be the probability that the software will perform its intended function for a specified period of time, under a set of specified environmental conditions. Software safety is the probability that the conditions that can lead to a mishap or hazard do not occur, whether or not the intended function is performed. Reliability requirements are concerned with making software failure free, whereas safety requirements are concerned with making software hazard free. These two concepts are not synonymous.

Failures of differing consequences are possible in any complex system. Reliability is concerned with every possible software error, whereas safety is concerned only with those errors that result in actual system hazards. Not all software errors cause safety problems, and not all software that functions according to its specification is safe. Severe mishaps have occurred while systems were operating exactly as intended, without failure.

System requirements can be separated into those related to the mission of the system and those related to safety while the mission is being accomplished. In general, some device requirements are not safety related at all, and some are related to the mission and can result in a hazard if they are not satisfied; others are related exclusively to the prevention of hazards. As the probability of safety-related requirements being satisfied increases, so does the overall safety of the system. Reliability can also be increased by similarly increasing the satisfaction of the non–safety-related requirements. However, in many complex systems, safety and reliability may imply conflicting requirements; the device is not usually built to maximize both.

In general, reliability models have merely counted failures, meaning that all failures are treated equally. In the 1980s, the concept of software reliability was perceptively altered in favor of including the relative severity of the consequences of failures into the software reliability determination (Cheung 1980; Littlewood 1980; Leveson 1981; Laprie and Coates 1982; Dunham 1984). Even if all failures cannot be prevented, it is possible to ensure that those that do occur have minor consequences and that the device will fail in a safe manner. There are, generally, three categories defined for deliberately engineered failure-severity systems:

1. Fail-safe or fail-passive procedures attempt to limit the amount of damage caused by the system through the failure, with no attempt to satisfy the functional specifications except where necessary to ensure safety.

2. Fail-operational or fail-behavior procedures provide full functionality during a fault situation.

3. A fail-soft system continues its operation but provides degraded performance or reduced functional capability until the fault is removed or the run-time conditions change.

Analytical procedures and approaches are useful when not all of the failures are of equal importance and consequence and when there is a relatively small number of failures that can lead to catastrophic results. Under these types of circumstances, the traditional reliability techniques can be augmented with techniques that concentrate on the high-cost failures. These types of software failure-severity approaches start with determining the unacceptable or high-cost failures, and then they ensure that these failures do not occur or, at least, minimize the probability of their occurrence. This approach and the traditional reliability approach are complementary, but their goals and appropriate techniques are different.

Software Safety

Most accidents in which software was involved can be traced to requirements flaws. More specifically, they result from incompleteness in the specified and implemented software behavior and incomplete, wrong assumptions about the operation of the controlled system or required operation of the computer, and controlled-system states and environmental conditions that were not accommodated in the implemented software. Although coding errors often get the most attention, they have more effect on reliability and other qualities than on safety (Ericson 1981; Lutz 1992).

Analysis of Software Safety Requirements

Determining the requirements for software is difficult, and it is a major source of software problems, especially with respect to safety. Many of the mishaps cited can be traced back to fundamental misunderstandings about the desired operation of the software, not unusual within the software industry. After studying mishaps in which computers were involved, safety engineers have concluded that inadequate design foresight and specification errors are the greatest cause of software problems (Ericson 1981; Griggs 1981). While software functional requirements often focus on what the system and its software will do, the safety requirements must also include what the system will not do. This includes the means of controlling and eliminating system hazards, as well as limiting the damage if a mishap occurs. An important part of the safety requirements is the specification of the ways in which the software and the system can fail safely and to what extent the failure is tolerable. In fact, some requirements specification procedures have noted the need for special safety requirements and include both specification of the undesired events and specification of the appropriate responses to those events.

An important issue then becomes how to identify and analyze software safety requirements. Several proposed techniques are used in limited contexts. They are fault-tree analysis, real-time logic, and time Petri nets. Fault-tree analysis, as discussed previously, is a technique used in the safety analysis of electromechanical systems. An undesired system state is specified, and the system is then analyzed in the context of its environment and operation, to find credible sequences of events that can lead to the undesirable event. The fault tree is a graphical model of the various parallel and sequential combinations of faults that result in the occurrence of a predefined undesired event. The faults can be events associated with component hardware failures, human errors, or any other type of pertinent event. The fault tree depicts the logical interrelationships of the basic events that lead to the hazardous event.

The success of fault-tree analysis is highly dependent on the ability of the analyst, who must thoroughly understand the system and its underlying scientific principles. However, fault-tree analysis does have the advantage that all of the system components, including human, can be considered during the analysis. This is extremely important, because a particular software fault may cause a mishap only if there is a simultaneous human and hardware failure. When the fault tree has been constructed down to the software interfaces, the high-level requirements for software safety can be derived in terms of the software faults and the failures that could adversely affect system safety. As the development of the software proceeds, additional fault-tree analyses can be performed on the emerging design as well as on the actual code.

Another method used to identify and analyze software safety requirements is the formalization of the safety analysis of timing properties in real-time systems by means of a formal real-time logic (Jahanian and Mok 1986). In this approach, the system designer first specifies the model of the system, including events and actions that describe the data dependency, as well as the temporal ordering of the computational actions that must take place in response to the real-time application. This model can then be translated into real-time logic formulas. The event-action model captures the timing requirements of the real-time system responses, and the real-time logic allows the specification of the absolute timing of the events as well as their order. This provides a uniform way of incorporating different scheduling disciplines.

To analyze the system design, the real-time logic formulas are transformed into predicates of Presburger arithmetic with uninterpreted integer functions. Decision procedures are then used to determine whether a given safety assertion is a theorem derivable from the system specification. If it is, then the system is safe with respect to the timing behavior denoted by that assertion, as long as the implementation satisfies the requirements specification. If the safety assertion is unsatisfiable with respect to the specification, then the system is inherently unsafe, because successful implementation of the requirements will cause the safety assertion to be violated. Alternatively, if the negation of the safety assertion is satisfiable under certain conditions, then additional constraints must be imposed on the system to ensure its safety. Although full Presburger arithmetic is inherently expensive computationally, a restricted set of Presburger formulas that allows for a more efficient decision procedure can be used.

Time Petri net models can also be used for software hazard analysis. Petri nets (Peterson 1981) allow the mathematical modeling of a discrete-event system in terms of its conditions and events and the relationships among them. Analysis and simulation procedures have been developed to determine the desirable and undesirable properties of the design, especially with respect to concurrent or parallel events. Analysis procedures have been derived to determine software safety requirements directly from the system design; to analyze a design for safety, recovery, and fault tolerance; and to guide the use of failure detection and recovery procedures (Leveson and Stolzy 1985, 1986). Faults and failures can then be incorporated into the Petri net model to determine their effects on the system.

Petri net backward analysis can be used to determine which failures and faults are potentially the most hazardous to the system and, therefore, which parts of the system need to be augmented with fault-tolerant and fail-safe mechanisms. Early in the design of the system, it is possible to treat the software parts of the design at a very high level of abstraction and consider only failures at the interfaces of the software and nonsoftware components. By working backward to this software interface, it is possible to determine software safety requirements and identify the most critical functions.

One possible drawback to the Petri net approach is that the construction of the model that represents the system is nontrivial. However, some of the effort may be justified by use of the model for other project objectives, such as performance analysis.

Software Safety Assessment

Software safety is not easily quantified, because mishaps or failures are almost always caused by multiple factors; the probabilities for success tend to be quite small. There are, however, three quantitative risk analysis methods: single-valued best estimate, probabilistic, and bounding. Single-valued best estimate is useful when a particular risk problem is well understood and enough information is available to build a determinate model that uses the best-estimate values for its parameters. If the science of the problem is reasonably well understood but only a limited amount of information is available about some of the important parameters, then probabilistic analysis can give an indication of the level of uncertainty in the answers. In this case, the single-valued best estimates of parameters are replaced by a probability distribution over the range of the values the parameters are expected to assume. If there is uncertainty about the functional form of the model that should be used, then this uncertainty can also be incorporated into the model. Some problems are so misunderstood that a probabilistic analysis is inappropriate. However, it is sometimes possible to use what little is known to at least bound the answer.

As with any quantitative analytical approach, there are advantages and disadvantages in using any of these assessment techniques. Quantitative risk assessment can provide the insight and the understanding that will allow various alternatives to be explored and compared. The need to calculate very low probability numbers usually forces the analyst to study the system in great detail. However, there is also the danger of placing implicit belief in the accuracy of a calculated number. It is also easy to overemphasize models and forget the many assumptions that are implied by the results of a model. In addition, quantitative risk assessment approaches can never capture all of the factors that are important in the problem to be solved, and they should not substitute for careful engineering judgment.

Another difficulty associated with formal software safety assessment is that some of the assumptions made in, and for, the analysis do not hold in practice. Although it can be argued that assumptions made during the analysis are the best possible, given the state of knowledge at the time, the mistake is in placing too much faith in assumptions and models, and not in taking corrective measures in case they are wrong. Effort is frequently diverted into proving theoretically that a system meets a stipulated level of risk when that effort could be used more profitably if applied to the elimination, minimization, and control of the hazards. Considering the inaccuracy of the present models for assessing software reliability, some of the resources applied to the modeling of the assessment might be more effectively used if they were applied to sophisticated software engineering and safety techniques. Models are important when used with care and judgment.

Because safety is a system quality, the models that assess it must consider all components of the system; few models currently do this when the system contains any programmable subsystems. In general, the expected probability with which a given mishap will occur is the product of the probability that the hazard will occur times the probability that the hazard will lead to a mishap. A more sophisticated model would also include such factors as the exposure time of the hazard or the average time needed to detect and correct the problem. The longer the exposure time, the more likely it is that other events or conditions will occur that cause the hazard to lead to a mishap. If an event sequence is involved, the exposure time for the first fault must be short or the fault must be rare, to minimize the probability of a mishap. Complex fault sequences are often analyzed by using fault trees, where probabilities are attached to the nodes of the tree; the probability of system or component failures can then be calculated as previously discussed.

In summary, the implications and ramifications of the various approaches used for assessment of software safety are still very much unresolved, although several techniques are emerging as preferred methods. High software reliability figures do not necessarily mean that the software is acceptable from a safety standpoint. The intent of software safety assessment approaches is to somehow combine software and hardware assessments to provide system safety measurements.

Software Safety Design

Preventing hazards through design involves designing the software so that faults and failures cannot cause hazards. This can be accomplished either by making the software design intrinsically safe or by minimizing the number of software hazards. Software can create hazards through omission or commission. Omission hazards are caused by failure to perform a required operation; commission hazards can occur when an operation is performed that should not be done or when an operation is performed at the wrong time or in the wrong sequence. Software is usually tested extensively to ensure that it performs only what it is specified to perform. Because of its complexity, however, software may be able to perform a lot more than what software engineers specified or intended, or what software V&V engineers anticipated and tested. In this case, design features can be used to limit the actions of the software.

As an illustration, it may be possible to use modularization and data access limitations to separate noncritical functions from critical functions and thereby ensure that the failures of noncritical modules do not place the device into a hazardous state. This strategy also ensures that noncritical modules cannot impede the operation of safety-critical functions. The goal of software safety design is to reduce the amount of software that affects the device safety and to change as many potentially critical faults into noncritical faults as possible. An added benefit of this goal is that it helps to reduce the verification effort, because it helps to reduce the volume of safety-related testing. As lofty as this goal is, it may be difficult to separate critical and noncritical functions; any software safety certification arguments based on this approach will need supporting analysis that proves it is impossible for the safety of the device to be compromised by faults in noncritical software.

Often in safety-critical software, some modules or data items must be carefully protected because their execution, destruction, or alteration at the wrong time can be catastrophic. For this type of situation, security techniques that involve authority limitation may be useful in protecting safety-critical functions and data. The same security techniques devised to protect against malicious actions can be used to protect against inadvertent but dangerous actions. In this case, the safety-critical parts of the software are separated, and an attempt is made to limit the authority of the rest of the software to do anything that is safety critical. The safety-critical routines can then be carefully protected. Inadvertent activation can also be limited by retaining a positive input from a human controller prior to execution of certain commands. In this case, the human will need some independent source of information on which to base the decision besides the information provided by the software.

In some systems, it may be impossible to always avoid hazardous states. In fact, hazardous states may be required for the device to accomplish its function. A general software design goal relative to safety is to minimize the amount of time that a potentially hazardous state exists. One simple way to accomplish this is to start in a safe state and require a change of the device state to a higher risk state. In this case, critical flags and conditions should be set and checked as close to the code they protect as possible; additionally, critical conditions should not be complementary. For example, the absence of the "arm hazard condition" should not mean safe.

Commonly, the sequence of events is critical to the operation of the device. In electromechanical applications, an interlock is used to ensure sequencing or to isolate two events in time. Equivalent design features are often available in software through the programming language facilities of concurrency and synchronization. These can be used to sequence the events, but they do not necessarily protect against inadvertent branches caused by either a software fault or a hardware fault. In fact, they are usually so complex in their implementation and use that they are prone to errors themselves; some protection can be afforded through the use of semaphores, batons, signals, and handshaking. In each of these applications, a parameter is checked prior to the function being executed, to assure that the previously required routines have concluded their processing and registered their completion. Another example of designing to protect against hardware failure is to ensure that bit patterns, used to satisfy a conditional branch to a safety-critical function, do not use common failure patterns, such as all zeros.

Operational Software Safety

Along with attempts to avoid and prevent hazards, it may be necessary to detect and treat hazards during execution of the software within the device. Ad hoc tests for unsafe software conditions can be programmed into any software and can be represented by exception handling, external monitors, and watchdog timers. In general, it is important that the software is able to detect unsafe states as quickly as possible, to minimize exposure time to the hazard. To implement this safeguard, software monitors independent from the application software can be used so that faults in one cannot disable the other; the monitor should add as little complexity to the system as possible. Although many mechanisms have been proposed to help implement fault detection, assistance with fault detection is harder to find than is help with the more difficult problem of formulating the content of fault checks or their placement.

From a safety standpoint, recovery routines and functions are frequently needed. For example, when an unsafe state is detected externally, when the software cannot provide a required output within a prescribed time limit, or when the continuation of regular processing would lead to a catastrophic system state, if there is no intercession, a recovery routine would be required. Recovery techniques are generally categorized as backward recovery or forward recovery.

Backward recovery techniques return the system to a prior state and then continue forward again with an alternative piece of code; there is no attempt to diagnose the particular fault that caused the error or to assess any other damage the fault may have caused. It is a tacit assumption with backward recovery techniques that the alternative code will work better than the original code. To ensure this, a different algorithm than was used in the normal code may be implemented in the alternative code, but there is still the possibility that the alternative algorithm will work no better than the original code, especially if the error originated from flawed specifications about the required operation of the software. Backward recovery is adequate if it can be guaranteed that software faults will be detected, and successful recovery completed, before the faults affect the external state. However, this cannot usually be guaranteed. Some control actions that depend on the incremental state of the device may not be recoverable by a checkpoint and a subsequent rollback; small errors may require hours to build up to a value that exceeds a prescribed safety limit. Even if backward recovery is attempted, it may be necessary to take concurrent action in parallel with recovery procedures. In these instances, forward recovery that would repair any damage or minimize the hazards may be required. Forward recovery techniques attempt to repair the faulty state, whether it is within the internal state of the microprocessor or computer or within the internal state of the controlled process. Forward recovery returns the device to a correct state, or it may contain or minimize the effects of the failure, if the correct state cannot be reached.

Most safety-critical systems and devices are designed to have a safe state that is reachable from any other state of the device or system; this state is always safe. There is usually a performance penalty associated with it, making it possible to require additional safety processing overhead to prevent the safe state from shutting down, or restricting the services or capabilities of the device. In more complex designs, there may be intermediate safe states that have limited functionality, particularly for those systems for which a shutdown would be hazardous in itself.

In general, the safe states for non-normal control modes are varied and provide differing levels of functionality. For example, partial shutdowns leave the system with partial or degraded functionality. In a hold state, no functionality is provided, but steps are taken to maintain safety or limit the extent of damage. In an emergency shutdown state, the system is shut down completely. A manual or externally controlled state allows the system to continue to function, but control is transferred to a source that is external to the computer or microprocessor, the computer commonly being responsible for a smooth transfer. In the restart state, such a system or device is in a transitional state from non-normal to normal.

Reconfiguration or dynamic alteration of the software control flow is a form of partial shutdown. In real-time systems or devices, the criticality of the tasks often changes during normal operations and may depend on the run-time environment conditions. If the peak system overload is increasing the response time above some critical threshold, for example, the run-time reconfiguration of the system may be achieved by delaying or temporarily eliminating noncritical system functions. The system overload itself may be caused or increased by internal conditions, such as excessive attempts to perform some form of recovery.

The design of the software can go a long way toward processing of run-time safety criticality. The safety requirements for the system should include the conditions that the software be able to respond within a few hundred milliseconds if overstressing or even catastrophic events are detected. Under no circumstances should other specified hazardous events be tolerated. The software could be designed as a two-level structure, the top level being responsible for the less important governing functions, as well as for the supervisory, coordination, and management functions. Loss of this upper level would not endanger the rest of the system, and it would not cause the system to shut down. The upper-level control could also reside on a separate processor from the base-level software.

The base-level software is, in effect, a secure core that can detect significant failures of the hardware that surrounds it. It would include self-checks to decide whether incoming signals are sensible and whether the processor itself is functioning properly. A failure of the self-check software would cause reversion of the output to a safe state through the action of fail-safe hardware. There are, of course, two potential software-related safety errors: (1) The code responsible for self-checking, validating incoming and outgoing signals, and promoting the fail-safe shutdown must be error free. (2) Corruption of this vital code must not cause a dangerous condition or allow a dormant fault to be manifested.

The organization of the base-level functional tasks is under the control of a comprehensive state table that determines the various self-check criteria appropriate under particular conditions. Furthermore, the state table defines the scheduling of the tasks themselves, allowing precise timing criteria to be applied to the execution time of certain sections of the most important code, such as the self-check code and the watchdog routines.

Safety Considerations of Unused Code

In the intense propagation of software control in systems that perform potentially life- or property-threatening operations, myriad issues associated with this software must be addressed. One of these issues is the safety implication of having software resident in memory with an operational program that is not intentionally executed. Unused software resident in memory in conjunction with a program load can generally be broken into two categories: *dead code* and *co-resident software*. Dead code is defined as software compiled and resident in a program or resident in memory in conjunction with a program executed only as a result of erroneous hardware or software actions. Dead code is usually unintentional in a system, and the software engineers often are not aware of its presence. This software can be either fully executable routines or merely a random collection of executable memory locations. Co-resident software is defined as multiple software packages resident on a single software load or end item, each of which is to be intentionally executed on a specified subset of host processors or under specific conditions. The presence of co-resident software in a system is intentional, and the execution control has been designed into the product. Examples include branches and procedures embedded in the software to allow execution of a unique superset or subset under specified conditions and multiple software programs combined into a common load of which any one is executed only on a specified subset of the host processors.

The safety concerns with dead code and co-resident software focus on unintentional access to and execution of the software and the resultant system-level actions. These actions can range from a minor inconvenience to an inadvertent catastrophic mishap. Dead code execution poses the hazard of unpredictable operation because the code is usually unexpected, its execution unplanned, and the resulting actions indeterminate and untestable. If fail-safe and error-handling features such as watchdog timers, command filtering, and exception handlers are incorporated in the design, unintended execution of dead code can usually be detected and acted upon. Co-resident code poses the same hazard as dead code, with the additional potential hazard of successful operation with undetected erroneous execution. Because the co-resident code is designed to execute, it will often satisfy the fail-safe and error-handling features incorporated into the system; consequently, it may execute for an extended period with resultant unexpected system interaction. On the positive side, because this code is designed to execute, entry conditions and system interaction can be understood and tested.

Execution in either case poses hazards that are essentially the same as those posed by inadvertent execution of the active code, in that operation is unpredictable and unanticipated. The concern is not the presence of this software; rather, it is unintentional access to and execution of this software. If the assumption is that this unintended execution does occur, then the increased quantity of executable software in fact increases the probability of unintended execution, because the target area has been expanded. However, the ratio of unused code to active code is usually so small that the increase in execution potential is negligible.

Dead code is created by a variety of actions, most of which can be traced to human errors. One of the causes of dead code is errors in software development that result in failure to invoke procedures or branch logic as designed. Dead code can be generated because of unreachable condition logic, improperly edited procedure names, unused standard case structure generated by the compiler, or simple actions such as a misplaced comment symbol. Another cause of dead code is the failure to remove test or debug routines. These routines are placed in the code during module or program-level testing as an aid in software development and are not intended to be part of the delivered product. Test routines often are deeply embedded in the software and only accessible by emulators or debug tools, so this software is considered to be transparent. Another type of dead code is erroneous, nonfunctioning code that remains after a software modification. This includes procedures no longer called, unused results of performed algorithms, and condition logic that cannot be satisfied. Still another type is old code, resident in computer memory, that is not entirely erased or overwritten by the new software load. This occurs when the new load is smaller than the old load and no actions are taken to purge the old load from memory. Nonoptimized code generated as a result of compiler or linker operation is a source of dead code. Standard libraries and link packages are often appended to a program during these operations, and code not needed for software execution is also loaded.

The action to be taken to mitigate dead code depends on how the code was generated; this usually falls into three categories: *design-induced code, load-induced code,* and *compile-induced code.* The cost and effort required to find and reduce or eliminate dead code must be carefully weighed against the potential gains of such actions. The effort should focus on software that controls systems that perform potentially life- or property-threatening operations and must address the potential impacts to that control by inadvertent execution of the dead code. In many cases, the presence of dead code is transparent to the program execution and requires no action. Dead code that results from a design, modification, or test routine error is generally not favored in a software system. Even when dead code is not executed, its presence consumes memory and impacts software load times. If executed, even with no effect, this code impacts program throughput. The majority of this code can be discovered by software test routines and branch testing, software tools that check reachability and connectivity, and compiler checks. The difficulty with design-induced dead code is that the code was developed for an intended purpose, and its failure to execute is usually indicative of a deeper design error. Discovered dead code should be documented in a software problem report, the underlying reason for its presence determined, and corrective action implemented. Design-induced dead code must not be blindly removed from the software.

Load-induced dead code is much easier to handle than design-induced dead code. Dead code that results from old programs left in memory can be mitigated by ensuring that every load overwrites all memory locations or by execution of security routines that purge all memory locations prior to a software load. Once the program load is performed or a purge routine executed, all memory locations not overwritten by the new software load will contain an established pattern. Data patterns left in unused memory locations as a result of a program load should be a known pattern that has acceptable execution consequences.

Inefficiencies in the compiler or in the granularity of the link can result in compiler-induced dead code. This form of dead code can be minimized by careful compiler manipulation and optimized link sets. Understanding how the compiler translates the source code allows the designer to influence the object code generated, but often at the cost of source code that is awkward and hard to maintain. The link can be screened and stripped of unused logic, which reduces the amount of loaded software. Although this optimization has the added benefit of reduced load image size, it poses potential problems during maintenance and upgrade.

Co-resident software usually evolves in an attempt to optimize the software design or the operating environment. Applications of co-resident software are considerable; three common examples are *multiple-use loads, common loads,* and *replacement loads.* A multiple-use load is a single program designed for differing functionality based on the operating environment. The functionality is altered by branch and procedure execution controlled by external stimulus. These branches and procedures are usually deeply embedded and form an integral part of the program. This technique is common in maintenance routines embedded in operational software. When executed, these routines execute in conjunction with the operational software to achieve the desired results. Common load software consists of multiple programs assembled into a common package to minimize the quantity of load sets and, consequently, the number of configurations to be maintained. These programs are usually stand-alone, only one program executing in a specific processor or environment, and are usually controlled by stimulus external to the software. Because the programs are stand-alone, the removal of one usually has no impact on the execution of the others. This technique is often used in systems that contain redundant processors or multiple common processors that perform installation-specific functions. Replacement load software consists of multiple programs designed to replace one another, depending on the operating environment. Design of these systems varies greatly; the programs are either stand-alone replacements or specified supersets or subsets, and execution is based on either internal or external stimulus. These programs are common in graceful degradation designs, in which a reduced capability subset can be executed upon detection of failure, and in designs in which programs share a common processor and each executes for a set period and is then swapped out. Many windowed applications rely on replacement load execution that allows each window's program a slice of the overall time line.

Co-resident software poses the unique risk of potential "successful" inadvertent execution, and special safety considerations are required in critical systems to minimize the consequences of such execution. One way to guard against this is to make program execution tightly controlled. In this approach, multiple hardware or software interlocks are required to prevent credible single-point failures from initiating erroneous execution. The level of interlocks should correspond to the relative hazard potential and should be very robust when loss of life or loss of the system is plausible. This is especially important in multiple-use systems in which execution of embedded routines in the wrong environment can have catastrophic consequences. Another guard is to consider operator interaction. When multiple operating modes are allowed, positive indications should be provided so that the operator can determine which mode is currently executing. Potentially hazardous systems should not rely solely on human actions to preclude inadvertent execution, and these systems should use keys and hardware interlocks for positive control.

Extensive exception testing must be specified and executed in dealing with co-resident software. Positive program load and execution control in normal and credible failure modes must be verified to ensure that the features designed into the system execute as planned. Software sneak circuit analysis or software reachability analysis should also be performed on the most critical systems to ensure no paths exist that would allow unintended software execution. These analyses should focus on the code branch points and common load boundaries. Automated tools available to perform both of these analyses should be used as much as possible to increase repeatability of regression testing.

Positive execution prevention should be considered for common load software. Examples include purge routines that delete all unused code following the software load and memory fences that limit access to a specified range of memory locations relating to the execution environment. However, care must be taken to ensure that such routines do not introduce greater hazards than they mitigate. For example, purge routines work well on independent programs packaged together, but they are less successful in cases where the branch logic is deeply embedded in the active code. Memory access control features are difficult to implement on dynamic programs and can induce problems during software upgrades, because the load image size and execution boundaries change. Replacement load software is prone to the generation of dead code. In the case of degraded mode replacement, this dead code can be of concern, because the software is executing in a suspect environment. Whenever possible, the new load should overwrite the entire replaced set or be invoked in concert with a purge routine that ensures that the old software is entirely replaced.

Dead code is undesirable in most systems but is not specifically a safety concern. Although the implications of dead code should always be addressed, its removal is not always practical or necessary. When elimination is deemed necessary, the dead code must not be blindly removed from the software. Disposition is required to ensure that any underlying problems are resolved. The identification and elimination of this code are best handled as a normal part of software development by the software development team. Co-resident software is a fact in many systems and requires special safety considerations to ensure that execution is adequately controlled. The level of control required to prevent inadvertent execution is a function of the hazard potential and design implementation; as such, it should be handled on a case-by-case basis. Hazard mitigation in co-resident code should be a normal part of the system safety, with an added emphasis on abnormal conditions and failure modes that might result in erroneous execution. The concern is not the presence of unused software but, rather, access to and unintentional execution of the unused software. As the use of software to control potentially hazardous systems continues to increase, software design groups must take a proactive role to ensure robust, fault-tolerant designs capable of preventing or recovering from unintentional software execution.

User Interface and Safety

Sometimes the worst accidents take place on perfectly functioning hardware and software that the operator simply misunderstood or misused because of a deficient user interface. When the safety properties of a system are analyzed, it is important to ensure that the design is both true to the safety requirements and robust enough to tolerate certain failures, particularly the design of the user-device interaction. Safety is a system property that resides in the device and in the individual(s) using the device. The safety of the device itself depends on sufficient testing and fail-safe mechanisms that protect the users and others when the software or hardware component, or both, does fail. Given a safe device, users can maintain that safety only if they act responsibly and can interpret the information displayed by the device. Users who disable sensors, ignore alarms, or use the device improperly can violate the device integrity; therefore, a system's safety depends fundamentally on the user taking ultimate responsibility.

However, although the operator is often a scapegoat for a badly designed user-machine interface, it would be unfair to blame an operator for ignoring an alarm from a device that issues several false alarms per day or for misinterpreting information that is displayed in a nonintuitive fashion. It is a flawed assumption that only trained personnel operate safety-critical devices. For example, consider driving a car. An automobile is a deadly weapon if not properly controlled. The law requires that you pass a test before you are permitted to drive, but the law does not require that you drive only the car that was used during the test, even though the interface in another car may be considerably different. Similarly, highly trained doctors and nurses use hospital equipment, but their training is mostly in the principles of medicine, not necessarily in the use of every brand of equipment. You can expect an educated and trained user to understand principles, but expecting that same user to know that the alarm volume control is located under menu item three on a device is not correct. Even a perfectly functioning device may contribute to a safety hazard if information is not presented intelligibly to the user. Three types of information must be presented clearly: direct feedback to actions implemented by the user; monitored parameters of the system; and alarms that alert the user to unusual patterns in the monitored data.

Increasing device safety often reduces the quality of other desirable properties of the system, such as cost, performance, and usability. Consequently, it is important that the person who is ultimately responsible for ensuring the safety aspects of a project has a minimal investment in the project's other properties, such as cost, timeliness, or usability of the system. Maintaining an organization in which this is the case is no trivial matter; in very small organizations, it just is not feasible to dedicate a person solely to safety, although in some cases it can be combined with testing. Safety goals are compatible with those of testing in that they both attempt to detect and eradicate any shortcomings of the product, and both may delay the launch date in return for increased quality. Testing, however, tends to emphasize finding areas where the implementation does not meet the specification, whereas safety engineering tries to ensure that the specification defines a system that is safe. Although software bugs make spectacular headlines and public perception may be that failures of implementation are the predominant cause of computer-related accidents, incorrect specifications have caused more accidents than software bugs have (Leveson 1995). The user interface is the place where unsafe actions can most effectively be rejected and unsafe states announced. If all of the safety mechanisms are buried deep within the system or product, it may be difficult for the user to diagnose the problem, and when an accident occurs, quick and accurate diagnosis of the failure may be vital.

Usability versus Safety Trade-off

Although it may seem intuitive that a device that is easy to use is safer than one that isn't, that is not always the case. To provide safety, the user may work harder, and many situations involve a direct trade-off between usability and safety. For example, the Therac-25 was a cancer irradiation device whose faulty operation led to some deaths. One of the safety features in the original design was that all of the settings for the device had to be entered through a terminal as well as on a control panel. Unfortunately, users of a prototype saw this as redundant, and the design was changed before release so that the settings could be entered on the terminal alone. Once the settings were accepted by selecting the Return key, the user was asked to confirm that the settings were correct by hitting the Return key a second time. It was judged that this extra step was a replacement for the original second interface. Users subsequently learned to press the Return key twice in succession, as a reflex. With repetition, the action became similar to double clicking a mouse, and the settings were never actually reviewed by the user. Because of a software bug, though, some settings were not properly recorded. The bug was a race condition created because proper resource locking of the data wasn't exercised. Because the independent crosscheck had been removed, the fault was not detected. This is a case in which the design was altered to favor usability but the safety of the device was fatally compromised.

If the rest of the design had been sound, removing the second set of inputs would not have been significant. The point of putting a safety infrastructure in place, however, is to allow for the times when something does go wrong. In the example above, the later design was more susceptible to the simple user error of entering a wrong value. If the user has to enter the value on two different displays, the chances that the same wrong value will be entered are greatly decreased. In fact, the software would detect the mismatch and not apply either setting. Often, safety measures can serve this dual purpose of protecting against device error and user error. In intensive-care medical ventilators, for example, the pressure rise in a patient's lung is a function of the lung volume and the volume of gas added. A pressure valve opens at a fixed pressure limit, and once the valve is open, an alarm sounds and the patient is exposed to room air pressure in the fail-safe state. This feature protects the patient against an electronic or software fault that may deliver a large volume of gas, as well as from a user accidentally setting the gas volume to be added higher than the threshold limit.

This does not mean that users should be required to enter data twice on all systems; in some cases, simpler measures will suffice. Limits can be placed on input values, or the values may be set on the basis of other known information. For example, a patient's weight may limit the amount of medication that can be delivered. A numeric keypad may allow the risk of a decimal point being entered in the wrong location; in turn, this might cause a setting to be wrong by a factor of ten. If the user were to rotate a dial to select the value, this error would be less likely to occur. If default values are presented to the user, then the user can be forced to select each of the defaults, which minimizes the chance that the user will proceed without considering whether each of the values is appropriate. Each of these steps will provide a more robust system, in that users are less likely to accidentally enter settings that they would never have consciously chosen. These types of approaches do sacrifice efficiency and expediency, however.

Validating Input

If the user can easily perform irreversible actions, then a mistake may have serious consequences. The system must make it obvious that an important or critical action is about to take place; asking the user to confirm an action is common, but it is not necessarily the best approach. It is sufficient to make the action different in some respect from the normal or usual user actions. For example, a medical device or equipment might have an "Apply to patient" button that would be pressed only when the adjusted settings are to be made active. This button can be physically separated from the other input controls, just as the power switch on a desktop computer is not placed on the keyboard. In other cases, the system can attempt to guarantee that risk has been removed before proceeding. For example, placing two buttons on either side of the machine can lower risk, because the user must press both simultaneously to operate the system; the user cannot press both buttons simultaneously if either hand is still in the process of readying the system. Another aspect of this problem is that the device must know when it is safe to continue operating in a certain mode in the absence of further instructions. Some devices employ a control that reverts to a safe state when force is removed. In the case in which an incapacitated operator can lead to a dangerous situation, this control can be implemented.

While some situations offer a neat solution, safety often depends on a sequence of actions, and the system should be capable of reminding users of incomplete actions. For example, the interface can appear different during a setup operation than during normal running, so that an incomplete setup will be immediately recognizable. If the user leaves a task incomplete, an audible tone can be used to attract the attention of the user, who must either complete the sequence or cancel the task to silence the tone. Some equipment can be made to time-out silently when an incomplete action is encountered. The time-out guarantees that the device isn't left waiting for a final key press to acknowledge an action that was partially completed at an earlier time, possibly by a different user. However, this type of time-out presents several problems. The initial steps may be canceled while the user is deciding which step to take next. Estimates for the time it takes to read a screen with English text may be optimistic, for example, if the designer assumes that users are native English speakers, but they are not. Even a time-out of several minutes is not long enough if the user decides to consult a manual or a colleague before selecting the next key. The user could place the device into a confusing or unknown state and have it cancel out of that state by the time the local expert sees it. Another danger is possible if the time-out occurs just as a user moves a finger toward the final key of a sequence. The user may not be sure which occurred first, the time-out or the completion of the sequence, and would not know whether the input changes have taken effect.

Dialogs should be clear and unambiguous. For example, the message "Press ACCEPT or CLEAR" is valuable feedback to the user when the user is offered the choice between confirming or rejecting a change. However, be sure that the physical location of the Clear key is not to the left of the Accept key, because this could lead to confusion, as the word Clear is to the right of the word Accept in the text message above. This example also breaks the earlier rule that the Accept and Clear keys should not be near each other (see Figure 10-12). Furthermore, there is the danger that the first-time user may press the wrong key once before learning the correct layout responses. Although the confusion caused in this example may seem slight, the greater danger occurs when a user reacts in an emergency, follows the wrong impulse, and presses the

Figure 10-12   User interface display example 1

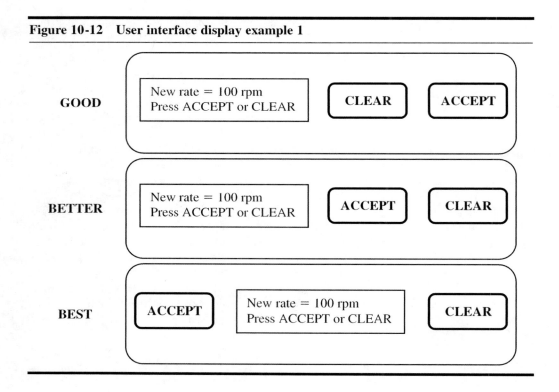

wrong key. A state of emergency is obviously the worst time to make a mistake; in this case, it is also the most likely.

Monitoring

Device values that are monitored are the user's window into the system; thus, the monitored values should tell the user the state of the system at a glance. An alarm that only detects whether the settings are being applied is not sufficient in a safety-critical system, because the parameter that is set may not be the appropriate value to monitor. For example, in a heart-lung machine, the user can set the speed of the pump that circulates and controls the flow of patient blood into and out of the body during heart bypass surgery. The volume of blood in the reservoir is monitored to inform the anesthesiologist of the blood level in the patient so that the patient does not bleed out or start to revive. Factors such as the amount of antibiotic infusion or intravenous infusion affect the volume of blood, however, and cannot be factored into the pump speed setting. Another difficulty with relying solely on settings and alarms is that alarms simply do not react quickly enough. If alarm thresholds or bands are set so tightly that a slight system anomaly causes an alarm to activate, then a large number of false alarms will be generated. This tends to lead to the cry-wolf scenario, so that alarms are discounted or ignored in emergency situations. On the other hand, if the bounds are set wide enough to avoid false alarms, then alarms will not occur as early as possible when a parameter slowly drifts out of range. The solution is to provide nonintrusive monitored information that allows the observation of the state of the system over time. Simple changes, such as a monitored temperature that rises slowly after the set temperature has been changed, can then be used to reflect the proper operation of the system.

Values displayed in an analog fashion, such as a bar graph or an analog needle indicator, are quicker to read and better at providing relative measures, especially if minimums and maximums are shown. Digital displays are more precise but require more concentration and interpretation by the user. The ideal application would be to provide both analog, with minimum and maximum, and the current digital value. If average or recent values are available, a trending bar graph can show the user sudden changes in behavior. These changes may be early warning signs of an impending problem. However, the difficulty is to determine how much information to present to the user and to avoid presenting too much information, because that could make important patterns difficult to decipher. As a guide, when safety is an issue, information from as many independent channels or locations as possible should be presented to the user. For example, consider a heater-cooler machine, used as a part of a heart-lung system that chills patient blood for bypass surgery, that has two monitoring thermistors positioned in different locations so the user can monitor how evenly the heater-cooler is performing. Suppose that the user can look at the average or current temperature on each thermistor. The two displays for this device shown in Figure 10-13 both have the same manufacturing cost, because they use the same components. In each case, the thermistor's average or current temperature is displayed, but in terms of safety Display 1 has a distinct advantage. In Display 2, if thermistor 1 fails and its data are unreliable, only information from the faulty sensor is displayed, whereas if Display 1 is chosen, data from each sensor are always visible. If a sensor is faulty, the values from the two sensors will diverge; if the user monitors all four values regularly, the problem will be noticed. However, with Display 2 the user may never bother to switch to the second thermistor and after a few weeks of using an apparently properly functioning system, the user may believe that the variation between the thermistors is not significant enough to affect normal operation. Users will always adapt their behavior to the normal situation, sometimes at great cost should a fault occur.

It could be argued that a simple alarm can check the difference between the two thermistors and annunciate if the difference becomes too large. If the second thermistor is added for redundancy alone and is located in the same part of the heater-cooler, then this system may be feasible. In many control systems, however, separate sensors monitor points that are expected to be different, and characterizing the differences can be difficult. During warm-up or cool-down,

Figure 10-13   User interface display example 2

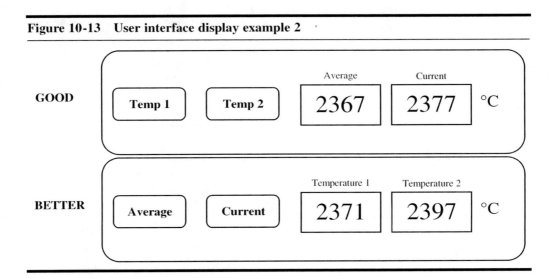

for example, the differences may be larger than those seen during steady-state conditions; an alarm's tolerance is set wide enough to cover all possible situations, it may be wide enough to allow a faulty sensor to pass its test. The result is that the user has not been helped and must evaluate the information. Furthermore, variations between the sensors may make the difference unsuitable as an alarm parameter, but the difference should be checked at some point when the system is stable, as a safety check that the components are functioning correctly.

Alarms

Safety-critical systems require both an alarm system and a monitoring system to provide warnings of device failure and to warn of possibly dangerous patterns in the monitored parameters. If a possibility exists that the user may not be directly observing the device during operation, an audible alarm should be included. For some classes of device, an audible warning is legally required. In some cases, the monitor and alarm can be combined as a single display, as shown in Figure 10-14. This illustrates a temperature bar graph that is labeled to show where the alarm is to be annunciated. Color coding can also be applied in order to emphasize the situation and provide clarity. This type of display has an added benefit in that it allows the user to anticipate the alarm before it occurs and to take evasive action.

Text Lists versus Dedicated Annunciators

Video display units (VDUs), whether LCD screens or cathode ray tube (CRT) screens, allow alarms to be displayed as text messages rather than requiring dedicated indicators. If the number of possible alarms is high, a VDU is probably the only option because of the amount of space that would be required for all of the individual annunciators. A VDU also has an added advantage if secondary information, such as a value for the monitored parameter, can be displayed along with the alarm. In addition, the alarms could be ordered either chronologically or by priority and displayed in sorted order on the VDU. The user could be given several filtering options, categories or characteristics that could provide several views of the system for extra insight into the cause of the alarms. This approach frequently helps to alleviate the difficulty encountered by a user trying to identify a real problem that is obscured by many nuisance alarms. On the other hand, individual annunciators, usually LEDs and a label, allow a visible pattern to emerge from the combination of conditions at any given moment. These annunciators are sometimes called tiles, because they may form a large area of small squares. Another advantage is that there is no competition for display space between alarms; consequently, one alarm never forces

Figure 10-14   User interface display example 3

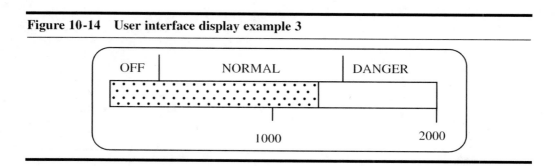

another off the VDU. Furthermore, the user knows which condition is associated with an indicator and does not have to read a lot of text to establish that relationship.

Text-based alarms on a VDU may cause confusion by giving the user too much information, because it is too easy for software developers to give a long and informative description of the condition. In an emergency, many conditions may be annunciated simultaneously, challenging the user's ability to read all of the generated text, and an LCD-based VDU may not be bright enough for an alarm to be noticed from the far side of the room. Furthermore, audible alarms are usually not directional enough, and the user may need to establish the alarm's source by glancing at many devices while trying to absorb the displayed information. This is particularly true in hospital intensive-care units, where each patient can be connected to several devices, each of which can generate audible alarms.

A viable approach is to use bright indicators for the most urgent alarm and include further data values or text information on a VDU. Alternatively, a small number of annunciators could be used for the most important conditions, while the less frequent or less urgent conditions can be displayed only on a VDU. Data suggest that individual annunciators generally outperform a VDU with text only, but VDUs surpass individual annunciators when they make use of color and graphics that allow the user to analyze the data (Stanton 1994).

Crying Wolf

Having many alarm conditions is not necessarily better than having just a few. Nuisance alarms may end up being ignored or disabled, which is worse than not having the alarm at all. If the alarm is absent, the user must accept the fact that the parameter simply isn't monitored. If the alarm is present but unreliable, it conveys to the user the superficial impression that a dangerous condition will be detected; in practice, the user may assume that an alarm is false, like many previous ones, and ignore it. In some cases, the nuisance alarm did not actually indicate a failure but was simply implemented with a too tight criterion. Criteria that seem reasonable during design aren't always so reasonable when manufacturing variability, real operating conditions, and years of wear and tear are factored into daily operation. An alarm sensor can be replaced or fixed if it fails, but if the design limits are wrong, the users may not be able to change them.

The number of false alarms can be reduced in several ways. First, reasonable limits for the parameter being monitored can be selected. This may not be enough, however, if the signal is noisy, for example. If noise is an issue, as is frequently the case, the signal can be filtered at several levels. For example, an analog signal can be electronically filtered to dampen some noise, or the software can specify that the alarm must be active for a specific period of time before the alarm sounds. If the condition is checked on a regular basis, several bad readings could be required before activating the alarm. A four-out-of-five reading rule may work better than a four-in-a-row rule, because the former would avoid the situation in which a genuine alarm condition occasionally spikes into the valid area and prevents the alarm from sounding at any other time.

There are times when some alarms should activate only in certain modes of operation. During startup or shutdown, for example, conditions may occur that are not conducive to or acceptable during normal operation. These alarms, sometimes referred to as *standing alarms,* can be avoided by widening the alarm limits or disabling some alarms during the changeover period. However, care should be exercised with this approach, to ensure that the disabled alarms aren't left disabled after the changeover is finished. It may not be prudent to filter out all standing alarms, particularly in the cases where a user expects alarms in certain phases of operation. In this instance the alarm reassures the user that the requested change is actually being implemented and that the alarm is functioning correctly. If there are few alarms and they do not disguise critical conditions, allowing the user to observe the alarms may be better than filtering them out completely. For example, a low-pressure alarm may be expected when a pneumatic component of a system is turned on; the alarm will automatically reset when the system has had time to reach the required pressure. This approach would reassure the user that the alarm is working and that the appropriate pressure change has taken place within the system.

Testing Alarms

Alarms should be tested regularly during the operational life of a device. Testing the alarm during design can verify that the system is capable of detecting the appropriate alarm conditions. However, it is also important that during the life of the product, alarm systems don't become ineffective because of component failure or unexpected environmental conditions. Other system features may be exercised so often that the user is aware if they fail, but alarms may not get exercised regularly, and they must work when needed. If alarms are not tested regularly and they fail silently, the operator may perform dangerous actions but believe them to be safe because no alarm occurred.

Two levels of testing, internal and external, are possible. Although external testing is more reliable, it may not always be a viable option. In the external method, the condition that the alarm is meant to detect is physically created external to the device. For example, pinching-off plastic tubing to reduce flow and therefore activate the low-flow alarm is performed external to the device. The external method usually tests the entire system to assure that the alarm will function properly when it activates normally. With the internal method, the system is considered to have a set of self-tests, and only certain parts of the full alarm system are tested. It is possible that the alarm will appear to work in test mode but could fail when running normally, because of a fault at any point in the alarm system. For example, a button on the device might test that the device is actively connected to the facility alarm because it causes the alarm to sound. Although this test ensures that the circuit to the facility alarm system is working correctly, it does not detect the clogged facility gas inlet that is the actual condition for the alarm. The point of this illustration is not trivial. The test demonstrated that the alarm warning was audible, and this informs the user that the facility alarm is working. This test is worthwhile in that the alarm itself can be a likely point of failure, but this test does not confirm that the entire warning system works. If the device's facility gas flow sensor, used to detect low gas flow, fails, the facility alarm test button does not detect failure.

Although the external method is obviously preferable to ensure reliability, in some cases generating the condition is too hazardous or too expensive for routine testing. For example, an automated system used to grow stem cells within controlled temperature and gas ratio ranges cannot be deliberately overheated or starved for gases to establish that the alarm systems are operating, because the hazards and costs would far outweigh the benefit of testing the alarm system. There are also cases in which the designers cannot depend on users to take the time to generate alarm conditions. In those cases, internal testing is the viable option.

Discovering Safety-critical Mistakes

Many accidents can be attributed to poor user interfaces, and accidents involving medical devices have been well documented. However, such accidents may be rare enough that establishing patterns is difficult, or the information may be heavily censored for liability reasons. Therefore, it is commonly advantageous to gather information on the near misses, especially if the user is available and can provide a full understanding of the aspect(s) of the interface that caused confusion. This exercise is not always a trivial one.

Neumann (1995) compiled descriptions of computer-related mishaps in many safety-critical areas. However, you will most likely have to gather your own information on your area of expertise to fully understand the risks for an individual device. More experienced users are often happy to discuss situations that involved less senior and, possibly, less well trained staff. The company's service and training groups may have many anecdotes of user mistakes. The biggest drawback with second-hand information is that you can't always find the person who made the mistake, to investigate the actions in question.

Imagine that you are part of a team that has just begun the development of a safety-critical device. As a team, you consider it important to discover where errors were common in the interfaces of your product's predecessors, especially if the errors were safety-critical. So you gather a cross-section of your user community and address them: "Please tell me about all the occasions in which you made serious errors using the current device. I am particularly interested if any mistakes put patients' lives in jeopardy." No matter how nicely you present this request, the users will be reluctant to reveal mishaps in which they were involved. In some cases, you will need to guarantee that the information will be confidential, especially from their employer.

11

The Software Quality
Assurance Program:
Software User Interface Activities

If your computer were a person, how long 'til you punch it
in the nose?

—Tom Carey

The Ubiquitous User Interface

In the past decade, the area of human-computer interaction has blossomed from being a gleam in the eye of a few researchers to becoming an integral part of many medical devices and, consequently, their user's daily working environment. Today, the user interface is among the first things that users ask about and marketing people demand when discussing new medical device software. To the user, the interface is the system. For today's medical device users, communication with the system has become at least as important as the functionality the system provides. Although a mind-boggling number of colors and new graphics and interaction styles are available, the problems of clumsy, difficult, and hard-to-use computers are still pervasive. All of the medical devices and systems using computers and containing microprocessors and microcontrollers are all undoubtedly computing well in their intended use but are they communicating? Users are less and less willing to accept anything that isn't "user friendly," because they have been spoiled by the natural, easy-to-learn, easy-to-use, direct manipulation interfaces they enjoy on nonmedical systems. From the user's perspective, usability has become a key issue.

From the interactive system developer's perspective, ensuring usability has become an overwhelmingly important issue. From the viewpoint of many software engineers, however, the user interface is not really an integral part of the interactive system but rather just a function that gets wedged between the user and the really important system functions. However, the emerging emphasis on usability is changing this perspective so much that the user interface is becoming a critical part of the whole system, and user interface development is an integral part of the overall software engineering process.

Ensuring usability is also a pressing issue for the organization developing the product. At one time, the cost of the hardware was the principal cost of developing a medical device. As hardware costs dropped, they were eclipsed by the costs to develop the new software for those devices. Today, the cost of creating the user interface can represent up to half of the total software development schedule and a major part of the cost. The initial cost of the system is paid only once by the manufacturer, but the cost of training and the user's time for using the system, including lost productivity in struggling with the system and recovering from errors, is paid every day.

What Is Usability?

Although users state that what they need is "user-friendly" software, what they mean is hassle-free productivity. The real issue, however, is *usability.* The difficulty is that, to the user, usability represents combinations of user-oriented features, but to the developer they are combinations of user-oriented characteristics; the features are easy to understand, but the characteristics are difficult to understand. Usability, from a slightly more technical viewpoint, is the combination of the following user-oriented characteristics (Shneiderman 1992).

- Ease of learning

- High speed of user task performance

- Low, preferably nonexistent, user error rate

- Subjective user satisfaction

- User retention over time.

Usability is related to the effectiveness and efficiency of the user interface and to the user's reaction to that interface. The naturalness of the interface for the user is also an important aspect of usability.

A discussion with a software engineer about user interfaces generates all sorts of high-technology terms about widgets, interaction styles, callbacks, and everything needed to build a user interface. The discussion may, in fact, generate a feeling of confidence that powerful and new interface software programming tools have transformed the software engineer into a real interface expert. However, just because software engineers know how to use an interface toolkit does not mean that they can design a highly usable interface. One of the reasons for this is that it has been difficult to convince system developers of the need for high usability, and software engineers and managers have not always believed that there was, or is, a problem. Moreover, product planners and marketing people sometimes see the user interface as a low-importance issue with no real effect on either the purchase or the acceptance of the product.

It is also easy to mistake various other positive signs as indicators that the interface is good or even adequate. Sales volume is not necessarily a valid measure; the product might be selling well because it is the only one of its kind, the product's sales group is much more effective than that of other products, or the marketing group has priced and bundled the product attractively. Under the "no news is good news" category, the software development managers may not ever hear about the usability complaints; some users simply won't complain. Sometimes the user's organization requires a cost-to-benefit analysis to be convinced of product features. In the case of usability, however, because the individual with the authority to purchase the product or sign a volume contract is not always the final user, the distance between cost and benefit is large and cannot be measured. Nevertheless, a case can be made to management that the cost of low usability can be measured in terms of training costs and lost productivity.

The usability of a product can be qualitatively ascertained, however. Interfaces having these types of characteristics are prime candidates for developing problems with usability:

- Software engineers and not human-computer interaction specialists designed it.

- It was developed by strict top-down, functional decomposition.

- It was not developed to meet written or measurable usability specifications.

- It was not prototyped as it was being developed.

- It was not developed by means of an iterative refinement process.

- It was not empirically evaluated.

A viable interface requires that these factors be present in the software development process.

Developing Human-Computer Interaction

Human-computer interaction, or HCI, is meant to encompass what happens when a human user and a computer system get together to perform tasks. The study of human-computer interaction, a relatively new field of endeavor, is devoted to answering the question of how best to make this interaction work. As a field, human-computer interaction includes user interface hardware and software, user and system modeling, cognitive and behavioral science, human factors, empirical studies, methodology, techniques, and tools. The goal of most of the work in human-computer interaction is, in one way or another, to provide a high degree of usability.

Just as there is a difference between product software engineering and user interface software engineering, there is a difference between developing the interaction design and developing the user interface. As shown simplistically in Figure 11-1, the user interface development process consists of two parts, the interaction development and the interface software development. The *interaction component* is how the user interface works, or its topology and behavior in response to what the user sees and hears and does while interacting with the device. The *interface software* is the means for implementing the code that represents the interaction component; both parts are necessary. Because interface software development can be fit into the discussions presented in previous chapters, this chapter focuses on interaction development. The interaction component process involves both art and science, but it also draws on the engineering idea of making things good enough and not necessarily perfect. Development of the interaction component helps specify the right content in the product. It includes a life cycle, methods, techniques, and tools that make up and support the interaction development process.

Behavioral and Constructional Domains

Because of the important difference between the development of the interaction component of an interface and the development of the user interface software that implements that interaction, the two kinds of development occur in different domains. Interaction design has special requirements that are not shared by software design. However, both historically and practically,

Figure 11-1   The parts of user interface development

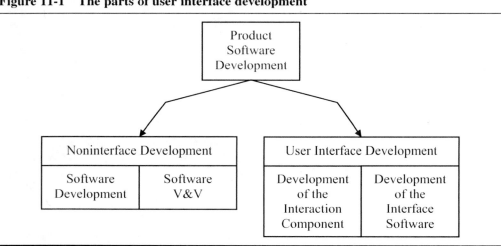

interactive systems have not always been designed and developed with this distinction between the interaction component and the interface software. The same software engineers who developed the software for the interactive system have commonly designed the interaction component. The result has been interfaces of varying quality and usability. Considerable work in the field of human-computer interaction has been directed toward new approaches to user interface development, with the hope of improving quality and usability.

The terms *behavioral domain* and *constructional domain* refer to, respectively, the working worlds of the individuals who design and develop the interaction component of user interfaces and the individuals who design and develop the user interface software. In the behavioral domain, interaction is described abstractly and independently of the software in terms of the behavior of the user and the interface as they interact with each other. Development in the behavioral domain involves human factor guidelines and rules, human cognitive limitations, graphic design, interaction styles, scenarios, usability specifications, rapid prototype development, and evaluation by human users. In the constructional domain, software engineers develop the software that implements the behavioral design. Constructional development involves widgets, algorithms, programming, procedure libraries, control and data flow, state transition diagrams, event handlers, callbacks, object-oriented representations, and user interface description languages. A comparison of the characteristics of the behavioral and constructional domains is shown in Table 11-1.

Approaching the user interface development in the behavioral domain from a user and task view results in higher usability than approaching user interface development from the constructional or software engineer view, where the software is the primary focus. This problem stems from the inherent and unavoidable conflict in developing a user interface; what is best for a user is rarely the easiest for a programmer. Both behavioral and constructional developments are necessary, and the behavioral design must be translated into a constructional design so that it can be implemented. Behavioral development does not replace constructional development; each serves different purposes. In the final product, of course, it is the merged results of both behavioral and constructional designs that determine usability. For example, a good behavioral design can run intolerably slowly, because of the implementation design, and this can adversely influence usability.

Table 11-1   Comparing the Behavioral and Constructional Domains

Criteria	Behavioral	Constructional
What is being developed	Interaction component of interface	Interface software implements interaction
What view is adopted	View of the user	View of the system
What is described	User actions, perceptions, and tasks	System actions in response to what the user does
What is involved	Human factors, scenarios, detailed representations, usability specifications, evaluation	Algorithms, callbacks, data structures, widgets, programming
The locale	Where interaction designers and evaluators do their work	Where interface software implementers do their work
The test	Procedures performed by the user	Procedures performed by the system

It is important to understand the distinction between the words *design* and *development*. In the context of user interface, these terms have a narrow and broad scope. The term *design*, which has a narrow scope, applies to the creative activity by which tasks, objects, and features are synthesized and melded to make up the user interface. The term *development*, which has a broader scope, refers to the activities of producing the user interface. This includes its own design activities, analysis, prototype development, evaluation, and iterative modification. Design is a major activity in the interaction development process because it is where the substance and appearance of the interface are synthesized; because of design's intimate relationship to other development activities, it is usually difficult to say when a developer is doing pure design.

Roles in User Interface Development

Human factor engineers have not always had a cooperating role in user interface development. For years, software engineers working in the constructional domain believed that they could design interactive systems without help from behavioral domain people. Some human factor engineers were not interested in interactive systems. Whether by edict or by guilt, constructional developers began to grudgingly let human factors engineers look at their designs. The problem with this was threefold. First, the human factor engineers could only apply human factors over the design after it was finished. Second, because they became involved in the middle of the project, they were committed just long enough to bless the design, which, in turn, caused the third problem. Regardless of whether the changes requested were major or minor, they were, in fact, major and unacceptable at this point of the project because the design had progressed too far and any change was, by definition, a significant change. In those instances where the human factor engineer did have enough authority to enforce changes, the role was viewed as that of an "inspector" who was looking for "violations" that had to be fixed. Fortunately, the situation has changed; now development projects feature teams that comprise engineers from both the behavioral and the constructional domains. However, the roles still are not always clear. For example, software engineers and computer scientists have adopted the view of the human user rather than the view of the system. Regardless of who performs the activities, the focus of user interface development is on two kinds of roles that logically correspond to the two domains of user interface development and to the involvement of human factors.

The behavioral domain is the human side of the interface. As discussed above, this broadly includes the areas of human factors, behavioral science, and cognitive psychology, and roles such as users, interaction designers and evaluators, and documentation specialists. The main role in the behavioral domain is that of the *user interaction developer,* the individual who carries out activities such as user class definition, interaction design, usability evaluation, and human factors engineering. It is the responsibility of individuals in this role to develop the content, behavior, and appearance of the interaction design. Interaction developers are directly responsible for ensuring usability, including user performance and satisfaction. They are also concerned with critical design issues such as functionality, sequencing, content, and information access, as well as such details as menu topology, forms format, input devices, and consistency across the interface. A major part of the interaction developer's job consists of setting measurable usability specifications, evaluating interaction designs with users, and redesigning based on analysis of the user evaluations of an interface.

The constructional domain is the software and computer side of the interface. This includes the areas of hardware and processors, computer science, and software engineering and roles such as software architect and designer and software engineer. The primary role in the constructional domain is the *user interface software developer.* Individuals in this role are responsible for translating the interaction design into an interface software design and then implementing that design. They are responsible for producing the algorithms, data structures, procedure calls, modules, and program code that implement the user interface, and they enable the appearance and behavior of the interaction. The software engineers work with user interface software toolkits, widgets, and other programmed interface objects.

A third distinct and important role is *problem domain expert,* a person who has in-depth knowledge of the area that an interactive application is being built to support. For example, this person is a physician if the system is a diagnostic device, a clinician if it is a clinical type of device, or a nurse if it is a patient point-of-care device. While this role typically falls into the behavioral domain, it is important enough to single out.

People in these three kinds of roles must work together and share in the design and development not just of the user interface but of the whole system, as depicted in Figure 11-2. While these roles correspond to distinguishable activities, they are mutually dependent aspects of the same effort, and they can, in fact, be performed by the same individual as long as one role does not supersede the others. These three roles represent essential ingredients in the development process; trade-offs concerning any one of them must be considered with regard to its impact on the other roles. In the past, the behavioral and constructional oriented engineers have not always worked together and didn't always seem compatible, because they usually have different goals, attitudes, skills, perspectives, philosophies, needs, techniques, and tools. However, they have cooperating and complementary roles that are essential to the development of high-quality user interfaces. The interaction developer and the interface software developer act as partners, along with the problem domain expert to produce the user interface. The three must communicate frequently during interface design and development, as they work across the behavioral, constructional, and problem domain boundaries within a team of closely coordinated peers. For example, the interface software developer communicates with the interaction developer about

Figure 11-2   Roles in an integrated team for user interface development

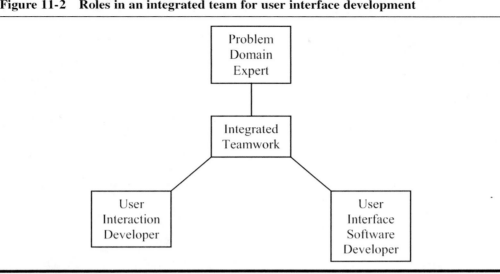

software constraints that affect the interaction design. The interface software developer may also act as liaison between the interaction developer and the interface software implementation engineer, as well as the software engineers who develop and implement the product noninterface software and mediate the interaction designs in response to their constraints.

The Value of User-friendly Medical Device Interfaces

The most difficult part of user interfaces is the feeling that there is not enough time and/or resources to use all the different techniques required to make the interface usable. At first, user interfaces will seem time-consuming and perhaps even daunting but, in reality, you do not have the time not to take the time. What frequently happens is that most of the development funds for the interactive part of the system are consumed by the implementation of a great deal of functionality that never makes it to the user because too little time was spent developing an interface that would make that functionality accessible and usable. It is better to reallocate some of those dollars and person-hours to developing an interface with high usability, even if it means somewhat lower product functionality. The funds spent on programming inaccessible functionality are essentially thrown away. To the user of an interactive system, communication is at least as important as the control and computational aspects of the product.

It is not altogether uncommon for medical device companies to spend several months developing a preliminary user-interface design, only to be dissatisfied with the result. Such organizations can come to regard a product's user interface as its Achilles' heel, especially when the competition has already brought a more user-friendly product to market. As a result, manufacturers may enlist the help and support of an objective third party such as a usability or human factors engineer, graphic designer, or marketing professional to enhance their product's usability and appeal without a major overhaul. This is certainly one approach that can be made to work. User-interface designs such as those associated with patient monitors, ventilators, blood chemistry analyzers, infusion pumps, and kidney dialysis machines often have superficial design problems that can negatively affect a device's usability and appeal but that are also relatively easy to remedy.

It is not uncommon for medical device displays to look crowded and jumbled with information and controls. Open space in displays is fundamentally important in a user interface because it helps to separate and catalog information into related groups and provides a resting place for the user's eye. Overly dense looking user interfaces can be initially intimidating to nurses, technicians, and physicians because of the difficulty in finding pertinent or specific information at a glance. What the design engineer does not put on the screen can be as important as what is put on it. To eliminate extraneous information, the user interface should present secondary information on demand via other screens. The size of graphics associated with brand identity such as logos and brand names can be reduced to provide more open areas, and simpler graphics can be used. For example, silhouette-styled icons can replace 3-D ones. Another approach that is easy to implement includes using empty space instead of lines to separate content and reducing the amount of text by stating information more simply.

Navigation among and through menus is frequently difficult and not necessarily intuitive even if the user is knowledgeable. Moving from one place to another in a medical device user interface, navigators can become lost, sometimes because they do not know where they are in the user-interface structure. For example, the end user's goal may be to set the alarm limits associated with a monitored parameter such as arterial blood pressure; instead, they become lost in a complex hierarchy of setup options that range from respiratory monitoring to reporting. At other times, the user may not understand how to move vertically or laterally within the menu structure because the methods of control are not apparent. A nurse or technician, for example, may find the way to an alarm setup screen but not recognize how to go back a step or leave the screen after making alarm-limit adjustments. Navigation options and controls, such as "Go to main menu," "Go back," "Previous," "Next," and "Help," should be grouped together in a single, consistent location on every screen. Furthermore, these types of navigation aids should be the same on every screen. The intent is that users can easily identify where and how to return to a previous screen or undo an action without concern for getting lost or causing irreparable harm. Placing meaningful titles on every screen and subcomponent, such as message boxes and other major elements, by means of a header is helpful. This can be effected as easily as providing a contrasting horizontal bar that includes text. For on-line help documents, numbering the pages can also benefit the reader. For example, each page of an eight-page electronic user's manual document could be marked "Page 1 of 8," "Page 2 of 8," and so on, for clarity.

Some medical device screens lack an orderly arrangement. In rare instances, such screens may actually appear stylish or refreshingly informal. However, most screens look and work better when they serve a utilitarian purpose and when their elements are aligned. Aligned screen elements seem less complex because they merge into a single, related set; moreover, the human eye can generally find information more quickly when scanning a straight path rather than an irregular or discontinuous one. Experienced graphic artists tend to align text on the left instead of centering it, because centered text makes the eye work harder to locate where the next line of text begins. Making the effort to fit on-screen elements into a grid pays off in terms of visual appeal and perceived simplicity. Grid-based screens also tend to be easier to implement in computer code, because the position of visual elements is predictable. Fitting these elements into a grid is fairly simple if the designer is working from scratch. However, converting an existing design that has no underlying grid structure into a more orderly arrangement is a bit more work.

When developing a grid structure, it helps to begin by defining the screen's dominant components and approximate space requirements. For example, the allotment of space for a title bar, a menu area, the body of the content, and a prompt can be achieved by dividing the screen vertically into four bands that are, respectively, 1/16, 2/16, 12/16, and 1/16 the height of the screen. Similarly, the variable content area can be divided into columns of field labels and data fields by sectioning the screen horizontally into bands that are 1/3 and 2/3, respectively, the width of the screen. The wider vertical band could also be subdivided into three additional bands, if necessary, to provide for fields with different widths. This sort of scheme can be used for displaying monitored parameter values as well as data input values. Keeping on-screen elements at a fixed distance, such as 10 pixels, from the grid lines can also provide visual appeal. The design creates margins around the grid lines, and the resulting space is a demarcation component that implies the grid and, therefore, eliminates the need for actual grid lines, which would add visual complexity to the screen. The margin width may also be used as a guide for spacing other composition elements, such as real time image displays and their caption. Most important, though, is to standardize the setback distance such that it is constant across all of the user interface screens.

Visual balance or symmetry should be created, especially around the vertical axis. This can be achieved by selecting or assuming where the vertical axis is or should be and then arranging the visual elements on either side so that each side has about the same amount of content or information as empty space. A balanced composition, whether it is an entire screen or a subcomponent, looks simple, uniform and whole; elements appear neither askew nor to be missing. It should be noted, however, that perfect symmetry might appear tedious, so the slight imbalances that are virtually inevitable should be tolerated. Perceived imbalances may be remedied by reorganizing information, adjusting the gaps between labels and fields, relocating elements to other screens, or displaying elements only on request.

Experienced designers suggest limiting the color palette of the user interface. The background and major on-screen components should be kept to between three and five colors, including shades of gray, while one-of-a-kind and small-scale elements may feature additional hues. These limits make the interface easier to look at and simpler to use. The user interface designer should also select colors carefully to be sure they are consistent with medical conventions. For example, red is commonly used to depict alarm information or to communicate arterial blood pressure values; certain secondary colors are associated with certain drugs and gases.

An efficient user interface is also based on uniform and consistent typographical rules that steer the user toward the most important information first and make screen content easy to read. The easiest way to achieve this result is to commit the user interface design to implementing a single font and just a few character sizes, such as 11-, 18-, and 24-point type. While characters should vary in size as necessary, the variations must not be so radical as to create a tense visual contrast. Another way to simplify typography is by eliminating excessive highlighting, such as underline, boldface, and italic. Because computer tools make it easy to highlight text in these ways, it becomes easy to overuse these features. In general, a single method, such as boldface, is enough to highlight information effectively when used in concert with different font sizes and extra line spaces.

Part of the difficulty with advanced technology fields is that several different terms and phrases are frequently used to describe the same physical reality. Sometimes the user interface result presents data information with all of its terminology. Redundant labeling leads to congested screens that take a long time to scan. For example, unnecessary indicators on a patient monitor that provides a summary of alarm limits associated with such patient parameters as heart rate and blood pressure could be time consuming and thus problematic for healthcare professionals. Excess visual congestion can make it difficult for users to pick out even the most salient details. However, hierarchical labeling can save space and speed scanning by displaying such items as heart rate (HR), respiratory rate (RR), pulmonary arterial pressure (PA), and arterial blood pressure (Art) more efficiently (see Figure 11-3).

Overly complex words, terms, and phrases often characterize medical device user interfaces. Despite the fact that medical workers consistently state a preference for simple language, product designers often write in a technical manner that compounds the complexity of the user interface. The user interface must be simple, because the communication of information is not only for healthcare professionals; the increasing number of patients and caretakers using devices at home may not have extensive education or training. User interface designers should assume that the user is a bright young person between the ages of 10 and 12 years old when they generate text for the user interface. Targeting this individual will usually provoke ideas on how to word things more simply and directly without compromising the user interface and turning it into automobile dashboard "idiot lights." Rules of thumb to achieve this include writing shorter sentences (one-half to no more than two lines), limiting paragraphs to two or three sentences, breaking complex procedures into ordered steps, using meaningful headings and subheadings, and using consistent syntax.

Many medical devices now employ relatively large displays with high resolution, presenting such functional options and actions as calibrating a device, setting alarms, or reading the user guide in the form of icons. This shift to an iconographic user interface style matches trends in the consumer and business software arenas. Unfortunately, medical device manufacturers do not match the major software developers in terms of their investment in icon quality, clarity, or representation. The icons that appear in most consumer and business applications are highly refined and tested by firms that employ usability engineers and graphic design professionals. Relatively speaking, a medical device company will have less time, money, and perhaps design talent to devote to icon design. Medical device manufacturers should be aware, however, that a limited investment in icon quality may produce a disproportionately large payoff, provided that talented designers are involved and icon testing is performed. In order to maximize icon comprehension and give the icons a family resemblance, a limited set of icon elements should be developed that represent nouns, such as patient, syringe, or EKG strip, there should be no cases of several

Figure 11-3   Typical example of hierarchical labeling

a. Redundant labeling

HR	Low	40	High	160
RR	Low	4	High	20
PA	Low	10	High	60
Art	Low	90	High	180

b. Hierarchical labeling

	Low	High
HR	40	160
RR	4	20
PA	10	60
Art	90	180

elements representing the same object. Further, the icon elements should be simplified to eliminate potentially confusing, misleading, and unnecessary details and accentuate the most significant aspects of the object or action. In addition, organizations should make similar-purpose icons the same overall size and should perform user testing to ensure that no two icons are so similar that they will he confused with one another. The same style should be used for similar-purpose icons, such as two- versus three-dimensional, detailed versus silhouetted, monochromatic versus multicolored, fine-lined versus bold-lined, outlined versus filled in, and so forth. The icons should also be backed up with text labels or tool tips that appear when the icon is in focus, selected, or highlighted, for example.

Design inconsistency is probably the single characteristic that defeats user interface appeal and usability and, for some medical devices, may compromise safety. For example, a user may be confused or, at the very least, annoyed by the use of the color red to communicate both critical and noncritical data. Similarly, the use of different words such as *enter, select, continue,* and *OK* to communicate the same basic function may confuse the user. To prevent such design inconsistencies, a style guide should be created and maintained. Standard existing graphical user interface (GUI) guides can be used as prototypes for style guides that are tailored to the organization's medical devices. The style guide need not necessarily start as a refined document, but merely as an organized collection of notes and rules that ensure consistent design practice at the project's early stages. Then, as a function of analyses and testing, the user interface design eventually becomes more refined, and the style guide is updated accordingly. Ultimately, the style guide can be integrated into final design specifications.

The success of most medical devices can be linked closely to the user interface quality. This is particularly true when there is substantial market competition and the associated technology has more or less matured and made user interface quality a prominent factor in product differentiation. The safety of most medical devices is also closely linked to user interface quality because design shortcomings in the user interface may lead directly or indirectly to use errors. There is no such thing as a perfect user interface; the imperfections arise from many sources, including technological limitations, incomplete understanding of user needs, and aesthetic decisions that may not match everyone's preferences. As a result, designers must aim for an optimal rather than a perfect user interface. Total user interface quality is found in the details of the superficial elements like navigation cues that, when used most appropriately, can help to create a more user-friendly design.

A Life Cycle for User Interaction Development

The life cycle concept presented here is especially suited for the needs of user interaction development. It is intended to be equally supportive of both top-down and bottom-up development, and to meet overall regulatory requirements for software V&V. Furthermore, it supports continual evaluation and iteration during interaction development and tighter, smaller loops of iteration than in the spiral methodology and minimizes the number of ordering constraints among the development activities. As shown in Figure 11-4, the phases of the life cycle are not ordered or connected in a sequence, which means that a user interaction developer can theoretically start with almost any development activity and move on to almost any other one. The various activities are highly interconnected, however, through the usability evaluation process in the center.

This life cycle is evaluation centered, and the results of each activity are evaluated before proceeding to the next activity. In general, a different type of evaluation is required after each different activity in this life cycle. The traditional noninterface life cycles lean toward a more

Figure 11-4   A typical life cycle of user interaction development

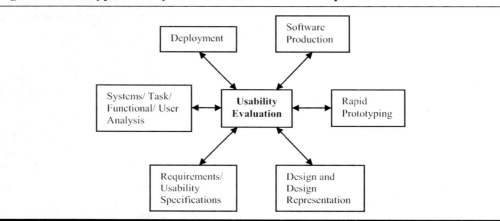

independent performance of each development activity, whereas the life cycle for user interaction development supports interdependent but distinct activities. The life cycle described here does not encompass deployment or the software production aspects. Discussions elsewhere in this book will assist the reader in determining how to implement these activities. The user interaction development activities presented in subsequent sections are representative development activities, common to almost any iterative approach; any that are currently implemented within the organization can be added or substituted. Much of the following discussion focuses on the development activities and not necessarily on the specific life cycle in which they can be set. The discussion also addresses how the activities fit together with each other and with the interface software life cycle to produce a user interface that can support specific, measurable usability claims.

The development activities of interest are predominantly in the behavioral domain. Although software production, final clean up and optimization of code, and deployment are important parts of the overall process, they are largely in the constructional domain, and those activities are not discussed. It is also important to remember that this representative life cycle for user interaction development is set within the larger and quite different noninterface software development life cycle. The highly iterative process shown in Figure 11-4 is one that potentially never ends. Some managers and organizations find this prospect frightening, but they must understand that the process must end if a product is to be shipped. The control mechanism that is used to decide when to stop iterating is based on establishing quantitative usability specifications with which to compare actual usability of the interaction design, as development progresses.

A Different Perspective of Noninterface Software Development

There are, of course, both parallels and differences between user interaction development and noninterface software engineering. The critical goals of noninterface software engineering as a technology are claimed to be software producibility and software quality. Software producibility addresses the difficulty and labor intensiveness of producing software and techniques that help with producibility, including high-level languages, abstraction, development environments, computer-aided software engineering (CASE) tools, and software reusability. Software quality usually means correctness, reliability, and maintainability. Techniques for formal specification and software V&V have been developed to verify that the implementation is faithful to the design. Very seldom does software quality include quality of the user interface. However, the critical goal for user interface development as a technology is software usability.

User interaction development and noninterface software development have many similarities. Fundamentally, they both produce parts of an interactive system and, because user interfaces are implemented with software, many software engineers believe that the well-established techniques for developing noninterface software will apply to user interface development. However, user interaction developers disagree. The real answer is that although noninterface software techniques do apply to the user interface software, they do not apply to designing the interaction with a user. Most significantly, the user is not a consideration of conventional software engineering as a discipline. To most software engineers, the system is the software, and possibly the hardware, but to a user interaction developer, the system includes the human user, and the connection to the rest of the system is the user interface. Because of this, user interaction development represents a domain with its own special problems, requiring its own skills and its own special development techniques. It turns out that noninterface software engineering development techniques do not transfer well to the engineering of user interaction, but the same types of concepts apply. However, requirements, specifications, design, metrics, evaluation, maintenance, documentation, and life cycle for user interaction must be done differently.

User interface development is a part of the larger set of development processes for an interactive system (Figure 11-5). The noninterface software referred to in Figure 11-5 is the software process and methodology discussed elsewhere in this book. The boundary between interface software development and noninterface software development is not as sharp as this figure indicates; there is unavoidable overlap between the two. The box on the left shows that users are part of the system, and their knowledge and understanding must be developed through training. The interactive medium and device development box has to do with the development of new hardware, which is outside the scope of this discussion. The hardware devices, of course, do have a strong influence on interaction styles used in development of the interaction. Interaction development is in the behavioral domain, whereas user interface software development is in the constructional domain.

A good way to view the relationship between user interaction development and software engineering is by examining how the development activities of each are modularized. In each case, the development process is divided into smaller subprocesses; through abstraction, all detail not germane to the domain of a given module is eliminated, and the developers in either domain can control complexity by limiting the amount of detail they must handle at any one time. The intention of this kind of compartmentalization is to try to separate issues by domain, so that they

Figure 11-5   Typical areas of device development

	Development of Overall System				
User Training	Development of Embedded System				
	User Interface Development			Noninterface Development	
	Interactive Medium and Interactive Device Development	Interaction Development	Interface Software Development	Device Hardware Development	Noninterface Software Development

can be considered independently of the other domains. Some issues tend to cross domains, preventing the creation of clean boundaries; this is why an integrated view is required of the development team. In any case, the boundaries introduce the need for formal communication, which, in turn, introduces new problems, such as how to handle incomplete or incorrect communication. As an example of this, examine the distinction between software design and software implementation in the noninterface software life cycle (see Figure 11-6). Some software development teams treat the communication between these activities very formally, while others resolve problems between design and implementation with less formality. The style of interaction has a large influence on how development gets done and how well it gets done in practice.

Within the domain of software design, a software designer usually works at a reasonably high level of abstraction, considering entities such as algorithms and data structures but not the details of coding. In contrast, the implementation domain requires concentration on coding; the software implementer takes the design as a given and is not concerned about analyzing the design. Consequently, the implementer avoids getting sidetracked with concerns over whether the software design should or can be improved. In reality, however, the coupling between these modules is not always as low as would be desirable. For example, limitations of the programming language selected for non-interface implementation may impose some very real constraints on what is practical in the design. Designers who take these limitations into account a priori will produce designs that are more likely to be implemented properly.

Although modularization solves some problems, it also introduces some new ones. With two modules instead of just one, a new communication need arises; the vehicle for communicating the design to the implementer is through specifications. The unfortunate thing about specifications is the difficulty in being sure they are complete and/or correct, but other formal methods provide a way to increase the likelihood of correctness and completeness. During the coding process, a skilled implementer will often know when something is missing or wrong in the specifications; there are at least two possible courses of corrective action. The implementer can try to fill in or modify the specifications or communicate the shortcomings to the designer. In the former case, the implementer is performing design, a violation of the distinction of design from implementation. More important, although the implementer may also have good design skills, the implementer is not in the best position to do this design. The implementer often will not have easy access to the design rules agreed on by the designers, the documentation of the design rationale that has guided design decisions, or methodology and structure used by the designers. The result will be ad hoc design decisions with a very high probability of introducing inconsistencies, exceptions, and deviations from acceptable design style. Furthermore, the same missing or incorrect specifications will be corrected in different ways by different implementers at different times, resulting in nonuniformity and inconsistency. Errors and other new problems may be introduced when solutions to problems do not take into account the global view used by designers to fit all the pieces of the puzzle together. As a result of these problems, most development projects have firm policies prohibiting implementers from doing on-the-fly design. As

Figure 11-6   Typical noninterface software design and implementation

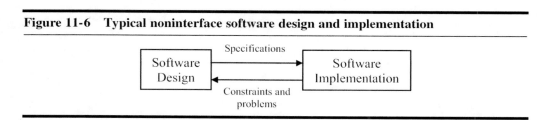

an alternative, it is important to establish an effective communication channel that feeds back design implementation issues from the implementer to the designer. In addition to this feedback, formal program verification techniques are available to confirm that the implementation meets design specifications.

In Figure 11-7, two more noninterface development activities have been added to Figure 11-6, providing a more complete picture of the process. Some of the activities having the most impact on the user interface are needs analysis, task analysis, and user class analysis. The result of systems analysis here is a set of design requirements for software designers that are high-level statements of system goals, needs, desired functionality, and features on which the software design is based. While some of the results from software testing are fed back to the implementation process, the main feedback path is to software design, where flaws and other problems are corrected, producing modifications to the specifications, which are then fed forward again to implementation. Some of the problems discovered in testing may be fundamental enough to require reconsideration in systems analysis.

To design the software in the software design box of Figure 11-7, the designer must know what the software is supposed to do. The problem domain of the system defines this. Problem domain design (see Figure 11-8) is abstract in the sense that it is independent of software design and implementation. The problem domain design is a formal model of the application that comprises theory, engineering concepts, and equations. The objective of software design is the design of data structures and algorithms that convert the problem domain design into an executable program. Inputs to problem domain design are from systems analysis, where it is decided what needs and features will be provided in the target system. This defines the underlying functionality of the developing system and the functionality that will also be supported in the user interaction design. Just as the software implementer gives feedback to the software designer about incomplete and incorrect specifications, the problem domain designer gives feedback to the systems analyst regarding missing and inconsistent requirements for the formal model. The problem domain designer also produces requirements for the software design that include algorithms, data structures, definition of modules and the calling structure, data flow, and operations. Although problem domain design and system analysis are two different roles, the activities are sometimes combined, because problem domain design is often viewed as a systems analysis resource rather than as a separate development role. The software designer provides feedback to the problem domain designer by reporting any inconsistencies, omissions, or ambiguities in

Figure 11-7   Typical noninterface software methodology

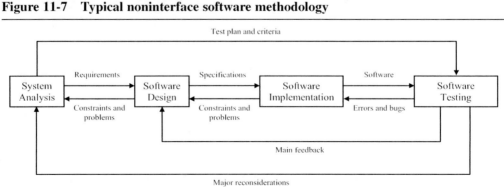

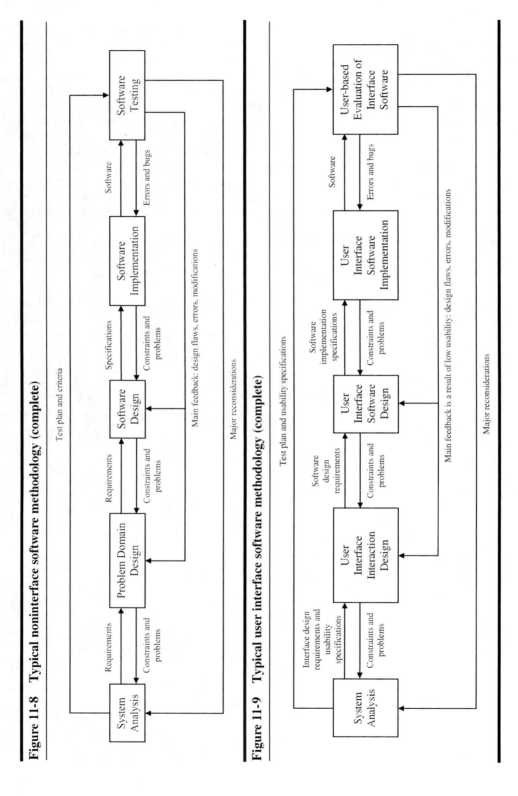

Figure 11-8   Typical noninterface software methodology (complete)

Figure 11-9   Typical user interface software methodology (complete)

the software requirements, and through verification that the software design meets the requirements. The software designer, in turn, provides specifications for software implementation, as discussed earlier.

User Interface Development

A set of activities for development of the user interface component is illustrated in Figure 11-9. The structure and labels in this figure exactly parallel those of Figure 11-8; it is important to understand that these figures are depictions of communication among development activities, not depictions of relative timing or sequencing between them.

User interface design consists of two parts; one involves software, and the other involves interaction that is independent of software, as described above. Although Figure 11-9 shows these two related activities in the context of other interactive system development activities, they are actually a connection between the two different domains. In particular, the left box corresponds to the behavioral domain and the right box to the constructional domain. Communication between these boxes is therefore the subject of representation of behavioral interaction design. Feedback of constraints and problems includes incomplete or incorrect requirements or specifications, infeasible design approaches, and limitations of development tools and environments. The left box in Figure 11-9 is different from the right, because as an activity, design of the interaction is very different from design of the interface software. As discussed in the opening sections of this chapter, interaction design involves user actions, feedback, screen appearance, and user tasks. It is also concerned with functionality, sequencing, content, and information access, as well as such details as designing interface objects, screen layout, and interaction styles.

Interface software design involves the same kinds of issues as does any other software design. If straight coding is used to implement the interface, the issues include algorithms, data structures, and the calling structure of modules. In practice, user interface software design will also involve widgets and calls to toolkit and library routines. The two kinds of design activity both contribute to the development of the user interface, but they require different skills, attitudes, perspectives, techniques, and tools. Design of software, even user interface software, is system centered, whereas interaction design is user centered and focuses on users' behavior as they perform tasks with the device.

Integration of Development Processes

In Figure 11-10, which shows the integration of the development processes in Figures 11-7 and 11-8, the far right-hand box encompasses the integrated testing, with users, of the noninterface software and interface software. The development picture is completed with the addition of rapid prototype development and formative, or usability, evaluation. The loop at the lower left corner of Figure 11-10 shows the short communication path for early evaluation of the interface prototype; design and prototype development are quickly followed by formative evaluation and then redesign, and so on. The communication distance between the user interface prototype (at the lower left) and the noninterface software implementation (upper right) indicates the gap between testing the functional software and the interface prototype as a whole-system prototype. Figure 11-10 depicts a clean separation between user interface software and the rest of the system software. In reality, such separation is usually not easy to achieve; therefore, these diagrams depict idealized distinction and communication paths among development activities and corresponding

Figure 11-10   Typical integrated software methodologies

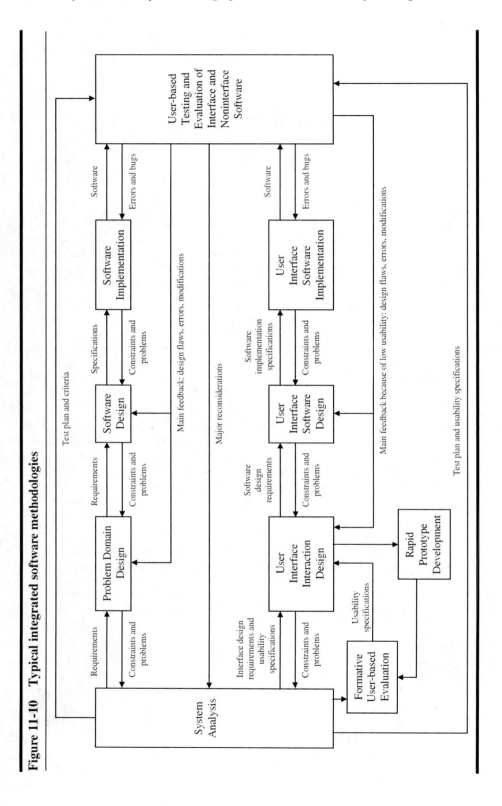

roles. As mentioned previously, many useful and even necessary paths of communication are not shown in these diagrams. The connections here, as in the previous diagrams, are not temporal and do not represent sequencing in time; the connections are communication paths (the arrows) among the various activities (the boxes) in the overall development processes. Just as some non-interface development teams treat communication formally and some treat it informally, user interface developers can be formal in their communication or they can discuss specifications and design informally.

Figure 11-10 shows the parallelism between interface and noninterface development activities in the lower and upper parts of the figure, respectively. It also shows the distinction between these parallel paths of development. In reality, there is a need for many vertical channels connecting the boxes of the two paths that represent the communication between developers of the interface and developers of the noninterface functionality connected to the interface. These interconnecting channels are essential to an integrated development team, but because these communication channels are too varied and extensive, they are not included in this diagram. Because Figure 11-10 is an idealized representation of communication paths, it does not express anything about how that communication should occur. For example, the figure shows the systems analysis group providing requirements to both the problem domain design and the user interface interaction design groups; this could be accomplished within a single, informal, highly interactive team or through formal specification documents.

Although Figure 11-10 seems to imply large development teams, this is not the case. None of the diagrams, Figures 11-6 through 11-10, are about individual versus team development; they are not about how many engineers are involved. These figures are about structuring the process with clearly defined roles and clear-cut lines of communication and about having the right abstractions and activities in the appropriate domains. How people are mapped to the roles is a function of the size of the project, the number of engineers involved, the management style, and project priorities. The most important thing is to keep the roles distinct, so that the activities, the communication lines, and the documentation are distinct. As the size of the system under development and the number of people working on it increases, communication must increase. In reality, much of this communication occurs via very informal channels; the engineers sometimes drift back and forth among roles in the process, but maintaining the distinction among roles can reduce side effects and unwanted dependencies.

Applied to the entire interactive system development process, distinguishable roles filled by people working as a team of closely integrated peers can lead to better designs, code, reliability, quality, and maintainability, and can ultimately ensure a more usable product. One way to achieve integration in practice is to have one engineer in the role of system architect, usually a senior-level engineer who understands the goals broadly and has invested heavily in achieving success. The system architect, who may not have all the needed expertise alone, will interact closely with all major contributors throughout the entire development process.

12

The Software Quality
Assurance Program:
Software Metrics

Count what is countable, measure what is measurable, and
what is not measurable, make measurable.

—Galileo Galilei

The ability to measure has fueled nearly all technological advances. Each new measurement
has given engineers and scientists ways to extend our natural abilities to better measure the physical properties inherent in objects. Measurement enhances our ability to sense things not accessible to our native intelligence. When we test and measure the phenomena around us, new vistas
of knowledge appear, and more pieces of the technical world fit into place. Each item of information concerning a technical discipline is compared to what is already known about the subject; the total knowledge about whatever had been measured is enhanced. For example, discovery
of small differences in the orbit of the planet Neptune led to the discovery of the planet Pluto,
because comparison of Neptune's predicted orbit to the measured, actual orbit led to the assumption that another planet was exerting an influence on Neptune. Mathematically, it was then
relatively easy to identify the location of the new planet, but finding Pluto would have been
impossible without the accuracy of modern astronomical telescopes and other related measuring
devices. There are instruments to measure almost every principle and practice in most technical fields, and nearly every one of them extends, refines, and improves human capabilities by
increasing sensitivity, range, speed, accuracy, precision, and consistency. Unfortunately, there
are no such instruments in software development.

Productivity, quality, and software measurement are all tied together inextricably. In retro-
spect, one of the major leaps in productivity and quality in software engineering came with the
introduction of and adherence to structured programming. Structured programming caused a significant improvement in software design quality, which was reflected in the quality of the code
and, ultimately, in the quality of the resulting system. The same quality improvements made by
structured programming also increased software productivity. The improvements reduced the

number of errors passed from the design process into the coding and testing process. Correcting an error in the design phase is less expensive than correcting it either in the coding and testing phases or after product release. Structured programming also reduced the errors passed from coding and testing into the released product. Correcting an error during the code and test phases is less expensive than correcting an error after product release.

Each of these software quality improvements depended heavily on methodology borrowed from industry. The design and software inspections favored today are both forms of measurement that were perfected in the industrial world. Although design and code walk-throughs are the formalization of the measurement process, they are manual and laborious, costly, and less than exact, and they consume valuable productive work time. Software metrics can automate much of the analysis normally performed in code walk-throughs and, thus, free the software engineer to identify quality problems quickly and take appropriate corrective action. Software quality measurement encourages quality improvement, which in turn affects the productivity of maintenance software engineers and, ultimately, end users.

High-quality software programs are easier to enhance and maintain because they are simpler and easier to understand; they also incur fewer costs relative to fixes. Quality measurement tools give the software engineer and software management immediate feedback about the quality of existing or emerging code. Measurement is the foundation of code quality. The only way to ensure software quality and productivity is to measure software products as they are produced; to measure quality and productivity effectively, the measurement process should be mechanized and automated wherever possible.

In software metrics, the measurements should provide information about software quality and productivity, but because these measurements are conceptual, they must be converted or translated into physical properties or familiar attributes. Few of these physical properties or attributes are directly measurable, but quality measurements can be inferred by combining other measurements. The collection of software metrics, then, must be broken down into simple steps that extract the needed data and combine it to produce the required measure. Although software metrics tools can measure precisely the content of software, or a software document, only recently has their accuracy been refined enough so that they have become predictors of software quality and productivity.

Software Metrics and Models

The field of software metrics is not really new. Metrics have been developed and used since the late 1960s; many metrics and methods to measure software complexity have been proposed and explored. In turn, this activity has led to and been fueled by interest in the various software development methodology and process models. Many of the proposed metrics can be obtained through algorithms, but some can only be determined subjectively. Several software development models have been constructed using various allegedly relevant factors that pertain to software size and complexity, programmer experience, and software development procedure, but none is currently in vogue or in use.

Software Complexity Metrics

The term *complexity* appears so often and in so many different contexts in software research that it is probably useful to examine its connotations. In theoretical environs, it is common to classify algorithms in terms of their computational complexity, implying the efficiency of the algorithm in its use of machine resources. The perceived complexity of software is usually referred to as psychological complexity, because it is concerned with the characteristics of the software that affect the software engineer's performance in the construction, comprehension, and modification of the software. In software, complexity is also a characteristic of the software interface that influences the resources another system will expend or commit while interacting with the software.

Software complexity implies a function of both the software itself and its interactions with various other systems, where systems are defined to include hardware, machines, people, and other software. This abstract concept of complexity can be made concrete and operational by defining and quantifying specific software metrics that are relevant to the phenomena under study. When these operational metrics are further combined according to some hypothesis or theory, a software complexity model is derived.

The specific types of complexity that have been considered include problem complexity, design complexity, and program or product complexity. For each of these complexity types, an appropriate metric accurately reflects the difficulty that a software engineer encounters in performing such routine tasks as designing, coding, testing, or maintaining the software. It is intuitive to assume that if one task is more difficult than another, it demands more skills or more effort to perform. Complexity metrics that can be obtained objectively and that can serve as the essential factors in models relating to important software development metrics, such as effort, are of paramount interest.

Objective and Algorithmic Measurements

It is possible to define software metrics that are subjective, but the disadvantages of subjective measurements are several. First, and probably foremost, is the difficulty with replication. By definition, subjective measurements are based on individual ideas and impressions about what the metric should be; this will differ with different observers. Second, even if the same observers are used, the method of assigning a value can change over time as the observer changes. Third, it is difficult to compare subjective measurements that were gathered in different studies. Last, it can be more costly to compute some subjective measurements, especially those based on the observations of several people and involving discussions among those people.

Objective or algorithmic measurement avoids many of these problems. An objective or algorithmic measurement is one that can be computed precisely according to an algorithm; its value does not change because of changes in time, place, or observer—there should be no question as to the replicability of an objective measurement. Software metrics that can be measured objectively should be comparable among several studies and allow the combination of data for research and analysis purposes. In addition, the measurement algorithm may be included in software analyzers that compute objective metrics, so that little human time is needed to obtain these values.

However, objective measurements also have inherent problems. First, in establishing computational algorithms, it can be very tedious to include all cases. For example, there is a software metric called "operand" and, intuitively, it is anything that is operated on. The question becomes, How does this apply to user-defined operands in languages that support such a capability, as well as allowing intrinsic operands to be redirected? Second, researchers differ in their opinion of the definition applied to specific metrics. For example, the most classical software metric is the number of lines of code, yet there is still no agreement on what constitutes a line of code. Last, there are some abstract concepts for which there are no attractive alternative algorithms. For example, the concept of "software complexity" has often defied agreement among researchers.

Intuitively, we know that some software is more complex than other software, but this knowledge is generally based on a combination of impressions of size, control structure, algorithms used, and data structures. Although it is possible to construct an algorithm that will measure these components, the question then becomes, How valid are the metrics?

Software quality could be based on items such as the number of errors uncovered in testing, defects discovered per thousand lines of code, defects removed per unit of time, or the elapsed time between the last two software failures; it is also possible to create functional combinations of these items. It can be argued that counting the number of errors discovered in testing is objective, but does that number bear any relation to the abstract concept of quality? Furthermore, because testing determines only the presence of errors, not the absence, does that number bear any relation to the overall totality of errors? Despite the difficulty in defining and applying software metrics, there is no shortage of complexity metrics to choose from. However, many of those that are proposed and fostered are very difficult to compute or have very little supporting evidence of their utility.

Process and Product Metrics

Measurements of software characteristics can be useful throughout the software life cycle. Software metrics are often classified as either process metrics or product metrics; they are applied to either the development process or to the software product that was developed. Process metrics quantify attributes of the software development process and environment. Product metrics are measures of the software product itself.

Process metrics include resource metrics, such as the experience of the software staff and the cost of development and maintenance. An illustration of the metrics representative of the levels of personnel experience includes the number of years a team has been using a programming language, the number of years a software engineer has been with the organization, the number of years a software engineer has been associated with a particular software team, and the number of years of direct experience constructing similar software. Other factors related to software development include items such as software development techniques, programming aids or tools, supervisory or managerial techniques, and quantity and availability of resources. In these instances, the value of the metric could be either a zero or a one, representing the absence or presence of a particular technique or process. A numeric value can also be used to represent the degree of usage for the attribute measurement. Although product metrics may reveal nothing about how the software has evolved into its current state, they do include the size of the product, the complexity of the logic and data structure, the function of the product, and a combination of these.

It may be difficult to classify certain metrics as either process or product related. For example, the number of defects discovered during formal testing depends on both the product as represented by the number of erroneous code segments and on the process that was used in the testing phase. In general, it is possible for a product metric to be influenced by the process used and vice versa, so a metric should be classified according to the factor that is believed to provide the major influence.

Metric and Model Limitations

Software metrics are currently receiving considerable attention, the hope being that management and software engineers will begin to use metrics more meaningfully in their work. The judicious use and interpretation of metrics cannot be emphasized strongly enough, particularly when attempts are made to use software metric models developed in one environment for use in a different and unsuitable environment, as well as when software metrics are used as personnel evaluation tools. There are several reasons for this caution.

First, data analysis can only be useful if the definitions of software metrics containing the data are the same. In comparing two different sets of data with items called lines of code, it is imperative that the items are really measuring the same thing. If one metrics set for lines of code excludes comment and declaration source lines while another set includes them, it will be difficult to draw conclusions from the combined data set without introducing bias. Second, most software metric models will require calibration through determination of the coefficients and constants from historical data gathered for a specific environment. Most software models cannot be transported directly from one environment to another without recalibrating; the result of violating this standard is erroneous and misleading predictions.

Third, the results of software models can support but not replace the decision-making process of experienced software engineering management. Metrics are valuable tools for decision makers, but they cannot replace managers, because, in general, metrics normally address only a small part of the development process or product; even when reasonably validated, metrics focus on only a small number of the variables involved. By their nature, product measures reflect an average of their respective software characteristics and, because of the extreme variations in human performance, such average measures may give distorted pictures when applied to specific projects. However, model and metric information, when combined with sound software engineering judgment, can help to provide greater precision for estimates and decisions. Last, software metrics and models are intended to be used for managing products and not for the evaluation of the performance of the software staff. However, metrics and models can be used to predict costs and development times for a project, as well as being a means to assess the relative performance of each software engineer.

In addition to the possible misuses of metrics, there are limitations inherent in the metric itself. Many of the predictive models rely on estimates of certain variables that may not be exactly known. For example, most predictive models use software or program size as an input parameter, yet the ability to estimate the size early in the development process is very poor. The predictive model can be no more accurate than the size prediction. Another limitation is the difficulty and cost of computing metrics where the cost of gathering them may outweigh their potential benefits. The most useful metrics are those that can be gathered automatically and with little extra effort by the software engineering staff. Some software tools tailored for specific languages can compute size, control structure, and other complexity metrics. Some companies automatically compute metrics on all code produced so that appropriate action may be taken when these metrics exceed certain prescribed limits or thresholds. Last, predictive models relating to software development should be treated as probabilistic models, because the inputs into these models are themselves subject to considerable variability. Some factors must inevitably be omitted from the model.

Metrics and Characteristics

Metrics should be objective and quantitative in the measurement of software products. Their goal is not only to improve software in general, but to help improve software despite declining resources. There are two ways to accomplish this: impose more rigorous testing and evaluate the software and its products. Although more rigorous testing is laudable, it, too, requires additional resources; frequently, the results are inadequate. Consequently, the measurement of software is a serious contender for the determination of software quality.

To measure and reflect the current state of software practice truly in an organization, a broad approach to the measurement of software should be undertaken, and the metrics should be classified into categories to ensure coverage of all facets of software engineering. Those categories should include (see Table 12-1) management, requirements, and quality metrics. When metrics are captured on a regular basis, an automated database and repository can be set up for managing and evaluating them. The data that are then collected can be used for trend analysis as well as historical analysis. As software engineers become more proficient with using metrics to manage software projects, changes and enhancements can be made to the process and

Table 12-1 Software Engineering Metrics and Characteristics

Category	Metrics	Objectives	Measurements	Apply To
Management	Software engineering environment	Quantify environment maturity	Computed maturity level	
Requirements	Traceability	Track requirements down to code	Percent requirements traced	System requirements to software requirements
				System requirements to code
				Software requirements to code
	Stability	Track changes to requirements	Number of requirements changes	Anomalies, errors, or bugs
				Change requests
Quality	Design stability	Track design changes	Stability index	Number of anomalies, errors, or bugs
				Number of change requests
	Complexity	Assess code quality	Complexity indices	
	Breadth of testing	Track testing of requirements	Percent of requirements tested	Development
				V&V
			Percent of requirements passed	Development
				V&V

Continued on next page.

Continued from previous page.

Category	Metrics	Objectives	Measurements	Apply To
	Depth of testing	Track testing of code	Degree of code testing	
	Fault profiles	Track open versus closed anomalies, errors, or bugs by type	Documentation	Open
				Closed
			Software	Open
				Closed
			Process	Open
				Closed
			Methodology	Open
				Closed
			Other	Open
				Closed
			Average open age	
	Reliability	Assess software failures		

methodology procedures. The idea to strive for with metrics is to standardize the measurement of software development and its processes, and thereby improve software quality.

Most of the metrics discussed in the literature are designed to shed light for software engineering researchers; the measurement needs of software practitioners differ from those of researchers in important ways and are based on experiences in a specific environment. Consequently, it is prudent for any organization to focus on a few key quality characteristics rather than attempt to measure everything. The organization should begin by relying on simple measures that are extractable from common design products and other sources. Many measurement schemes require more detail than is usually practicable for the typical software project, and the leap from zero or a few metrics to hundreds is too large a step. Figure 12-1 shows a basic set of software metrics that cover essential elements of cost, quality, and product attributes. The data items in the figure are metric primitives that can be combined in other ways to form rates or percentages.

Software Size Metrics

Software programs have been written in all types of languages for all kinds of applications. Some were developed with the most archaic procedures, and some used the latest and greatest

Figure 12-1   Basic software measurement set

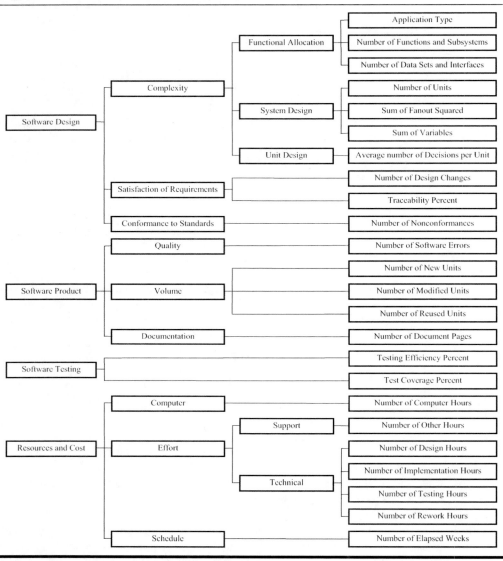

processes. Some are well documented with carefully crafted internal comments, and some have little or no documentation. The one characteristic that all software programs have in common, however, is size. The size of a program is an important measure for three reasons:

1. Size is easy to compute after the program has been completed.

2. Size is the most important and common factor used in many models of software development.

3. Software productivity is normally based on size.

The program listings generated by most compilers and assemblers have a serial number printed for each line of the program. This feature is included to provide a quick way of finding individual program lines in case there are errors in the program. An added advantage of such line numbers is that, after a program is compiled, the software engineer immediately knows the total number of lines in the program. Because nearly everyone agrees that, to a large extent, the amount of effort necessary to construct a program depends on the number of lines written, this size measure naturally becomes a dominating factor in effort-related metrics.

However, the lines of code measure may not be satisfactory for modern programming languages, because some lines or groups of lines of code are more difficult to produce than other lines in the same program. Such concerns have led to two opposing approaches to program size: (1) Refine the size measure by counting basic tokens on all lines and ignore the lines themselves. (2) Generalize the measure by grouping together the lines of code that support well-defined logical functions. Measures that relate to the lines of code, the count of tokens, and the count of functions have all been used for cost estimation, comparison of products, and productivity studies. The only method of system sizing that can be applied to any type of software, regardless of its functionality, is lines of code. Despite all of the reservations about its applicability, and all the other limitations, source lines of code are still viable as a system-sizing metric. They are still the only sizing metric that can be applied in many software activities.

Lines of Code

The most familiar software measure is the count of the *lines of code,* usually represented by the symbol S_s; its unit is LOC. For large programs, it is more appropriate to measure the size in thousands of lines of code (KLOC; symbol S). Although this may seem to be a simple metric that can be counted algorithmically, there is no general agreement about what constitutes a line of code.

For example, in the FORTRAN routine shown in Table 12-2, if S_s is simply a count of the number of lines of code, then the table contains 21 LOC. Most, but not all, researchers agree that the line of code measure should not include comments or blank lines, because these really represent internal documentation; their presence or absence does not affect the functioning of the code. More important, comments and blank lines are not as difficult to construct as program lines. However, some researchers insist that time and effort are expended on comments and blank lines, and therefore they should be counted, albeit at a lower measure; they should not count against the productivity measure of the code. The inclusion of comments and blank lines in the line count may tend to encourage software engineers to introduce artificially many such lines to create the illusion of high productivity, which is normally measured as LOC per person-month.

As another illustration, if the main interest is the size of the program that supports a certain function, it is reasonable to include only executable statements in the S_s count. This seems to be a fair alternative to the above situation, particularly, as some researchers have argued, since this represents the direct part of the code that the software engineer will really test and debug. However, this count neglects the effort that data initialization and data structure creation represents. Therefore, the productivity measure will potentially be very low, because it neglects another significant part of the software development process. Others argue that to include these types of statements is an arbitrary inflation of the lines of code, because these types of statements appear in multiple code modules and will, therefore, be counted more than once. For example, the routine in Table 12-2 has 21 lines of code, 18 lines excluding comments and blank lines, and

Table 12-2   A FORTRAN Subroutine That Sorts an Array into Ascending Order

Listing Line Number	Nesting Level	Code Listing
1		SUBROUTINE SORT(ARRAY, ENTRYS)
2		C * * SORT AN INTEGER ARRAY INTO ASCENDING ORDER
3		INTEGER ARRAY
4		INTEGER ENTRYS
5		INTEGER SAVE
6		DIMENSION ARRAY(ENTRYS)
7		C * * ONLY SORT WITH 2 OR MORE ARRAY ELEMENTS
8	1	IF (ENTRYS .GE. 2) THEN
9	2	DO 20 I = 1, (ENTRYS - 1)
10	3	DO 10 J = (I + 1), ENTRYS
11		C * * SWAP ARRAY ELEMENTS
12	4	IF (ARRAY(I) .GT. ARRAY(J)) THEN
13	5	SAVE = ARRAY(I)
14	5	ARRAY(I) = ARRAY(J)
15	5	ARRAY(J) = SAVE
16	4	END IF
17	3	10 CONTINUE
18	2	20 CONTINUE
19	1	END IF
20	1	RETURN
21		END

12 lines if only executable code is counted. It is easy to see the potential for major discrepancies in large programs with many comments, or for programs written in languages that allow for, or even require, a large number of descriptive but nonexecutable statements. Furthermore, some languages allow source code compounding, so that two or more statements can be placed on one line or a single statement can be extended over two or more lines, thus creating another problem.

The consequence of these inconsistencies is a standard definition for lines of code. In general, a line of code is any line of program text that is not a comment or blank line, regardless of the number of statements or statement fragments on the line. This specifically includes all lines containing program headers, declarations, and executable and nonexecutable statements. This is probably the predominant definition currently in use for lines of code. The count of lines of code, S_s in LOC or S in KLOC, is the total of the program lines of code.

Token Count

Another solution to the difficulty of defining the lines of code is to give more weight to the lines that have more information in them. For example, if a line of code contains a two-dimensional array, pointers, qualified names, or a function call, then it is intuitively more complex than a line that merely increments a single variable. A natural weighting scheme to handle this problem involves using the number of basic syntactic units or *tokens* that are distinguishable by a compiler. This type of scheme was devised by Halstead (1977) in his family of metrics that is commonly referred to as Software Science.

A computer program is considered to be a collection of tokens classified as either *operators* or *operands*. The Halstead measures are functions of the counts of these tokens. The basic metrics are defined as follows:

η_1 = the number of unique operators

η_2 = the number of unique operands

N_1 = the total occurrences of operators

N_2 = the total occurrences of operands.

Any symbol or keyword in a program that specifies an action is considered an operator, a symbol used to represent data is considered an operand, and most punctuation marks are also categorized as operators. Variables, constants, and even labels are operands. Operators consist of arithmetic symbols, command names, special symbols, and even function names. Table 12-3 shows a sample operator and operand analysis of the routine shown in Table 12-2. The size of a program in terms of the total number of tokens used is defined as follows:

$$N = N_1 + N_2, \tag{12.1}$$

where N is the length of the code. The metric N may be converted to an estimate of S_s by using the relationship $S_s = N/c$, where the constant c is language dependent. In Table 12-3, $N_1 = 45$ and $N_2 = 36$; the length of the routine is, therefore, $N = N_1 + N_2 = 81$.

Just as there are variations in counting the lines of code, there are also variations in the classification of operators and operands. Originally, declaration statements, such as lines 3 through 6 in Table 12-2, and input/output (I/O) statements were not counted. Furthermore, statement labels were not counted as operands, but rather were considered a part of direct transfers and were counted as two unique operators. In current practice, the tokens in I/O and declaration statements are counted, and statement labels are counted as operands wherever they are found. However, there is currently no general agreement on what is the most meaningful way to classify and count these tokens. In fact, their classification is usually determined at the convenience of the software engineer who is building the counting tool. The rules are also largely language dependent, and ambiguities in the counting of unique operators and operands are common. For example, in some languages, the "−" symbol can denote either the unary operator of negation or the binary operator of subtraction. If both uses occur in a program, are there two unique operators or two instances of one operator?

Table 12-3 A Token Analysis of Subroutine SORT

Operators		Operands	
Token Symbol	**Occurrence**	**Token Symbol**	**Occurrence**
SUBROUTINE	1	SORT	1
,	3	ARRAY	9
INTEGER	3	ENTRYS	6
DIMENSION	1	SAVE	3
IF	2	2	1
.GE.	1	20	2
THEN	2	I	5
DO	2	1	3
=	5	10	2
–	1	J	4
+	1		
.GT	1		
END IF	2		
CONTINUE	2		
RETURN	1		
end-of-line	17		

Additional metrics can be defined by using these basic terms. The *vocabulary* is defined as

$$\eta \;=\; \eta_1 + \eta_2. \tag{12.2}$$

The term *vocabulary* emphasizes the concept that if you have a programming vocabulary that consists of these η operators and operands, then the program can be successfully constructed. This means that from the large vocabulary of operands and operators the software engineer could potentially use, these η have been selected as the set to be used in the construction of the software. This leads to another measure of the size of a program, *volume,* defined as

$$V \;=\; N \times \log_2 \eta. \tag{12.3}$$

The unit of measure for volume is the bit, the common unit for measuring the actual size of a program in a computer if a uniform binary encoding for the vocabulary is used.

For the routine shown in Table 12-2 and analyzed in Table 12-3, $N = 81$ and $\eta = 26$. If a binary number scheme is used to represent each of the 26 items in the vocabulary, it would take 5 bits per item, since a 4-bit scheme leads to a maximum of 16 unique codes (not enough), and a 5-bit scheme leads to 32 unique codes (more than sufficient). Each of the 81 tokens used in the routine could be represented in order by a 5-bit code, which leads to a string of $5 \times 81 = 405$ bits that would allow the complete storage of the entire routine in memory. However, because a 5-bit scheme allows for 32 tokens instead of just the 26 that are needed, the volume uses the noninteger $\log_2\eta = 4.70$ to arrive at a slightly smaller volume of 381.

The variables S_s, N, and V are linearly related and are equally valid as the relative measures of the software size. S_s measures the same software characteristic as N, which in turn seems to be measuring about the same software characteristic as V. The size characteristics N and V are robust enough so that even a significant variation of the rules in the classification of operators and operands has virtually no effect on the resulting size.

Function Count

Units larger than the LOC are useful measures for characterizing the size of large software programs and projects. For these larger programs, it may be easier to predict the number of modules, which are independently compatible segments of the program. However, unless there are strict guidelines about the way a program is divided into modules, this metric may give little information. For example, if modules are required to be nearly x lines in length, then a prediction of m modules will lead to a projected size of $(m \times x)$ lines of code. So if a module is supposed to be 50 lines long and a software engineer reports that the program will require 100 modules, then the size of the program will be approximately 5000 LOC.

However, the definition of a module varies greatly; a more useful term is function. A *function* is defined as a collection of executable statements that performs a certain logical task, together with the declarations of the formal parameters and local variables manipulated by those statements. This approach is based on the observation that software engineers tend to think in terms of building a program from functions rather than from modules or even statements. Thus, the routine shown in Table 12-2 does not contain several lines of code but a single function called an interchange or bubble sort.

The number of lines of code for any particular function will usually not be very large. This is based on the observation that a software engineer cannot mentally manipulate information efficiently when the lines of code are greater than the limit of one's mental capacity. It has been advocated that the size of functions should be limited to the range 50 to 200 LOC, since sizes within this range tend to maximize understandability and minimize errors. However, the mental and syntactic overhead involved with the coding of a function discourages the definition of functions that are too small. It is probably easier to construct a program with three 40-line functions than it is to put together twelve 10-line functions or 120 one-line functions. The variation of the size in LOC for functions may not be as great as that for modules, because software engineers tend to use a similar number of functions to solve a given problem, but a different number of modules.

Equivalent Size Measures

Much software development consists of the modification of existing code. There are many reasons why a project may include reused code, but the fact is that for many programs, there are two components of size. The newly written code has size S_n and the adapted or reused code has size S_u. These components of size may be expressed in any of the previously discussed units, but there is an equivalent size measure, S_e, that is a function of S_n and S_u. This means that the effort required to develop the software with new and reused code is equivalent to the effort required to develop a product that has all new code and no reused code. Intuitively, S_e should not be greater than the simple sum of S_n and S_u, but there are situations in which it will actually cost more to put together several existing program segments than it would be to construct the equivalent software from scratch.

Usually, reused code consists of code adapted to fit the form and function of the program into which it is being merged. To do this, it is sometimes necessary to write some new code to be included in the existing code or to delete some existing code not needed. This makes the determination of S_n and S_u more difficult, but it is possible to delineate the new code from the reused code. Three such computations have been used frequently.

One function of the equivalent size measure used in effort estimation models (Boehm 1981a) is

$$S_e = S_n + [(a/100) \times S_u], \tag{12.4}$$

where the adjustment factor a is determined by the percentage of modification required of the design (*DM*) and of the code (*CM*) and the percentage of the effort necessary for integration of the modified code (*IM*). This adjustment factor is defined as

$$a = (0.4 \times DM) + (0.3 \times CM) + (0.3 \times IM). \tag{12.5}$$

The maximum value of a is 100, which corresponds to the case in which it is just as difficult to adapt the used code as it is to rewrite it completely. The second function, of a similar formula (Bailey and Basili 1981), is given by

$$S_e = S_n + (0.2 \times S_u). \tag{12.6}$$

The constant 0.2 was derived from an analysis of the projects studied and may not always be appropriate. The third function assumes that the contribution of the adapted code is nonlinear (Thebaut 1983). This function is given as

$$S_e = S_n + S_u^k, \tag{12.7}$$

where k is a positive constant that is no greater than 1. Through regression analysis, the value of $k \approx 6/7$ was derived, and for values of S_u up to about 98,000,

$$S_u^{6/7} > 0.2 \times S_u. \tag{12.8}$$

It is interesting to observe the behavior of these formulas on the equivalent size count if the sum of $(S_n + S_u)$ is kept constant and the proportion of new code to used code is changed. Conte, Dunsmore, and Shen (1986) made a comparison of these models and showed that all three formulas have a decreasing S_e as S_n decreases. Although there is no consensus about how to compute equivalent size, intuitively, these formulas seem very appropriate.

Function Point Analysis

A count of the source lines of code (SLOC) is a measure of the size of the user requirements for the system after decisions have been made about how to construct the system and what basic software to use, and the requirements have been translated into logic expressions in the syntax of the programming language(s) used. The one great merit of the SLOC metric is that the source lines of code can be counted objectively and automatically. However, the list of disadvantages is quite lengthy. Albrecht (1979), faced with the problem of measuring software performance and helping to improve software estimating in an environment that was already using at least three programming languages, developed an index for the functionality of a system as a measure of its size; this method is called *function point analysis*. Albrecht's original approach has undergone refinements, and it is now in wide use primarily in the information system organizations, although this method does have application to code that uses mathematical algorithms, real-time systems, and process control systems.

Mark (Mk) II Function Points have the same basic structure as those of the Albrecht method. They are obtained as the product of the measure of the information processing size and the technical complexity adjustment. In the Mk II model, the system is a collection of logical transactions. Each transaction consists of an input, a process, and an output component. It is triggered by a unique event of interest to the user. The Mk II method for determining the information processing size of a logical transaction is expressed in *unadjusted function points* (UFPs) and is based on the assumption that

$$\text{UFP} = [W_I \times (\text{number of input data type elements}) + W_E \times (\text{number of entity types referenced}) + W_O \times (\text{number of output data type elements})] \times [0.65 + C \times (\text{total degree of influence})],$$

where the weights (W_I, W_E, and W_O) of the respective types of component and the coefficient C can be determined by calibration within the organization using the UFP. The UFPs for a total system are obtained by summing the UFPs for all of the logical transactions. The process of calibration (Symons 1991) has been attempted to determine the weights by finding out how time was spent on the various components in the development of a system; values of C = 0.005 have been derived. The calibration process was extended to take the work hours used for the information processing size and break them down into the effort required to deal with the input, processing, and output; the industry average weights turn out to be $W_I = 0.58$, $W_E = 1.66$, and $W_O = 0.26$.

Although the strength of function point analysis is in business transaction application systems, two borderline applications have met with varying degrees of success. The first such application is software concerned with mathematical algorithms. Capers Jones (1986b) developed an extension of function point analysis known as *feature point analysis;* the only difference between the two methods is the introduction of the algorithm component, which can be classified as simple, average, or complex and weighted appropriately. Another borderline category for the applicability of function point analysis is real-time systems, such as process control systems, which function point analysis does not directly address. However, Reifer (1987) extended function point analysis to scientific and real-time systems with the ASSET-R method, and DeMarco's (1982) Bang metric is based on counts of the number of functional primitives on a data flow diagram of the system and the number of objects and interobject relationships in the data model diagram.

Structured analysis methods describe two approaches for determining the logical transactions of a scientific, engineering, or real-time system: the functional decomposition approach and data analytic approach; in theory, they will ultimately derive the same result for a system. In the *functional decomposition method,* system functions are repeatedly broken down or refined until unique stand-alone input, process, and output combinations at the lowest level are obtained. In function point analysis, these represent the logical transactions. In the *data analytic method,* a transaction is a process triggered by an event in the real world that transforms an entity from one state to another, updates one or more attributes of an entity, or retrieves one or more attributes of an entity. In this approach, logical transactions are the entities. Although each method will yield the same results, agreeing on when to distinguish one logical transaction from another is the toughest part of function point analysis. The decision will depend on the software engineer's perspective as to what gives rise to separately distinguishable processing as seen in the system requirements of the user.

Data Structure Metrics

A count of the amount of data input to, processed in, and output from the software is called a data structure metric. Some of these metrics concentrate on the variables and constants within each module and ignore their I/O dependencies, while others concentrate primarily on the I/O characteristics. As with the count of the lines of code, there are various methods for measuring data structures as well.

The Amount of Data

Most compilers and assemblers have an option to generate a cross-reference list that indicates the printed line number where a certain variable is declared, used, and referenced. One method for determining the amount of data is to count the number of data entries in the cross-reference list. However, care should be exercised to eliminate from this count those variables that are defined but never used. The definitions of these variables may be made for future reference, but they do not affect the operational characteristics of the software or the difficulty of development.

The *count of variables* is referred to as *VARS*. For example, a compiler cross-reference listing of the routine in Table 12-2 identified ARRAY, ENTRYS, I, J, and SAVE as variables and therefore *VARS* = 5. In general, a *variable* is a string of alphanumeric characters defined by a software engineer; it is used to represent some value during either code compilation or code execution. Although a simple way to obtain *VARS* is from a cross-reference list, it can also be generated by using a software analyzer that counts the individual tokens as described above. Just as with the counting of the lines of code, the algorithmic approach to determining the value of *VARS* is, in fact, somewhat subjective. For example, language-specific items like eof, input, output, PRINT, TYPE, WRITE, READ, or even the name of the routine or function can appear as variable names. However, because none of these is a variable, in the sense of variables that are created to produce a program, they should be excluded from the *VARS*.

Another consideration in the *VARS* deals with constants. For example, in Table 12-2, the constant 2 is used to avoid the sorting of arrays that have fewer than two elements; in addition, the constant 1 is used to provide control of the array element range during comparison processing. Neither of these constants is in the *VARS*, but they nonetheless serve special purposes in the routine. Furthermore, mathematical constants, such as pi, are important for trigonometric or logarithmic applications. Even array references that have explicit indices, such as A(11), may indicate some special meaning for that particular location.

The metric η_2, introduced previously as the count of the operands in the software, included all variables, constants, and labels. Therefore, the count of the operands can be redefined as

$$\eta_2 = VARS + \text{unique constants} + \text{labels}. \qquad (12.9)$$

For example, the SORT routine shown in Table 12-2, and analyzed in Table 12-3, has five variables (ARRAY, ENTRYS, I, J, and SAVE), two constants (1 and 2), and three labels (SORT, 10, and 20); therefore, $\eta_2 = 10$. The name of the routine is counted as a label, because it is the label that will be used by any other routine that wants to access SORT. Note that η_2 is the count of the number of unique operands and fails to capture the total operand usage. Consequently, the metric N_2 captures the total number of occurrences of all operands in the software. For the routine in Table 12-2, $N_2 = 36$.

The metrics *VARS*, η_2, and N_2 are probably the most popular data structure measures; they seem to be robust. Slight variations in the algorithm computation schemes for computing them do not seem to affect inordinately any other measures based on them.

Live Variables

A software engineer must constantly be aware of the status of several data items during the programming process. Intuitively, the more data items that a programmer must keep track of when constructing an individual statement within the program, the more difficult the program will be to construct. Another data metric of interest is the size of the set of those data items that are *live variables* (*LV*) for each statement in the program.

The set of live variables for a particular statement is not limited to the number of variables referenced in that statement. For example, the particular statement being considered may be just one of several that set up the parameters for a complex procedure. The software engineer must be aware of the entire list of parameters to know that they are being set up in an orderly fashion, so that any statement within the group disturbs no variables needed later in the program. Consequently, a variable is live from its first to its last references within a procedure (Dunsmore and Gannon 1981); a software analyzer can be constructed to produce live variable counts for all statements in a program or procedure. Table 12-4 lists an example of live variable counting for the routine shown in Table 12-2.

From this, it is possible to define the *average number of live variables* (LV_{avg}) as the sum of the count of live variables divided by the count of executable statements in a procedure. This is a complexity measure for data usage in a program or procedure. The average number of live variables for the routine in Table 12-2 is $LV_{avg} = 20/12 = 1.7$. Although this discussion is relative to a single procedure or module, it can be extended into a program metric. For example, the *average number of live variables for a program* ($LV_{p\text{-}avg}$) of *m* modules is given by

$$LV_{p\text{-}avg} = \sum^{m} LV_{i\text{-}avg}/m, \tag{12.10}$$

where $LV_{i\text{-}avg}$ is the average live variable metric that was computed for the *i*th module.

Live variables depend on the order of the statements in the source code and not on the dynamic, run-time order in which they are encountered. A metric based on the run-time order

Table 12-4   Live Variables Analysis for Subroutine SORT

Executable Code Line Number	Cumulative Live Variables	Count
8	ENTRYS	1
9	ENTRYS, I	2
10	ENTRYS, I, J	3
12	I, J, ARRAY	3
13	I, J, ARRAY, SAVE	4
14	I, J, ARRAY, SAVE	4
15	J, ARRAY, SAVE	3
16		0
17		0
18		0
19		0
20		0

would be more precisely related to the life of the variable and would be much more difficult to define algorithmically.

Variable Spans

Two variables can be alive for the same number of statements, but their use within those statements can be markedly different. A metric that captures some of the essence of how often a variable is used within the software is called the *span (SP)*. This metric is the number of statements between two successive references to the same variable (Elshoff 1976). For a program that references a variable in n statements, there are $(n - 1)$ spans for that variable.

The size of the span indicates the number of statements that pass between the successive uses of the variable. A large span can require that the software engineer remember a variable that was last used far back in the program. This increases the amount of information the software engineer must remember during the construction of the program. The *average span size* (SP_{avg}) of a variable with n spans is

$$SP_{avg} = \sum{}^{n}SP_i/n, \tag{12.11}$$

where SP_i is the span size of the ith span. For example, if a variable has four spans of 10, 12, 7, and 6 statements, then it has an average span of 8.75. Although this discussion is relative to a single procedure or module, it can be extended into a program metric. For example, the average span size of a variable for a program $(SP_{p\text{-}avg})$ of n spans is given by

$$SP_{p\text{-}avg} = \sum{}^{n}SP_{i\text{-}avg}/n, \tag{12.12}$$

where $SP_{i\text{-}avg}$ is the average span size computed for the ith span.

Logic Structure Metrics

The logic structure of a program allows the software to perform different operations dependent on different input data, intermediate calculations, or various physical states. The ability to test data and take action dependent on the outcome of the test severely complicates the difficulty and comprehension of the software, because the branching that takes place is based on the test outcomes that create new pathways through the software. The tests made and the actions taken in a branch after a test are often grouped together and compose a separate logic structure. As with all the metrics presented so far, there is no agreement on which logic metric is the most important. Even for metrics with the same name and intention, different counting schemes have been used.

Decision Count

The flow of control in a program is normally sequential, but it can be interrupted in three possible situations:

1. It can branch forward on the basis of a conditional test that leads to a choice between at least two possible actions.

2. A backward branch can be used to create loops, which may be unconditional or may follow a conditional test that allows another iteration or the termination of the loop.

3. A horizontal branch is typically a transfer of control to a procedure or routine and is not normally considered an interruption, because when the invoked procedure terminates, it is supposed to return control to the statement immediately following the branch.

A simple control structure metric is called the *decision count* (*DE*) (Shen et al. 1985); it is the count of the number of IF, DO, WHILE, UNTIL, CASE, and any other conditional and loop control statements. For example, in the routine in Table 12-2, $DE = 4$. Software with a larger *DE* value is considered to be more complex than software with a lower *DE*. Many programming languages allow the use of compound conditions in IF and other conditional and loop control statements; to accommodate this, an IF statement with two simple conditions is counted as contributing two to the count of decisions. Thus, the number of conditions within the IF statement are counted, rather than merely the number of occurrences of the keyword for the particular conditional statement. Similarly, the CASE statement is considered to be a statement with multiple predicates, and it is the predicates that are counted.

A more sophisticated and better known metric based on the number of decisions is the *cyclomatic complexity number*, $v(G)$ (McCabe 1976). The cyclomatic complexity number is defined in a manner similar to that of the cyclomatic number in a directed graph. In a directed graph

$$v(G) = e - n + p, \tag{12.13}$$

where e is the number of edges, n is the number of nodes, and p is the number of connected components in the flow graph. The cyclomatic complexity number, however, has a branch from the exit node to the entry node in a flow graph before computing the measure so that $p = 2$. Therefore, a flow graph with e edges and n nodes is defined as

$$v(G) = e - n + 2. \tag{12.14}$$

As with the count of *DE*, the higher the cyclomatic complexity number, the more difficult and complex the module becomes. Available commercial packages will calculate the cyclomatic complexity number. A computationally more attractive formula for $v(G)$ is

$$v(G) = DE + 1; \tag{12.15}$$

this calculation can be easily obtained by an automated software analyzer.

The cyclomatic complexity number for a multimodule program is simply the sum of the value of $v(G)$ for the individual modules. For example, for a program with m modules,

$$v(G_{\text{program}}) = \sum^m v(G_i) = \sum^m e_i - \sum^m n_i + (2 \times m), \tag{12.16}$$

where $v(G_i)$ is the cyclomatic complexity number of the ith module. Since $v(G_i) = DE_i + 1$,

$$v(G_{\text{program}}) = \sum^m DE_i + m. \tag{12.17}$$

Nesting Levels

Another important complexity metric is the *depth of nesting*. For example, a simple statement in the sequential part of a program, such as line 8 in Table 12-2, may be executed only once. A similar statement, such as line 12, is executed on the order of $ENTRYS^2$ times, because it is a part of the inner loop. The higher the nesting level, the more difficult it is to assess the entrance conditions for a certain statement. Such difficulty leads to the definition of the metric *average nesting level* (NL_{avg}) (Dunsmore and Gannon 1980).

In order to compute this metric, every executable statement in a program must be assigned a nesting level. Most compilers will produce a nesting level indicator along with the printed line number for each line of source code that is listed. Because this is not always generated, however, a simple, three-step recursive procedure for generating the nesting level is useful:

1. The first executable statement is assigned nesting level *l*.

2. If statement *a* is at level *l* and statement *b* simply follows sequentially the execution of statement *a*, then the nesting level of statement *b* is also *l*.

3. If statement *a* is at level *l* and statement *b* is within the range of a loop, or a conditional transfer governed by statement *a,* then the nesting level of statement *b* is *l* + 1.

In Table 12-2, all executable statements have been assigned a nesting level on the basis of this procedure. The average nesting level (NL_{avg}) is the sum of all the executable statement nesting levels divided by the sum of the number of statements. For Table 12-2, the number of executable statements is 12, the sum is 36, and the average nesting level is 3.0.

Transfer Usage

A metric for the use of GOTO statements is the measure *knots* (Woodward, Hennell, and Hedley 1979). To define the knots metric, assume that the lines in a program are numbered sequentially. Let an ordered pair of integers (*a, b*) indicate that there is a direct transfer from line *a* to line *b.* Given two pairs (*a, b*) and (*c, d*), there is a knot if one of the following two cases exists: (1) min(*a, b*) < min(*c, d*) < max(*a, b*) and max(*c, d*) > max(*a, b*), or (2) min(*a, b*) < max(*c, d*) < max(*a, b*) and min(*c, d*) < min(*a, b*). The knot count reflects the concept that an inappropriate use of the conditional statement may increase the logical complexity of the software.

For languages that permit multiple statements on one line, the source code probably should be reformatted so that all direct transfers are on individual lines before applying this definition to determine the number of knots. In certain situations, this rearrangement of some of the statements in the program will not change the function of the program, but it will alter the knot count. For these equivalent programs, the one with the lower knot count is believed to be better designed.

Composite Metrics

The metrics presented so far are basic count metrics and, other than the minor variations in their definition, are noncontroversial. Additional software metrics are functions of the four basic metrics η_1, η_2, N_1, and N_2. Many of these composite metrics have been met with some degree of controversy and opposition concerning their theoretical basis and empirical support; consequently, they are used sparingly. Some of the composite metrics are described here to complete the metrics philosophy, to show that they are of interest, and to demonstrate some degree of usefulness.

Estimated Program Length

One measure of the size of a program is the total number of tokens, or length *N,* which was defined previously as the sum of the total operator and operand occurrences ($N = N_1 + N_2$). In reality, though, the length of a well-structured program is a function of only the number of unique operators and operands. This function is called the *length equation* and is defined as

$$N_{hat} = \eta_1 \times \log_2\eta_1 + \eta_2 \times \log_2\eta_2. \qquad (12.18)$$

For example, the SORT routine in Table 12-2 has 16 unique operators and 10 unique operands, as shown in Table 12-3.

If these numbers had been known before the completion of the program, possibly through the use of a programming design language, and knowing the programming language to be used, then it is possible to estimate the length N_{hat} of the program in number of tokens by using this equation. Using the token counts from Table 12-3, $N_{hat} = 16 \times \log_2 16 + 10 \times \log_2 10 = 98.2$. This indicates that if the total number of operands and operators could be predicted before the coding actually started, then there will be about 98 tokens used in the completed program.

While it may not be a precise equality for a specific program, N_{hat} may be considered statistically valid over a large collection of many programs (Shen, Conte, and Dunsmore 1983). The length equation can be viewed as a relationship that explains typical performance, even though it fails to achieve precision in specific instances. It is also known that certain poor programming practices can make the length equation a poor predictor of N (Halstead 1977).

Potential Volume and Difficulty

An algorithm may be implemented by many different but equivalent programs. Among these programs, the one that has minimal size is said to have the *potential volume* V^*. The minimal implementation of any algorithm is through a reference or a call to a procedure that has been previously written, because the implementation of this algorithm requires nothing more than invoking the procedure and supplying the operands for its parameter list. The potential volume of an algorithm implemented as a procedure call is expressed as

$$V^* = (2 + \eta_2^*) \times \log_2(2 + \eta_2^*). \tag{12.19}$$

The first term in the parentheses represents the two unique operators for the procedure call itself, the procedure name and the grouping symbol that separates the procedure name from its parameters. The second term in the parentheses represents the number of conceptually unique input and output parameters. For the SORT routine in Table 12-2, these conceptual parameters are shown in the header of line 1 as ARRAY, the array holding the integers to be stored, and ENTRYS, the number of array elements to be sorted. From this, $\eta_2^* = 3$, because ARRAY is used as both input and output, and the potential volume V^* of the sorting routine is $V^* = 5 \times \log_2 5 = 11.6$. While η_2^* can probably be determined for small application programs, it is much more difficult to compute for large complicated programs.

Any program with volume V is considered to be implemented at the *program level L,* as defined by

$$L = V^*/V. \tag{12.20}$$

The value of L for a program is a maximum of 1, which represents a program written at the highest possible level or minimum size. The sorting routine in Table 12-2 is implemented at level $L = 11.6/381 = 0.030$. The inverse of the program level is the *difficulty D,* defined as

$$D = 1/L. \tag{12.21}$$

As the volume V of an implementation of a program increases, the program level L decreases and the difficulty D increases. Programming practices such as the redundant usage of operands or the failure to use high-level control constructs will tend to increase the volume metric as well as the difficulty metric. For the sorting routine, $D = 1/0.030 = 33.33$.

The program level L of a particular implementation of an algorithm depends on the ratio of the potential volume V^* and the actual volume V. The potential volume metric is usually very hard to determine, however, so an alternate formula that estimates the program level is defined as

$$L_{hat} = 1/D_{hat} = (2/\eta_1) \times (\eta_2/N_2). \tag{12.22}$$

An intuitive argument for this formula is that programming difficulty increases if additional operators are introduced and if an operand is used repetitively. Each of the parameters used to compute L_{hat} can be obtained by counting the operators and operands in a finished program. Using the sorting routine, $\eta_1 = 16$, $\eta_2 = 10$, and $N_2 = 36$, so that $L_{hat} = (2/16) \times (10/36) = 0.035$. An alternate formula to determine an estimate of the potential volume is

$$V_{hat}^* = V \times L_{hat}. \tag{12.23}$$

Using the sorting example, $V_{hat}^* = 381 \times 0.035 = 13.34$.

Effort and Time

The effort required to implement a computer program increases as the size of the program increases. It also takes more effort to implement a program at a lower level and higher difficulty than an equivalent program at a higher level and lower difficulty. *Effort* is defined as

$$E = V/L_{hat} = D_{hat} \times V = (\eta_1 \times N_2 \times N \times \log_2\eta)/(2 \times \eta_2). \tag{12.24}$$

The unit of measurement for E is *elementary mental discriminations*. Using the sorting routine again, $E = 381/0.035 = 10,886$. This means that 10,886 elementary discriminations are required by the software engineer to construct this routine.

The human mind is capable of making a limited number of elementary discriminations per second and this number, β, ranges between 5 and 20. Because the effort E uses elementary mental discriminations as its unit or measure, the programming time T of a program in seconds is

$$T = E/\beta. \tag{12.25}$$

The value of β is usually set to 18, determined through experiments to correlate with observed programming times.

This formula can be used to estimate the programming time when a problem is solved by one proficient, concentrating software engineer writing a single-module program. For the sorting routine, $T = 10,866/18 = 605$ seconds < 10 minutes. Although a formula for estimating the time to write a software program seems like a valuable tool, it is currently not in favor, because the original work by psychologists on the number of elementary discriminations per second lacks good empirical evidence, and there is a poor analogy between the domain of that work and that of software engineering.

Language Level

There are hundreds of programming languages that can be used to create a software program. It is not unusual for several to be in use within any company at the same time. Each language has its supporters and advocates, who argue that their favorite language is the best to use; these arguments tend to suggest a metric that expresses the power of a language. If the programming language is kept fixed as V^* increases, then L decreases in such a way that the product $(L \times V^*)$ remains constant. This product, called the *language level* λ, can be used to characterize a programming language:

$$\lambda = L \times V^* = L^2 \times V. \tag{12.26}$$

When several programs were examined that had been written in different languages, the average language level metrics were determined to be 1.53 for PL/1, 1.21 for Algol, 1.14 for FORTRAN, and 0.88 for assembly languages in general (Halstead 1977).

Although these average λs follow the intuitive rankings by most software engineers for these languages, they all have large variances. These fluctuations are not entirely unexpected, because the language level metric depends on the language itself, the nature of the problem being programmed, and the proficiency and style of the software engineer. Nevertheless, studies have failed to confirm that λ is statistically constant for any language; what the studies do show is that λ is a decreasing function of program size.

If equation 12.26 for λ was valid, then it could be useful in the selection of a programming language for a particular application area. For a given problem with fixed V^*, the programming effort is inversely proportional to the square of the language level, or

$$E = V^{*3}/\lambda^2.$$
(12.27)

This relationship, for example, may help project software engineers to decide, on the basis of the availability, reliability, and efficiency of various compilers, the appropriate language to be used for a given problem or application.

Software Defects

Despite recent advances in software engineering technology, it is not yet possible for software engineers to produce error-free software consistently. As a result, a significant amount of effort is typically allocated to testing and correcting software before its delivery. A software product is considered defective when it does not perform according to the user's expectations. However, defects can be divided into several types. A fault is an error in the software that causes the software to produce an incorrect result from valid input. Software may fail for several distinct input sets because of the same fault; a single input set may reveal several different faults. Although it is difficult to identify and fix all of the faults in a program, one can concentrate on the evidence of the presence of faults by counting the number of defects. A defect is the evidence that a fault exists.

The actual number of defects can only be determined dynamically by fixing an error. If the input set(s) that caused earlier failures now yield correct results, there was only one defect. If an input set still yields incorrect results, then there were originally at least two defects, or fixing the first defect has created a second defect. It is desirable that the input sets used to test the software are independent in the sense that the failure or success of one test run does not necessarily imply the success or failure of another. To manage the testing and maintenance phases of the software life cycle, it is often desirable to estimate the number of defects in the software.

Defect Metrics and the Software Life Cycle

There are four software life cycle phases that are logically similar from the standpoint of introducing, discovering, and fixing defects: the design, coding, testing, and maintenance phases. In the design phase, defects can be caused by a poor understanding of the requirements or specifications as well as by unclear requirements or specifications. This can lead to an incorrect design that will later lead to incorrect code. Defects can be fixed in this phase by recognizing that the design does not fully satisfy the specifications. In the coding phase, defects can be caused by poor understanding of the design, poor choices of data structures or algorithms, or errors in the logic or syntax of the software. Defects are fixed in this phase by changing the code or by altering the design to match the code already in place.

During the testing phase, defects may not be caught without appropriate test data being used and some formalized method, such as verification, being employed. Furthermore, some defects will be created during the correction of other defects. Defects are generally fixed in this phase by code changes. In the maintenance phase, every execution of the software constitutes a new "test" case, and the defects found are fixed in a manner similar to that of the testing phase. However, there is usually a reluctance to change the software as long as the software is reliable, in which case the documentation may be changed instead. Inadequate performance of the software in this phase may result from many causes other than incorrect code, including poor documentation or poor understanding of the software or documentation by the user.

Because it is often easier to change the documentation than to change the software, it is not uncommon to remove software defects by making a change. As there is no easy way to determine which documentation changes are results of genuine documentation errors, the study of software defects usually concentrates on errors that lead to design and code changes. There are three typical metrics for assessing the defects in software.

The metric *number of changes required in the design* begins with the design phase and results from a faulty understanding of the specifications. Excluded from this metric are those design changes made because of dynamic requirements or specification changes. The counted design changes can occur anywhere in the software life cycle from the design phase on, whenever a defect is discovered. The method of computing the number of changes required in the design is subject to a count based on the software analyst's assessment of the number of items changed.

The metric *number of errors* counts the defects when they are discovered from the coding phase on, and especially during the testing phase. After a program reaches the point where it is written, any errors uncovered via hand checking, walk-throughs, or testing can be counted in this metric. In many instances, formal software error reports are generated whenever errors are found; a count of the different error reports can be used as a defect metric.

The *number of program changes* is an algorithmic defect metric based on the fact that defects are usually fixed by means of alterations to the code. In this case, the code changes can be observed to determine where defects must have been present. This metric depends on the ability to exclude any code changes related to changed specifications and to include only those involved in fixing errant software.

The difficulty with the number of program changes metric is that it is not nearly so cut and dried as the previous two types of changes, especially when it deals with a contiguous set of statements that represent a single abstract action to be corrected. In this case, for example, each of the following code text changes represents a single program change: (1) one or more changes to a single code statement; (2) one or more statements being inserted between existing statements; and (3) a change to a single statement that is followed by the insertion of new statements. The last instance represents the situation in which an existing statement is insufficient and must be altered and supplemented by additional statements to implement the abstract action intended. The insertion and deletion of debugging statements, comments, and blank lines are not counted as program changes because they do not directly relate to program defects. Simple deletions of statements are not counted because they are normally counted by insertions elsewhere in the code. A defect report may lead to more than one program change, so the complexity and seriousness of a defect may be reflected by the number of program changes it takes to correct the defect.

It is reasonable to expect that larger software programs will have more errors and, therefore, more changes. The raw count of the number of errors or program changes is not very meaningful for discerning whether the software has a lot of defects or just a few. For example, a 17-line program requiring three program changes is a poor software development performance, but three program changes for a 1000-line program is good. To compare the defects in software meaningfully, the raw counts are normalized by the size of the software. The most common metric for defect comparison is the defect density, defined as

$$\text{defect density} \ = \ \text{number of defects}/S, \qquad (12.28)$$

where S is the program size in thousands of lines of code. However, the defect density will vary as a function of the program size.

There are other characteristics of defects than just the number or the density of them. It is possible to consider defects in terms of their severity. If a severity number or index is desired, this metric can be obtained by running the software with a set of test cases, and the percentage of runs judged as failures can be used as a severity metric, assuming that the test cases are independent. Another way to account for the differing severity of defects is to count the number of changed lines of code, which is conceptually thought of as the weighted sum of the metric of program changes. For example, a 100-statement change is counted as 100 times more severe than a single-statement change.

Another concern with defects, the difficulty of actually fixing them, is usually independent of their severity. A very serious error may require a single statement change and only a few minutes of time to accomplish. Less severe defects may require person-hours of analysis to determine the particular set of circumstances that caused the defect. Defects can be characterized by either the time required to repair them or the estimated time for defects not yet repaired. As before, this time can be normalized by the number of thousands of lines of code or even the number of defects, to be made comparable.

Discovering and Correcting Defects

Whenever a defect enters the software, it may not be discovered until late in the process. To help discover defects earlier, regular design and code reviews and inspections are held on a formal and informal basis. During this process, the reviewers are "walked" through the software structure in detail so that the concerns of reviewers are either explained away, or identified as action items. The number of recorded action items can be considered as the number of defects in the design or code. In fact, all three of the defect metrics discussed can be used to capture the results of the walk-through.

Toward the end of the coding phase, the software engineer is expected to test separate modules by using appropriate data according to the I/O specifications of the modules. This activity is commonly called unit testing; the number of defects found and the number of program changes can be recorded as the code is changed to make the module work correctly.

The number of defects discovered during the design and coding phases is represented by d_0. However, in addition to the inherent quality of the design, d_0 depends on several other factors; many changes may be the normal consequence of the evolutionary nature of the design process. If the software engineer attempts to construct a complete program during the design and coding phases, with the intention that it should run correctly without effort, then d_0 may be an accurate measure for the quality of the code. If the software engineer prefers to let the code evolve into the final state through successive testing and changes, then d_0 may not be meaningful. Because it is difficult to record consistently and algorithmically the reasons for changes that are made, defect measures during the design and coding phases will not have been thoroughly investigated. However, if the verification and validation group generates defect or error reports during these phases, it is reasonable to use these as a measure of defects.

During the testing phase, most software is tested before release by groups independent of the software development team. During this phase, the number of defects found and the number of program changes can be especially useful. Frequently, this testing group assembles a large number of test cases based on the specifications for a product. When the product is a revised version of a previous product, many of the test cases assembled for the earlier version are reused for the current version. In either case, defects that are found during this testing are normally sent back to the designers and software engineers to be fixed; these defects are recorded as a part of the software metrics.

The number of defects discovered during the testing phase is represented by d_1. To make sure that all defect reports are handled promptly, they are usually documented on a formal test report that is maintained either manually or electronically on-line. In either case, the defect report can be resolved by changing the code or the documentation or by identifying the defect to be a duplicate of some previously reported problem. The defect may also be categorized as invalid if the software engineer cannot reproduce the problem with the same test case, or if the defect is due to erroneous application of the test case. The existence of this defect-reporting mechanism provides an objective measure for d_1. The type of resolution for the defect also provides a meaningful measure; it is a natural by-product of the defect-capturing mechanism. However, the total number may not be appropriate unless the invalid reports or duplicate reports are removed from the count.

The maintenance phase of the product's life cycle begins at the point of the product's external release. During this phase, all three of the defect metrics are still applicable, because the product will be undergoing error correction, feature addition, and performance improvement. These three metrics can be tracked not only by means of the defect-reporting mechanism, but also from the count of error reports made by the product's customers. Generally, customers discover a relatively large number of defects shortly after product release; when a certain threshold of usage is reached, fewer and fewer errors are discovered thereafter. The number of defects discovered after release and during the maintenance phase is represented by d_2.

For the rest of this discussion, the following designations will be used for the number of defects found in the various software development phases. Given that d_0 represents the defects discovered during the design and coding phases, that d_1 represents the defects discovered during the testing phase, and that d_2 represents the defects discovered after release and during the maintenance phase, the total number of defects is defined as

$$d_{\text{tot}} = d_0 + d_1 + d_2. \tag{12.29}$$

Software Defect Models

Methodologies such as structured design, design reviews and code walk-throughs, and conventions for module interfaces are attempts to reduce the probability of human error in software development. It is impossible, however, to enforce earlier software design decisions in the same way as physical constraints are used to enforce hardware design decisions. Because there is an almost infinite number of ways to do something, and many of those ways can result in a catastrophe, there are defects in most software systems. It is surprising that even under these circumstances, software products can be as reliable as they sometimes are.

Since a significant amount of effort is often allocated to the testing of software, a priori knowledge of the error proneness of the software being tested could make the testing process more efficient and effective. Accurate knowledge of the number of defects that remain in the software can make the decision on the software release date more rational. Two types of models assess some quality aspects of the software. A static model uses software metrics to estimate the number of defects in the software. A dynamic model uses the past defect discovery rate to estimate this rate for the future.

Static Models of Defects

A static model of software defects assumes the general form

$$y = f(x_1, x_2, \ldots, x_n).$$

(12.30)

The dependent variable y is the defect metric, such as any of those presented above. The independent variables $x_1, x_2, \ldots, x_n$ can be either product or process related. The model is static in the sense that it estimates the dependent variable on the basis of current values of the independent variables and ignores, for example, the rate of change of the metric over time. A reasonable predictive model for a certain defect count depends only on metrics measured before the defect count itself can be measured. For example, a predictive model of postrelease defects (d_2) based on product metrics is reasonable, because all of the product metrics can be objectively measured before the product is released. However, a model of the number of defects found during the testing phase (d_1) cannot use the number of postrelease defects (d_2) as an independent variable, even though both sets of data may be available at some later date when the analysis is made. Models whose independent variables can be measured much earlier than the dependent variable have the potential of being used to guide the release, testing, and maintenance processes.

Defect Model Studies

The defect counts used in the models discussed in this section may be either the number of defects found or the number of changes. The metric number of defects found is used when the analysis is performed at the product level, where the defects are measured for completed programs or systems. The metric number of changes is often used when the analysis is performed at the module level. When both metrics are available, the latter count is at least as large as the former, because a defect may require changes in more than one module.

One of the first studies (Akiyama 1971) of the relationship between defects and product metrics examined data from a software product developed at Fujitsu, Ltd. of Japan. The system consisted of 10 modules, one of which was considered unusual in its structure and was excluded from later analysis. The metrics used in the analyses included the program size in steps or lines of code (S_s) and the count of decisions (DE). The number of subroutine calls, J, was also recorded for each module. A composite metric, C, was called the nature of the program and was defined as the sum of DE and J. The dependent variable was the total number of bugs found, and it included all of the defects found during the testing phase (d_1) and those found during the first two months after release (d_2). The result of the study showed that linear models of several simple metrics provide reasonable estimates for the total number of defects.

Motley and Brooks (1977) of IBM's Federal Systems Division were commissioned in 1976 by the Rome Air Development Center to develop multilinear regression models for program defects. Two large Department of Defense command and control software projects, totaling nearly 300 KLOC, were studied. The first project consisted of 534 modules with more than 181 KLOC; the second contained 249 modules of more than 115 KLOC. In addition to the error data collected during the testing phase (d_1), some 53 variables were counted in the first project and 15 in the second; several items that were collected were related to S_s and DE. Motley and Brooks also collected metrics related to the number of comment statements, the number of variables referenced but not defined, the number of source instructions in all second-level DO loops, and the number of data handling statements; through factor analysis, they were able to eliminate those metrics that provided minimal contribution to the dependent variable. Through multilinear regression, they derived a 10-variable function for predicting the test phase defects. Motley and

Brooks discovered that many of the collected metrics were linearly related to each other. This study is one of the most thorough ever made and has the largest volume of data. The results are typical of those studies that use regression analysis, in which the goodness of fit may be reasonable, but the potential use as a predictive model is very limited.

Halstead (1977) and Ottenstein (1979) attempted to create models with some theoretical basis and with support from empirically collected data, by extending the theories developed in Software Science. Software Science suggests that the programming process is a selection process, in which a program is constructed by selecting tokens from a set of unique operators and unique operands. As previously discussed, the volume metric V measures the number of mental comparisons needed to write a program of length N. Halstead and Ottenstein hypothesized that the total number of defects for a program with volume V could be estimated as

$$d_{tot} = V/3000. \tag{12.31}$$

The constant 3000 was defined as the mean number of elementary mental discriminations between potential errors in programming; it was not derived through regression analysis, but rather from other assumptions related to potential volume, such as program level and language level. No published data on the defects included the basic parameters of η_1, η_2, N_1, and N_2, which are needed to compute V directly. However, when only the size in LOC (S_s) was given for a program, a simple procedure could be followed to obtain V. Eventually, two commercial products were analyzed for which complete Software Science metrics and defects were generated. Nineteen data points were generated from the first product and 108 data points from the second product. The correlation for both products was significant at the 0.01 level and demonstrated that the hypothesized value of 3000 was valid. Variations for the determination of V were made by Lipow (1982) and Gaffney (1984). Lipow used a series function of S_s to approximate V, and Gaffney showed that V increases as a function of $S_s^{4/3}$.

Potier, Albin, Ferreol, and Bilodeau (1982) studied the error data of a family of compilers for the purpose of identifying the metrics that can be used to discriminate between modules with defects and modules with no defects. The compiler consisted of 11 subsystems, called compiling units, that had a total of about 62 KLOC; it was divided into 1,106 procedures, of which 606 were without errors. The measurements accumulated were for the basic token metrics, program volume, potential volume and difficulty, effort and time, the cyclomatic complexity number, and paths and reachability. In addition, because many of these metrics are related to a program of length N, a set of normalized metrics was defined by dividing the individual metrics by N.

The approach was to compute the mean values of the complexity metrics for the set of procedures that had errors and for the set that had no errors. The discriminant effect of a metric was defined as the ratio of these mean metric values. The analysis of the distribution of these defects produced results comparable to those of Motley and Lipow. However, the analysis also pointed out that it is very difficult to find values that correctly discriminate error-free and error-prone procedures; the metric that was most effective for discrimination at the first level is η (defined as $\eta_1 + \eta_2$), and the η metric has the potential to be available early in the development process.

A technique that facilitates early detection of the majority of software defects should be very useful. One approach is to identify those software components that are believed to have the highest concentration of defects early, so that more testing and correcting resources can be directed at them. Therefore, it is of interest to study the metrics available during the development phases to see if any metric, or any combination of metrics, can be used to guide the testing process. One such study is of products developed at IBM's Santa Teresa Laboratory and released between the years 1980 and 1983 (Shen et al. 1985). These products consisted of a software metrics counting tool, a compiler that had three releases, and a software database system. The number of program changes was recorded as defect data during the testing and maintenance phases, all metrics related to Software Science were generated, and the number of decisions (DE) were available for analysis.

The authors of that study were interested in regression models that could be used to predict the total number of defects (d_{tot}) at the end of all phases. Because most modules did not have any defects after product release ($d_2 = 0$), and those that did typically had only one or two, Shen et al. were also interested in a binary dependent variable $P(d_2 > 0)$ whose value is zero if the module has no postrelease defects and one otherwise. A regression-derived estimator for $P(d_2 > 0)$ has a potentially useful interpretation because it represents the expected probability that a particular module will have one or more defects after release. A search procedure for all possible regressions was used to identify the best set of one, two, and three independent variables from the pool of variables available at the end of each phase.

The metrics found to be the best single predictors of d_{tot} and $P(d_2 > 0)$ at the end of the design phase were the number of unique operands (η_2) and the number of decisions (DE). In those cases where DE was the best predictor, the difference in performance between η_2 and DE was not significant at the 0.01 level. At the end of the coding phase, the best predictors were the same as those that remained at the end of the design phase, namely η_2 and DE. This finding is consistent with Akiyama's results and lends some support to the finding by Motley and Brooks, but it differs from the finding by Halstead and Ottenstein. At the end of the testing phase, d_1 becomes an independent variable and only $P(d_2 > 0)$ is considered a dependent variable. The best predictors of $P(d_2 > 0)$ at the end of testing were η_2 and d_1, and the issue of how soon these metrics can be accurately estimated becomes quite important. Because η_2 can be useful in identifying at an early stage those modules most likely to contain errors, it may be used to target certain modules for early or additional testing, to increase the efficiency of the defect removal process.

Defect Density

The one finding with regard to program defects that all studies tend to agree on is that larger modules have more defects. Correlation analysis of published data shows that a linear relationship between defects and size is significant at the 0.01 level. Halstead's (1977) model hypothesizes a perfect correlation between defects and the volume, V, which is also a metric of program size. It is not unreasonable to consider a normalized metric for program quality defined as

$$\text{defect density} \;=\; (\text{number of defects in a module})/\text{module size.} \quad (12.32)$$

The intent of this calculation is that after the size component has been extracted by division, the resultant density metric will be independent of module size and will serve as a useful measure of the module's quality. In a similar way, many of the metrics discussed so far that are linearly related to module size can also be normalized before analysis.

An interesting phenomenon related to size was observed independently by several researchers: Larger modules seem to have lower defect densities. Because larger modules are generally more complex, a lower defect density was unexpected. There are several explanations for this.

- Some researchers admitted tacitly that the longer programs were less thoroughly tested.

- There may have been a large number of interface errors that were distributed more or less evenly across all modules and thus biased the measurement against the smaller modules.

- The larger modules might have been coded with more care than the smaller modules precisely because of their size.

These explanations, however, are attempts to support the intuition that defect density should be independent of module size, even though such independence has not been observed.

Plots of (d_{tot}/N) versus N for the Shen et al. (1985) defect study show that there is a higher defect density in smaller modules than larger ones. Whatever the reasons for this, it implies that $(d_0 + d_1N)$ is a better model for d_{tot} than is d_1N, which is consistent with this result. If

$$d_{tot} < d_0 + d_1N, \tag{12.33}$$

then the defect density becomes

$$d_{tot}/N < d_0/N + d_1. \tag{12.34}$$

So as N increases, (d_{tot}/N) decreases asymptotically to d_1. Further analysis of the data showed that the minimum size beyond which the error density could reasonably be considered unrelated to module size was $N = 2500$, or approximately 500 lines of code.

An analysis by Conte, Dunsmore, and Shen (1986) led to the conclusion that error density is generally a poor size-normalized index of program quality. Using it to compare the quality of programs, without regard to related factors such as complexity and size, is ill advised. Similarly, normalizing other metrics by division by a size metric should be examined carefully. Even if the metric in question is linearly correlated with the size metric, such normalization is meaningful only if the constant term d_0 in the regression model is approximately zero.

Dynamic Models of Defects

A dynamic model of software defects includes the component of time, which is the interval between successive detections of defects. Most dynamic models consider software to be a black box, where the reliability and MTTF (mean time to failure) is estimated without regard to the complexity of the program. Many dynamic models are called reliability growth models. The general assumption is that all defects detected during the development and testing phases are corrected and that corrections do not introduce any new defects. This ideal process allows the reliability to increase; therefore, the cost of testing and fixing may be balanced against the increase in reliability to produce a software system at minimal cost while still meeting reliability objectives. Other models do not consider the correction of defects after detection, and they assume that the software is being tested for the purpose of estimating its reliability. These models can be used to show that the software is highly reliable without having to prove its correctness by analytic methods. All dynamic models include some constraint on the distribution of defects or the hazard rate.

To use dynamic models, the parameters must frequently be estimated by means of some other methods. In fact, a dynamic model cannot be accurate unless it incorporates an accurate static model that produces d_{tot}. The other parameters are then determined by observation of the defect history or a similar program. The difficulty with dynamic models is that software processes occur in real time, and capturing metrics is difficult. Defects can sometimes be detected faster than predicted by a particular model and slower at other times. Depending on resource limitations, the software may not be actively tested while waiting for the correction to take place. Therefore, it is usually necessary to convert the execution time t commonly used in the dynamic models to a calendar time t'.

A good comparison of the dynamic models that can be used is found in Ramamoorthy and Bastani (1982) and in Lyu and Nikora (1992). The Musa (1980a) model, the Jelinski and

Moranda (1972) linear model, the Shooman (1983) model, and the Schick and Wolverton (1978) model all share some common assumptions, such as that test input sets should be selected randomly from the complete set of input sets anticipated in actual operation, all software failures are observed, failure intervals are independent of each other, the distribution function assumes the form $F(\tau) = 1 - e^{-\lambda t}$, and the density function assumes the form $f(\tau) = \lambda e^{-\lambda t}$. These models can be generalized and called general Poisson models where the hazard rate is of the form

$$h_j = (d_{\text{tot}} - M_j)\phi, \tag{12.35}$$

where M_j is the number of defects corrected before the jth failure and after the $(j-1)$th failure. All of the Poisson models have the simple property that MTTF $= 1/h_j$. However, lack of reliable data makes the validation of any of these model types difficult.

Because there appear to be no error-free software development techniques in use, the testing phase cannot be eliminated. Any technique that identifies error-prone modules that may require more testing should be very useful. Because of the uncertainties involved with defect detection, models that accurately reflect the total number of defects are difficult to formulate and validate. However, it may be a moot point, because knowing that a module will almost certainly have errors in it is enough to guide the testing process. Some studies have provided methods to set threshold values for certain metrics so that modules with measurements higher than the threshold are more likely than others to have errors. If the threshold values can be determined for a wide range of programs and applications, they may be included in software programming standards and conventions. Programs with measurements that exceed the threshold values would receive extra attention.

Static models, rather than dynamic ones, can be used to determine threshold levels. Before more supporting evidence becomes available, dynamic models of software reliability or MTTF will remain primarily of academic interest. However, the recording of defects and their times of discovery are still very valuable. The data on discovery times may be combined with other product and process metrics to construct a hybrid model that assesses the reliability of the software during the various phases of the software life cycle.

Software Reliability and Reliability Growth Models

Software is an essential component of many systems, and the reliable operation of such systems depends critically on the reliable operation of their software components. A program will always produce the same answer for the same input as long as the hardware does not fail, since there is no physical deterioration of the software and the fabrication or duplication of the code is a trivial process. Software failures are normally due to the presentation of an input that finally reveals a defect present since software inception. There is no random malfunction in software, other than defects revealed by random inputs.

The history of defect detection for a program is represented by a dot on the line of the defect history. Assuming that the detection of software defects is a stochastic process, the distribution of the time interval between defect recordings may be represented by the function $F(\tau)$ for $\tau \geq 0$. This function is interpreted to be the probability that a defect is detected by time τ. The reliability, $R(\tau)$, of the software is the probability that there are no failures during the time interval of length τ, or

$$R(\tau) = 1 - F(\tau). \tag{12.36}$$

This definition assumes that the software being studied is in continuous use during the time interval.

For some applications, it may be more appropriate to use the number of runs instead of real time, because no defects can be detected unless the program is executed. In this case, the reliability is the probability that there is no failure over n runs, or

$$R(n) = 1 - (d_n/n), \qquad (12.37)$$

where d_n is the number of defects detected over the n runs. If $f(\tau)$ is the probability density function

$$f(\tau) = dF(\tau)/d\tau, \qquad (12.38)$$

then $f(\tau)d\tau$ is the probability that the software fails during the semi-open interval $(\tau, \tau + d\tau]$. The hazard rate $h(\tau)$ is defined as the probability that the software fails during the interval $(\tau, \tau + d\tau]$, given that it has not failed before τ and

$$h(\tau) = f(\tau)/[1 - F(\tau)]. \qquad (12.39)$$

The right-hand side of equation 12.39 is actually the derivative of $\ln(1 - F(\tau))$, so that

$$h(\tau) = -d\ln[1 - F(\tau)]/d\tau, \qquad (12.40)$$

and as a result,

$$\ln R(\tau) = -\int_0^\tau h(x)dx. \qquad (12.41)$$

Therefore, another way to represent the reliability, $R(\tau)$, is

$$R(\tau) = e^{-\int h(x)dx}, \qquad (12.42)$$

from time 0 to time τ. Another measure is the mean time to failure (MTTF), defined as

$$\text{MTTF} = \sum^n t_i/n, \qquad (12.43)$$

where t_i is the time interval between the $(i - 1)$th and ith failures. As n approaches infinity, this mean value converges to the expected value of the random variable

$$\text{MTTF} = \int^\infty \tau dF(\tau) = \int^\infty \tau f(\tau)d\tau. \qquad (12.44)$$

It is possible to compute MTTF from $R(\tau)$ by substituting $F(\tau) = 1 - R(\tau)$ into equation 12.44 and integrating by parts to obtain

$$\text{MTTF} = \int^\infty \tau d(1 - R(\tau)) = \int^\infty R(\tau)d\tau. \qquad (12.45)$$

The reliability of a software component can be represented by $R(\tau)$ or by MTTF. Both can be derived if we know the distribution of the time interval between defect recordings $F(\tau)$ by using equations 12.36 and 12.45. They can also be derived if the hazard rate calculated by equation 12.39 is known, by using equations 12.42 and 12.45. In addition to the count of defects, it is important to record the times of their detection, so that a reliability measure may be computed.

Reliability is usually concerned with the time between failures or its reciprocal, the failure rate. However, most data come from a test environment; consequently, a defect detection rate is often more informative than the failure rate. Although defect detection is usually a failure during a test, it turns out that test software may also detect a defect even though the test continues to operate. Defects can also be detected during design reviews and code inspections. The assumption is that each defect is fixed when it is discovered, and this decreases the number of defects in the code except for defects that may be introduced by the repair itself. As the number of defects decreases, so does the defect discovery rate, or, alternatively, the length of time between defect discoveries should increase and when the defect-discovery rate reaches an acceptably low value, the software is deemed suitable to release.

It is difficult to extrapolate from the defect-discovery rate in the test environment to the failure rate during system operation because it is hard to extrapolate from test time to system operation time. A way around this is that the expected number of remaining or residual defects can provide an upper limit on the number of unique failures that could be encountered in field use. Knowing the number of residual defects helps determine whether the code is suitable for release, as well as how much more testing is required if it is not. It also provides an estimate of the number of failures that customers will encounter when operating the software in the field. This estimate helps define the appropriate levels of support that will be required for defect correction after the software has been released and shipped.

Software reliability growth models are mathematical functions that describe defect detection rates. There are two major classes: *concave models* and *S-shaped models* (Figure 12-2). As illustrated, concave models bend downward whereas S-shaped models are initially convex and then become concave. This geometry reflects the underlying assumption that early testing is not as efficient as later testing, so that there is a ramping-up period during which the defect detection rate increases. This period terminates at the inflection point in the S-shaped curve. The most important thing about both models is that they have the same *asymptotic behavior,* in that the defect detection rate decreases as the number of defects detected increases and the total number of defects detected asymptotically approaches a finite value. For a third, less-common class of models, *infinite failure models,* the assumption is that the code has an infinite number of failures. Of course, defect repair can introduce new defects, and some models explicitly account for this during test by modifying the mathematical form of the model, while in others new defects are accounted for by the statistical fit of the model to the data. In practice, either method works, as long as the model does a good job of fitting the data.

Software reliability growth models predict the expected number of defects μ at test time t, or $\mu(t)$. For example, the Goel and Okumoto (1979) exponential model expresses this as

$$\mu(t) = a \times (1 - e^{-bt}), \tag{12.46}$$

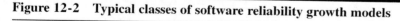

Figure 12-2   Typical classes of software reliability growth models

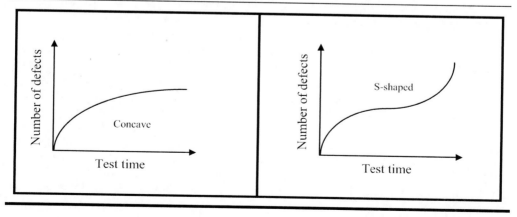

where *a* is the expected total number of defects and *b* is the *shape factor* or the rate at which the defect detection rate decreases. The Goel and Okumoto model has two parameters; other models can have three or more parameters (Table 12-5).

Maintainability Metrics Models

As the software development community becomes aware of the practical application of software, metrics approaches have been found to be especially useful for understanding and improving software maintainability through the application of maintainability metrics models. Historically speaking, software practitioners interested in measuring software maintainability have struggled in their attempt to gather and understand meaningful metrics. Many traditional software metrics have come under academic scrutiny, and although many of the objections to traditional metrics are valid, there is still significant data to support application of most of these metrics; some interesting results have been achieved through the application of composite software metrics models.

In an effort to better quantify software maintainability, Oman and Hagemeister (1994) and Zhuo et al. (1993) have defined two polynomial regression models that predict software maintainability. These models use a combination of predictor variables in a polynomial equation to determine a *maintainability index* (*MI*). The predictor variables are a combination of a weighted coefficient and an independent metric and have shown strong correlation between Halstead's metrics, McCabe's cyclomatic complexity, lines of code, and number of comments to the maintainability of the software system. The original polynomial equations were defined in two forms as a three-metric and four-metric version. The equations are

$$MI3 = 171 - 3.42 \times \ln(aveE) - 0.23 \times aveV(g')$$
$$- 16.2 \times \ln(aveLOC) \qquad (12.47)$$

where *MI*3 is the three-metric *MI* value, *aveE* is the average Halstead effort per module, *aveV*(g′) is the average extended cyclomatic complexity per module, and *aveLOC* is the average lines of code per module, and

$$MI4 = 171 - 3.42 \times \ln(aveE) - 0.23 \times aveV(g') - 16.2$$
$$\times \ln(aveLOC) + 0.99 \times aveCM, \qquad (12.48)$$

where *MI*4 is the four-metric *MI* value, *aveCM* is the average number of lines of comments per module, and the remaining variables are the same as defined for equation 12.47.

Data have been used to construct the polynomial equations to provide an appropriate fit of *MI* to software systems and to validate the models' predictive capacity for measuring the maintainability of those same software systems. In applying the four-metric *MI*, two quality cutoffs for analyzing systems with the polynomial metrics have been derived. Values above 85 indicate that the software is highly maintainable, values between 85 and 65 suggest moderate maintainability, and values below 65 indicate that the software is difficult to maintain. Although hard quality cutoffs are not always appropriate, they do establish a general context for rating maintainability, and the cutoffs provide a frame of reference. Since their initial publication, the polynomial equations have been fine-tuned so that the *MI* better represents system maintainability. For example, Halstead's volume measure has more academic support for predictive capability than the effort metric. In addition, the original model was overly sensitive to the comment predictor variable of the four-metric equation and, therefore, the comment predictor has been

Table 12-5   Models of Software Reliability Growth

Model Description		Prediction Formula	Comments
Name	**Type**		
Goel-Okumoto (G-O)	Concave	$a \times (1 - e^{-bt})$ $a \geq 0, b > 0$	Also called the Musa model or exponential model
G-O S-Shaped	S-shaped	$a \times [1 - (1 + bt) \times e^{-bt}]$ $a \geq, b > 0$	Modification of G-O model to make it S-shaped
Hossain-Dahiya/G-O	Concave	$a \times (1 - e^{-bt}) / (1 + c \times e^{-bt})$ $a \geq, b > 0, c > 0$	Solves a technical condition with the G-O model; becomes same as G-O as c approaches 0
Gompertz	S-shaped	$a \times (b^d)$ where $d = c^t$ $a \geq 0, 0 \leq b \leq 1, 0 < c < 1$	
Pareto	Concave	$a \times [1 - (1 + t/\beta]^{(1 - \alpha)}$ $a \geq 0, \beta > 0, 0 \leq \alpha \leq 1$	Assumed failures have different failure rates and failures with highest rates are removed first
Weibull	Concave	$a \times (1 - e^{-d})$ where $d = bt^c$ $a \geq 0, b > 0, c > 0$	Same as G-O for c = 1
Yamada exponential	Concave	$a \times (1 - e^{-r\alpha \times d})$ where $d = (1 - e^{-\beta t})$ $a \geq 0, r\alpha > 0, \beta > 0$	Attempts to account for testing effort
Yamada Raleigh	S-shaped	$a \times (1 - e^{-r\alpha \times d})$ where $d = (1 - e^c)$ and $c = -\beta t^2/2$ $a \geq 0, r\alpha > 0, \beta > 0$	Attempts to account for testing effort

modified to include a comments-to-code ratio, which has a maximum additive value to the overall *MI*. Consequently, the modified definitions are

$$MI3 = 171 - 5.2 \times \ln(aveV) - 0.23 \times aveV(g') - 16.2 \\ \times \ln(aveLOC) \tag{12.49}$$

where *MI3* is the three-metric *MI* value, *aveV* is the average Halstead volume per module, *aveV*(g') is the average extended cyclomatic complexity per module, and *aveLOC* is the average lines of code per module, and

$$MI4 = 171 - 5.2 \times \ln(aveV) - 0.23 \times aveV(g') - 16.2 \\ \times \ln(aveLOC) + 50 \times \sin\sqrt{2.4 \times perCM} \tag{12.50}$$

where *MI4* is the four-metric *MI* value, *perCM* is the average percent of lines of comments per module, and the remaining variables are the same as defined for equation 12.49.

To determine which polynomial equation is the most appropriate fit to measure the *MI* of a given software system, some analysis of the comments in the code must be performed. If any of the following criteria are true, then the three-metric *MI* may be a better fit than the four-metric *MI* for measuring maintainability.

1. The comments do not accurately match the code.

2. There are large, company-standard comment header blocks, copyrights, and disclaimers.

3. There are large sections of code that have been commented out.

Generally speaking, if it is believed that the code comments significantly contribute to understanding and maintainability, then the four-metric *MI* is the best choice. Otherwise, the three-metric MI will be more appropriate.

As new code is developed, it is easy to see how a metrics assessment capability can lead to the development of more maintainable software. For example, after a module has been designed and coded, its maintainability can be measured and, should the *MI* evaluation predict maintenance difficulty, the module may be redesigned and coded to achieve better maintainability. The real value of using the *MI* is that it provides an unbiased second opinion on the state of the software module and thereby gently reminds and encourages the software developer to improve software engineering skills that lead to the development of higher quality code. Applying the *MI* during software maintenance also is useful. Traditionally, when metrics are determined for a software system, they have been used to target modules for maintenance, and the most grievously offending routines are targeted for redesign or restructuring. This approach works well if an organization has enough time to make perfective maintenance changes based on the singular merits of developing higher quality software. However, in most maintenance environments, the software engineers do not have sufficient time to use this approach fully, and they spend more time fixing software defects or making enhancements than they do improving the system, while making no functional change. Furthermore, by using *MI* analysis to quantify the maintainability of modules scheduled for change, either to fix defects or to make enhancements, a decision can be made about the most appropriate type of change to make to the module. For example, modules having low maintainability are candidates for a complete redesign. For modules that are moderately maintainable, it may be advantageous to perform some restructuring, whereas for modules that have high maintainability, it may make sense to just make the change without any additional considerations. After modifying the module scheduled for change, an assessment should be made to again determine if the code is maintainable or if further work should be performed.

Software Statistical Process Control

Most hardware manufacturers and service suppliers have made statistical process control part of their development regimen. Although a few practitioners have attempted to use statistical process control in software engineering applications, the opinion of many academics and the remaining practitioners is that statistical process control does not fit into a software environment. Many tend to dismiss it simply because software cannot be measured; when properly applied, statistical process control can flag potential process problems even though it cannot supply absolute scores or goodness ratings.

Statistical process control is founded on the principle that as long as a process is performed consistently, it will demonstrate consistent results in measures such as productivity, error rate, and cycle time. Within this meaning, however, consistent does not mean identical; the results will vary somewhat, although the variation will be minor. If the principle is that consistent process execution yields consistent measured performance, then a basis for using measurement to manage process is established. If the performance level differs substantially from the capability level, then the assumption can be made that the process has probably changed in some way; a significant difference between the two indicates the need to investigate the reason for the discrepancy and to take corrective action, if necessary.

In implementing statistical process control, begin with a model of the process and then select techniques to monitor performance. For example, Table 12-6 shows a simple software process model and its associated quality performance parameters. The performance measures for each activity in the model indicate the success of that activity in achieving its quality goal. Because the quality goal of design and code is to not introduce errors into the software, a good performance indicator is the error insertion rate expressed as errors per line of code. The quality goal of inspections and testing is the discovery of errors so that they can be removed. A good performance measure for this activity is error detection rate expressed as the percentage of errors found. In practice, the actual values shown in the table can be determined after the project's completion, after each build, or after each release.

Control charts are often used to monitor process performance. In Figure 12-3, an expected performance, based on data from prior releases as well as upper and lower control limits and current performance, is indicated. As the data show, the testing process is generally stable. Testers find a relatively fixed proportion of errors, 50–60 percent in this case. To change this proportion,

Table 12-6   A Simple Process Control Model with Performance Parameters

Performance Parameters		Error Distribution	
Construction Activities (Errors inserted per thousand lines)	**Evaluation Activities (Percentage of errors present that are found)**	**Percentage of all errors inserted in this phase**	**Percentage of all errors detected in this phase**
Design (20)	Inspect (50)	67	33
Code (10)	Inspect (50)	33	33
	Test (75)	0	25
	Operate (100)	0	8

Figure 12-3   Process control chart to track testing efficiency

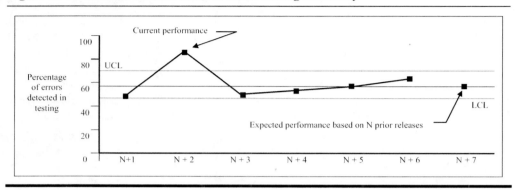

the process can be changed by any of the normal and usual methods, such as allocating more resources and acquiring better methods and better tools. Analysis should then be performed whenever any release exceeds the control limits, just as it is in the real world hardware counterpart, to understand what has happened to the process, whether good or bad. The efficiency of each project can also be compared to the organization's baseline. For example, the testing efficiency of the project in Figure 12-3 does not compare favorably with the organizational parameter of 75 percent in Table 12-6. This implies that the project's testing activity could be improved, even though it is stable.

Control charts are not the only way of approaching process control. Current project results can be compared with historical profiles or theoretical distributions by examining the distribution of errors rather than the number or rate of errors. For example, assume that past projects have found about as many errors during design as during coding. The percentage of errors found in a phase is the net effect of insertion and detection activities during that phase, as well as the preceding phases (see the last column in Table 12-6). If the current project finds twice as many errors during coding as during design, then the design process, and one or more of its activities, has most likely changed. It might be possible to detect this during coding, but it will certainly be noticed when coding is complete. This type of analysis can easily be accomplished with a Pareto diagram or histogram.

Although this concept of statistical process control is simple, it is rarely straightforward to implement for the following reasons:

1. Unless the software process is documented and generally complied with, there is no reason to expect measurably consistent performance.

2. If selecting one or two measures that offer insight into the performance of a process or activity is correct, the cost of tracking them should also be considered.

3. The control charts or distributions should be constructed with a view toward detecting process trends rather than identifying individual nonconforming events.

4. Several formulas exist for computing control limits and analyzing distributions in different situations; although they are straightforward, it is easy to make implementation mistakes without the proper background.

5. Statistical process control merely signals that a problem may exist. If a detailed investigation or audit is not performed, along with follow-up corrective action, there will be no benefit to using it.

6. Most of these problems of process control implementation can be overcome with effective training, but the training must focus on software engineering examples rather than on examples from other disciplines.

Because software maintenance is usually a series of small and frequent deliveries, it is probably worthwhile for an organization to start applying and learning about statistical process control within that environment. In addition, maintenance processes are often more mature than development processes and are more limited in scope; consequently, these activities are usually performed in a more consistent way.

Decision Making with Metrics

In general, the predictions made from metrics data have no element of statistical confidence; metrics are first and foremost design tools. As tools, they are used to compare plans to actual results, to identify overly complicated parts of the software and system, and to serve as input to risk analysis, evaluation, and management. The metrics and the models that use the metrics need not be exact to be useful. In fact, many exact models are so cumbersome and intractable that they are often useless to managers who need to make decisions on the basis of their results. Excellent and useful results are regularly obtained from simple models like those described earlier.

However, at times, these simple models yield results that do not make sense in the environment of an organization. For example, a software reliability estimate may be predicated on the fact that the number of lines of code in test is stable, but its predictions do not match the observed failure rates in the project. An investigation may lead to the discovery that the size of the software under test is actually increasing incrementally, so a model that accommodates software growth during testing should be used. The new model's output and predictions should then be closely monitored relative to the project actuals. If they correspond, then the new model can be useful for predictions and for management decision making. The important point is that when the results from a model are not reasonable, those results still convey some very pertinent information; either a mistake has been made in the mathematics, or the assumptions that define the model are incorrect. At times, an incorrect assumption is difficult to notice, and the model must be worked backward, manipulating the assumptions to give the best results, or a new approach must be taken.

Metrics analysis begins with a fundamental understanding and insight into the workings of the software development and maintenance processes. The analysis continues with calculations from the conceptual models that reflect that insight; it results in answers that may affect decisions and ultimately change processes. Those parts of the metrics task that are computationally intensive are best done by support tools and automated analyzers, but some are best done by individuals. The people-related parts of the metrics task are those that involve insight into the internal workings of the organization's processes. The insights gained by performing a Pareto analysis or the debugging of a model can result in improvements to the subject process as well as the model of that process. There is value to the organization in performing some of the metrics tasks by hand, because the integrity of the system cannot be achieved without sound engineering applied to established software development and maintenance tasks.

13

The Software Quality Assurance Program: Productivity and Capability Maturity Measurement

If you cannot repeat a process and get the same results, other problems pale by comparison.

—Randall R. Macala

While software measurement is becoming an integral part of software development, software process assessment is becoming an integral part of the measurement activities. The approach to software process-assessment measurement requires documented software engineering procedures and processes, along with a defined software metrics process. This is followed by the establishment of goals to improve the software engineering processes over a specified period of time. Relative to those goals, measures are then defined, collected, and used to gauge periodically the progress toward achieving the specified improvement goals. When the process-related data that have been collected indicate that software engineering process problems exist, the organization formulates actions to correct the situation. The results are compared over time to determine the best improvement solution. Figure 13-1 shows the fundamental software process-assessment and measurement approach used for incremental improvements to the software process. The cumulative, net result of these improvements is to attain higher quality products and increase the competitiveness of the organization and its software.

Overview of Software Process Improvement Measurement

To observe and quantify the impact of software process improvement, the performance of the software engineering organization must be measured over time as well as between groups or projects. Comparisons of performance across a software organization are very difficult, however,

Figure 13-1   The typical software measurement approach

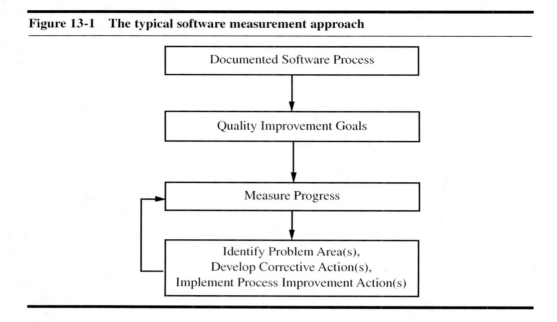

because the organization typically defines measures and collects performance data in different ways. However, performance improvement can be tracked separately in each group or project if the measures are defined consistently, and if similar end products are produced. As a consequence, a set of basic measures for the performance of a software engineering organization should be defined and limited to a small number of simple measures. This strategy will reduce the complexity of collecting, analyzing, maintaining, and comparing the performance data.

Improving the software engineering process improves the quality of the software products and the overall performance of the software engineering group. However, process is only one of several controllable factors in improving software quality and the performance of the software group. Other factors include the skills and experience of the software engineering staff; the technology and tools used to implement the software; the complexity of the product itself; and environmental characteristics, such as schedule, communications, and regulatory requirements. For example, different productivity performance should be expected from projects developing new products, enhancing existing products, and maintaining existing products. Furthermore, business environmental factors, such as whether the business is profitable, regulatory requirements, and the type of device, will also affect performance. Consequently, rather than try to establish what good performance is, or compare the performance of one organization with that of another, changes in performance over time within a specific organization, group, or project should be tracked.

Many software engineering groups want to improve their software processes to improve product quality, increase productivity, and reduce development time, but few know how to improve the software process. A wide assortment of available methods for process improvement include configuration management, defect prevention, function point analysis, quality function deployment, software quality assurance, software reliability engineering, and total quality management, but confusion is common about which methods to introduce at what time. Although the motivation to improve the software process usually results from a business need, such as strong competition, external regulation, or a dictate for increased profitability, sometimes the software engineering group voluntarily attempts to improve their process.

Regardless of the origin of the motivation, the software engineering group must assess its current practices and process maturity, and then initiate approaches to improve the software process (see Figure 13-2). The selection and successful implementation of the proposed method improvements depend on several variables, including current process maturity, resource skill base, organization and organizational dynamics, and business issues such as cost, risk, and implementation speed. Being able to predict a priori the success of a specific improvement is difficult because of environmental variables external to the proposed improvement method, such as staffing skills, acceptance of or reluctance about change, training effectiveness, and implementation efficiency. After the improvement method has been installed, the organization must then determine whether the method was implemented successfully, whether the process is mature enough to consider implementing additional methods, and whether the selected method is appropriate, given the current process maturity level and environment.

In general, a software process improvement method is an integrated collection of procedures, tools, and training used for increasing software product quality, improving software productivity, or reducing software product development time. A software process improvement method can either support a process area or improve the effectiveness of key practices in an existing process area. Software process improvement methods often require a significant investment in training and effort, and considerable barriers must often be overcome before a measurable impact results from the improved process. However, improved software process benefits include fewer product defects discovered by customers, earlier identification and correction of defects, fewer defects being introduced during the development effort, faster time to market, and better predictability of project schedules and resources.

Figure 13-2   The typical approach to measurement of software process improvement

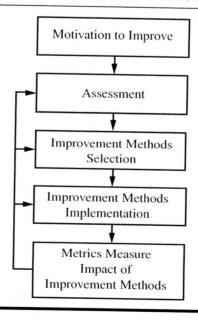

Productivity Differentials in Software

An undisputed difference in productivity among practicing software engineers represents a commentary on the ability to measure and enforce software productivity standards. Programming is a problem-solving activity, and individuals differ greatly in their ability to solve problems of the kinds found in programming. The software engineering industry tolerates this differential because programming productivity is extremely difficult to measure. Although lines of source code written and debugged per day are easy to measure, they are distantly related to real productivity. Depending on the project, for example, the highest real productivity may be the result of determining how to reuse programs that have already been written, possibly for a radically different purpose. Another form of high productivity might be manifested in finding how to solve problems with preexisting programs and rewriting them as subprograms. In short, there are no objective ways to measure programming productivity except by results, and the results must be measured in value to the organization, not in lines of code. The difficulty is that to decide in each case what exactly is the value to the organization requires time and effort, the two quantities that are usually in short supply.

Not only are there differences among individual software engineers on a project, there are also differences in productivity among software organizations; the individual differences do not average out across different software organizations. There are two main reasons for this.

1. Individual software productivity is not naturally additive in a software organization; trying to make it additive takes good technology and even better management.

2. Individual software engineers do not join software organizations at random.

Organizations that have good technology and good management can attract better software engineers, and vice versa, so the better organizations tend to attract individuals with higher productivity, and those individuals, in turn, tend to make the productivity more additive.

The fallacy of this discussion is that the best performing software groups are typically held in no higher esteem by other software organizations within the same company than the lowest performing software groups. This tends to make sense for two reasons. First, each software organization knows only how well it does, not how well the other group does, because every attempted comparison ends up evaluating different problems, different enterprises, and different situations; no two comparisons are identical. Second, the low-productivity performers usually make software development appear to be difficult, whereas the high-productivity achievers tend to make it look easy. Consequently, an organization cannot readily distinguish between performing hard tasks easily and making an easy task look hard. There is no simple and objective way to know software engineering productivity.

Judging the productivity of the software organization to which an individual belongs is both difficult and frustrating, but the high-productivity performers do get separated from the low-productivity performers. The discriminant is organizational survival; the organizations that produce timely, reliable, and quality software survive to do it again on another project. In the long run, there is no problem in identifying the productive software organizations, but the essence of management is to anticipate and improve the productivity of its software organization in the short run. Because no simple measurements will suffice, productivity indicators are available and useful, but none is numerical, objective, or additive, and they do not have a fixed role of importance; every indicator requires management assessment and judgment. However, management measurements based on a numerical and objective form can be devised that reflect the productivity indicators, but such measurements must be devised by an organizational management that knows the special circumstances of the indicators, the limitations and fallibilities of the measurements, and software engineering intimately.

Exceptional software engineering productivity begins with the minimization of reinvention and the development of new software. However, when new software is required, exceptional performers find the simplest and most direct way of producing that software. The most cost-effective way to get a new software system operational is to discover that it already exists. This may take some effort, and there is some degree of risk associated with the effort because it may only reveal that no such software exists; in exceptional performance, reinvention is minimized. The next most effective way to get new software operational is to uncover a large number of existing components that can be integrated with minimal effort into the required system.

Exceptional performance also reduces by large factors the amount of work required in software development. In fact, exceptional performance can reduce the amount of work required in subsequent phases by a factor of three or more (Mills 1988). For example, a good requirements analysis can reduce the design effort by a factor of three; a good design effort can reduce the implementation effort by a factor of three; and a good implementation effort can reduce the operations and maintenance activities by a factor of three. The opportunities for productivity decay exponentially throughout the product life cycle, and the cost of the software often reflects more directly the capability of the team than it does the size of the job to be done.

Another key to exceptional performance is that it requires more powerful techniques, both conceptual and organizational. The key to exceptional performance is intellectual control, not by the individual software engineer, but by the entire organization. Consequently, techniques of work structuring are as important as conceptual techniques of program structuring. As a comparison, sports franchises spend nearly all of their time rehearsing and practicing plays, not only so they know what to do, but also to understand what the other teammate will be doing. In software engineering terms, software teams are productive because they know what the process is, who is doing what, and when to deliver what as outputs.

Exceptional performance is also characterized by working smart and minimizing rework. Program debugging is rework, and it tends to reflect a lack of concentration and design integrity. Regardless of why debug must occur, it results in lower productivity. For example, if a software engineer writes 100 lines of code in one day and then takes two weeks to debug it, that engineer has actually averaged 10 lines a day in productivity. Debugging, as much as possible, should be the exception, to recover from an untenable situation. Professional golfers, as another comparison, make fewer bad shots than amateurs, but when they do get that occasional bad lie, they more often than not make a solid recovery shot.

Software Assessment Standards and Models

The currently available software assessment standards and models represent a wide variety of interests and concerns. For example, the emphasis of the U.S. Food and Drug Administration (FDA) and the German Electrotechnical Commission (TÜV) is on the safety of medical devices; the guidance for applying ISO 9000 standards to software is governed by ISO 9000-3, and it defines a general quality assurance program. The Software Process Improvement Capability Determination (SPICE) model, the Software Engineering Institute (SEI) Capability Maturity Model (CMM), and the TickIT program were created specifically to support software process assessment. These standards and models represent a wide variety of interests and concerns, and the scope of each differs; the FDA, SEI, SPICE, ISO, and TickIT models are applicable to software systems in general, while the TÜV model targets embedded system software.

The FDA has documented the failures of medical devices that are controlled by software and, in particular, failures that resulted from unstructured software development and implementation practices. As a consequence, the FDA produced the *Reviewer Guidance for Computer-Controlled Medical Devices Undergoing 510(k) Review* to provide more stringent guidelines for the evaluation of software. This document emphasizes the definition of software product documentation and software development procedures, but provides minimal advice relating to specific implementation controls. However, the document does provide flexibility in the development of software documentation that is a function of the risk level of the device. Furthermore, the document emphasizes safety and hazard analysis activities and end products that augment the software engineering activities.

The ISO 9000-3 document provides guidance for software quality systems and is primarily concerned with situations in which software is developed under a contractual relationship. Since it is an integral part of the ISO standards, its requirements for a software quality assurance framework are essentially the same as those provided in ISO 9001. However, it addresses software activities and plans that are developed from a software life cycle perspective, as well as software support activities, such as configuration management, software engineering measurement, and procedures. This document also emphasizes the development of software quality management plans and quality assurance controls, the need for software quality assurance reviews during software development, and subcontractor management and tracking.

The SEI initially provided a process framework and questionnaire to help government organizations improve their software development processes and to provide a method for evaluating the capability of software development contractors. Eventually, this framework evolved into the CMM, which is the basis of two SEI assessment methods. The first assessment method is the Software Process Assessment, which helps an organization determine its software process strengths, weaknesses, and areas of improvement; the second is the Software Capability Evaluation method, which helps an organization evaluate the software processes of its suppliers. In addition, the SEI provides process, definition, and measurement techniques and tools that help an organization improve its software process. The CMM defines five levels of maturity in a software development organization, from chaotic (Level 1) to optimized (Level 5); for each level, the CMM defines key process areas and key activities or practices within each area (see Table 13-1). The CMM provides detailed guidance in its descriptions of the key software practices to implement so as to reach the next maturity level. This model is probably the most widely used assessment model in the United States.

The German Electrotechnical Commission (TÜV) publishes *Principles for Computers in Safety-Related Systems* (DIN V VDE 0801), which is applied by TÜV when approving a medical device. The document primarily addresses the implementation of embedded software and does not address software process methods or provide for process improvement activities. Device software and hardware control measures are graded and assigned to different safety requirements classes to determine the appropriateness of the design strategy; requirements classes are ranked and categories of design controls are then defined. As a consequence, according to the document, additional software controls will be required if hardware architecture redundancies are not implemented. This document also defines other trade-offs that specify varying levels of system controls based on the types of failures experienced when the device is in operation. In particular, this document requires mechanisms to ensure that if a component fails, software controls are in place that will allow the system to fail to a safe state.

TickIT, formally known as the *Guide to Software Quality Management System Construction and Certification Using EN 29001,* was created by the British Computer Society. The TickIT guide provides a certification scheme for software quality management systems, and it addresses

Table 13-1 SEI Process Maturity Levels

Level	Characteristics	Process Area
5. Optimizing	Improvement fed back to process	Defect prevention Technology change management Process change management
4. Managed	Measured process (quantitative)	Quantitative process management Software quality management
3. Defined	Process defined, institutionalized	Organization process focus Organization process definition Training program Integrated software management Software product engineering Intergroup coordination Peer reviews
2. Repeatable	Process dependent on individuals	Requirements management Software project planning Software project tracking and oversight Software subcontractor management Software quality assurance Software configuration management
1. Initial	Ad hoc	None

the application of ISO 9000 and EN 29001 to software. This document provides valuable quality systems guidance for software purchasers by defining activities for management and quality oversight, for software suppliers by defining quality systems and control elements for successful software development, and for auditors by defining methods used to assess software development organizations. TickIT does not provide guidance relative to defining and applying a consistent process-measurement framework.

SPICE is intended to provide an internationally recognized standard for the conduct and assessment of software development organizations, and it combines the most successful elements of the previous assessment models. This model emphasizes software engineering and management practices, as well as the application of software process improvement principles, but it does not list specific documentation required for a software development project. SPICE features a flexible scoring system that allows it to be tailored to address a user's or an organization's specific application.

The software assessment standards and models followed by medical device software developers will usually not be a single model but a collection of models determined by the device's target market and expectations relative to the device capabilities. There is so much commonality among all of these standards and models that meeting the requirements of one does not preclude use of another. As these standards and models evolve, they can be expected to become more closely aligned; therefore, the task of conformance will become easier and more consistent. At the same time, the standards and models will also evolve, to maintain pace with the state of the art in software engineering and escalating technology.

Software Metrics and Process Maturity

As evidenced in Chapter 12, dozens, if not hundreds, of metrics have been described in the software engineering literature, and the metrics chosen for a particular project play a major role in the degree to which the project can be controlled, but deciding which metrics to use is difficult. The purpose and utility of each metric can only be evaluated in light of the needs and desires of the software engineering organization and within the overall organization of the product development group. Consequently, data should be collected and software metrics analyzed in the broad context of the software engineering processes, the intent being to understand and improve those processes and their results. The concept of software process maturity originated at the SEI; it has evolved into a set of maturity levels in which a software organization's development processes take place. Only when the development process has sufficient structure and procedures does it make sense to collect certain metrics.

Rather than recommend a large and probably unwieldy set of metrics to collect for each project, SEI proposes that metrics be divided into five levels. Each level's metrics are based on the amount of information made available by the development process. As the development process matures and improves, additional metrics can be collected and analyzed, and the information derived from those metrics allows the process to be controlled and enhanced. Metrics collection, in the SEI framework, begins at the lowest maturity level and moves on to the higher levels only when it is indicated that the process can support that evolution.

Process Maturity Levels

The concept of process maturity levels is based on the notion that some software development processes provide more structure or control than others do. In effect, as certain characteristic process problems are solved by process methods and tools, the process matures and begins to focus on other problems. Maturity also provides a framework in which to depict the types of software processes and to evaluate what kinds of metrics are best suited for collection in each process type. The metrics are then used in concert with a variety of tools, techniques, and methods to improve the software engineering process, increase the software engineering maturity level, and allow for the collection of additional software metrics. Table 13-2 shows the five SEI maturity levels of process and their fundamental characteristics.

The first, termed initial, is characterized by an ad hoc approach to the software development process. In this maturity level, the inputs to the process are not well defined and the outputs are

Table 13-2   SEI Process Maturity Levels Related to Metrics

Level	Characteristics	Metrics to Use
5. Optimizing	Improvement fed back to process	Process and feedback for changing process
4. Managed	Measured process (quantitative)	Process and feedback for control
3. Defined	Process defined, institutionalized	Product
2. Repeatable	Process dependent on individuals	Project
1. Initial	Ad hoc	Baseline

expected, but the transition from inputs to outputs is undefined and uncontrolled. In this level, projects that are similar may vary widely in their productivity and quality characteristics because of inadequate structure and control; the collection of metrics for this process maturity level is difficult at best. Elementary project metrics should be gathered to form a baseline for comparisons as improvements are made and the maturity level increases. The degree of improvement at this level can be demonstrated by comparing new project measurements with the baseline measurements. For example, initial measurements can be made relative to product size and software engineering effort, and from this a development rate can then be calculated and compared to similar rates on subsequent projects. At this level, rather than concentrate on the metrics and their meaning, the software engineering staff should focus on imposing more structure and control on the process itself.

The second maturity level is termed repeatable, in that proper inputs produce proper outputs, but there is no visibility of how the outputs are produced. For example, requirements are input to software development and the output is the software, but the activities that produced the software are not particularly well known. Only project-level metrics make sense at this maturity level, because the activities within the transition from input to output are not available for measurement. The types of measurements that can be made at this maturity level are the number of lines of source code, function point count, object and method count, number of requirements changes (the process inputs), the size of the project staffing, actual person-months of effort, reported person-months of effort, the size of the budget (the process controls), and the size of the code and the time required to produce the code (the process outputs). For a repeatable process in general, the amount of effort needed to produce the software, the duration of the project, the size and volatility of the requirements, and the overall project cost should be available for measurement. The output can be measured in terms of its physical or functional size, and the resources used to produce that output can be viewed relative to the size measurement, to compute the productivity. Additional metrics may be desirable; they depend on the characteristics of the project and the needs of project management. These would include software experience with the domain or application, the architecture, the tools and methods, and the overall years of programming experience.

The third process maturity level is termed "defined" because the activities of the process are clearly defined with entry and exit conditions. For example, in the prior level, there was no visibility of how the output was produced; in this level, the output is typically the result of known stages and activities such as design, code and test, and integrate and test. The additional structure in this level means that the inputs to, and the outputs from, each well-defined software development functional activity can be examined, and the intermediate product's characteristics can be measured. The key to this maturity level is that the activities are delineated and distinguished from one another, and the products of each activity can be measured and assessed. In particular, the complexity of the requirements, design and code, and the test results can be examined, and the quality of the requirements, design, code, and testing can be assessed.

In terms of complexity, the following items can be measured for a defined process: the number of distinct objects and actions addressed in the requirements, the number of design modules, the design cyclomatic complexity, the McCabe design complexity, the number of code modules, the code cyclomatic complexity, the number of test paths to test, and the number of interfaces to test. An additional quality view of the software at this level is an examination of the number of defects in each product, the density of those defects overall, and the thoroughness of testing. These types of metrics might include the number of defects discovered, the number of defects discovered per unit size, the number of requirements faults discovered, the number of design faults discovered, the number of code faults discovered, and the fault density for each product.

This metrics set does not represent the full spectrum of quality measures that can be employed. For example, issues such as maintainability, utility, ease of use, and other aspects of quality software are not necessarily addressed by defect counts. However, defect counts and analysis are relatively easy to implement, and they do provide useful information about the reliability of the software and the thoroughness of the software testing. A final metric that might be desirable is the total number of pages of documentation. As defect density decreases, a meaningful metric might be how succinctly the requirements or design were specified. This measure indicates the proficiency and productivity of the software development group in system specification.

The fourth level of process maturity is the managed process. In this level, feedback from early project activities, such as the number of problem areas discovered in design, can be used to set priorities for later project activities, such as more extensive review and testing of certain parts of the code. Because activities can be compared and contrasted, the effects of changes in one activity can be tracked in other activities at this maturity level. In a managed process, the feedback helps to allocate resources, while the basic activities do not change; this allows for measurements to be made across process activities. For example, measurement and evaluation can be made relative to code reuse, defect-driven testing, and configuration management. The measures that are collected are then used to control and stabilize the process so that productivity and quality match expectations. As an illustrative example, metrics can be used in feedback loops that report on the number of design defects and on the number and types of problems encountered with specific versions of the software. Project management then uses these metrics to make decisions about project level corrections, directions, or emphasis.

If the software process has reached the managed maturity level, then process-wide metrics can be collected and analyzed. These metrics reflect the characteristics of the overall software processes, and of the interaction among the major activities in the process. Therefore, a distinguishing characteristic of a managed process is that software development can be carefully controlled, and a major characteristic of the metrics in this level is that they help management control the development process. For example, project management would use current design defects and problems with earlier software versions to alter the project's emphasis so that a redesign would be initiated or the software integration sequence would be altered from its original plan. The following types of data should be collected and analyzed in a managed process: process data specific to the particular process model in use; the amount of requirements, design, code, and testing reuse; defect identification by how and when defects are discovered; the use of defect density modeling to determine when testing is complete; the use of configuration management for traceability links to assess the impact of alterations or proposed changes; and module completion rate. An important point is that when this level is reached, the metrics gathered, collected, and analyzed for the previous maturity levels are used in concert with the continuing metrics. Relationships can then be determined between product characteristics and process variables to assess whether certain processes or aspects of a process are effective in meeting productivity or quality goals. This list of process metrics is not complete, and they are presented as an example for the initial attempt at capturing important information about the process itself.

The ultimate level of process maturity is the optimized process in which measures from ongoing activities are used to change and improve the process. At this level, a process change will effect the organization and project as well, because results from one or more ongoing or completed projects may lead to a refined, different development process for future projects. In addition, a project may change its process before project completion in response to feedback from early activities. As an example of this dynamic process tailoring, the project manager may begin development with a standard waterfall approach. As the requirements are defined and the design is begun, metrics may indicate a high degree of uncertainty in the requirements. On the basis of this information, the project may change its process to one that prototypes the requirements and the design, to resolve some of the uncertainty before a substantial investment is made in the implementation of the current design. In this way, an optimizing process gives the greatest flexibility to the development effort. At this level, metrics act as sensors and monitors, and not only is the process under control but it is also dynamic, flexible, and adaptive.

Achieving Higher Maturity Levels

Many organizations use the SEI CMM to improve their software engineering processes by setting goals to achieve higher maturity levels. To that end, an instrument and a process are needed that can be used to evaluate an organization's status relative to these goals. SEI provides services to help evaluate an organization's current level, as well as measure the progress toward achieving higher levels. Whether provided by SEI or developed internally, the method for assessing progress to higher maturity levels must let software engineers and management evaluate the organization's current status and identify those areas that need attention and improvement. The identified method for process assessment serves as the means to ensure continuous improvement as well as provide grass-roots participation and support in achieving higher maturity levels.

If the assessment process is developed in-house, it should not necessarily be intended as a replacement for any formal assessment instruments developed or provided by the SEI or any other process assessment service organization, but rather as an internal tool that can be used to prepare for a formal assessment at a later date. An in-house developed process assessment method offers several benefits to the organization. First, it can empower software engineers and managers working in an organization, product group, or project to conduct a self-evaluation relative to a maturity level and create their own list of findings and action plans. This ensures a grassroots involvement in the process and an institutionalization of the resultant improvements. Second, the process assessment facilitates communication among those involved in it and ensures that important information regarding processes and tools used in the software development groups is disseminated at assessment meetings. Third, the process assessment helps to educate software engineers and managers regarding key process areas and practices relative to the specifics of their software engineering process. This increases their understanding of topics in which they may not have been involved in the past, and it also increases the capability of practitioners in terms of the overall software engineering process, methods, tools, and technology. Last, the process assessment prepares the overall organization for a formal assessment.

Each level of maturity should be associated with several key process areas, and the process assessment instrument should let the organization determine scores associated with the level the organization is striving to achieve. In each key process area, there should be several pertinent activities that can be used for measuring how well an organization implements specific process activity. These process areas should reflect the organization's commitment to process performance, its ability to perform that process, the process activities performed, monitoring of software implementation, and verification of that implementation. In general, these dimensions attempt to capture the criteria relating to the organization's commitment to and management's support of the software practices, as well as the organization's ability to implement the process and practices. These dimensions also indicate the breadth and consistency of the implementation across all project areas and the demonstration of positive results over time and across all projects.

The assessment instrument usually takes the form of a survey or worksheet and an accompanying guideline. The intent of the guideline is to provide a framework to rate the designated activities specified on the worksheet and ensure that the participant addresses the spirit and themes of the evaluation. Scoring for an activity is accomplished by examining the worksheet evaluation dimensions and their guideline criteria simultaneously. The scoring values used on the worksheet are usually even-numbered integers, and the guideline would suggest values such as 0, 2, 4, 6, so that odd-numbered scores are possible if some, but not all, of the criteria for the next higher level have been met. For example, if some of the dimensions for a key process area are rated as 4 at the current level, while others are rated as 6 at the next higher level, a score of 5 would be appropriate. The worksheet is used to summarize the score determined for the activities of a given process area.

To calculate the score for a specific process area, the score for each activity as entered on all of the worksheets would be added together, and the average for the activity would be calculated from the individual activity scores for that process area. An average score of 7 or higher, for example, for all process areas within a specific level would indicate that the organization has achieved the goal of the next higher maturity level. The average of the process area scores for a specific level indicates how well the process areas and their activities have been implemented within the organization. Low scores identify those activities and process areas that need attention, to raise the organization's software process capability.

The organization's status can then be summarized on a bar chart, although a Kiviat plot is generally more dramatic. The bar chart summarizes the overall status of the process area implementation for a specific level only, and not for all levels at the same time. The Kiviat plot, or chart, summarizes the status for all process areas of a specific level. Figure 13-3 is an example of an organization's progress in implementing an arbitrary level. Each axis starts at the center of the circle and represents a process area at the specified level. In this mythical example, the chart indicates that progress was achieved in advancing from the lower level to the higher level in four of the six process areas and that two process areas still require attention.

Suppose that the organization is not satisfied with the progress made in a specific process area—for example, Project Tracking and Oversight in Figure 13-3—and wants to obtain additional information about the key activities that must be immediately addressed. Information about the implementation status can be presented in a bar chart showing the average of the individual activity scores from the worksheets used to generate the status summary. The lower bars on this chart will indicate the key activities of the process that need improvement, and addressing these items will then lead to better performance and, subsequently, the attainment of the higher maturity level.

To be effective, process assessment must be championed, used, and understood by all members of the organization. Senior management is primarily responsible for understanding what is involved in a process assessment, indicating their support for the whole process, committing resources to implement the action plans created, and following up to ensure the completion of the assessment. A single individual is responsible for championing the whole process for at least one assessment period, ensuring management support, identifying who should participate in the assessment, taking care of administrative items, and championing action-plan implementation. This individual should be technically competent, in a middle management position, and well respected by the organization as a whole. This position will require a great deal of work, because the individual is responsible for all aspects of the assessment, as well as the assessment of his or her own group. In addition, this individual initiates the organization improvement plans after the areas needing that improvement are identified.

An assessment facilitator is primarily responsible for ensuring that the assessment operates smoothly. This person must also provide consulting support when necessary. The process assessment includes not only assessment meetings, but also the creation and implementation of action plans that result from those meetings. It is possible that the assessment facilitator may be involved in several assessments simultaneously. The facilitator's background should include experience

Figure 13-3   A Kiviat plot of a typical summarized process area progress for a specific maturity level

Status of Implementation for Level *N*
Process Maturity

Organization: Software Development Engineering   **Date:** 1 Jan 2002

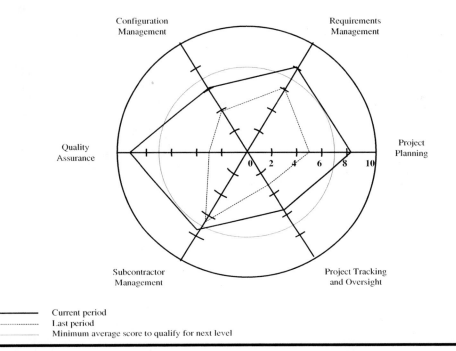

Current period
Last period
Minimum average score to qualify for next level

in conducting assessments and audits of software organizations, and he or she should be able to work closely with the assessment champion. The assessment participants are primarily technical individuals and middle-management personnel who are involved in day-to-day software engineering development and maintenance activities. To assure a complete and well-rounded view of the process being evaluated, other participants should be involved, such as product management, marketing, and hardware engineers, as long as those individuals have at least a working knowledge of the overall software process.

The Steps in Using Maturity Metrics

Metrics are most useful only when implemented in a careful sequence of activities for which the groundwork has been laid. This foundation is laid by evaluating the needs and characteristics of the software engineering processes before identifying the appropriate metrics to collect. In the first step, the current process maturity level should be established, and a determination of the process maturity level desired should be made by working with a set of metrics guidelines or with an assigned process and metrics team. When the current process maturity level is known, the next step is to decide on the metrics to be collected. Using the SEI CMM model as an example, if Level 2 is indicated as the process level desired, but ongoing projects currently collect no metrics at all, then Level 1 metrics may be suggested as a starting point, and Level 2 metrics would be added later.

When the types of metrics to be collected have been determined, in step three the tools and techniques to be used for metrics collection are identified. The collection of the metrics can be targeted for a proposed project, an ongoing project, or both, but the overall goals of the project(s) need to be assured and not compromised. Thus, whenever possible, automated support for metrics collection and analysis should be implemented as a part of the project development environment. It is essential that metrics collection and analysis do not impede the primary project development activities. When the current and proposed process levels have been determined and the development environment selected, the cost and schedule of the project(s) can be estimated, as step four. The intent of this measurement is to establish an initial baseline of productivity that will be used to gauge future project efforts. These two estimates will always be performed regardless of any other metrics that are to be collected.

In step five, the actual project cost and schedule are continuously monitored, and the metrics determined to best measure the maturity level are collected. The frequency of collection is variable; it should not be done too often or too seldom. Too frequent measuring might disrupt the normal project activities and process flow and, therefore, skew the metrics results; too seldom measuring might not capture a true reflection of the project activities and process flow. A convenient time to collect metrics is immediately after a major project deliverable, at a milestone, or when one phase of the project ends and the next one begins, and metrics should always take place as an integral part of the project postmortem. In the meantime, a project database of metrics data should be created and maintained. The database repository will facilitate the storage, handling, analysis, and archiving of the project metrics information. These data are used for analysis on the current project, as well as for tracking the value of the metrics over time to determine trends and to understand how project and product characteristics change.

When the project is complete, the last step is to evaluate the initial estimates of cost and schedule for accuracy and determine which of the factors may account for discrepancies between the predicted and actual values. In addition, an overall evaluation of the project productivity and product quality, based on the metrics that were collected during the project, should be made. On the basis of metrics evaluation, further changes to the process implementation can then be proposed, and the procedure begins again. When the analysis and evaluation have been completed, the project metrics should be incorporated into a corporate or organizational database of metrics. This larger database can then be used to provide historical information as a basis for estimation on future projects, and the database can be used to suggest the most appropriate tools and techniques for proposed projects.

Identifying and Managing Risks
for Software Process Improvement

It is well documented that quality improvement programs and business process reengineering projects fail for a broad range of reasons (Bashein et al 1994; Masters 1996). Software project data indicate that these programs fail to meet their target cost, schedule, and content (Johnson 1995). Implementing a new *software process improvement* (SPI) program can be risky, and the chance of failure in an SPI program is also significant. Handling SPI risks requires the same careful identification and analysis of the work environment that is needed for software projects; SPI work must be carefully run as a project. Successful SPI projects must

- Have the support of the organization's management
- Have experienced people be responsible and accountable for success
- Be carefully planned and tracked
- Have clearly identified and usable deliverables
- Suit the goals and mission statement of the organization
- Identify and manage the risks to success
- Be staffed by teams with change management expertise.

To ensure an SPI program's success, the organization must understand the risks to that program and mitigate them as early and completely as possible. In fact, the risks to the overall SPI program must be analyzed well before any individual SPI project is undertaken, or the project may never get started. Organizations need to deal with risks at three key points in an SPI program: (1) the initiation of the overall SPI program, (2) planning and defining a specific process, measure, or other work items for the SPI program, and (3) analyzing lessons learned from the SPI project activity or from the program as a whole. During initiation, SPI teams must analyze the organization with regard to known critical success factors and failure points for an SPI program. Subsequently, for each project activity in the SPI program, the project team should identify and manage project risks as part of its standard project planning and tracking. It must examine how well the risk handling worked during its learning phase, using a post-project or post-phase review.

Risk Factors for Software Process Improvement

To identify the significant risks at any of the above three points, it is useful to have a knowledge base of risks experienced by past SPI projects. Available literature contains useful information about the enablers and roadblocks to process improvement from organizations that are either engaged in or have implemented an SPI program. Typical categories of SPI risk factors include budget and cost, content of deliverables, culture, maintenance of SPI deliverables, mission and goals, organization management, organization stability, and process users. The typical risk factors for SPI as a managed project include the development schedule, environment, and process, project management, and staffing. For each risk factor within each category, the organization should construct a factor chart (Table 13-3) that has cues for low, medium, and high risk for the SPI program. The chart is tailored for the organization or group, but it evolves as new risks are encountered, forming a living repository of the group's known SPI risks. When identifying risks, the SPI team members can examine the chart to see if it suggests a specific risk in their situation. If it does, they rate the project's exposure to risks suggested by that factor, perhaps on a scale of 1 to 5. As they progress farther into the risk identification, they describe the specific risk suggested by the factor.

This examination is the beginning of the risk management process. As the team reviews the factor chart, it develops a consensus on the overall exposure represented by each factor. The team then details the specific risk to the project or program for each high-ranking factor. After establishing a ranked list, the team decides what to do about each risk: accept it and go forward,

Table 13-3   Typical Chart of Risk Factors for Software Process Improvement

Risk Category	Risk Factor	Cues for Low Risk	Cues for Medium Risk	Cues for High Risk	Rating
Budget and cost					
Content of deliverables					
Culture					
Maintenance of SPI deliverables					
Mission and goals					
Organization management					
Organization stability					
Process users					
Schedule for SPI development					
SPI development environment					
SPI development process					
SPI project management					
SPI staff					

develop a mitigation strategy, or drop the effort. In the latter case, the team might conclude that the project as currently defined has no chance of success, and serious changes are needed. If this is the SPI initiation risk assessment, the conclusion may be to put the SPI program on hold until critical success factors can be established.

Identifying Risks during Initiation

Before investing time and resources in the venture, it is first prudent to have an objective review of the organization's status to see if conditions are favorable for an SPI program to proceed. When an SPI program is initiated, a risk assessment should include participation by someone experienced with SPI in other organizations. Although a new SPI team may identify risks using the list of risk factors, it will likely need help selling management on the organization factors that generally impede SPI program startup. Some obvious risk factors include:

- Organization instability, such as high rates of employee turnover
- Frequent organic or structural changes in the organization
- Significant change in business focus within the past three to six months
- Threat of or impending sale or merger of the organization

- Lack of management commitment
- Lack of personal time invested in SPI
- Unfounded expectation of fast-paced changes
- Lack of knowledge about how to proceed.

Where such threats are present, the SPI program generally cannot obtain the organizational focus and support needed to ensure success. Management teams in crisis-stricken organizations need all the organization's members to help deal with those crises. In instances of high organizational instability, it is usually too difficult to dedicate resources to establish and manage a process improvement program; such organizations should resolve those problems before continuing with SPI.

To perform an assessment of SPI initiation risk, an evaluation team should both formally and informally examine the state of the organization. Formal techniques ensure that all generally relevant areas are covered, whereas informal techniques gather supporting information unique to the organization. The SPI risk factors chart can be used as a trigger for interview questions or to survey project members and thereby derive consensus on how much risk the organization faces for each risk factor. It is useful to combine surveys and interviews into a coordinated effort for a team composed of external SPI experts and internal SPI team members, with steps such as the following:

1. The SPI experts meet with management and describe the approach to be taken.

2. The organization builds a risk team composed of external and internal members.

3. Management endorses the effort and communicates the request for the organization to be involved.

4. The risk team agrees on the content of the risk survey.

5. The organization members complete the survey, and the results are compiled and used by the risk team to generate interview scripts.

6. The risk team interviews a subset of the organization in depth, selecting interviewees on the basis of which factors have been identified as high risks.

7. The risk team compiles the interview results showing the key risk factors, summaries of the evidence supporting those factors, and the specific risks identified for the SPI program.

8. The SPI experts deliver the recommendations to management, including guidance on whether risk factors that threaten the SPI program are present, what actions are needed to prepare for the SPI program, and when the SPI program might he started.

9. Management makes the decision to proceed or to delay initiation of the SPI program.

Managing Risks during Software Process Improvement Activities

As the team that manages the SPI program begins its work, it builds an SPI project plan that describes its goals and objectives, technical approach, management approach, communication plan, and approach to risk management. The team considers the risks identified during the initiation of the SPI program to see if any are still relevant. The team also reviews the chart of SPI risk factors to see what risks may be present for the project activity being planned. After identifying the factors that appear relevant, the team crafts clear statements of risk for each highly rated factor, using the traditional $<$*risk condition, risk consequence*$>$ format. For example, in an organization in which there has been little experience with defined processes, the statement might be worded "Because few in the organization have experience using defined processes and are concerned that new processes will stifle creativity, individuals will actively oppose introduction of documented processes." After building the specific risk statements, an SPI project team may have many risks on its list. Team members then estimate the likelihood of occurrence for each risk and its possible consequences. Losses from specific risks can be represented in terms of financial impact, time impact, or overall level of loss. In practice, loss levels can range from 1 to 10, where 1 is a minor delay or small amount of change to the SPI project and 10 is total SPI project failure. A narrower assessment range can be used, such as 1 to 5, but this restricts possible interpretations of the loss risk. The total risk exposure for each risk is then computed as the product of probability and loss.

Using this information, the team would organize a chart in the form shown in Table 13-4, with specific risks ordered by level of risk exposure. Generally, a team will see several risks that rank near the top and need to be mitigated. Just as with a software project, if there are more than a half dozen serious risks, then the project is seriously challenged and needs to be re-planned. Throughout the project, the team must monitor the serious risks to ensure that their mitigation actions keep each risk in check. The team must also continue to watch for other serious risk conditions that arise during the project's execution and add those risks to the list to monitor and mitigate. The overall approach is fundamentally much like the approach recommended for a software development project. The SPI project team would use action teams for specific efforts in the SPI program; each action team would take on part of the overall SPI project. For each of these action teams, there is a similar risk management effort for that subproject. Subproject risks tend to be concerned with elements such as available time and expertise, methods to deploy the results effectively, and methods to measure impact on the organization. The action team develops its list of top risks, with associated mitigation actions, and monitors progress with that risk in the same manner as with the overall SPI project.

An especially critical point for risk management is when the improvement team has completed its work, has piloted the improvement, and is prepared for organization rollout. There is a whole new set of risks to manage once the team starts to stage the improvement into projects, to implement appropriate management reviews and training, and to provide any necessary tools or consulting. The process owners must handle these risks, perhaps through a software engineering process group or managers whose business efforts require effective use of the new process. Common risk elements at this point include project management resistance to change, project

Table 13-4   Typical Chart of Risk and Loss in a Software Process Improvement Project

Item	Risk Item	Probability	Loss	Exposure	Mitigation Approach
1					
2					
3					
4					
5					

team resistance to change, project schedules that restrict time for learning about new processes, and difficulty in measuring the impact of changes because of a previously chaotic environment.

Process owners need to employ risk identification, analysis, and mitigation techniques like those for any other project as part of their implementation planning and support. Those who ultimately own the responsibility for effective use of the processes and those who maintain the process collaborate on a rollout plan, which includes its own risk management approach. At this point, some risks can be handled only by managers who have access to the resources and means of enforcement, while other risks must he mitigated by the process owners as they deal with improvements suggested by those who use the process.

Learning from the Risk Management Efforts

After each action team develops its process change, it conducts a post-project review of its work products and processes. As part of that review, the team examines how well it identified and managed its risks to success. For items that were successfully managed, the organization's chart of SPI risk factors might be annotated with a description of the methods that helped counteract those risks. For problems that were not anticipated but did arise, the chart might also be extended to include telltale risk factors and the evidence to watch for in the future. Similarly, when the overall SPI project finishes a phase or completes the overall plan, the SPI team conducts a post-project review of its work and considers its performance against the risk items, as well as the organization's ability to absorb the changed processes from the action teams. Learning, in the form of what worked well and what new risks arose, is incorporated into the organization's chart of risk factors. As they examine the chart from improvement project to improvement project, the SPI team can see what factors can be removed because they did not recur. They also can ensure that all new factors are incorporated, to ensure that they will be considered when launching new SPI activities.

In practice, teams can predict their chances for success on the basis of the risks they identify. To optimize their chances of success, SPI project teams should consider what has been learned about risk by those who have conducted similar programs. Teams can minimize problems by identifying and managing risks before starting a risk program, by making risk management an integral part of every SPI project, and by learning after deployment of organization change. A collection of risk factors in a chart of SPI risk factors can be a powerful and simple tool to identify risks and to provide a means to accumulate learning. Analyzing the risks identified, establishing a plan to manage them, and monitoring the most important risks throughout a project allow the project team to minimize the impact of those risks.

Software Process Improvement Scope Based on Organizational Goals

The CMM developed by the SEI is a model to help software organizations improve their development capability. Acceptance and use of the CMM for process improvement varies among organizations, some using it as an optional guideline and others revering it as gospel. When used appropriately, CMM can help organizations develop software with predictable cost, schedule, and quality. When used inappropriately, it can waste time and demoralize an entire organization. Many organizations approach process improvement by simply documenting each and every process. This process-centric approach may be amplified when an organization attempts to adopt a more sweeping and systematic technique for improvement, such as ISO 9001 or the CMM. Despite the process-centric goal "Be SEI CMM Level 3 by December," the approach of documenting all processes is reinforced and might even appear natural. A process-centric approach can work, but it has a high risk of failure because most people mistake documentation for progress. In this case, the improvement effort is not particularly integrated with the organization's product development goals, and this usually results in a large stack of unused process documents.

The CMM version 1.1 consists of five levels of engineering and management process maturity, in which each level builds on the next. CMM Level 1 has no criteria and represents projects that typically have large amounts of rework, numerous technical surprises, frustrated customers, and significant cost and schedule overruns. Although good software can come from a CMM Level 1 organization, this result is not easy to achieve or sustain. CMM Level 2 comprises sound project management, negotiations with the customer, version control, vendor management, and simple process and product assurance. Organizations at CMM Level 3 can focus on product development rather than day-to-day crises. CMM Level 4 focuses on organization-wide engineering skills, basic systems engineering, advanced project management, and an infrastructure to support sustained improvement. Organizations at CMM Level 5 consistently produce reliable software on time.

An alternative to the process-centric approach of improvement is to scope the improvement program on the basis of the problems and goals of the organization. Adopting this approach enables significant progress to be made on real issues and headway to be made using the CMM. Examples of an organization's business goals might include the delivery of a product, the completion of a software project, or the completion of software upgrades. The goal could also be the desired outcome when a critical problem has been solved. For example, an organization may be unable to hit delivery deadlines, or it might spend 75 percent of its resources on rework; the goals related to these problems would be meeting deadlines 100 percent of the time or reducing rework to 25 percent. To use the goal-problem approach, the first step is to determine the organization's business goals and problem areas and then compare these to the elements of the SEI CMM. The second step is to select the appropriate elements of the CMM that address these problems and help to move toward the organization goals. For example, suppose the company is planning an improvement program and the organization was about to form six teams. The teams are to work on the six key process areas (KPA) of CMM Level 2, which are requirements management (RM), software project planning (SPP), software project tracking and oversight (SPTO), software configuration management (SCM), and software quality assurance (SQA). As a reference for this example, the key process areas of CMM Level 3 are training programs (TP), software product engineering (SPE), peer reviews (PR), intergroup coordination (IC), and integrated software management (ISM). Rather than embarking on an effort to reach CMM Level 2, the organization begins by stating all of the major product development problems that are currently being faced and then lists the business goals to be achieved over the next six to 18 months. The problems and goals are compared with the practices in SEI CMM Levels 2 and 3. The related KPA names and activities are then paired with each item (see Tables 13-5 and 13-6). The activities represent smaller and more manageable solutions that address the problems and support the goals. If the company had been using ISO 9001 or the Malcolm Baldrige Award, their activities would have mapped the problems and goals to those criteria.

The scope of the improvement program is to address the problems and the goals of the organization. As shown in Tables 13-5 and 13-6, 21 of the 23 items, or 91 percent, map to CMM Level 2 practices and activities. This also means that when all the problems and goals have been addressed, 46 percent of the CMM Level 2 activities will have been addressed. The essential difference between this approach and addressing the six KPAs in parallel is that the problems and goals indicate which part of each KPA should be addressed first. Regardless of whether the organization is using SEI CMM, ISO 9001, or another model or standard, the problem-goal approach will help scope and sequence the improvement program. Of course, not every problem

Table 13-5   Typical Organizational Problems and Capability Maturity Model Solutions

Problem		CMM Solution	
Number	**Description**	**Level**	**Area**
1	Need better requirements; requirements tracking not in place; changes to requirements are not tracked; code does not match specifications at test time	2	Requirements Management activities 1, 2, and 3
2	Management direction unclear for version 2.3; goals change often	2	Requirements Management activities 1 and 3 and verification 1
3	Hard to revise project plan; items drop off, new items are added, plan is out of date	2	Software Project Tracking and Oversight activities 2, 8, and 9
4	Wrong files get put on CD-ROM; do not know what the correct ones should be	2	Software Configuration Management activities 4, 7, 8, 9, and 10
5	Defect repairs break essential product features	2	Software Configuration Management activities 5, 6, 7, 9, and 10; abilities 1, 2, 4, and 5; verifications 3 and 4
6	Customers are unhappy; approximately 75 outstanding defects have not been addressed	2	Software Configuration Management verification 1
			Requirements Management activity 3
		3	Intergroup Coordination activity 3
7	Difficult to find time to do critical activities (product development) versus crisis activities	2	Software Project Planning activities 4, 10, and 12
8	Lack of resources and skills allocated to software design	2	Software Project Planning activity 10
9	Quality department needs team training on product and test skills	2	Software Quality Assurance abilities 2, 3, and 4
10	Changes to specifications and documentation aren't communicated effectively to documentation and test groups	2	Requirements Management activities 1, 2, and 3
			Software Configuration Management activities 5, 6, 7, and 9 and ability 1

Continued on next page.

Continued from previous page.

Problem		CMM Solution	
Number	**Description**	**Level**	**Area**
11	Unreliable project schedule estimates	2	Software Project Planning activities 5, 9, 10, 12, 13, and 14 and ability 4
12	Unclear status of software changes	2	Software Configuration Management activities 8 and 9
13	Testing doesn't necessarily comprehend things that matter to the customer	3	Software Product Engineering activities 5, 6, and 7

Table 13-6   Typical Organizational Goals and Applicable Capability Maturity Model Solutions

Problem		CMM Solution	
Number	**Description**	**Level**	**Area**
1	Orderly plans for development	2	Software Project Planning activities 2, 5, 6, 7, 8, 13, and 14
2	Understand what our capacity is; develop one list of all the work to be done	2	Software Project Planning activity 7 and ability 1
3	Improve schedule tracking and communication of changes to impacted groups	2	Software Project Tracking and Oversight activities 3 and 4
4	Successfully deliver new product	2	Requirements Management activities 1, 2, and 3
			Software Project Planning activities 6, 10, and 13
5	Improve performance of core software product	2	Software Project Planning activity 11
			Software Project Planning activity 7
6	Identify needed skills for new designers and hire, promote, and train accordingly	3	Software Product Engineering activity 3 and ability 2
7	Identify tools to support software developers	2	Software Project Planning activity 14
		3	Software Product Engineering activity 1

Continued on next page.

Continued from previous page.

Problem		CMM Solution	
Number	**Description**	**Level**	**Area**
8	Keep making a profit, and keep customers happy	2	Requirements Management activities 1 and 2
			Software Project Planning activities 10, 12, and 13
			Software Project Tracking and Oversight activities 4, 6, 8, and 10
			Software Quality Assurance activity 5
		3	Software Product Engineering activities 2 and 7
			Intergroup Coordination activity 1
			Peer Review goal 2
9	Identify tools to support software testers	2	Software Project Planning activity 14
		3	Software Product Engineering activity 1
10	Empower Quality Department to have final say on product shipment	2	Software Quality Assurance activities 6 and 7

listed in Tables 13-5 and 13-6 exactly matches the key process areas of CMM Level 2. For example, the CMM does not specifically address the fifth goal, which is to improve the performance of the core software product. In this situation, the organization must determine which areas it is most important to fix now; serious problems should be worked on first, regardless of whether they relate to the CMM. Solutions to this specific goal will likely come from other technical sources.

Five lessons can be learned from adopting the goal-problem approach. First, and fundamentally, all process improvement can be meaningful. Second, the problems and goals can help identify that part of the SEI CMM that should be worked on first. The CMM should not be seen as an all-or-nothing approach, in which all parts should be attempted at once. Rather, it should be treated as a large toolbox of smaller actions, ideas, and solutions, each of which is useful at different times. Third, any process document developed to solve a problem will be meaningful and useful; therefore, a process improvement team will be more focused on the process, because its scope is defined by a problem. Four, the group's motivation to work on improvement is increased when its problems and goals are the primary focus of the improvement program. Last, focusing on goals and solutions to problems prevents the organization from creating academic process documents.

One of the primary concerns that has been expressed about the goal-problem approach is that an organization will not achieve its initial goal of CMM Level 3 or ISO 9001, because attention will be diverted to the business goals and problems lists. The solution is to repeat the cycle to determine the next set of problems and goals when the first set of problems and goals has been addressed. This new set can then be compared to the remaining elements in the CMM, and, over a one-to three-year period, each section of the CMM can be matched with a problem or goal. As an example, assume that the company that owned the problems and goals listed in Tables 13-5 and 13-6 conducted an informal process assessment after nine months of improvement work. Suppose the assessment showed that 50 percent of CMM Level 2 practices had been adopted, and many of the initial problems had been fixed. At the end of the assessment, the company could revise its problem list for the next phase of the improvement program so that, again, each one of these problems maps specifically to practices in the SEI CMM. To be sure, there are situations in which some of the elements of the CMM are not used when solving a problem or achieving a goal. In this instance, these elements should be left until the end of the improvement cycle, when either the outstanding elements are put to good use or are considered not applicable. CMM elements are put to good use by asking the question, "What problem do we have where this element could help?" This question frequently elicits project team experiences in which the project problems have been solved but some lingering difficulties still exist.

The goal-problem approach also helps an organization avoid prematurely using practices from the CMM. Process auditing is an example of a practice that is sometimes adopted prematurely. Process audits verify that the correct process steps have been carried out when performing engineering activities such as schedule estimation, testing, peer reviews, and SCM. Process audits identify and eliminate engineering mistakes before they cause large, unnecessary costs in the project's later phases. In the beginning of an improvement program, there is usually little benefit in performing process audits. However, the need for the process becomes apparent when it has been defined, used, and proven effective. Defining the scope of an improvement program can be difficult and frustrating; moreover, the task becomes daunting when a process model, such as the CMM, is adopted wholesale. However, a simple, immediately available solution is to use the goals and problems of the organization to provide a timeless and effective scope for any improvement program and to apply a model or standard that can be used as a source of ideas, solutions, and actions to achieve this scope.

Bibliography

Aas, E. J. 1996. Design quality metrics based on an event-oriented design process model: Theory and example of use in electronic design. *Quality Engineering* 8 (4).

Abdel-Hamid, T. K. 1993. Adapting, correcting, and perfecting software estimates: A maintenance metaphor. *Computer* 26 (3).

Abdel-Hamid, T. K., and S. E. Madnick. 1983. The dynamics of software project scheduling. *Communications of the ACM* 26 (5).

Abdel-Hamid, T. K., and S. E. Madnick. 1990. The elusive silver lining: How we fail to learn from software development failures. *Sloan Management Review* (Fall).

Abe, J., K. Sakamura, and H. Aiso. 1979. An analysis of software product failure. In *Proceedings of the Fourth International Conference on Software Engineering.* Los Alamitos: Computer Society Press.

Abelson, H., and G. Sussman. 1985. *The structure and interpretation of computer programs.* New York: McGraw-Hill.

Adam, J. A., and R. C. Eberhart. 1994. Medical electronics: Surgery simulated, wireless house call. *IEEE Spectrum* 31 (1).

Addelman, S. 1962. Orthogonal main effect plans for asymmetrical factorial experiments. *Technometrics* 4.

Akiyama, F. 1971. An example of software engineering debugging. *Information Processing* 71.

Alavi, M. 1984. An assessment of the prototyping approach to information systems development. *Communications of the ACM* 27 (6).

Albrecht, A. J. 1979. Measuring application development productivity. In *Proceedings of the Joint GUIDE/SHARE/IBM Application Development Symposium.* Monterey: International Business Machines.

Albrecht, A. J., and J. E. Gaffney. 1983. Software function, source lines of code and development effort prediction: A software science validation. *IEEE Transactions on Software Engineering* 9 (6).

Allworth, S. T. 1981. *Introduction to real-time software design.* New York: Springer-Verlag.

Allworth, S. T., and R. N. Zobel. 1987. *Introduction to real-time software design,* 2nd ed. New York: Springer-Verlag.

Altmayer, L., and J. DeGood. 1986. A distributed software development case study. In *HP Software Productivity Conference Proceedings*. Palo Alto: Hewlett-Packard.

Alunkal, J. M. 1993. Designing an integrated corporate test strategy. *Electronic Design* (March).

Anderson, J., F. Fleek, K. Garrity, and F. Drake. 2001. Integrating usability techniques into software development. *IEEE Software* 17 (1).

Anderson, T., and R. W. Witty. 1978. Safe programming. *Biomedical Instrumentation and Technology* 18.

Anderson, T., and P. A. Lee. 1981. *Fault tolerance: Principles and design*. Englewood Cliffs: Prentice-Hall.

Andriole, S. J., ed. 1986. *Software validation, verification, testing, and documentation*. Princeton: Petrocelli Books.

Andriole, S. J., and P. A. Freeman. 1993. Software systems engineering: The case for a new discipline. *Software Engineering Journal* (May).

Aron, J. D. 1969. *Estimating resources for large programming systems*. Rome: NATO Science Committee.

Arthur, J. 1984. Software quality measurements. *Datamation* (December).

Arthur, L. J. 1985. *Measuring programmer productivity and software quality*. New York: John Wiley & Sons.

Asada, T., et al. 1996. The quantified design space. In *Software architecture*, ed. M. Shaw and D. Garlan. Englewood Cliffs: Prentice-Hall.

Association for the Advancement of Medical Instrumentation. 1988. *Human factors engineering guidelines and preferred practices for the design of medical devices*. AAMI Publication HE-1988. Arlington: Association for the Advancement of Medical Instrumentation.

Austin, R. D. 1996. *Measuring and managing performance in organizations*. New York: Dorset House.

Babel, P. 1997. Software development capability evaluation: An integrated systems and software approach. *CrossTalk: The Journal of Defense Software Engineering* 10 (4).

Bach, J. 1997. Good enough quality: Beyond the buzzword. *Computer* (August).

Bach, J. 1998. A framework for good enough testing. *Computer* 31 (10).

Bailey, J. W., and V. R. Basili. 1981. A meta-model for software development resource expenditures. In *Proceedings of the 5th International Conference on Software Engineering*. Los Alamitos: Computer Society Press.

Baker, A. L., and S. H. Zweben. 1980. A comparison of measures of control flow complexity. *Transactions on Software Engineering* 6 (6).

Baker, F. T. 1972. Chief programmer team management of production programming. *IBM Systems Journal* 11 (1).

Baker, F. T., and H. D. Mills. 1973. Chief programmer teams. *Datamation* 19 (12).

Baldwin, J. T. 1995. Predicting and estimating real-time performance. *Embedded Systems Programming* 8 (2).

Balzer, R., T. E. Cheatham, and C. Green. 1983. Software technology in the 1990s: Using a new paradigm. *Computer* (November).

Barnard, K., and A. Price. 1994. Managing code inspection information. *IEEE Software* 11 (2).

Barnes, B. H., and T. B. Bollinger. 1993. Making reuse cost-effective. In *Software management,* ed. D. Reifer. Washington, D.C.: IEEE Computer Society Press.

Barnes, D. 1983. Special series on system integration. *Electronic Design* 31 (8).

Baronas, A., and M. Louis. 1988. Restoring a sense of control during implementation: How user involvement leads to system acceptance. *MIS Quarterly* 12 (1).

Bashein, B. J., et al. 1994. Preconditions for bpr success. *Information Systems Management* (Spring).

Basili, V. R., and J. D. Musa. 1991. The future engineering of software: A management perspective. *IEEE Computer* (September).

Basili, V. R., and B. T. Perricone. 1984. Software errors and complexity: An empirical investigation. *Communications of the ACM* 27 (1).

Basili, V. R., and R. W. Reiter. 1979a. Evaluating automatable measures of software development. In *Proceedings of the Workshop on Quantitative Software Models.* Los Alamitos: Computer Society Press.

Basili, V. R., and R. W. Reiter. 1979b. An investigation of human factors in software development. *Computer* 12 (12).

Basili, V., and H. D. Rombach. 1987. Tailoring the software process to project goals and environments. In *Proceedings of the Ninth International Conference on Software Engineering.* Los Alamitos: Computer Society Press.

Basili, V. R., and H. D. Rombach. 1991. Support for comprehensive reuse. *Software Engineering Journal* (September).

Basili, V. R., and R. W. Selby. 1983. Metric analysis and data validation across FORTRAN projects. *IEEE Transactions on Software Engineering* 9 (6).

Basili, V. R., and A. J. Turner. 1975. Iterative enhancement: A practical technique for software development. *IEEE Transactions on Software Engineering* 1 (4).

Basili, V. R., and D. M. Weiss. 1981. Evaluation of a software requirements document by analysis of change data. In *Proceedings of the Fifth International Conference on Software Engineering.* Los Alamitos: Computer Society Press.

Basili, V. R., and D. Weiss. 1984. A methodology for collecting valid software engineering data. *IEEE Transactions on Software Engineering* 10 (6).

Basili, V., et al. 1996. The empirical investigation of perspective-based reading. *Empirical Software Engineering: An International Journal* 1 (2).

Bassen, H., J. Silberberg, F. Houston, W. Knight, C. Christman, and M. Greberman. 1985. Computerized medical devices: Usage trends, problems, and safety technology. In *Proceedings of the 7th Annual Conference of IEEE Engineering in Medicine and Biology Society.* Los Alamitos: Computer Society Press.

Bear, S., and T. Rush. 1991. Rigorous software engineering: A method of preventing software defects. *Hewlett-Packard Journal* 42 (5).

Behrens, C. A. 1987. Measuring the productivity of computer systems development activities with function points. *IEEE Transactions on Software Engineering* 13 (1).

Beizer, B. 1983. *Software testing techniques.* New York: Van Nostrand Reinhold.

Beizer, B. 1984. *Software system testing and quality assurance.* New York: Van Nostrand Reinhold.

Belady, L., and M. Lehman. 1976. A model of large program development. *IBM Systems Journal* 15 (3).

Belady, L., and M. Lehman. 1979. The characteristics of large systems. In *Research directions in software technology,* ed. P. Wegner. Cambridge: MIT Press.

Bell, T. E., and T. A. Thayer. 1976. Software requirements: Are they really a problem? In *Proceedings of the Second International Conference on Software Engineering.* Los Alamitos: Computer Society Press.

Bennatan, E. 1992. *On time, within budget: Software projects management practices and techniques.* Wellesley: QED Publishing Group.

Bennington, H. D. 1956; 1983; 1987. Production of large computer programs. In *Proceedings of the ONR Symposium on Advanced Programming Methods for Digital Computers.* Los Alamitos: Computer Society Press. *Annals of the History of Computing.* Los Alamitos: Computer Society Press. In *Proceedings, International Conference on Software Engineering 9, IEEE-Computer Society.* Los Alamitos: Computer Society Press.

Berard, E. V. 1993. *Essays on object-oriented software engineering, Vol. I.* Englewood Cliffs: Prentice-Hall.

Berard, E. V. 1996. Bringing testing into the fold. *IEEE Software* 13 (3).

Berdichevsky, D., and E. Neunschwander. 1999. Toward an ethics of persuasive technology. *Communications of the ACM* 42 (5).

Berlack, H. R. 1992. *Software configuration management.* New York: John Wiley & Sons.

Berlack, H. R. 1995. Evaluation and selection of automated configuration management tools. *CrossTalk: The Journal of Defense Software Engineering* 8 (11).

Berns, G. M. 1984. Assessing software maintainability. *Communications of the ACM* 27 (1).

Bernstein, A., and P. K. Hart. 1981. Proving real time properties of programs with temporal logic. In *Proceedings of the 8th ACM Symposium on Operating Systems.* New York: Association for Computing Machinery.

Bernstein, L. 1995. Where to invest your software bucks. *IEEE* (February).

Bernstein, L., and A. Lubashevsky. 1995. Living with function points. *CrossTalk: The Journal of Defense Software Engineering* 8 (11).

Bernstein, L., and C. M. Yuhas. 1993. Testing network management software. *Journal of Network and System Management* 1 (1).

Bersoff, E. H. 1988. Elements of software configuration management. In *Tutorial: Software engineering project management,* ed. R. H. Thayer. Washington, D.C.: IEEE Computer Society Press.

Bersoff, E. H., and A. M. Davis. 1993. Impacts of life cycle models on software configuration management. In *Software management,* ed. D. Reifer. Washington, D.C.: IEEE Computer Society Press.

Betteridge, R., D. Fisher, and P. Goodman. 1990. Function points vs. lines of code. *System Development* (August).

Beyer, H., and K. Holtzblatt. 1997. *Contextual design: A customer-centered approach to systems design.* San Francisco: Morgan Kaufmann.

Bias, R. G., and D. J. Mayhew, eds. *Cost-justifying usability.* Boston: Harcourt Brace and Company.

Biffl, S. 2000. Using inspection data for defect estimation. *IEEE Software* 17 (6).

Birrell, N. D., and M. A. Ould. 1985. *A practical handbook for software development.* New York: Cambridge University Press.

Black, R. K. D., R. P. Curnow, R. Katz, and M. D. Gray. 1977. *BCS software production data.* Final Technical Report, RADC-TR-77-116, Boeing Computer Services, Inc. NTIS Number AD-A039852.

Blair, S. 1986. A defect tracking system for the Unix environment. *HP Journal* 37 (3).

Blank, J., M. M. H. Drummen, H. Gerstling, T. G. M. Janssen, M. J. Krijer, and W. D. Pelger. 1983. *Software engineering: Methods and techniques.* New York: John Wiley & Sons.

Boar, B. 1984. *Application prototyping.* Reading: Addison-Wesley.

Boehm, B. W. 1975. Software design and structuring. In *Practical strategies for developing large software systems,* ed. E. Horowitz. Reading: Addison-Wesley.

Boehm, B. W. 1976. Software engineering. *IEEE Transactions on Computers* (December).

Boehm, B. W. 1981a. *Software engineering economics.* Englewood Cliffs: Prentice-Hall.

Boehm, B. W. 1981b. An experiment in small-scale application software engineering. *IEEE Transactions on Software Engineering* 7 (5).

Boehm, Barry. 1984. Prototyping versus specifying: A multiproject experiment. *IEEE Transactions on Software Engineering* (May).

Boehm, B. W. 1984. Software engineering economics. *IEEE Transactions on Software Engineering* 10 (1).

Boehm, B. W. 1988a. A spiral model of software development and enhancement. In *Tutorial: Software engineering project management,* ed. R. H. Thayer. Washington, D.C.: IEEE Computer Society Press.

Boehm, B. W. 1988b. Improving software productivity. In *Tutorial: Software engineering project management,* ed. R. H. Thayer. Washington, D.C.: IEEE Computer Society Press.

Boehm, B. W. 1990. Verifying and validating software requirements and design specifications. In *Milestones in software evolution,* eds. P. W. Oman and T. G. Lewis. Washington, D.C.: IEEE Computer Society Press.

Boehm, B. W. 1991. Software risk management: Principles and practice. *IEEE Software* (January).

Boehm, B. W. 1993. Software risk management: Principles and practices. In *Software management,* ed. D. Reifer. Washington, D.C.: IEEE Computer Society Press.

Boehm, B. W., J. R. Brown, and M. Lipow. 1976. Quantitative evaluation of software quality. In *IEEE 2nd International Conference on Software Engineering.* Los Alamitos: Computer Society Press.

Boehm, B. W., J. R. Brown, H. Kaspar, M. Lipow, G. J. MacLeod, and M. J. Merrit. 1978. Characteristics of software quality. *TRW Series of Software Technology,* Vol. 1. Amsterdam/New York: North-Holland.

Boehm, B. W., J. F. Elwell, A. B. Peyster, E. D. Stuckle, and R. D. Williams. 1982. The TRW software productivity system. In *Proceedings of the 6th International Conference on Software Engineering.* Los Alamitos: Computer Society Press.

Boehm, B. W., T. E. Gray, and T. Seewaldt. 1984. Prototyping vs. specification: A multi-project experiment. In *Proceedings of Seventh International Conference on Software Engineering.* New York: Association of Computing Machinery and Institute of Electronic and Electrical Engineers.

Boehm, B. W., M. H. Penedo, R. D. Stuckle, R. D. Williams, and A. B. Peyster. 1984. A software development environment for improving quality. *Computer* (June).

Boehm, B., et al. 1995. Cost models for future software life cycle processes: COCOMO 2.0. *Annals of Software Engineering 1.* Los Alamitos: Computer Society Press.

Boehm, B. W., and H. In. 1996. Identifying quality-requirements conflicts. *IEEE Software* (March).

Boehm, B. W., and T. DeMarco. 1997. Software risk management. *IEEE Software* 14 (3).

Boehm, B., et al. 2000. *Software cost estimation with COCOMO II.* Upper Saddle River: Prentice-Hall.

Bollinger, T. B., and C. McGowan. 1991. A critical look at software capability evaluations. *IEEE Software* 8 (4).

Booch, G. 1990. *Object-oriented design with applications.* Redwood City: Benjamin/Cummings.

Bouldin, B. M. 1989. *Agents of change.* Englewood Cliffs: Yourdon Press.

Bowen, J., and M. G. Hinchey. 1994. Formal methods and safety-critical standards. *IEEE Computer* (August).

Bowen, J. P., and V. Stavridou. 1992. Safety-critical systems, formal methods, and standards. *IEE/BCS Software Engineering Journal* 8 (4).

Bozoki, G. J. 1991. Performance simulation of SSM (software sizing model). In *Proceedings of 13th Conference, International Society of Parametric Analysts*. New Orleans: International Society of Parametric Analysts.

Breton, E. J. 1981. Reinventing the wheel. *Mechanical Engineering* (March).

Briand, L., K. El Emam, and B. Freimut. 1998a. A comparison and integration of capture-recapture models and the detection profile method. In *Proceedings of the Ninth International Symposium on Software Reliability Engineering*. Los Alamitos: IEEE Computer Society Press.

Briand, L., K. El Emam, and B. Freimut. 1998. *A comprehensive evaluation of capture-recapture models for estimating software defect content*. Technical Report ISERN-98-31. Germany: International Software Engineering Research Network.

British Computer Society. 1990. *Guide to software quality management system construction and certification using EN 29001*. Swindon: British Computer Society.

Brocklehurst, S., and B. Littlewood. 1992. New ways to get accurate reliability measures. *IEEE Software* 9 (4).

Brodman, J. G., and D. L. Johnson. 1995. Return on investment (ROI) from software process improvement as measured by US industry. In *Software process improvement and practice*. Sussex: John Wiley & Sons.

Brooks, F. P. 1975. *The mythical man-month*. Reading: Addison-Wesley.

Brooks, W. D. 1981. Software technology payoff: Some statistical evidence. *Structured Programming, The Journal of Systems and Software* 2.

Brubaker, D. 1992. Fuzzy-logic basics: Intuitive rules replace complex math. *Electronic Design News* (June 18).

Brubaker, D. 1995a. Design and simulate your own fuzzy setpoint controller. *Electronic Design News* (January 5).

Brubaker, D. 1995b. Embedding a fuzzy design. *Electronic Design News* (September 1).

Buck, R. D., and J. H. Robbins. 1984. Application of software inspection methodology in design and code. In *Software validation*, ed. H. L. Hausen. New York: Elsevier.

Buckley, F. J. 1993. *Configuration management: Hardware, software, and firmware*. New York: IEEE Press.

Budlong, F. C., and J. A. Peterson. 1996. Software metrics capability evaluation methodology and implementation. *CrossTalk: The Journal of Defense Software Engineering* 9 (1).

Bunyard, J. M., and J. M. Coward. 1988. Today's risks in software development—Can they be significantly reduced? In *Tutorial: Software engineering project management*, ed. R. H. Thayer. Washington, D.C.: IEEE Computer Society Press.

Bureau of Medical Devices, Office of Small Manufacturers Assistance. 1982. *Regulatory requirements for marketing a device*. Washington, D.C.: U.S. Department of Health and Human Services.

Burrows, P. 1991. In search of the perfect product. *Electronic Business* (June 17).

Butler, K. 1995. The economic benefits of software process improvement. *CrossTalk: The Journal of Defense Software Engineering* (July).

Canadian Standards Association. 1985. *One step guide—Your roadmap for getting help when you need it.* Toronto: Canadian Standards Association.

Canadian Standards Association. 1989. *Quality assurance program for the development of software used in critical applications.* Toronto: Canadian Standards Association.

Caplan, F. 1980. *The quality system: A source book for managers and engineers.* Radnor: Chilton.

Card, D. 1992. Capability evaluations rated highly variable. *IEEE Software* 9 (5).

Card, D. 1994. Statistical process control for software? *IEEE Software* 11 (3).

Card, D. N., V. E. Church, and W. E. Agresti. 1986. An empirical study of software design practices. *IEEE Transactions on Software Engineering* 12 (2).

Card, D. N., and R. L. Glass. 1990. *Measuring software design quality.* Englewood Cliffs: Prentice-Hall.

Carleton, A. D., R. E. Park, and W. B. Goethert. 1994. The SET core measures: Background information and recommendations for use and implementation. *CrossTalk: The Journal of Defense Software Engineering* (May).

Carroll, J. M., and M. B. Rosson. 1985. Usability specifications as a tool in iterative development. In *Advances in human-computer interaction,* ed. H. R. Hartson. Norwood: Ablex.

Center for Devices and Radiological Health. 1987. *Device good manufacturing practices manual.* Washington, D.C.: U.S. Department of Health and Human Services.

Charette, R. N. 1989. *Software engineering risk analysis and management.* New York: McGraw-Hill.

Charette, R. 1991. The risk with risk analysis. *Communications of the ACM* 34 (6).

Chen, E. T. 1978. Program complexity and programmer productivity. *IEEE Transactions on Software Engineering* 4 (3).

Chernak, Y. 2001. Validating and improving test-case effectiveness. *IEEE Software* 17 (1).

Cheung, R. C. 1980. A user-oriented software reliability model. *IEEE Transactions on Software Engineering* 6 (2).

Chevlin, D. H., and J. Jorgens, III. 1996. Software requirements: Definition and specification. *Biomedical Instrumentation and Technology* 30 (2).

Chidarnber, S., and Chris Kemerer. 1994. A metrics suite for object-oriented design. *IEEE Transactions on Software Engineering* (June).

Christensen, K., G. P. Fitsos, and C. P. Smith. 1981. A perspective on software science. *IBM Systems Journal* 20 (4).

Coad, P., and E. Yourdon. 1991a. *Object-oriented analysis.* Englewood Cliffs: Yourdon Press.

Coad, P., and E. Yourdon. 1991b. *Object-oriented design.* Englewood Cliffs: Yourdon Press.

Cobb, R., L. Smeraglinolo, and D. Wood. 1999. Determining the completed effort of adapting existing software. *CrossTalk: The Journal of Defense Software Engineering* (November).

Cobb, R. H., and H. D. Mills. 1990. Engineering software under statistical quality control. *IEEE Software* 7 (6).

Cohen, B., W. T. Harwood, and M. J. Jackson. 1986. *The specification of complex systems.* Reading: Addison-Wesley.

Coleman, D., D. Ash, B. Lowther, and P. Oman. 1994. Using metrics to evaluate software system maintainability. *IEEE Computer* 27 (8).

Coleman, D., B. Lowther, and P. Oman. 1995. The application of software maintainability models on industrial software systems. *Journal of Systems and Software* 29 (1).

Collins, W. R., K. W. Miller, B. J. Spielman, and P. Wherry. 1994. How good is good enough? An ethical analysis of software construction and use. *Communications of the ACM* 37 (1).

Connell, J. L., and L. B. Shafer. 1989. *Structured rapid prototyping.* Englewood Cliffs: Yourdon Press.

Conner, D. 1993. Designing a fuzzy-logic control system. *Electronic Design News* (March 31).

Connolly, B. 1993. A process for preventing software hazards. *Hewlett-Packard Journal* 44 (3).

Conover, W. J. 1971. *Practical nonparametric statistics.* New York: John Wiley & Sons.

Constantine, L. L. 1967. *Concepts in program design.* Cambridge: Information and Systems Press.

Constantine, L. L., and L. A. D. Lockwood. 1999. *Software for use: A practical guide to the models and methods of usage-centered design.* Reading: Addison-Wesley Longman.

Conte, S. D., H. E. Dunsmore, and V. Y. Shen. 1986. *Software engineering metrics and models.* Menlo Park: Benjamin/Cummings.

Cook, J. E., and A. L. Wolf. 1999. Software process validation: Quantitatively measuring the correspondence of a process to a model. *ACM Transactions on Software Engineering and Methodology* 8 (2).

Cook, M. L. 1982. Software metrics: An introduction and annotated bibliography. *ACM SIG-SOFT Software Engineering Notes* 7 (2).

Cooper, A. 1995. *About face: The essentials of user interface design.* Foster City: IDG Books Worldwide.

Corbi, T. 1989. Program understanding: Challenge for the 1990s. *IBM Systems Journal* 28 (2).

Coté, V., P. Bourque, S. Oligny, and N. Richard. 1988. Software metrics: An overview of recent results. *The Journal of Systems and Software* 8.

Cougar, J., and H. Adelsberger. 1988. Comparing motivation of programmers and analysts in different socio/political environments: Austria compared to the United States. *Computer Personnel* 11 (4).

Coulter, N. 1983. Software science and cognitive psychology. *IEEE Transactions on Software Engineering* 9 (2).

Cox, E. 1994. *The fuzzy systems handbook.* San Diego: Academic Press.

Crosby, P. B. 1979. *Quality is free.* New York: McGraw-Hill.

Crosby, P. B. 1988. *Quality without tears.* New York: McGraw-Hill.

Currit, P. A., M. Dyer, and H. D. Mills. 1986. Certifying the reliability of software. *IEEE Transactions on Software Engineering* 12 (1).

Curtis, B., H. Krasner, and N. Iscoe. 1988. A field study of the software design process for large systems. *Communications of the ACM* 31 (11).

Cusumano, M. A. 1991. *Japan's software factories: A challenge to U. S. management.* New York: Oxford University Press.

Dahl, O. J., E. W. Dijkstra, and C. A. R. Hoare. 1976. *Structured programming.* New York: Academic Press.

Daly, E. B. 1977. Management of software development. *IEEE Transactions on Software Engineering* (May).

Daly, E. B. 1979. Organizing for successful software development. *Datamation* 25 (10).

Daskalantonakis, M. K. 1994. Achieving higher SEI levels. *IEEE Software* 11 (4).

Daskalantonakis, M. K., R. H. Yacobellis, and V. R. Basili. 1990. A method for assessing software measurement technology. *Quality Engineering* 3 (1).

Davis, A. M. 1993. *Software requirements: Objects, functions and states.* Englewood Cliffs: Prentice-Hall.

Davis, A. M., and P. Hsia. 1994. Giving voice to requirements engineering. *IEEE Software* 11 (2).

Davis, R., P. Samuelson, M. Kapor, and J. Reichman. 1996. A new view of intellectual property and software. *Communications of the ACM* 39 (3).

Davis, T. 1994. Adopting a policy of reuse. *IEEE Spectrum* (June).

Dean, E. S. 1981. Software system safety. In *Proceedings of the 5th International System Safety Conference,* Vol. 1, Pt. 1. Newport Beach: System Safety Society.

DeGrace, P., and L. H. Stahl. 1990. *Wicked problems, righteous solutions: A catalogue of modern software engineering paradigms.* Englewood Cliffs: Prentice-Hall.

Dekkers, C. A. 1999. Managing (the size of) your projects: A project management look at function points. *CrossTalk: The Journal of Defense Software Engineering* (February).

DeMarco, T. 1978. *Structured analysis and system specification.* New York: Yourdon Press.

DeMarco, T. 1982. *Controlling software projects: Management, measurement and estimation.* New York: Yourdon Press.

DeMarco, T. 1984. An algorithm for sizing software products. *SIGMETRICS Performance Evaluation Review* 12 (2).

DeMarco, T., and T. Lister. 1985. Programmer performance and the effects of the workplace. In *IEEE Proceedings of the Eighth International Conference on Software Engineering.* Los Alamitos: Computer Society Press.

DeMarco, T., and T. Lister. 1987. *Peopleware: Productive projects and teams.* New York: Dorset House.

DeMillo, R. A., et al. 1978. Hints on test data selection: Help for the practicing programmer. *Computer* (April).

DeMillo, R. A., W. M. McCracken, R. J. Martin, and J. F. Passafiume. 1987. *Software testing and evaluation.* Menlo Park: Benjamin/Cummings.

Department of Industry. 1981. *Report on the study of an ADA-based system development methodology,* Vol. 1. London: Department of Industry.

DeSain, C., and C. V. Sutton. 1994. *Validation for medical device and diagnostic manufacturers.* Buffalo Grove: Interpharm Press.

Deutsch, M. S. 1982. *Software verification and validation: Realistic project approaches.* Englewood Cliffs: Prentice-Hall.

Digital Equipment Corporation. 1989. *The digital guide to software development.* Bedford: Digital Press.

Dijkstra, E. W. 1965. Programming considered as a human activity. In *Proceedings of the 1965 IFIP Congress.* Amsterdam: North-Holland.

Dijkstra, E. W. 1968a. GO TO statement considered harmful. *Communications of the ACM* 11 (3).

Dijkstra, E. W. 1968b. Structure of "the"—multiprogramming system. *Communications of the ACM* 11 (5).

Dijkstra, E. W. 1969. *Notes on structured programming.* Rome: NATO Science Committee.

Dijkstra, E. W. 1970. *Structured programming.* Technische Hogeschool Eindhoven, Report No. EWD-248.

Dijkstra, E. W. 1976. *A discipline of programming.* Englewood Cliffs: Prentice-Hall.

Dion, R. 1992. Elements of a process improvement program. *IEEE Software* 9 (4).

Dion, R. 1993. Process improvement and the corporate balance sheet. *IEEE Software* 10 (4).

Doerflinger, C., and V. Basili. 1985. Monitoring software development through dynamic variables. *IEEE Transactions on Software Engineering* 11 (9).

Donahue, G. M. 2001. Usability and the bottom line. *IEEE Software* 17 (1).

Donaldson, S. E., and S. G. Siegel. 1997. *Cultivating successful software development: A practitioner's view.* Upper Saddle River: Prentice-Hall PTR.

Donaldson, S. E., and S. G. Siegel. 1998. Measurement in everyday language. *CrossTalk: The Journal of Defense Software Engineering* (February).

Donnelly, M., W. Everett, J. Musa, and G. Wilson. 1995. Best current practice in software reliability engineering. In *Handbook of software reliability engineering,* ed. M. R. Lyu. New York: McGraw-Hill.

Dorofee, A. J., J. A. Walker, and R. C. Williams. 1997. Risk management in practice. *CrossTalk: The Journal of Defense Software Engineering* 10 (4).

Douglass, B. P. 1999a. Safety-critical embedded systems. *Embedded Systems Programming* 12 (11).

Douglass, B. P. 1999b. *Doing hard time: Developing real-time systems with UML, objects, frameworks and patterns.* Reading: Addison-Wesley.

Drake, D. 1986. A pre-release measure of software reliability. In *HP Software Productivity Conference Proceedings.* Palo Alto: Hewlett-Packard.

Dreger, J. B. 1989. *Function point analysis.* Englewood Cliffs: Prentice-Hall.

Drucker, P. F. 1999. *Management challenges for the 21st century.* New York: HarperCollins.

Dumaine, B. 1989. How managers can succeed through speed. *Fortune* (February 13).

Dumas, J. S., and J. C. Redish. 1993. *A practical guide to usability testing.* Norwood: Ablex.

Dunham, J. R. 1984. Measuring software safety. *Proceedings of Compcon '84.* New York: IEEE.

Dunn, R. 1984. *Software defect removal.* New York: McGraw-Hill.

Dunn, R., and R. Ullman. 1982. *Quality assurance for computer software.* New York: McGraw-Hill.

Dunsmore, H. E., and J. D. Gannon. 1980. Analysis of the effects of programming factors on programming effort. In *Tutorial on models and metrics for software management and engineering,* ed. V. R. Basili. New York: Computer Society Press.

Dunsmore, H. E., and J. D. Gannon. 1981. Data referencing: An empirical investigation. In *Human factors in software development,* ed. B. Curtis. Silver Spring: Computer Society Press.

Dyer, J. L. 1984. Team research and team training: A state-of-the-art review. In *Human factors review.* Santa Monica: The Human Factors Society.

Dyer, M. 1992. *The cleanroom approach to software quality.* New York: John Wiley & Sons.

Eastwick, M. 1995. Verification and validation of off-the-shelf software. *Medical Device and Diagnostic Industry* 17 (4).

Ehn, P. 1990. *Work oriented design of computer artifacts.* Hillsdale: Eribaum.

Ehrlich, W. K., S. K. Leer, and R. H. Molisani. 1993. Applying reliability management: A case study. In *Software management,* ed. D. Reifer. Washington, D.C.: IEEE Computer Society Press.

El Emam, K., O. Laitenberger, and T. Harhich. 1999. *The application of subjective estimates of effectiveness to controlling software inspections.* Technical Report ISERN-99-09, Fraunhofer Institute for Experimental Software Engineering. Germany: International Software Engineering Research Network.

Elshoff, J. L. 1976. An analysis of some commercial PL/1 programs. *IEEE Transactions on Software Engineering* 2 (2).

Emam, K. E., B. Shostak, and N. Madhavji. 1996. Implementing concepts from the personal software process in an industrial setting. In *Proceedings 4th International Conference on Software Process.* Los Alamitos: Computer Society Press.

Endres, A. 1975. An analysis of errors and their causes in system programs. *IEEE Transactions on Software Engineering* 1 (2).

Ericson, C. A. 1981. Software and system safety. In *Proceedings of the 5th International System Safety Conference.* Denver: System Safety Society.

Escala, D., and M. Morisio. 1998. A metric suite for a team PSP. In *Metrics 98.* Los Alamitos: IEEE Computer Society Press.

Fagan, M. E. 1976. Design and code inspection to reduce errors in program development. *IBM Systems Journal* 15 (3).

Fagan, M. E. 1986. Advances in software inspections. *IEEE Transactions on Software Engineering* 12 (7).

Fairley, R. 1978. Tutorial: Static analysis and dynamic testing of computer software. *Computer* 11 (4).

Fairley, R. 1985. *Software engineering concepts.* New York: McGraw-Hill.

Fairley, R. E. 1992. Recent advances in software estimation techniques. In *Proceedings of the 14th International Conference on Software Engineering.* New York: Association of Computing Machinery Press.

Fathi, E. T., and C. V. W. Armstrong. 1985. *Microprocessor software project management.* New York: Marcel Dekker.

Fayad, M. E., L. J. Hawn, M. A. Roberts, and J. R. Klatt. 1993. Using the Shlaer-Mellor object-oriented analysis method. *IEEE Software* (March).

Fayad, M., W. Tsai, and M. Fulghum. 1996. Transition to object-oriented software development. *Communications of the ACM* 39 (2).

Federal Information Processing Standards Publications. 1976. *Guidelines for documentation of computer programs and automated data systems.* FIPS PUB 38. Washington, D.C.: National Bureau of Standards.

Federal Information Processing Standards Publications. 1979. *Guidelines for documentation of computer programs and automated data systems for the initial phase.* FIPS PUB 64. Washington, D.C.: National Bureau of Standards.

Federal Information Processing Standards Publications. 1983. *Guidelines for life-cycle validation, verification and testing of computer software.* FIPS PUB 101. Washington, D.C.: National Bureau of Standards.

Feigenbaum, A. V. 1983. *Total quality control.* New York: McGraw-Hill.

Felder, M., D. Mandrioli, and A. Morzenti. 1994. Proving properties of real-time systems through logical specifications and Petri net models. *IEEE Transactions on Software Engineering* 20 (2).

Fenton, N. E. 1990. Software measurement: Theory, tools and validation. *Software Engineering Journal* 5 (1).

Fenton, N. E. 1991. *Software metrics: A rigorous approach.* London: Chapman and Hall.

Fenton, N. E., and S. L. Pfleeger. 1998. *Software metrics: A rigorous and practical approach.* Stamford: Brooks/Cole Publishing Company.

Ferguson, P., et al. 1997. Introducing the personal software process: Three industry cases. *Computer* 30 (5).

Ferré, X., N. Juristo, H. Windl, and L. Constantine. 2001. Usability basics for software developers. *IEEE Software* 17 (1).

Fetcke, T., A. Abran, and T. H. Nguyen. 1998. Mapping the OO-Jacobsan approach into function point analysis. In *Proceedings TOOLS-23 '97*. Piscataway: IEEE Press.

Fisher, R., and W. Ury. 1981; 1983. *Getting to yes*. Boston: Houghton Mifflin; New York: Penguin Books.

Fogg, B., and C. Nass. 1997. Silicon sycophants: The effects of computers that flatter. *International Journal of Human-Computer Study* 46.

Food and Drug Administration. 1979. *Federal food, drug, and cosmetic act, as amended, January 1979*. Washington, D.C.: U.S. Government Printing Office.

Food and Drug Administration. 1982. *Computerized drug processing: CGMP applicability to hardware and software*, Compliance Policy Guide 7132A.07. Washington, D.C.: U.S. Government Printing Office.

Food and Drug Administration. 1984. *Computerized drug processing: Input/output checking*, Compliance Policy Guide 7132A.08. Washington, D.C.: U.S. Government Printing Office.

Food and Drug Administration. 1987a. *Computerized drug processing: Source code for process control application programs*, Compliance Policy Guide 7132A.15. Washington, D.C.: U.S. Government Printing Office.

Food and Drug Administration. 1987b. *Software development activities—Reference material and training aids for investigators*. Washington, D.C.: U.S. Government Printing Office.

Food and Drug Administration. 1988. *Reviewer guidance for computer controlled devices*. Washington, D.C.: U.S. Government Printing Office.

Food and Drug Administration. 1989. *Preproduction quality assurance planning: Recommendations for medical device manufacturers*. Final draft. Washington, D.C.: U.S. Government Printing Office.

Food and Drug Administration. 1990. *Application of the medical device GMPS to computerized devices and manufacturing processes*. Washington, D.C.: U.S. Government Printing Office.

Fowler, P., and S. Przybylinski. 1988. *Transferring software engineering tool technology*. Washington, D.C.: IEEE Computer Society Press.

Freedman, D. P., and G. M. Weinberg. 1990. *Handbook of walk-throughs, inspections, and technical reviews*. New York: Dorset House.

Freeman, P., and A. I. Wasserman. 1982. *Software development methodologies and ADA (Methodman)*. Arlington: Department of Defense ADA Joint Program Office.

Friedman, M., and J. Voas. 1995. *Software assessment: Reliability, safety, testability*. New York: John Wiley & Sons.

Fries, R. C. 1991a. *Software quality assurance and reliability: Developing safe, effective and reliable medical software.* Arlington: Association for the Advancement of Medical Instrumentation.

Fries, R. C. 1991b. *Reliability assurance for medical devices, equipment, and software.* Buffalo Grove: Interpharm Press.

Fries, R. 1992. Human factors and system reliability. *Medical Device Technology* (March).

Fries, R. C., P. J. Pienkowski, and J. Jorgens, III. 1996. Safe, effective, and reliable software design and development. *Biomedical Instrumentation and Technology* 30 (2).

Fuget, C. 1986. Using quality metrics to improve life cycle productivity. In *HP Software Productivity Conference Proceedings.* Palo Alto: Hewlett-Packard.

Gabel, D. A., and R. Troy. 1994. Software engineering: Objects desired, clients to be served. *IEEE Spectrum* 31 (1).

Gaffney, J. E. 1984. Estimating the number of faults in code. *IEEE Transactions on Software Engineering* 10 (4).

Gamma, E., R. Helm, R. Johnson, and J. Vlissides. 1995. *Design patterns: Elements of reusable object-oriented software.* Reading: Addison-Wesley.

Gannon, C. 1979. Error detection using path testing and static analysis. *Computer* 12 (8).

Ganssle, J. 1990. The Zen of diagnostics. *Embedded Systems Programming* 3 (6).

Ganssle, J. 1990. Self-calibrating systems. *Embedded Systems Programming* 3 (10).

Garmus, D. 1996. Function point counting in a real-time environment. *CrossTalk: The Journal of Defense Software Engineering* 9 (1).

Gause, D. C., and G. M. Weinberg. 1989. *Exploring requirements: Quality before design.* New York: Dorset House.

Gehani, N., and A. D. McGettrick, eds. 1986. *Software specification techniques.* Wokingham: Addison-Wesley.

General Accounting Office. 1989. *Medical device recalls: Examination of selected cases.* GAO/PEMD-90-6-B-233199. Washington, D.C.: U.S. Government Printing Office.

General Electric Company. 1986. *Software engineering handbook.* New York: McGraw-Hill.

Gerhart, S., D. Craigen, and T. Ralston. 1994. Experience with formal methods in critical systems. *IEEE Software* 11 (1).

German Electrotechnical Commission. 1990. *Principles for computers in safety-related systems* (VDE-0801). Frankfurt am Main: German Standards Institute.

Gersick, C., and J. Hackman. 1990. Habitual routines in task-performing groups. *Organizational Behavior and Human Decision Processes* 47 (1).

Ghezzi, C., D. Mandrioli, S. Morasca, and M. Pezzè. 1991. A unified high-level Petri net model for time-critical systems. *IEEE Transactions on Software Engineering* 17 (2).

Gibbs, W. W. 1994. Software's chronic crisis. *Scientific American* (September).

Gilb, T. 1985. Evolutionary delivery versus the "waterfall model." *Software Engineering Notes (ACM SIGSOFT)* (July).

Gilb, T. 1987. *Principles of software engineering management.* Reading: Addison-Wesley.

Gilb, T., and D. Graham. 1993. *Software inspection.* Reading: Addison-Wesley.

Gill, G. K., and C. F. Kemerer. 1991. Cyclomatic complexity density and software maintenance productivity. *IEEE Transactions on Software Engineering* 17 (12).

Gillies, A. C. 1992. *Software quality: Theory and management.* London: Chapman and Hall.

Glass, R. 1992. *Building quality software.* Englewood Cliffs: Prentice-Hall.

Glass, R. L. 1993. The "software crisis"—Is it a matter of "guts management"? In *Software management,* 4th ed., ed. D. J. Reifer. Washington, D.C.: IEEE Computer Society Press.

Glass, R. L. 1994. From wonderland to the real problem. *IEEE Software* 11 (3).

Glass, R. L. 1999. *Computing calamities—lessons learned from products, projects, and companies that failed.* Englewood Cliffs: Prentice-Hall.

Goel, A. L., and K. Okumoto. 1979. A time dependent error detection model for software reliability and other performance measures. *IEEE Transactions on Reliability* (August).

Goldberg, E. A. 1988. Applying corporate software development policies. In *Tutorial: Software engineering project management,* ed. R. H. Thayer. Washington, D.C.: IEEE Computer Society Press.

Good, M., et al. 1986. User-derived impact analysis as a tool for usability engineering. In *Proceedings of the CHI Conference on Human Factors in Computing Systems.* New York: Association of Computing Machinery Press.

Gordon, F., and R. Isenhour. 1989. Simultaneous engineering. *Engineering Manager* (January 30).

Gordon, V. S., and J. M. Bieman. 1994. Rapid prototyping: Lessons learned. *IEEE Software* 12 (1).

Gould, J. D., and C. Lewis. 1985. Designing for usability: Key principles and what designers think. *Communications of the ACM* 28 (3).

Gould, J. D., S. J. Bojes, and C. Lewis. 1991. Making usable, useful, productivity-enhancing computer applications. *Communications of the ACM* 34 (1).

Grady, R. B., and D. L. Caswell. 1987. *Software metrics: Establishing a company-wide program.* Englewood Cliffs: Prentice-Hall.

Grady, R. 1992. *Practical software metrics for project management and process improvement.* Englewood Cliffs: Prentice-Hall.

Grady, R. B. 1993a. Work-product analysis: The philosopher's stone of software? In *Software management,* ed. D. Reifer. Washington, D.C.: IEEE Computer Society Press.

Grady, R. B. 1993b. Measuring and managing software maintenance. In *Software management,* ed. D. Reifer. Washington, D.C.: IEEE Computer Society Press.

Grady, R. 1994. Successfully applying software metrics. *IEEE Computer* 27 (9).

Gregory, S. T. 1984. On prototype vs. mockups. *SIGSOFT Software Engineering Notes* 9 (5).

Grey, S. 1995. *Practical risk assessment for project management.* New York: John Wiley & Sons.

Griggs, J. G. 1981. A method of software safety analysis. In *Proceedings of the 5th International System Safety Conference,* Vol. 1, Pt. 1. Newport Beach: System Safety Society.

Gruman, G. 1989. Major changes in federal software policy urged. *Software* (November).

Haag, S. H., M. K. Raja, and L. L. Schkade. 1996. Quality function deployment usage in software development. *Communications of the ACM* 39 (1).

Haase, V., R. Messnarz, and R. Cachia. 1992. Software process improvement by measurement. In *Shifting paradigms in software engineering,* ed. R. Mittermeir. Berlin: Springer-Verlag.

Haase, V., R. Messnarz, G. Koch, H. J. Kugler, and P. Decrinis. 1994. Bootstrap: Fine-tuning process assessment. *IEEE Software* 11 (4).

Hackos, J. T., and J. C. Redish. 1998. *User and task analysis for interface design.* New York: John Wiley & Sons.

Halang, W. A., and A. D. Stoyenko. 1991. *Constructing predictable real time systems.* Boston: Kluwer.

Halasey, S. 1996. Software development. *Medical Device and Diagnostic Industry* 18 (6).

Hall, J. A. 1990. Seven myths of formal methods. *IEEE Software* 7 (5).

Halstead, M. H. 1977. *Elements of software science.* New York: Elsevier.

Halstead, M. H. 1979. Advances in software science. *Advances in Computers* 18.

Hamilton, W. R. 1995. How to construct a basic quality manual. *Quality Progress* 28 (4).

Hamlet, D. 1992. Are we testing for true reliability? *IEEE Software* 9 (4).

Haque, T. 1997. Processed based configuration management: The way to go to avoid costly product recalls. *CrossTalk: The Journal of Defense Software Engineering* 10 (4).

Harrell, C. 1994. Tame project management software. *Electronic Design* (October 14).

Harris, L. N., and C. J. Dale. 1982. Approaches to software reliability prediction. *Proceedings of the Annual Reliability and Maintainability Symposium.* New York: IEEE.

Harrison, W. A., K. I. Magel, R. Kluczny, and DeKrok. 1982. Applying software complexity metrics to program maintenance. *Computer* 15 (9).

Hartson, H. R., and D. Hix. 1989. Toward empirically derived methodologies and tools for human-computer interface development. *International Journal of Man-Machine Studies* 31.

Hartson, H. R., and E. C. Smith. 1991. Rapid prototyping in human-computer interface development. *Interacting with Computers* 3 (1).

Hartson, H. R., J. L. Brandenburg, and D. Hix. 1992. Different languages for different development activities: Behavioral representation techniques for user interface design. In *Languages for developing user interfaces,* ed. B. A. Myers. Boston: Jones and Bartlett.

Hatley, D., and I. Pirbhai. 1988. *Strategies for real-time system specification.* New York: Dorset House.

Haynes, J. L. 1993. The attribute-driven specification. *Medical Device and Diagnostic Industry* 15 (5).

Hect, H. 1977. Measurement, estimation, and prediction of software reliability. *Software Engineering Technology,* Vol. 2. Maidenhead: Infotech International.

Heller, R. 1995. An introduction to function point analysis. *CrossTalk: The Journal of Defense Software Engineering* 8 (11).

Helmer, O. 1966. *Social technology.* New York: Basic Books.

Henry, S., and D. Kafura. 1981. Software structure metrics based on information flow. *IEEE Transactions on Software Engineering* 7 (5).

Herrmann, D. S. 1995. A preview of IEC safety requirements for programmable electronic medical systems. *Medical Device and Diagnostic Industry* 17 (6).

Hetzel, W. 1984. *Complete guide to software testing.* Wellesley: QED Information Science.

Hihn, J., and H. Hahibagahi. 1991. Cost estimation of software intensive projects: A survey of current practices. In *Proceedings of the 13th International Conference on Software Engineering.* Los Alamitos: IEEE Computer Society Press.

Hix, D., and H. R. Hartson. 1993. *Developing user interfaces: Ensuring usability through product and process.* New York: John Wiley & Sons.

Holloway, C., and R. Butler. 1996. Impediments to industrial use of formal methods. *Computer* 29 (4).

Holmblad, L. P., and J. J. Ostergaard. 1982. *Fuzzy information and decision process.* Denmark: North-Holland.

Hölscher, H., and J. Rader. 1986. *Microcomputers in safety technique: An aid to orientation for developer and manufacturer.* München: Verlag TüV Bayern.

Hossain, S., and R. Dahiya. 1993. Estimating the parameters of a non-homogeneous Poisson-process model of software reliability. *IEEE Transactions on Reliability* (December).

Houston, D., and J. B. Keats. 1998. Cost of software quality: A means of promoting software process improvement. *Quality Engineering* 10 (3).

Howard, J. M. 1991. *Analysis of hazards of computerized medical devices. Developing safe, effective and reliable medical software.* Arlington: Association for the Advancement of Medical Instrumentation.

Howell, C. C., and G. J. Vecellio. 1995. Developing safety-critical software: The role of software error handling. *Medical Device and Diagnostic Industry* 17 (6).

Hsia, P., J. Samuel, J. Gao, D. Kung, Y. Toyoshima, and C. Chen. 1994. Formal approach to scenario analysis. *IEEE Software* 11 (2).

Huff, K. E., J. V. Sroka, and D. D. Struble. 1986. Quantitative models for managing software development processes. *Software Engineering Journal* 1 (1).

Humphrey, W. S., and W. L. Sweet. 1987. *A method for assessing the software engineering capability of contractors.* SEI Technical Report CMU/SEI-87-TR-23. Pittsburgh: SEI.

Humphrey, W. S. 1989. *Managing the software process.* Reading: Addison-Wesley.

Humphrey, W. S., and B. Curtis. 1991. Comments on "a critical look." *IEEE Software* 8 (4).

Humphrey, W. S. 1995. *A discipline for software engineering.* Reading: Addison-Wesley.

Humphrey, W. S. 1996. Using a defined and measured personal software process. *IEEE Software* 13 (3).

Humphrey, W. S. 1997. *Managing technical people: Innovation, teamwork, and the software process.* Reading: Addison-Wesley.

Humphrey, W. S. 1998. Three dimensions of process improvement, Part III: The team process. *CrossTalk: The Journal of Defense Software Engineering* 11 (4).

Humphrey, W. S. 2000. *Introduction to the team software process.* Reading: Addison-Wesley.

Huskey, V. R., and H. D. Huskey. 1990. Lady Lovelace and Charles Babbage. *Annals of the History of Computing* 2 (4).

Iivari, J. 1996. Why are CASE tools not used? *Communications of the ACM* 39 (10).

Inglis, J. 1985. Standard software quality metrics. *AT and T Technical Journal* 65 (2).

Institute of Electrical and Electronics Engineers. 1992. *IEEE standard for a software quality metrics methodology.* IEEE Standard 1061-1992. New York: IEEE Press.

International Organization for Standardization. 1991. *ISO 9000-3, quality management and quality assurance standards—Part 3: Guidelines for the application of 9001 to the development, supply and maintenance of software.* Geneva: International Organization for Standardization.

International Organization for Standardization. 1998. *Ergonomic requirements for office work with visual display terminals,* ISO 9241-11. Geneva: International Organization for Standardization.

Ireson, W. G., C. F. Coombs, and R. Y. Moss. 1996. *Handbook of reliability engineering and management,* 2nd ed. New York: McGraw-Hill.

Iyer, R. K., and P. Velardi. 1985. Hardware related software errors: Measurement and analysis. *IEEE Transactions on Software Engineering* 11 (2).

Jackson, M. A. 1975. *Principles of program design.* New York: Academic Press.

Jacky, J. 1991. *Safety of computer-controlled devices: Developing safe, effective and reliable medical software.* Arlington: Association for the Advancement of Medical Instrumentation.

Jaffe, M. S., N. G. Leveson, and M. P. E. Heimdahl. 1991. Software requirements analysis for real-time process-control systems. *IEEE Transactions on Software Engineering* 17 (3).

Jahanian, F., and A. K. Mok. 1986. Safety analysis of timing properties in real-time systems. *IEEE Transactions on Software Engineering* 12 (9).

Jeffery, D. R., and G. Low. 1990. Generic estimation tools in management of software development. *Software Engineering Journal* 5 (4).

Jelinski, Z., and P. Moranda. 1972. *Software reliability research. Statistical computer performance evaluation,* ed. W. Freiberger. New York: Academic Press.

Jensen, H. A. 1985. An experimental study of software metrics for real-time software. *IEEE Transactions on Software Engineering* 11 (2).

Jobson, J. D. 1992. *Applied multivariate data analysis,* Vol. II: *Categorical and multivariate methods.* New York: Springer-Verlag.

Johnson, J. 1995. Chaos: The dollar drain of IT project failures. *Application Development Trends* (January).

Johnson, P. M., and A. M. Disney. 1998. The personal software process: A cautionary case study. *IEEE Software* 15 (6).

Johnson, P. M., and A. M. Disney. 1999. A critical analysis psp data quality: Results from a case study. *Empirical Software Engineering* 4 (4).

Jones, C. 1976. *Program quality and programmer productivity.* San Jose: International Business Machines.

Jones, C. 1986a. *Programming productivity.* New York: McGraw-Hill.

Jones, C. 1986b. *The SPR feature point method.* Cambridge: Software Productivity Research.

Jones, C. 1994a. *Assessment and control of software risks.* Englewood Cliffs: Prentice-Hall.

Jones, C. 1994b. Software management: The weakest link in the software engineering chain. *Computer* (May).

Jones, C. 1994c. Economics of software reuse. *Computer* (July).

Jones, C. 1996. By popular demand: Software estimating rules of thumb. *Computer* 29 (3).

Jones, C. B. 1980. *Software development: A rigorous approach.* Englewood Cliffs: Prentice-Hall.

Jones, P. L., W. T. Swain, and C. J. Trammell. 1999. Engineering in software testing: Statistical testing based on a usage model applied to medical device development. *Biomedical Instrumentation & Technology* 33 (4).

Jones, T. C. 1978. Measuring programming quality and productivity. *IBM Systems Journal* 17 (1).

Jones, T. C. 1991. *Applied software measurement.* New York: McGraw-Hill.

Jorgens, J., III. 1991. *The purpose of software quality assurance: A means to an end. Developing safe, effective and reliable medical software.* Arlington: Association for the Advancement of Medical Instrumentation.

Joyce, E. D. 1989. Is error free software achievable? *Datamation* (February).

Joyce, E. J. 1987. Software bugs: A matter of life and liability. *Datamation* (May).

Juran, J. M. 1974. *Quality control handbook.* New York: McGraw-Hill.

Juran, J. M., and F. M. Gryna. 1988. *Juran's quality control handbook,* 4th ed. New York: McGraw-Hill.

Juran, J. M., and F. M. Gryna. 1993. *Quality planning and analysis.* New York: McGraw-Hill.

Kafura, D., and G. R. Reddy. 1987. The use of software complexity metrics in software maintenance. *IEEE Transactions on Software Engineering* 13 (3).

Kahan, J. S. 1987. Validating computer systems. *Medical Device and Diagnostic Industry* (March).

Kahan, J. S. 1989. The 510(k) notice and device software: What is required? *Medical Device and Diagnostic Industry* (January).

Kaminsky, F. C., R. A. Dovich, and R. J. Burke. 1998. Process capability indices: Now and in the future. *Quality Engineering* 10 (3).

Kaner, C., J. Folk, and N. Q. Nguyen. 1993. *Testing computer software,* 2nd ed. Boston: International Thompson Computer Press.

Kaner, C. 1998. *Bad software: What to do when software fails.* New York: John Wiley & Sons.

Kaposi, A. A., and B. Kitchenham. 1987. The architecture of system quality. *Software Engineering Journal* 2 (1).

Karjalainen, J., M. Mäkäräinen, S. Komi-Sirviö, and V. Seppänen. 1996. Practical process improvement for embedded real-time software. *Quality Engineering* 8 (4).

Karlsson, J. 1996. Software requirements prioritizing. In *Proceedings of the 2nd IEEE International Conference on Requirements Engineering.* Los Alamitos: IEEE Computer Society Press.

Karlsson, J., and K. Ryan. 1997. A cost-value approach for prioritizing requirements. *IEEE Software* 14 (5).

Karunanithi, N., D. Whitley, and Y. K. Malaiya. 1992. Using neural networks in reliability prediction. *IEEE Software* 9 (4).

Kearney, J. K., R. L. Sedlmeyer, W. B. Thompson, M. A. Gray, and M. A. Adler. 1986. Software complexity measurement. *Communications of the ACM* 29 (11).

Kececioglu, D. 1991. *Reliability engineering handbook,* Vol. 2. Englewood Cliffs: Prentice-Hall.

Keller, M., and K. Humate. 1992. *Software specification and design disciplined approach for real-time system.* New York: John Wiley & Sons.

Kemeny, J. G., and J. L. Snell. 1960. *Finite Markov chains.* Princeton: Van Nostrand.

Kemerer, C. F. 1987. An empirical validation of software cost estimation models. *Communications of the ACM* 30 (5).

Kemmerer, R. A. 1985. Testing formal specifications to detect design errors. *IEEE Transactions on Software Engineering* 11 (1).

Kemmerer, R. 1990. Integrating formal methods with the development process. *IEEE Software* 7 (5).

Kempthorne, 0. 1979. *The design and analysis of experiments.* New York: Robert E. Krieger.

Kernighan, B. W., and P. J. Plauger. 1974. *The elements of programming style.* New York: McGraw-Hill.

Kernighan, B. W., and P. J. Plauger. 1976. *Software tools.* Reading: Addison-Wesley.

Khoshgoftarr, T. M., et al. 1992. Predictive modeling techniques of software quality from software measures. *IEEE Transactions on Software Engineering* 18 (11).

Khoshgoftarr, T. M., and P. Oman. 1994. Software metrics: Charting the course. *IEEE Computer* 27 (9).

King, W. R., and T. A Wilson. 1967. Subjective time estimates in critical path planning—A preliminary analysis. *Management Science* 13 (6).

King, W. R., D. M. Witterrongel, and K. D. Hezel. 1967. On the analysis of critical path time estimating behavior. *Management Science* 14 (1).

Kitchenham, B. A. 1987. Towards a constructive quality model. *Software Engineering Journal* 2 (4).

Kitchenham, B. A., and J. A. McDermid. 1986. Software metrics and integrated project support environments. *Software Engineering Journal* 1 (1).

Kitchenham, B. A., and J. G. Walker. 1989. A quantitative approach to monitoring software development. *Software Engineering Journal* 4 (1).

Kitchenham, B. A., L. M. Pickard, and S. J. Linkman. 1990. An evaluation of some design metrics. *Software Engineering Journal* 5 (1).

Kleiman, S., D. Shah, and B. Smaalders. *Programming with threads.* Mountain View: SunSoft Press.

Kleinbaum, D. G., and L. L. Kupper. 1978. *Applied regression analysis and other multivariate methods.* North Scituate: Duxbury Press.

Klir, G., and D. Schwartz. 1992. Fuzzy logic flowers in Japan. *IEEE Spectrum* (July).

Knox, S. T. 1993. Modeling the cost of software quality. *Digital Technical Journal* 5 (4).

Knuth, D. E. 1974. Structured programming with GOTO statements. *ACM Computing Surveys* 6 (4).

Kolb, D. A. 1973. *On management and the learning process.* Working Paper 652-673. Cambridge: MIT Sloan School.

Krasner, H., et al. 1992. Lessons learned from a software process modeling system. *Communications of the ACM* 35 (9).

Krasner, H. 1998. Using the cost of quality approach for software. *CrossTalk: The Journal of Defense Software Engineering* (November).

Kraut, R. E., and L. A. Streeter. 1995. Coordination in software development. *Communications of the ACM* 38 (3).

Kyper, C. H. 1992. The 510(k) route to the marketplace. *Medical Device and Diagnostic Industry* (January).

Lakos, J. 1996. *Large scale C++ software projects.* Reading: Addison-Wesley.

Langer, E. 1983. *The psychology of control.* Thousand Oaks: Sage Publications.

Lanning, D. L., and T. M. Khoshgoftarr. 1994. Modeling the relationship between source code complexity and maintenance difficulty. *Computer* 27 (9).

Lantz, K. S. 1986. *The prototyping methodology.* Englewood Cliffs: Prentice-Hall.

Laprie, J. C., and A. Coates. 1982. Dependability: A unifying concept for reliability computing. In *Proceedings of the 12th International Symposium on Fault Tolerant Computing.* New York: IEEE.

Larsen, P. G., J. Fitzgerald, and T. Brookes. 1996. Applying formal specification in industry. *IEEE Software* 13 (3).

Lawrence, M. 1981. Programming methodology, organizational environment and programming productivity. *The Journal of Systems and Software* (September).

Leffingwell, D., and D. Widrig. 2000. *Managing software requirements: A unified approach.* Reading: Addison-Wesley.

Legg, G. 1994. Fuzzy tools help build embedded systems. *Electronic Design News* (July 21).

Lehman, M. 1980. Programs, life cycles and laws of software evolution. *Proceedings of the IEEE* 68 (9).

Leveson, N. G. 1981. *Software safety: A definition and some preliminary ideas.* Technical Report 174. University of California, Irvine, Computer Science Department.

Leveson, N. G. 1984. Software safety in computer-controlled systems. *IEEE Computer* (February).

Leveson, N. G. 1986. Software safety: Why, what, and how. *Computing Surveys* 18 (2).

Leveson, N. G. 1989. Safety as a software quality. *IEEE Software* 6 (3).

Leveson, N. G. 1991. Software safety in embedded computer systems. *Communications of the ACM* 34 (2).

Leveson, N. G. 1995. *Safeware: System safety and computers.* Reading: Addison-Wesley.

Leveson, N. G., and P. R. Harvey. 1983. Analyzing software safety. *IEEE Transactions on Software Engineering* 9 (5).

Leveson, N. G., and J. L. Stolzy. 1985. Analyzing safety and fault tolerance using time Petri nets. In *TAPSOFT: Joint Conference on Theory and Practice of Software Development.* Berlin/New York: Springer-Verlag.

Leveson, N. G., and J. L. Stolzy. 1986. Safety analysis using Petri nets. *IEEE Transactions on Software Engineering* 13 (3).

Leveson, N. G., and C. S. Turner. 1993. An investigation of the Therac-25 accidents. *IEEE Computer* (July).

Levkoff, B. 1996. Increasing safety in medical device software. *Medical Device and Diagnostic Industry* 18 (9).

Lew, K. S., T. S. Dillon, and K. E. Forward. 1988. Software complexity and its impact on software reliability. *IEEE Transactions on Software Engineering* 14 (11).

Li, H. F., and W. K. Cheung. 1987. An empirical study of software metrics. *IEEE Transactions on Software Engineering* 13 (6).

Linger, R. C. 1994. Cleanroom process model. *IEEE Software* 11 (2).

Linger, R. C., H. D. Mills, and R. L. Witt. 1979. *Structured programming: Theory and practice.* Reading: Addison-Wesley.

Lipow, M. 1982. Number of faults per line of code. *IEEE Transactions on Software Engineering* 8 (4).

Littlewood, B. 1980. Theories of software reliability: How good are they and how can they be improved? *IEEE Transactions on Software Engineering* 6 (September).

Littlewood, B. 1981. Stochastic reliability growth: A model for fault removal in computer programs and hardware design. *IEEE Transactions on Reliability* (December).

Littlewood, B., and L. Strigini. 1998. The risks of software. *Scientific American* (November).

Lloyd, D., and M. Lipow. 1992. *Reliability: Management, methods, and mathematics.* Englewood Cliffs: Prentice-Hall.

Lorenz, M. 1993. *Object-oriented software development: A practical guide.* Englewood Cliffs: Prentice-Hall.

Lorenz, M., and J. Kidd. 1994. *Object-oriented software metrics.* Englewood Cliffs: Prentice-Hall.

Lund, A. M. 1997. Another approach to justifying the cost of usability. *Interactions* 4 (3).

Lutz, R. R. 1992. Analyzing software requirements errors in safety-critical, embedded systems. *Software Requirements Conference.* IEEE (January).

Lyu, M., ed. 1995. *Software fault tolerance.* New York: John Wiley & Sons.

Lyu, M., ed. 1996. *Handbook of software reliability engineering.* New York: McGraw-Hill, and Los Alamitos: IEEE Computer Society Press.

Lyu, M. R., and A. Nikora. 1992. Applying reliability models more effectively. *IEEE Software* 9 (4).

Macala, R. R., L. D. Stuckey Jr., and D. C. Gross. 1996. Managing domain-specific, product-line development. *IEEE Software* 13 (3).

MacKenzie, D., Microsafe Systems, and Noblitt and Rueland, Inc. 1991. *Hazard analysis and medical device safety.* Del Mar: Microsafe Systems, and Irvine: Noblitt and Rueland.

Mackey, K. 1996. Why bad things happen to good projects. *IEEE Software* 13 (3).

Madhavji, N. H. 1991. The process cycle. *IEE/BCS Software Engineering Journal* 6 (5).

Magers, C. S. 1978. Managing software development in microprocessor projects. *IEEE Computer* 11 (6).

Maguire, S. 1993. *Writing solid code.* Redmond: Microsoft Press.

Mallory, S. R. 1990. A hybrid software development model for medical instruments. *Medical Device and Diagnostic Industry* 12 (11).

Mallory, S. R. 1992a. Using prototyping to develop high-quality medical device software. *Medical Device and Diagnostic Industry* (June).

Mallory, S. R. 1992b. Integrating software prototyping with software QA and product development. *Medical Device and Diagnostic Industry* (September).

Mallory, S. R. 1993a. Building quality into medical product software design. *Biomedical Instrumentation and Technology* (March/April).

Mallory, S. R. 1993b. The use of rapid prototyping techniques for medical device software. In *Health Industry Manufacturers Association (HIMA) Annual Proceedings, Software Quality Assurance Session*. Washington D.C.: HIMA.

Mandel, T. 1997. *The elements of user interface design*. New York: John Wiley & Sons.

Mandeville, W. A. 1990. Software costs of quality. *IEEE Journal on Selected Areas in Communications* 8 (2).

Mandl, R. 1985. Orthogonal Latin squares: An application of experiment design to compiler testing. *Communications of the ACM* 28 (10).

Mantei, M., and T. Teorey. 1989. Incorporating behavioral techniques into the systems development life cycle. *MIS Quarterly* 13 (3).

Marick, B. 1995. *The craft of software testing*. New Jersey: Prentice-Hall.

Maring, B. 1996. Object-oriented development of large applications. *IEEE Software* 13 (3).

Masters, R. J. 1996. Overcoming the barriers to TQM's success. *Quality Progress* (May).

Mataban, B. A. M. 1994. Prototype expert system for infusion pump maintenance. *Biomedical Instrumentation and Technology* 28 (1).

Matsubara, A. 1990. Project management in Japan. *American Programmer* 4 (6).

Mayhew, D. J. 1999. *The usability engineering lifecycle*. San Francisco: Morgan Kaufmann.

Mayrhauser, A. 1990. *Software engineering: Methods and management*. New York: Academic Press.

Mays, R. G., C. L. Jones, G. J. Halloway, and D. P. Studinski. 1990. Experiences with defect prevention. *IBM Systems Journal* 29 (1).

McBride, S. 1989. *The guide to biomedical standards*. Brea: Quest.

McCabe, T. J. 1976. A complexity measure. *IEEE Transactions on Software Engineering* 2 (4).

McCall, J., P. Richards, and G. Walters. 1977. *Factors in software quality,* Vols. 1, 2, and 3. NTIS Report No. AD-A049-014, -015, -055.

McConnell, S. 1997. Gauging software readiness with defect tracking. *IEEE Software* 14 (3).

McCracken, D. D. 1980. Software in the 80s: Perils and promises. *Computerworld* (September).

McCracken, D. D. 1981. *A maverick approach to systems analysis and design*. In *Systems analysis and design: A foundation for the 1980s*. Amsterdam: Elsevier–North Holland.

McCracken, D. D., and M. A. Jackson. 1982. Life cycle concept considered harmful. *Software Engineering Notes*. ACM (April).

McCullough-Graham, A. 1994. Software test and evaluation panel. *CrossTalk: The Journal of Defense Software Engineering* 7 (6).

McFarland, M. C. 1991. Ethics and the safety of computer systems. *IEEE Software* 24 (2).

McGowen, C. L., and J. R. Kelly. 1975. *Top-down structured programming techniques*. Princeton: Petrocelli/Charter.

McNeill, M., and E. Thro. *Fuzzy logic—A practical approach*. San Diego: Academic Press.

Meyer, B. 1988. *Object-oriented software construction.* Hempstead: Prentice-Hall International.

Mili, A., N. Boudriga, and F. Mili. 1989. *Towards structured specifying: Theory, practice, applications.* Chichester: Ellis Horwood.

Miller, B. 1995. Fuzzy logic case study. *Embedded Systems Programming* (December).

Miller, B. 1997. *The design and development of fuzzy logic controllers.* Minneapolis: Impatiens Publications.

Miller, G. A. 1956. The magical number seven, plus or minus two: Some limits on our capacity for processing information. *The Psychological Review* 63 (2).

Miller, J., M. Wood, and M. Roper. 1998. Further experiences with scenarios and checklists. *Empirical Software Engineering: An International Journal* 3 (1).

Mills, H. D. 1971. Top-down programming in large systems. In *Debugging techniques in large systems,* ed. R. Ruskin. Englewood Cliffs: Prentice-Hall.

Mills, H. D. 1976. Software engineering. *IEEE Transactions on Software Engineering* 2 (4).

Mills, H. D. 1988. *Software productivity.* New York: Dorset House.

Miranda, E. 2001. Improving subjective estimates using paired comparisons. *IEEE Software* 17 (1).

Misra, P. N. 1983. Software reliability analysis. *IBM Systems Journal* 22 (3).

Möller, K. H., and D. J. Paulish. 1993. *Software metrics: A practitioner's guide to improved product development.* London: Chapman and Hall.

Mood, A., F. Graybill, and D. Boes. 1974. *Introduction to the theory of statistics.* New York: McGraw-Hill.

Mori, G. 1987. The Japanese Standards Association (JSA)—Its role in the standardization activity in Japan. *ASTM Standardization News* (October).

Morris, D. C., and J. S. Brandon. 1989. *Relational systems development.* New York: McGraw-Hill.

Morzenti, A., and P. S. Pietro. 1994. Object-oriented logical specification of time-critical systems. *ACM Transactions on Software Engineering and Methodology* 3 (1).

Mosteller, F., and J. W. Turkey. 1977. *Data analysis and regression.* Reading: Addison-Wesley.

Motley, R. W., and W. D. Brooks. 1977. *Statistical prediction of programming errors.* RADC-TR-77-175. Griffiss AFB: Rome Air Development Center.

Mullet, K., and D. Sano. 1994. *Designing visual interfaces: Communication oriented techniques.* Upper Saddle River: Prentice-Hall.

Mullet, K., and D. Sano. 1995. *Designing visual interfaces.* Mountain View: SunSoft Press.

Munson, J., and T. Khoshgoftarr. 1992. The detection of fault-prone programs. *IEEE Transactions on Software Engineering* 18 (5).

Murphy, N. 1995. Designing user interfaces. *Embedded Systems Programming* 8 (2).

Murphy, N. 1998. Safe systems through better user interfaces. *Embedded Systems Programming* 11 (8).

Murphy, N. D. 1998. *Front panel: Designing software for embedded user interfaces.* Lawrence: R&D Books.

Musa, J. D. 1975. A theory of software reliability and its application. *IEEE Transactions on Software Engineering* 1 (3).

Musa, J. D. 1980a. Software reliability measurement. *The Journal of Systems and Software* 1 (3).

Musa, J. D. 1980b. The measurement and management of software reliability. *Proceedings of the IEEE* 68 (9).

Musa, J. D. 1993. Operational profiles in software reliability engineering. *IEEE Software* 10 (March).

Musa, J. D. 1996. Software-reliability-engineered testing. *Computer* 29 (11).

Musa, J. D. 1998. *Software reliability engineering.* New York: John Wiley & Sons.

Musa, J. D., A. Iannino, and K. Okumoto. 1987. *Software reliability: Measurement, prediction, application.* New York: McGraw-Hill.

Myers, G. J. 1976. *Software reliability: Principles and practices.* New York: John Wiley & Sons.

Myers, G. J. 1979. *The art of software testing.* New York: John Wiley & Sons.

Mylopoulos, J., L. Chung, S. S. Y. Liao, H. Wang, and E. Yu. 2001. Exploring alternatives during requirements analysis. *IEEE Software* 17 (1).

National Bureau of Standards. 1980. *Validation, verification, and testing for the individual programmer.* NBS Special Publication 500-56. Washington, D.C.: National Bureau of Standards.

National Bureau of Standards. *Validation, verification, and testing of computer software.* NBS Special Publication 500-75. Washington, D.C.: National Bureau of Standards.

National Bureau of Standards. *Planning for software validation, verification, and testing.* NBS Special Publication 500-98. Washington, D.C.: National Bureau of Standards.

National Bureau of Standards. *Structured testing: A software testing methodology using the cyclomatic complexity metric.* NBS Special Publication 500-99. Washington, D.C.: National Bureau of Standards.

National Fire Protection Agency. 1987. *NFPA 99 Health Care Facilities.* Washington, D.C.: National Fire Protection Agency.

National Institute of Standards and Technology. *A framework for the development and assurance of high integrity software.* NIST Special Publication 500-223. Washington, D.C.: National Institute of Standards and Technology.

Neuman, P. G. 1989. Illustrative risks to the public in the use of computer systems and related technology. *Software Engineering Notes* 14 (1).

Neumann, P. C. 1995. *Computer related risks.* Reading: Addison-Wesley.

Niehoff, K. 1994. Designing reliable software. *Medical Device and Diagnostic Industry* (September).

Nielsen, J. 1993. Is usability engineering really worth it? *IEEE Software* 10 (6).

Nielsen, J. 1994. *Usability engineering.* San Francisco: Morgan Kaufmann.

Nintzel, J. S. 1991. *Verifying purchased software. Developing safe, effective and reliable medical software.* Arlington: Association for the Advancement of Medical Instrumentation.

Noble, W. B. 1984. Developing safe software for critical airborne applications. In *Proceedings of the 6th Digital Avionics Systems Conference.* New York: IEEE.

Norman, D. A. 1988. *The psychology of everyday things.* New York: Basic Books.

Norman, D. A. 1990. *The design of everyday things.* New York: Doubleday.

O'Connor, P. D. T. 1991. *Practical reliability engineering.* New York: John Wiley & Sons.

O'Day, D. 1998. This old house. *IEEE Software* 15 (2).

Office of Compliance and Surveillance. 1989. *Preproduction quality assurance planning: Recommendations for medical device manufacturers.* Washington, D.C.: U.S. Department of Health and Human Services.

Office of Compliance and Surveillance. 1990. *Application of the medical device GMPS to computerized devices and manufacturing processes: Medical device GMP guidance for FDA investigators.* Washington, D.C.: U.S. Department of Health and Human Services.

Office of Device Evaluation. 1991. *Reviewer guidance for computer controlled medical devices undergoing 510(k) review.* Washington, D.C.: Center for Devices and Radiological Health.

Office of Standards and Regulations. 1987. *Medical devices standards activities report.* Washington, D.C.: U.S. Department of Health and Human Services.

Olivier, D. P. 1992. Inspections: A successful approach to achieving high-quality software. In *Designer's handbook: Medical electronics.* Santa Monica: Canon Communications.

Olivier, D. P. 1994. IEEE software engineering standards: Medical device applications. In *Designer's handbook: Medical electronics.* Santa Monica: Canon Communications.

Olivier, D. P. 1996. Implementation of design controls offers practical benefits. *Medical Device and Diagnostic Industry* (July).

Olivier, D. P., M. D. Konrad, and M. Weber. 1994. Comparing software assessment standards. *Medical Device and Diagnostic Industry* 16 (6).

Oman, P., and J. Hagemeister. 1994. Constructing and testing of polynomials predicting software maintainability. *Journal of Systems and Software* 24 (3).

Onel, S. 1997. Draft revision of FDA's medical device software policy raises warning flags. *Medical Device and Diagnostic Industry* 19 (10).

Onoma, A. K., W. Tsai, M. H. Poonawala, and H. Suganuma. 1998. Regression testing in an industrial environment. *Communications of the ACM* 41 (5).

Orlikowski, W. 1993. CASE tools as organizational change: Investigating incremental and radical changes in systems development. *MIS Quarterly* 17 (3).

Oshana, R. 1997. Software testing with statistical usage-based models. *Embedded Systems Programming* 10 (January).

Otis, D. L., et al. 1978. Statistical inference from capture data on closed animal populations. *Wildlife Monographs,* No. 62.

Ottenstein, L. M. 1979. Quantitative estimates of debugging requirements. *IEEE Transactions on Software Engineering* 5 (5).

Ould, M. A., and C. Unwin. 1986. *Testing in software development.* Cambridge: Cambridge University Press.

Ozog, H. 1997. Risk management in medical device design. *Medical Device and Diagnostic Industry* 19 (10).

Page-Jones, M. 1988. *The practical guide to structured systems design.* New York: Yourdon Press.

Parikh, G., and N. Zvegintzov. 1983. *Tutorial on software maintenance.* Los Alamitos: IEEE Computer Society Press.

Parnas, D. L. 1972. On the criteria to be used in decomposing systems into modules. *Communications of the ACM* 15 (12).

Parnas, D. L. 1977. *Use of abstract interfaces in the development of software for embedded computer systems.* Report 8047. Washington, D.C.: Naval Research Laboratory.

Parnas, D. L., A. J. von Schouwen, and S. P. Kwan. 1990. Evaluation of safety-critical software. *Communications of the ACM* 33 (6).

Parr, F. N. 1980. An alternative to the Rayleigh curve model for software development effort. *IEEE Transactions on Software Engineering* 6 (3).

Paulish, D. J. 1990. Methods and metrics for developing high quality patient monitoring system software. In *Proceedings of the Third IEEE Symposium on Computer-Based Medical Systems.* Los Alamitos: Computer Society Press.

Paulish, D. J., and A. D. Carleton. 1994. Case studies of software process improvement measurement. *IEEE Computer* 27 (9).

Paulk, M., et al. 1993. Capability Maturity Model for software (version 1.1). *IEEE Software* 10 (4).

Paulk, M. C., et al. 1995. *The Capability Maturity Model: Guidelines for improving the software process.* Reading: Addison-Wesley.

Paulk, M. C., and M. D. Konrad. An overview of ISO's SPICE project. *American Programmer* 7 (2).

Peters, T., and R. Waterman. *In search of excellence.* New York: Harper and Row.

Peterson, G. E. 1990. *Object-oriented computing:* Vols. 1 and 2. Los Alamitos: IEEE Computer Society Press.

Peterson, J. L. 1981. *Petri net theory and the modeling of systems.* New Jersey: Prentice-Hall.

Pfleeger, S. L., and C. McGowan. 1993. Software metrics in the process maturity framework. In *Software management,* ed. D. Reifer. Washington, D.C.: IEEE Computer Society Press.

Pfleeger, S. L., N. Fenton, and S. Page. 1994. Evaluating software engineering standards. *IEEE Computer* 27 (9).

Phadke, M. S. 1989. *Quality engineering using robust design.* New Jersey: Prentice-Hall.

Piaget, J. 1950. *The psychology of intelligence.* Orlando: Harcourt Brace Jovanovich.

Poore, J. H., H. D. Mills, and D. Mutchler. 1993. Planning and certifying software system reliability. *IEEE Software* 10 (January).

Poore, J. H., and C. J. Trammell. 1997. Bringing respect to software testing through statistical science. *American Programmer* 10 (August).

Poore, J. H., and C. J. Trammell. 1998. Engineering practices for statistical testing. *CrossTalk: The Journal of Defense Software Engineering* 11 (4).

Porter, A., and L. Votta. 1994. An experiment to assess different defect detection methods for software requirements inspections. In *Proceedings of the 16th International Conference on Software Engineering.* Los Alamitos: IEEE Computer Society Press.

Poston, R. M. 1991. A complete toolkit for the software tester. *American Programmer* (April).

Potier, D., J. L. Albin, R. Ferreol, and A. Bilodeau. 1982. Experiments with computer software complexity and reliability. In *Proceedings of the Sixth International Conference on Software Engineering.* Los Alamitos: Computer Society Press.

Potter, N., and M. Sakry. 2001. Practical CMM: Scoping your improvement program based on the problems and goals of your organization allows you to make significant headway. *Software Development* 9 (3).

Potts, C. 1993. Software engineering research revisited. *IEEE Software* (September).

Potts, C., K. Takahashi, and A. I. Antón. 1994. Inquiry-based requirements analysis. *IEEE Software* 11 (2).

Preece, J., et al. 1994. *Human-computer interaction.* Reading: Addison-Wesley Longman.

Pressman, R. S. 1987. *Software engineering: A practitioner's approach.* New York: McGraw-Hill.

Pressman, R. S., and S. R. Herron. 1991. *Software shock: The danger and the opportunity.* New York: Dorset House.

Prieto-Díaz, R. 1993. Status report: Software reusability. *IEEE Software* (May).

Prowell, S. J., C. J. Trammell, R. C. Linger, and J. H. Poore. 1998. *Cleanroom software engineering: Technology and process.* Reading: Addison-Wesley Longman.

Putnam, L. 1980. *Tutorial on software cost estimating and life cycle control: Getting the software numbers.* Los Alamitos: IEEE Computer Society Press.

Putnam, L. 1991. Trends in measurement, estimation and control. *IEEE Software* (March).

Putnam, L. H. 1978. A general empirical solution to the macro software sizing and estimating problem. *IEEE Transactions on Software Engineering* 4 (4).

Putnam, L. H. 1989. Analyzing productivity using function points. In *Proceedings of the International Function Points User Group (IFPUG).* Los Alamitos: Computer Society Press.

Putnam, L. H., and A. Fitzsimmons. 1979. Estimating software costs. *Datamation* 25 (10), 25 (11), and 25 (12).

Pyzdek, T. 1992. To improve your processes: Keep it simple. *IEEE Software* 9 (5).

Quirk, W. J., ed. 1985. *Verification and validation of real-time software.* New York: Springer-Verlag.

Rabbitt, J. T., and P. A. Bergh. 1993. *The ISO 9000 book.* White Plains: Quality Resources.

Raghavrao, D. 1971. *Construction of combinatorial problems in design experiments.* New York: John Wiley & Sons.

Rakos, J. J. 1990. *Software project management: For small to medium sized projects.* Englewood Cliffs: Prentice-Hall.

Ramamoorthy, C. V., and F. B. Bastani. 1982. Software reliability—Status and perspectives. *IEEE Transactions on Software Engineering* 8 (4).

Ramamoorthy, C. V., A. Prakash, W. Tsai, and Y. Usuda. 1988. Software engineering: Problems and perspectives. In *Tutorial: Software engineering project management,* ed. R. H. Thayer. Washington, D.C.: IEEE Computer Society Press.

Ranganathan, K. 2001. How to make software peer reviews work: Simple enhancements can turn every peer review into a success. *Quality Progress* 34 (2).

Rapps, S., and E. J. Weyuker. 1985. Selecting software test data using data flow information. *IEEE Transactions on Software Engineering* 11 (4).

Rauscher, T. G. 1978. A unified approach to microcomputer software development. *IEEE Computer* 11 (6).

Rechtin, E. 1991. *Systems architecting: Creating and building complex systems.* Englewood Cliffs: Prentice-Hall.

Reifer, D. J. 1987. Predicting the size of software for real-time systems. In *NASA/GSFC Twelfth Annual Software Engineering Workshop.*

Reifer, D. J., B. W. Boehm, and S. Chulani. 1999. The Rosetta stone: Making COCOMO 81 estimates work with COCOMO II. *CrossTalk: The Journal of Defense Software Engineering* (November).

Reliability Analysis Center. 1976. *Reliability design handbook.* RDH-376. Griffiss AFB: Rome Air Development Center.

Richards, J. T., S. J. Boies, and J. D. Gould. 1986. Rapid prototyping and system development: Examination of an interface toolkit for voice and telephony applications. In *Proceedings of CHI Conference on Human Factors in Computing Systems.* New York: Association of Computing Machinery Press.

Rieger, W. B. 1997. Safety considerations of unused code: Its causes and implications. *CrossTalk: The Journal of Defense Software Engineering* 10 (1).

Robertson, J., and S. Robertson. 1994. *Complete systems analysis,* Vols. 1 and 2. New York: Dorset House.

Robertson, S., and J. Robertson. 1999. *Mastering the requirements process.* New York: Association of Computing Machinery Press.

Rogers, E. 1995. *Diffusion of innovations,* 4th ed. New York: Free Press.

Rombach, H. D. 1987. A controlled experiment on the impact of software structure on maintainability. *IEEE Transactions on Software Engineering* 7 (5).

Rook, P. 1993. Controlling software projects. In *Software management,* ed. D. Reifer. Washington, D.C.: IEEE Computer Society Press.

Rosenberg, L. H., and L. E. Hyatt. 1997. Software quality metrics for object-oriented environments. *CrossTalk: The Journal of Defense Software Engineering* 10 (4).

Rosenblatt, A., and W. George, eds. 1991. Special report: Concurrent engineering. *IEEE Spectrum* 28 (7).

Rosson, M. B., S. Maass, and W. A. Kellogg. 1987. Designing for designers: An analysis of design practice in the real world. In *Proceedings of CHI+GI Conference on Human Factor in Computing Systems.* New York: Association of Computing Machinery Press.

Royce, W. W. 1970. Managing the development of large software systems: Concepts and techniques. In *Proceedings, WESCON.*

Rubin, J. 1994. *Handbook of usability testing: How to plan, design, and conduct effective tests.* New York: John Wiley & Sons.

Rubin, R. 2000. Complex drug labels bury safety message. *USA Today* (May 3).

Rumbaugh, J., et al. 1991. *Object oriented modeling and design.* Englewood Cliffs: Prentice-Hall.

Russell, G. W. 1993. Experience with inspection in ultralarge-scale developments. In *Software management,* ed. D. Reifer. Washington, D.C.: IEEE Computer Society Press.

Ryan, L. 1998. Software usage metrics for real-world software testing. *IEEE Spectrum* 35 (4).

Saaty, T. L. 1980. *The analytic hierarchy process.* New York: McGraw-Hill.

Sabbagh, K. 1996. *21st-century jet.* New York: Scribner.

Saiedian, H., and R. Kuzara. 1995. SEI capability maturity model's impact on contractors. *IEEE Computer* 28 (1).

Sammet, J. E. 1969. *Programming languages: History and fundamentals.* Englewood Cliffs: Prentice-Hall.

Samson, W. B., D. G. Nevill, and P. I. Dugard. 1990. Predictive software metrics based on a formal specification. *Software Engineering Journal* 5 (1).

Santic, J. S. 1995. Watchdog timer techniques. *Embedded Systems Programming* 8 (4).

Savitzky, S. 1985. *Real-time microprocessor systems.* New York: Van Nostrand Reinhold.

Schach, S. 1990. *Software engineering.* Boston: Aksen Associates.

Schafer, W., R. Prieto-Díazand, and M. Matsumoto. 1993. *Software reusability.* Chichester: Ellis Horwood.

Schick, G. J., and R. W. Wolverton. 1978. An analysis of competing software reliability models. *IEEE Transactions on Software Engineering* 4 (2).

Schneider, G., and J.P. Winters. 1998. *Applying use cases: A practical guide.* Reading: Addison-Wesley Longman.

Schneidewind, N. F., and H. Hoffmann. 1979. An experiment in software error data collection and analysis. *IEEE Transactions on Software Engineering* 5 (3).

Schneidewind, N. F. 1992a. Minimizing risks in applying metrics on multiple projects. In *Proceedings of the Third International Symposium on Software Reliability.* Los Alamitos: IEEE Computer Society Press.

Schneidewind, N. F. 1992b. Methodology for validating software metrics. *IEEE Transactions on Software Engineering* 18 (5).

Schneidewind, N. F. 1993. Software reliability model with optimal selection of failure data. *IEEE Transactions on Software Engineering* 19 (11).

Schulmeyer, G. G. 1990. *Zero defect software.* New York: McGraw-Hill.

Schulmeyer, G. G., and J. I. McManus. 1987. *Handbook of software quality assurance.* New York: Van Nostrand Reinhold.

Schulmeyer, G. G., and J. I. McManus, eds. 1992. *Total quality management for software.* New York: Van Nostrand Reinhold.

Sharp, J. K. 1999. Validating software requirements. *CrossTalk: The Journal of Defense Software Engineering* (November).

Sheldon, F. T., K. M. Kavi, R. C. Tausworthe, J. T. Yu, R. Brettschneider, and W. W. Everitt. 1992. Reliability measurement: From theory to practice. *IEEE Software* 9 (4).

Shen, V. Y., S. D. Conte, and H. E. Dunsmore. 1983. Software science revisited: A critical analysis of the theory and its empirical study. *IEEE Transactions on Software Engineering* 9 (2).

Shen, V. Y., T. J. Yu, S. M. Thebaut, and L. R. Paulsen. 1985. Identifying error-prone software— An empirical study. *IEEE Transactions on Software Engineering* 11 (4).

Shepperd, M. J. 1988a. A critique of cyclomatic complexity as a software metric. *Software Engineering Journal* 3 (2).

Shepperd, M. J. 1988b. An evaluation of software product metrics. *Journal of Information and Software Technology* 30 (3).

Shepperd, M. J. 1990. Design metrics: An empirical analysis. *Software Engineering Journal* 5 (1).

Shepperd, M. 1993. *Software engineering metrics volume 1: Measures and validation.* London: McGraw-Hill Book Company.

Sherer, S., A. Kouchakdjian, and P. G. Arnold. 1996. Experience using cleanroom software engineering. *IEEE Software* 13 (3).

Sherif, Y. S., and D. C. Ince. 1986. Computer software quality measurements and metrics. *Microelectronics Reliability* 25 (6).

Sherman, R. W. 1995. Shipping the right products at the right time: A view of development and testing at Microsoft. *CrossTalk: The Journal of Defense Software Engineering* 8 (10).

Shiba, S., A. Graham, and D. Walden. 1993. *A new American TQM: Four practical revolutions in management.* Portland: Productivity Press.

Shina, S. G. 1987. *Concurrent engineering and design for manufacture of electronics products.* New York: Van Nostrand Reinhold.

Shlaer, S., and S. J. Mellor. 1988. *Object-oriented systems analysis: Modeling the world in data.* Englewood Cliffs: Prentice-Hall.

Shlaer, S., and S. J. Mellor. 1991. *Object lifecycles: Modeling the world in states.* Englewood Cliffs: Prentice-Hall.

Shneiderman, B. 1980. *Software psychology: Human factors in computer and information systems.* Cambridge: Winthrop Publishers.

Shneiderman, B. 1992. *Designing the user interface: Strategies for effective human-computer interaction.* Reading: Addison-Wesley.

Shneiderman, B. 1998. *Designing the user interface: Strategies for effective human-computer interaction,* 3rd ed. Reading: Addison-Wesley.

Shooman, M. L. 1983. *Software engineering—Design, reliability, management.* New York: McGraw-Hill.

Shooman, M. L. 1984. Software reliability: A historical perspective. *IEEE Transactions on Reliability* 33 (1).

Siddiqi, J. 1994. Challenging universal truths of requirements engineering. *IEEE Software* 11 (2).

Siddiqi, J., and M. C. Shekaran. 1996. Requirements engineering: The emerging wisdom. *IEEE Software* (March).

Silver, B. 1992. TQM vs. SEI Capability Maturity Model. *Software Quality World* 4 (2).

Simpson, H., and S. M. Casey. 1988. *Developing effective user documentation: A human factors approach.* New York: McGraw-Hill.

Smith, D. J., and K. B. Wood. 1989. *Engineering quality software.* New York: Elsevier.

Smith, P. G., and D. G. Reinertsen. 1991. *Developing products in half the time.* New York: Van Nostrand Reinhold.

Software Engineering Institute. 1987. *A method for assessing the software engineering capability of contractors.* SEI Technical Report CMU/SEI-87-TR-23. Pittsburgh: Software Engineering Institute.

Software Engineering Institute. 1991. *Capability maturity model for software.* SEI Technical Report CMU/SEI-91-TR-24. Pittsburgh: Software Engineering Institute.

Sorenson, R. 1995. A comparison of software development methodologies. *CrossTalk: The Journal of Defense Software Engineering* 8 (1).

Sorensen, R. 1999. CCB—An acronym for "chocolate chip brownies"? A tutorial on control boards. *CrossTalk: The Journal of Defense Software Engineering* (March).

Sroka, J. V., and R. M. Rusting. 1992. Medical device computer software: Challenges and safeguards. *Designer's handbook: Medical electronics.* Santa Monica: Canon Communications.

Stamatis, D. H. 1995. *Failure mode and effect analysis: FMEA from theory to execution.* Milwaukee: ASQC Quality Press.

Stankovic, J. A. 1988. Misconcepts about real-time computing: A serious problem for next-generation computing. *IEEE Computer* 21 (10).

Stanton, N. 1994. *Human factors in alarm design.* London: Taylor and Francis.

Start, G., R. C. Durst, and C. W. Vowell. 1994. Using metrics in management decision making. *IEEE Computer* 27 (9).

Statz, J., and S. Tennison. 1995. Getting started with software risk management. *American Programmer* (March).

Statz, J., D. Oxley, and P. O'Toole. 1997. Identifying and managing risks for software process improvement. *CrossTalk: The Journal of Defense Software Engineering* 10 (4).

Stetter, F. 1984. A measure of program complexity. *Computer Languages* 9 (3).

Stoddard, R., and J. Hedstrom. 1995. A Bayesian approach to deriving parameter values for a software defect predictive model. In *Proceedings of the Sixth Annual Conference on Applications of Software Measurement.* Los Alamitos: Computer Society Press.

Storey, N. 1996. *Safety-critical computer systems.* Reading: Addison-Wesley.

Sullivan, J. W., and S. W. Tyler, eds. 1991. *Intelligent user interfaces.* New York: Association of Computing Machinery Press.

Sunazuka, T., M. Azuma, and N. Yamagishi. 1985. Software quality assessment technology. In *Proceedings Eighth International Conference on Software Engineering.* Los Alamitos: IEEE Computer Society Press.

Sundararajan, C. (Raj). 1991. *Guide to reliability engineering: Data, analysis, applications, implementation, and management.* New York: Van Nostrand Reinhold.

Suzuki, J. K. 1996. Documenting the software validation of computer-controlled devices and manufacturing processes: A guide for small manufacturers. *Medical Device and Diagnostic Industry* 18 (1).

Swartout, W., and R. Baizer. 1982. On the inevitable intertwining of specification and implementation. *Communications of the ACM* 25 (7).

Swezey, R. W., and E. Salas, eds. 1992. *Teams: Their training and performance.* Norwood: Ablex.

Symons, C. R. 1988. Function point analysis: Difficulties and improvements. *IEEE Transactions on Software Engineering* 14 (1).

Symons, C. R. 1991. *Software sizing and estimating: Mk II FPA (function point analysis).* New York: John Wiley & Sons.

Taguchi, G. 1986. *Introduction to quality engineering: Designing quality into products and processes.* New York: UNIPUB/Kraus International Publications.

Tate, G., and J. M. Verner. 1990. Software sizing and costing models: A survey of empirical validation and comparison studies. *Journal of Information Technology* 5.

Tausworthe, R. C. 1977a. *Stochastic models for software project management.* Deep Space Network Progress Report Number 42-37. Pasadena: Jet Propulsion Laboratory.

Tausworthe, R. C. 1977b. *Standardized development of computer software.* Englewood Cliffs: Prentice-Hall.

Tausworthe, R. C. 1988. The work breakdown structure in software project management. In *Tutorial: Software engineering project management,* ed. R. H. Thayer. Washington, D.C.: IEEE Computer Society Press.

Tausworthe, R., and M. Lyu. 1996. A generalized technique for simulating software reliability. *IEEE Software* 13 (2).

Taylor, E. W. 1911. *The principles of scientific management.* New York: Harper and Row.

Thadhani, A. J. 1984. Factors affecting programmer productivity during application development. *IBM Systems Journal* 23 (1).

Thayer, R. H., A. Pyster, and R. C. Wood. 1980. The challenge of software engineering project management. *IEEE Computer* 14 (8).

Thebaut, S. M. 1983. *The saturation effect in large-scale software development: Its impact and control.* Ph.D. diss., Purdue University.

Thomson, W. 1995. Managing firmware development by contract. *Embedded Systems Programming* 8 (5).

Thorp, J. 1998. *The information paradox.* New York: McGraw-Hill.

Tian, J., P. Lu, and J. Palma. 1995. Test-execution-based reliability measurement and modeling for large commercial software. *IEEE Transactions on Software Engineering* (May).

Tian, J., and J. Palma. 1998. Analyzing and improving reliability: A tree-based approach. *IEEE Software* 15 (2).

Trenner, L., and J. Bawa. 1998. *The politics of usability.* London: Springer-Verlag.

Troy, R. 1994. Software reuse: Making the concept work. *Engineering Software* (June).

Turner, J. 1980. The structure of modular programs. *Communications of the ACM* 23 (5).

Turski, W. M., and T. S. E. Maibaum. 1987. *The specification of computer programs.* Wokingham: Addison-Wesley.

Verner, J. M., G. Tate, B. Jackson, and R. G. Hayward. 1989. Technology dependence in function point analysis: A case study and critical review. In *Proceedings of the 11th International Conference on Software Engineering.* Los Alamitos: Computer Society Press.

Voas, J. 1992. PIE: A dynamic failure-based technique. *IEEE Transactions on Software Engineering* (August).

Wallace, D. R., and R. U. Fujii. 1993. Software verification and validation: An overview. In *Software management,* ed. D. Reifer. Washington, D.C.: IEEE Computer Society Press.

Wallace, D. R., and L. M. Ippolito. 1994. *A framework for the development and assurance of high integrity software,* NIST SP 500-223. Washington, D.C.: U. S. Government Printing Office.

Wallace, R. H., J. E. Stockenberg, and R. N. Charette. 1987. *A unified methodology for developing systems.* New York: Intertext Publications.

Ward, P. T., and S. J. Mellor. 1985. *Structured development for real-time systems,* Vol. 1, 2, and 3. New York: Yourdon Press.

Warnier, J. D. 1974. *Logical construction of programs.* New York: Van Nostrand Reinhold Company.

Wasserman, A. I. 1990. Tool integration in software engineering environments. In *Software engineering environments,* ed. F. W. Long. Berlin: Springer-Verlag.

Wasserman, A. I., P. A. Pircher, and R. J. Muller. 1990. The object-oriented structured design notation for software design representation. *IEEE Computer* 23 (3).

Wasserman, A. I., and D. T. Shewmake. 1985. The role of prototypes in the user software engineering methodology. In *Advances in human-computer interaction,* ed. H. R. Hartson. Norwood: Ablex.

Webb, D., and W. S. Humphrey. 1999. Using the TSP on the task view project. *CrossTalk: The Journal of Defense Software Engineering* 12 (2).

Weide, P. 1994. Improving medical device safety with automated software testing. *Medical Device and Diagnostic Industry* (August).

Weidenhaupt, K., K. Pohl, M. Jarke, and P. Haumer. 1998. Scenarios in system development: Current practice. *IEEE Software* 15 (2).

Weinberg, G. M. 1971. *The psychology of programming.* New York: Van Nostrand Reinhold.

Weinberg, G. M. 1988. *Understanding the professional programmer.* New York: Dorset House.

Weiss, D. M., and V. R. Basili. 1985. Evaluating software development by analysis of changes: Some data from the software engineering laboratory. *IEEE Transactions on Software Engineering* 11 (2).

Welker, K. D., and P. W. Oman. 1995. Software maintainability metrics models in practice. *CrossTalk: The Journal of Defense Software Engineering* 8 (11).

Weller, E. F. 1994. Using metrics to manager software projects. *IEEE Computer* 27 (9).

Wexelblat, R. L. 1981. *History of programming languages.* New York: Academic Press.

Weyuker, E. J. 1988. Evaluating software complexity measures. *IEEE Transactions on Software Engineering* 14 (9).

Wheelwright, S. C., and K. B. Clark. 1992. *Revolutionizing product development.* New York: Free Press.

Whiteside, J., and D. Wixon. 1985. Developmental theory as a framework for studying human-computer interaction. In *Advances in human-computer interaction,* Vol.1, ed. H. R. Hartson. Norwood: Ablex.

Whiteside, J., J. Bennett, and K. Holtzblatt, 1988. Usability engineering: Our experience and evolution. In *Handbook of human-computer interaction.* Amsterdam: Elsevier North-Holland.

Whittaker, J. A., and J. H. Poore. 1993. Markov analysis of software specifications. In *ACM Transactions on Software Engineering and Methodology* 2. New York: Association of Computing Machinery Press.

Whittaker, J., and M. Thomason. 1994. A Markov chain model for statistical software testing. *IEEE Transactions on Software Engineering* 30 (October).

Whittaker, J. A., and J. Voas. 2000. Toward a more reliable theory of software reliability. *Computer* 33 (12).

Whitten, W. 1990. *Managing software development projects.* New York: John Wiley & Sons.

Wiegers, K. 2000. Stop promising miracles. *Software Development* 8 (2).

Wiener, L. R. 1994. *Digital woes: Why we should not depend on software.* Reading: Addison-Wesley.

Wiklund, M. E. 1992. Human error signals opportunity for design improvements. *Medical Device and Diagnostic Industry* 14 (2).

Wiklund, M. E. 1994a. Usability considerations in selecting user interface hardware. In *Designer's handbook: Medical electronics.* Santa Monica: Canon Communications.

Wiklund, M. E. 1994b. *Usability in practice: How companies develop user-friendly products.* Boston: Academic Press.

Wiklund, M. E. 1998. Making medical device interfaces more user-friendly. *Medical Device & Diagnostic Industry* (May).

Williams, L. G. 1994. Assessment of safety-critical specifications. *IEEE Software* 11 (1).

Wirfs-Brock, R., B. Wilkerson, and L. Wiener. 1990. *Designing object-oriented software.* Englewood Cliffs: Prentice-Hall.

Wirth, N. 1971. Programming development by stepwise refinement. *Communications of the ACM* 14 (4).

Wirth, N. 1977. Toward a discipline of real-time programming. *Communications of the ACM* 20 (8).

Wohlwend, H., and S. Rosenbaum. 1994. Schlumberger's software improvement program. *IEEE Transactions on Software Engineering* 20 (11).

Wolverton, R. W. 1974. The cost of developing large-scale software. *IEEE Transaction on Computers* (June).

Wood, B. J., and J. W. Ermes. 1993. Applying hazard analysis to medical devices, part II: Detailed hazard analysis. *Medical Device and Diagnostic Industry* 15 (3).

Woodward, M. R., M. A. Hennell, and D. Hedley. 1979. A measure of control flow complexity in program text. *IEEE Transactions on Software Engineering* 5 (1).

Wright, J. F. 1993. Designing for compliance: Medical equipment. *Compliance Engineering* (Spring).

Yamada, S., M. Ohba, and S. Osaki. 1983. S-shaped reliability growth modeling for software error detection. *IEEE Transactions on Reliability* (December).

Yamada, S., H. Ohtera, and H. Narihisa. 1986. Software reliability growth models with testing effort. *IEEE Transactions on Reliability* (April).

Yourdon, E. 1975. *Techniques of program structure and design.* Englewood Cliffs: Prentice-Hall.

Yourdon, E. 1989. *Modern structured analysis.* Englewood Cliffs: Yourdon Press.

Yourdon, E., and L. L. Constantine. 1979. *Structured design: Fundamentals of a discipline of computer program and systems design.* Englewood Cliffs: Prentice-Hall.

Yung, W. K. C., and C. Y. Tang. 1998. Finance-driven maintenance system with failure mode consideration. *Quality Engineering* 10 (3).

Zhuo, F., et al. 1993. Constructing and testing software maintainability assessment models. In *Proceedings of the First International Software Metrics Symposium.* Washington, D.C.: IEEE Computer Society Press.

Zultner, R. E. 1993. TQM for technical teams. *Communications of the ACM* 36 (10).

Index

acceptance criteria. *See also* Software End-Product
    Acceptance Plan (SEAP)
  determination of, 272–273
  governing policies, 59
  risk management and, 330
  software safety and, 310–311
  test execution and, 286
acceptance testing, 126, 275–276
accident prevention
  discovering safety-critical mistakes, 372–373
  hazard analysis and, 336
  requirement flaws and, 356
accuracy, 344, 448
active redundancy, 353–354
adaptive reuse, 252
ad hoc tests, 360
ADR. See Architecture Design Review (ADR)
ADS. *See* Architecture Design Specification (ADS)
Advise, A. M., 207, 237–238, 240
Akiyama, F., 421, 423
alarms, 195–196, 365, 368, 370–372
Albin, J. L., 422
Albrecht, A. J., 408
algorithmic estimation models, 128–129, 132
algorithmic measurements, 397–398
algorithms
  constructional domain and, 378
  feature point analysis, 409
  software metrics and, 396–398
allocated baseline, 319
analog to digital converter (ADC), 217–218
analogy methods, 132, 134–135

analysis phase, 45–48
analysis tools, 312–313
analytic models, 43, 128–129
Anderson, T., 310–311
AND gate, fault-tree analysis, 346
anomalies
  impact of, 174
  SEAP and, 158
  Software Anomaly Report, 201
  in software life cycle, 227–229
  software metrics and, 95
  SVTP and, 166–167
  SVVP and, 172–173
  verification and validation, 79–80
Anomaly Reporting and Resolution policy, 72, 79
ANSI/IEEE Std 730-1989, 26–27
ANSI/IEEE Std 829-1016-1987, 27–29
ANSI/IEEE Std 829-1983, 26–27
ANSI/IEEE Std 830-1984, 26–27
ANSI/IEEE Std 1012-1986, 28, 299
A-1 matrix, SQFD and, 214–215
Architecture Design Phase
  document elements, 24
  IDS support for, 202–203
  object-oriented model and, 47
  in software life cycle, 225
  Verification and Validation policy, 72, 75
  WBS and, 114–115
Architecture Design Review (ADR)
  elements of, 65–67
  review process and, 243
  in software life cycle, 224–225

software reviews, 245–246
Software User's Manual policy and, 68
SVTP and, 78, 163
SVVP and, 71
Architecture Design Specification (ADS)
ADR and, 245
elements of, 63–65
features of, 177–182
physical model and, 176
review process and, 243
SRS and, 202–203
Aron, J. D., 129
assembly language, 119, 311, 416
assessment methods, 439–441, 445–446
ASSET-R method, 409
asymptotic behavior, 427
auditing. *See also* Software Configuration Audit
  Report (SCAR)
code audits, 269
configuration management policies, 82–83
DTIS, 68
incremental model and, 41
off-the-shelf software and, 309–310
process audits, 458
SCAR and, 77
software quality assurance and, 8
software reviews and, 248–249
SQAP and, 160
SVVP and, 171
system testing and, 275
of VTIS, 197
automated tools. *See also* software development tools
software librarian, 321
SVVP and, 171
test coverage and, 291
test preparation and, 285

backward recovery, 360
Baker, F. T., 39
Balzer, R., 42
baselines
ADS as, 181–182
configuration management and, 316
CRAs and, 228
operational prototypes and, 239–240
planning documents and, 146
purpose of, 318–320
regression testing and, 284–285
SCMP and, 149
software reuse and, 252
software validation testing and, 200
Bashein, B. J., 448
Basic COCOMO, 129–130
Bastani, F. B., 424
behavioral domain, 377–380
Bennington, H. D., 38
Berard, Edward V., 259
Bernstein, L., 135

Bersoff, E. H., 237–238, 240
Bieman, J. M., 237
Bilodeau, A., 422
Birrell, N. D., 42
Black, R.K.D., 129
black-box analysis, 51, 291
Blank, J. M., 42
blood chemistry analyzers, 381–382
Boar prototype, 233–234
Boehm, B. W., 40, 42–43, 124–125, 408
Boeing model, 129
bottom-up methods, 133–134, 385–386
boundary conditions, 268, 304, 338–339
boundary tests, 262–263
bounding analysis, 358
breach of contract, 11–12
Breton, E. J., 12
Brooks, F. P., 40, 105, 107
Brooks, W. D., 421–423

C++ language, 45
calibration
algorithmic estimation models and, 132
boundary tests and, 262
error calibration, 268
software metric limitations and, 399
table models and, 129
Capability Maturity Model (CMM)
maturity metrics and, 448
process assessment, 439–440
process maturity and, 445
SPI scope based on, 453–458
Carey, Tom, 375
CASE. *See* computer-aided software engineering
  (CASE)
cathode ray tube (CRTs), 370
centralized teams, 121–122
certification
cleanroom model and, 48–50
embedded software and, 276
methods of, 286–287
software reuse and, 251
SVVR and, 80
testing for, 281, 286
TickIT program, 440–441
validation testing and, 272
change control
documentation structure for, 54–55
revisions and, 35
software development and, 324–326
tracking feature, 33
Change Request/Approval (CRA)
change control and, 324–325
elements of, 81–82, 84–86
operational prototypes and, 241
in software life cycle, 224, 226–229
software metrics and, 95
SVTP and, 163

Charette, R. N., 351
Cheatham, T. E., 42
checksums, software quality assurance and, 6
Cheung, R. C., 355
chief programming team, 121–122
cleanroom model, 47–50
CMM. *See* Capability Maturity Model (CMM)
Coates, A., 355
Cobb, R. H., 9
code-and-fix model, 42
Code and Test Phase Verification and Validation
    policy, 72–73, 76
code walk-throughs
    defects and, 420
    purpose of, 269–270
    software metrics and, 396
    software reviews and, 247
    testing allocation and, 279–280
cognitive dissonance, 54
Collins, W. R., 10
color palette, patient monitors and, 383
commission hazards, 359
common loads, 363
common mode analysis, 311–312
communication
    development processes and, 391–393
    importance of, 25
    patient monitor considerations, 384
    planning documents and, 146
    in programming teams, 122
comparator capability, 33
complexity and precision. *See also* cyclomatic
    complexity number, v(G)
    defined, 127, 396–397
    function point analysis and, 135–137
    fuzzy logic and, 50
    microprocessor and, 5–6
    pass-fail acceptance test and, 126
    requirements engineering and, 207–208
    underestimating software development, 119
composite estimation models, 129–131
compositional reuse, 252
computer-aided software engineering (CASE)
    automation and, 42, 223
    capabilities of, 24
    software producability and, 386–387
    tool examples, 33–34
concave models, 427, 429
conditional statements, decision count metric and, 413
configuration management. *See also* Software
    Configuration Audit Report (SCAR); Software
    Configuration Management Plan (SCMP)
    activities for, 315–327
    cleanroom model and, 48
    policies for, 55, 92, 94–95
    process infrastructure and, 31–32
    prototypes and, 237–240
    reporting configuration changes, 225

software policies, 80–86
software validation testing and, 200
Software Verification and Validation Anomaly
    Report, 167
SQAP and, 160
SVTP and, 163
Configuration Manager, 164, 174–175
consistency index (CI), 213
consistency ratio (CR), 213
Constantine, L. L., 39, 42
constants, data structure metrics and, 410
constructional domain, 377–379
Constructive Cost Model (COCOMO), 129–131
constructs, programming, 52, 260
Conte, S. D., 408, 415, 424
Control Data Corporation, 12
control flow paths
    constructional domain and, 378
    interruptions in, 412–413
    testing, 261
    unit testing and, 268
copyrights, product release policies, 87–88
co-resident software, 361–365
cost-benefit analysis, 376–377
costs
    cost-value requirements, 210–214
    effectiveness of code inspections, 270
    integrated testing strategy and, 292–293
    maturity metrics and, 448
    meeting project commitments, 216
    number of test cases and, 284
    risks in software requirements, 309
    software quality and, 396
    software reuse, 252–253
    verification and validation considerations, 308
CRA. *See* Change Request/Approval (CRA)
CRTs (cathode ray tubes), 370
Curfew, R. P., 129
cyclic redundancy checks (CRCs), 6
cyclomatic complexity number, v(G), 413, 430, 443

Dally, E. B., 120
Data Analysts, 164
data element types (DETs), 138–140
Data Integrity and Retention policy, 56, 87
Data Security policy, 87–88
data structures, 24, 409–412
DDR. *See* Detailed Design Review (DDR)
dead code, 361–365
debugging
    certification testing and, 281
    productivity measurement and, 439
    static analysis and, 269
    testing allocation and, 279–280
decay rate, 273
decision count, 412–413, 423
defect density, 423–424
defects. *See also* faults

analysis tools displaying, 312–313
breach of contract action and, 11–12
change requests and, 324
dynamic model of defects, 420, 424–425
elements of software, 417–420
hardware quality assurance and, 8
impact on product lines, 14
installed variants and, 326–327
software metrics and, 19
static models of defects, 420–421
testing, 262–266
during validation testing, 272
zero defects, 252–253
degradation
design considerations, 21
of hardware over time, 6
degree of influence (DI), 141
Delphi technique, 133
DeMarco, T., 42, 409
demonstration
IDS and, 186
as verification method, 154, 165, 190
Department of Defense, 2, 42, 421
design-to-cost methodology, 216–217
design walk-throughs, 279–280, 396
DET (data element type), 138–140
Detailed COCOMO, 129–130
Detailed Design Phase
ANSI/IEEE Std 1016-1987, 29
estimations and, 124–125
IDS support for, 202–203
object-oriented model and, 47
review process and, 243
Verification and Validation policy, 72, 75–76
Detailed Design Review (DDR)
elements of, 63–64, 66–68
software reviews, 246–247
SVTP and, 163
Detailed Design Specification (DDS)
ADS, 202–203
DDR and, 246
development flow, 176–177
DTP and, 155–156
elements of, 65
features of, 177–178, 180, 182–183
product release policies, 87
review process and, 243
RTM and, 192
in software life cycle, 224
software quality and, 306
SVTPR and, 167
SVVP and, 71
verification and validation review, 76
VTIS and, 78, 198
Development Practices policy, 61–62
Development Test Information Sheet (DTIS)
elements of, 63–64, 68
purpose of, 155

RTM and, 188
safety testing and, 278
SRS and, 189
testing process and, 196–197
verification and validation review, 76–77
development testing, 281–282, 285
deviation
policies for, 103–104
from standards, 18–19
test execution and, 285
DI (degree of influence), 141
Dijkstra, E., 39
Dijkstra, E. W., 39–40
DIN V VDE 0801, 440
directed graphs, 260–261
documentation. *See* software documentation
double-mode faults, 267
Drummen, M. H., 42
DTIS. *See* Development Test Information Sheet (DTIS)
due diligence, 57–59
Dunham, J. R., 355
Dunsmore, H. E., 408, 411, 413, 415, 424
dynamic model of defects, 420, 424–425

EEPROM. *See* erasable electronically programmable read-only memory (EEPROM)
efficacy, of tools, 265–266
efficiency
quality software and, 305
statistical process control and, 432
usability and, 376
effort estimation models, 408
EI. *See* external input (EI)
EIF. *See* external interface files (EIFs)
Einstein, Albert, 315
electronically programmable read-only memory (EPROM), 190
electronic reliability, 20
Elshoff, J. L., 412
embedded software
Principles for Computers in Safety-Related Systems, 440
system testing and, 275–276
TÜV model, 439
embedded systems, 23, 186–187
EN 29001, 440–441
end-product baseline, 319
engineers. *See* software engineers/engineering
EO. *See* external output (EO)
EPROM. *See* electronically programmable read-only memory (EPROM)
EQ. *See* external inquiries (EQ)
equivalent size measures, 407–408
erasable electronically programmable read-only memory (EEPROM), 179, 321
Ericson, C. A., 356

errors
  causes of, 24–25
  defect metrics and, 418
  error detection, 162, 181, 194–196, 216, 306
  error tolerance, 5, 9
  factors affecting estimations, 109
  fault tree examples, 345–347
  hardware errors, 344–345
  reasons for, 299
  structured programming and, 39
  testing paths and, 261–262
  user error, 366
  validation testing and, 272
estimation. *See also* function point analysis (FPA)
  Gantt charts and, 125
  methods for, 132–135
  models for, 128–132, 152, 289, 408
  overestimates, 106
  project management, 108–110
  underestimates, 106, 119
ethical considerations, 9–11
event handlers, 378
evolutionary design, prototypes and, 233–234
evolutionary development model, 42, 44
evolutionary prototypes, 231, 237–239
exception testing, 364
exhaustive theory, 260–261
external consistency, 308
external input (EI)
  depicted, 142
  FTRs and, 139
  functional complexity and, 137
  ILFs and, 136
external inquiries (EQ)
  counting, 140
  depicted, 142
  FPA and, 137
  functional complexity and, 137
external interface files (EIFs)
  defined, 136
  depicted, 142
  examples of, 139
  functional complexity and, 137
  weighting, 140
external output (EO)
  depicted, 142
  FPA and, 136
  functional complexity and, 137
  transactional function matrix, 140
extraction by interview, 51
extraction by observation, 51, 129

Fagan, M. E., 270
failure intensity, 281–283, 285–286
failure modes and effects analysis (FMEA). *See also*
    software FMEA (SFMEA)
  hazard analysis and, 337–341, 351
  risk assessment and, 352–353

  risk management and, 330, 333
  safety requirements and, 23
failure rates
  device reliability and, 20–21
  fault-tree analysis and, 348
  and redundancy, 353–354
failures
  defect detection and, 425
  defined, 282
  fault-tree analysis and, 342
  FMEA and, 338–340
  medical devices and, 9–11, 440
  region faults and, 267
  software and, 6–7
  test execution and, 285
failure-severity systems, 282, 355–356
false alarms, 371
faults
  defined, 282
  isolated faults, 287
  region faults, 267–268
  removal as reliability strategy, 283
  statistical testing and, 289
fault-tree analysis (FTA)
  complex triggering mechanisms and, 337
  features of, 342–348
  probabilities, 348–351
  risk management and, 332–333
  safety requirements and, 23, 356–357
  software safety and, 311, 352–353
FDA. *See* Food and Drug Administration (FDA)
feature point analysis, 409
feature sets, 14–16
feedback
  importance of presenting clear information, 365
  process maturity and, 444
  waterfall model and, 39
Ferreol, R., 422
file management, as software tool feature, 33
file types referenced (FTRs), 139–140
firmware, configuration management and, 321–322
Fitzsimmons, A., 109–110, 130–131
501(k) review, 440
510(k) reviewer guidance requirements, 29
flammability, as potential hazard, 331
FMEA. *See* failure modes and effects analysis
    (FMEA)
Fogg, B., 11
Food and Drug Administration (FDA)
  assessment standards, 439
  510(k) reviewer guidance requirements, 29
  IEEE standards and, 26
  medical device failures, 440
  off-the-shelf software and, 309
  *Reviewer Guidance for Computer-Controlled
      Medical Devices Undergoing 510(k) Review,* 440
  risk analysis and, 330
formal notation, 52

Freeman, P., 42
FTA. *See* fault-tree analysis (FTA)
FTR. *See* file types referenced (FTRs)
Fujitsu, Ltd., 421
function, 407
functional decomposition method, 409
functional manager, 120–121
functional modularity, 259–260
functional specifications, 48, 146
functional testing
    defined, 153–154
    examples of, 263
    quality assurance and, 304
    SRS and, 190
    as validation test, 164
function count, 407
function point analysis (FPA), 135–143, 408–409
function points per hour (FP/hr), 137
fuzzy-logic model, 50–52

Gaffney, J. E., 422
Galilei, Galileo, 395
Gannon, C., 269–270
Gannon, J. D., 411, 413
Gantt charts, estimation and, 125
General Accounting Office (GAO), 12
general system characteristics (GSCs), 141–142
German Electrotechnical Commission (TÜV),
    439–440
Gerstling, H., 42
Goel, A. L., 427–429
Gompertz model, 429
good enough testing, 293–294
Gordon, V. S., 237
GOTO statements, 39, 414
Graham, R. M., 329
graphical user interface (GUI), 385
Gray, M. D., 129
Green, C., 42
Griggs, J. G., 356
growth testing, 154, 165, 190
GSC (general system characteristics), 141–142
guidelines. *See* policies
Guide to Software Design Descriptions (IEEE Std
    1016.1-1993), 27, 29
*Guide to Software Quality Management System
    Construction and Certification Using EN 29001,*
    440

Haag, S. H., 214
Hagemeister, J., 428
Halstead, M. H., 129, 405, 415–416, 422–423, 428,
    430
handshaking, protection through, 359–360
hardware design/development, 23, 52, 184–185
hardware engineer, as software engineer, 115–117
hardware errors, 344–345
hardware quality assurance, 6–8, 20–21

Hardware Tools policy, 63, 68
Harvey, P. R., 311
hazard analysis
    difficulties in, 351–352
    models and techniques, 337–351
    safety requirements and, 23
    software design and, 359
    software hazards and, 333–337
hazard and operability (HAZOP) study, 332–333
hazards and effects table, 333, 335–336
Hedley, D., 414
Helmer, O., 133
Hennell, M. A., 414
heuristics, *versus* rigor, 215–216
Hezel, K. D., 106
Hossain-Dahiya model, 429
human-computer interaction (HCI), 377
human factors, 378–381
Huskey, H. D., 10
Huskey, V. R., 10

IBM
    Federal Systems Division, 421
    Santa Teresa Laboratory, 422
icon elements, patient monitors and, 384–385
IDS. *See* Interface Design Specification (IDS)
IEEE. *See* Institute of Electrical and Electronic
    Engineers (IEEE)
IEEE Std 1016.1-1993, 27, 29
ILF. *See* internal logical files (ILFs)
implementation
    errors during, 299
    IDS and, 184
    object-oriented model and, 47
    primary goal of, 88
    of quality control, 3
    of software, 34
    of software quality assurance, 31–35
implementation phase, 52
incremental model, 40–41
infinite failure models, 427
input/output
    code inspections and, 270
    data structures and, 409–410
    Halstead measures and, 405
    off-the-shelf software and, 310
    tasks and, 181–183
    user interface and, 194–195
    validation of, 367–368
input variables, 284
inspection
    of code, 269–270
    quality assurance as, 2
    SVVP and, 171
    test execution and, 285
    as verification method, 154, 165, 190
Institute of Electrical and Electronic Engineers
    (IEEE), 25, 260. *See also* ANSI/IEEE standards

Integration, Test, Operations policy, 61–62
Integration and Test Phase
  baselines and, 319
  fuzzy-logic model and, 52
  IDS support for, 202–203
  specifics, 270–271
  Verification and Validation policy, 72–73, 77
Interface Design Phase, 24, 72–74
Interface Design Specification (IDS)
  features of, 184–186
  phase support, 202–203
  policy elements, 62–64
  product release policies, 87
  purpose of, 175
  RTM and, 188
  SDP and, 153
interfaces. *See also* User Interface Specification
    (UIS); user-machine interface
  code inspections and, 270
  environmental risks and, 309
  integration testing and, 270
  obscurity of, 206
  potential hazards and, 331
  software safety and, 365–373
  user interfaces, 379–385
Intermediate COCOMO, 129–130
intermediate event, 346
internal consistency, 308
internal logical files (ILFs), 136–137, 139–140
internal testing, 372
interrupts, testing and, 278
interviews, 51
invariant functionality, 251–252
isolated faults, 267
ISO 9000 standard, 439, 441
ISO 9000-3 standard, 439–440
ISO 9001 standard, 440, 453–454, 458
iterative approach
  object-oriented model and, 45–47
  software engineering and, 53
  validation with fuzzy-logic model, 52
  waterfall model and, 39

Jackson, M. A., 42
Jahanian, F., 357
Janssen, T.G.M., 42
Jelinski, Z., 424–425
Johnson, J., 448
Jones, C., 253, 269, 305, 409
Jones, C. B., 42

Katz, R., 129
KDSI (thousands of source instructions), 130–131
King, W. R., 106
Kiviat plot, 446–447
KLOC. *See* thousand lines of code (KLOC)
knowledge extraction, 51
Knuth, D. E., 39

Krijer, M. J., 42
Kwan, S. P., 10

labeling practices, 322–323, 383–384
languages. *See* programming languages
Laprie, J. C., 355
legal considerations
  copyrights, 87–88
  software quality and, 11–12
length equation, software metrics, 414–415
lessons learned. *See* postmortems
Leveson, N. G., 10, 311, 355, 357, 366
librarians
  program librarians, 122
  software librarian, 321
life cycle. *See* software life cycle
linear development estimating models, 128
linearity, fuzzy logic and, 50
lines of code (LOC), 403–405, 422
Lipow, M., 422
Littlewood, B., 355
live variables (LV), 410–412
loads/load testing
  certification testing and, 281
  co-resident software and, 363–364
  purpose of, 284
  SDP and, 150
  test execution and, 285
logical models, 175
logic structures, 412–414
loop control statements, 413
Lutz, R. R., 356
LV (live variables), 410–412
Lyu, M. R., 424

Macala, Randall R., 435
maintainability
  measuring, 31
  metrics models for, 428–431
  object-oriented model and, 45
  quality software and, 305
maintainability index (MI), 430
maintenance cycle/phase, 95–104, 417
Malcolm Baldridge Award, 454
malfunctions. *See* failures
Mallory, S. R., 3
management
  awareness of policy circumvention, 103–104
  educating, 35–36
  functional manager, 120–121
  lack of understanding, 119
  overseeing productivity, 438–439
  planning documents and, 146
  software development crisis and, 13
  software metrics and, 399–400
  SVVP and, 172
  wariness toward projects, 19
Mandl, R., 266

manpower. *See* resources
Mark (MK) II Function Points, 408–409
Markov chain, 287–289
Martin prototype, 233
Masters, R. J., 448
matrix organization, 121
maturity metrics, 447–448
McCabe, T. J., 413, 428, 443
McCabe complexities, 95
McCall, J., 305
McCracken, D., 233–234
McCracken, D. D., 42
McFarland, M. C., 10
mean time between failures (MTBF), 18, 353
mean time to failure (MTTF), 6, 49, 424–426
measurement. *See also* lines of code (LOC); unit
    of measure
  of changes, 7
  defining, 31
  FPA and, 137
  fuzzy logic and, 50
  objective measurements, 397–399
  of process improvements, 435–437
  process maturity and, 437, 441, 444–445
  productivity measurement, 438–439
  program size, 401–409
  software metrics and, 395–396
  software quality and, 18, 399–401
medical devices
  boundary conditions for, 338–339
  discovering mistakes, 372–373
  evolution of software, 1
  FDA failure documentation, 440
  hazard analysis example, 333–334
  misuse, 354–355
  need for quality assurance, 3–5
  object-oriented model and, 45
  off-the-shelf software and, 309–310
  *Principles for Computers in Safety-Related
      Systems,* 440
  reliability in, 20
  *Reviewer Guidance for Computer-Controlled
      Medical Devices Undergoing 510(k) Review,* 440
  robustness of hardware testing, 7
  role of quality assurance program, 17–18
  software development crisis and, 12–13
  user-friendly interfaces, 381–385
Mellor, S. J., 42
menus
  navigating, 382
  UIS and, 195–196
methodology, 37–38
MI (maintainability index), 430
microprocessors, 4–5, 117–119
milestones
  baselines as, 318
  criteria for, 106
  estimation and, 125

Project Preparation policy, 61–62
  SDP and, 150, 152
  software quality assurance and, 18
  WBS and, 112–114
Miller, K. W., 10
Mills, H. D., 9, 39–40, 439
misrepresentation (doctrine of), 12
modeling/models. *See also specific models*
  basic tasks in, 288
  difficulty in, 51
  object-oriented model, 45–47, 378
modules
  integration testing and, 270
  LOC and, 403–405
  purpose in testing, 268
  software reuse and, 250–252
  specifications for, 146
Mok, A. K., 357
monitors. *See* patient monitors
Moranda, P., 424–425
Motley, R. W., 421–423
MTBF. *See* mean time between failures (MTBF)
MTTF. *See* mean time to failure (MTTF)
multimode faults, 267
Musa, J. D., 424

NASA, 2
Nass, C., 11
negligence (doctrine of), 12
nesting levels, 413–414
Neumann, P. C., 373
Neumann, P. G., 9
New York Times project, 39
Nikora, A., 424
Noble, W. B., 311
nodes, testing, 260–262
Norris, William, 12
North Atlantic Treaty Organization (NATO), 39
"Notes on Structured Programming," 39
nuclear magnetic resonance (NMR), 1

objective measurements, 397–399
object-oriented model, 45–47, 378
observation, 51, 129
off-the-shelf software, 309–310
Okumoto, K., 427–429
Oman, P., 428
omission hazards, 359
operands, 405, 414–415
operation, 283
operational modes, 195, 283, 285
Operations policy, 61–62
operators, 405, 414–415
organization. *See also* team organization
  differences in productivity, 438
  of documentation, 54–56
  functional organization, 119–121
  software process improvement and, 450–451

SPI scope based on goals, 453–458
structured programming and, 38
organizational efficiency, 120
OR gate, fault-tree analysis, 346
orthogonal array testing, 266–268
Ossher, Harold, 37
Ottenstein, L. M., 422–423
Ould, M. A., 42
overall profiles, 283
overestimates, 106

Pareto's law, 127, 429, 432–433
Parkinson principle, 132
Parnas, D. L., 10
pass-fail criteria
precision and, 126
RTM and, 192
SVTPR and, 165
path testing, 260–262, 270–271
patient monitors, 368–370, 381–382
Paulsen, L. R., 413, 422, 424
Pelger, W. D., 42
performance
measuring, 435–437
as module specifications, 146
object-oriented model and, 47
reliability processes and, 20
requirement considerations, 24
stress testing and, 262
PERT (Program Evaluation Report Technique), 125,
130–131, 312
Peterson, J. L., 357
Phase Verification and Validation Task Summary
Report, 171
physical model, 175–176
physical testing, 154, 165, 190, 262
pilot projects, 31–35
planning documents, 146–175
Poisson models, 425
policies. *See also specific policies*
configuration management, 80–86
development documentation, 61–70
directory documentation, 59–61
governing policies, 56–59
guidelines for, 88–95
IDS verification, 203
implementing, 31–32
incorporating lessons learned, 35
organizing, 54
product releases, 87–88
Reviews policy, 61–62
for software metrics, 92, 94–103
SQAP and, 160
used in postmortems, 256–257
verification and validation, 70–80
VTIS and, 78, 197
polynomial regression models, 430
postmortems

as implementation step, 34–35
planning documents and, 146
from risk management efforts, 453
software development, 253–257
potential difficulty, 415
potential volume, 415–416
Potier, D., 422
power tests, 278–279
precision. *See* complexity and precision
predictive models, 399
Presburger arithmetic, 357
price-to-win methods, 132
Principles for Computers in Safety-Related Systems
(DIN V VDE 0801), 440
priority matrix, 212–213
probabilities
fault-tree analysis, 348–351
fuzzy logic and, 51
probability distribution, 288, 358
problem domain expert, 380–381
process. *See* review process
process improvement. *See* software process
improvement (SPI)
processor environment model, 175–176
product definition phase, 110, 146
product design specification, 124
productivity. *See* programming productivity
productivity rates, 117–118, 129, 137
product life cycle, 17–18, 26
Product Management and Acceptance policy, 61–62
products
classification and testing, 291–292
complexity of, 397
configuration management and integrity, 315–316
metrics for, 398
software quality dimensions and, 14–16
professional malpractice (doctrine of), 12
program librarians, 122
programming constructs, 52, 260
programming languages
assembly language, 119, 311, 416
C++ language, 45
limitations of, 388
object-oriented model and, 45–47
programming productivity, 118
SDP and, 152
software metrics and, 414, 416–417
programming productivity
differentials in software, 438–439
estimation and, 108–110
function point analysis and, 135–136
measurement and, 395–396
productivity rates and factors, 117–118
software reuse, 249–253
Programming Standards and Conventions policy, 63,
67
programming teams. *See also* team organization
characteristics of, 115–123

members of, 223–225
ownership and, 352
planning documents and, 146
resistance to change, 452–453
roles in, 393
SDP and, 150
software postmortems and, 255
support of review process, 243
program size, 401–409
project management
data usage by, 312–313
estimations for, 108–110
process maturity and, 444
resistance to change, 452
statistical process control and, 432
Project Preparation policy, 61–62
PROM devices, 276, 321
prompts, 196
proof by contradiction, 311
proof of adequacy, 311
proof of correctness, 311
prototypes
behavioral domain and, 378
cleanroom model and, 48
construction considerations, 231–233
development policies, 56
documentation for, 241–242
evolutionary design and, 233–234
GUI style guides and, 385
hazard analysis and, 331–332
as models, 229–231
object-oriented model and, 47
operational prototypes, 230, 239–241
as risk management technique, 43–44
spiral model and, 42–43
stagewise process and, 38
structured design and, 234–236
throwaway prototypes, 236–237
waterfall model and, 39
pseudocode, as semiformal notation, 52
Putnam, L. H., 109–110, 129–131
Pyster, A., 119

quality
aspects of, 18–22
defined, 18, 211
dimensions of, 14–16
quality assurance. *See* software quality assurance
(SQA)
quality control, 2–3
quality engineers, 29–30
Quality Function Deployment (QFD), 214–215
quantitative criteria, 289, 399

radiation therapy, 9–10, 366
Raja, M. K., 214
RAM (random-access memory), 179, 279
Ramamoorthy, C. V., 424

Rand Corporation, 133
random index (RI), 213
random testing, 287
Rayleigh distribution function, 109–110
reactivity, as potential hazard, 331
read-only memory (ROM), 87, 179, 276, 321
*Recommended Practice for Software Design
Descriptions* (ANSI/IEEE Std 1016-1987),
27–29
record element types (RETs), 139
redundancy, 6, 353–354
region faults, 267–268
regression analysis/models, 408, 430
regression testing
defined, 154
purpose of, 284–285
software and, 7
SRS and, 190
SVTP and, 164
usefulness of, 276
validation testing and, 165, 272–273
as verification method, 165–166
regulatory affairs/agencies, 15, 23, 59, 98
Reifer, D. J., 409
reliability
criticality of failure and, 340–341
defined, 18
fault-tree analysis, 342
measuring, 31
quality software and, 305
role of, 20–21
of software, 425–429
software quality dimension, 14–16
software safety *versus,* 355–356
strategies for, 283
testing alarms, 372
testing and, 282
reliability bathtub-curve model, 21–22
reliability demonstration chart, 286
reliability engineering, 20
reliability growth models, 425–429
requirements definition, 44, 51
requirements engineering, 207–214
requirements management (RM), 25, 454
Requirements Phase
fuzzy-logic model and, 52
IDS support for, 202–203
requirements analysis, 208–210, 231
requirements document, 51–52
Task Summary Report, 73–74
Verification and Validation policy, 72, 74
requirements specifications, 306
Requirements Traceability Matrix (RTM)
elements of, 72–74, 77–78
features of, 191–192
SQAP and, 160
SRS and, 188–190
verification and validation policies, 75–76

rescheduling, 107
resource engineering feasibility, 308
resources
    demands on, 1
    developing products, 15
    programming productivity estimations and, 109
    project scheduling and, 106–107
    SDP and, 150
    software quality assurance, 29–30
    SVVP and, 71
    usage model and, 289
    user interface development, 379–381
    WBS and, 111, 114–115
responsibilities
    of Configuration Manager, 164
    of Data Analyst, 164
    directory documentation, 61
    organizational efficiency, 120
    for product acceptance, 2
    programming team members, 122
    SCMP and, 147
    during software development process, 10
    software policies and, 64
    SQAP and, 159–160
    SVTP and, 161
    SVVP and, 170
    of Test Administrator, 164
    for testing, 156
    of Test Team, 164
    verification and validation policy, 73
RET (record element types), 139
reusability
    code reusability, 19
    object-oriented model and, 45, 47
    reused code, 407–408
    software and, 249–253
    software producibility and, 386–387
    of test cases, 420
Reviewer Guidance for Computer-Controlled Medical Devices Undergoing 510(k) Review, 440
review process
    cleanroom model and, 47
    design phases and, 23–24
    incremental model and, 41
    planning documents and, 146
    software development and, 243–249
    spiral model and, 44
    SQAP and, 160
    SVVP and, 171, 174–175
    VTIS and, 197
Richards, P., 305
rigor, *versus* heuristics, 215–216
risk assessment
    safety requirements and, 23
    in software requirements, 308–309
    software safety and, 352–353, 357–358
    spiral model and, 42–43
    SVVP and, 71–74

risk management
    SDP and, 150, 152
    software hazards and, 330–333
    software process improvement and, 448–458
    software reuse and, 249
    spiral model and, 42–43
RM (requirements management), 25, 454
robustness
    quality software and, 305
    software requirements and, 23
robustness testing
    defined, 154
    examples of, 264
    SRS and, 190
    as validation test, 164
    as verification method, 165
ROM. *See* read-only memory (ROM)
Rome Air Development Center, 421
Royce, W. W., 39
RTM. *See* Requirements Traceability Matrix (RTM)
run, 284
Russell, G. W., 269

Sabbagh, K., 12
safety engineering, 329–373
safety/safeguards
    considerations, 356–365
    FMEA and, 339
    hazard analysis and, 336
    Principles for Computers in Safety-Related Systems, 440
    versus reliability, 355–356
    review process, 23
    software hazards and, 352–355, 359–360
    techniques used, 23
    user interface and, 365–373
    verification and validation of, 310–312
safety testing
    defined, 154
    features of, 276–279
    SRS and, 190
    as validation test, 165
scatter plots, system linearity and, 50
scenario analysis, 208–210, 378
schedules
    and development pressures, 13
    maturity metrics and, 448
    meeting project commitments, 216
    Project Preparation policy, 61–62
    project scheduling, 106–107
    risks with, 309, 453
    SDP and, 150, 152
    software quality dimension, 14–16
    SVTP and, 161
    usage model and, 289
Schick, G. J., 425
Schkade, L. L., 214

SCMP. *See* Software Configuration Management Plan (SCMP)

scripts. *See* test cases

SDP. *See* Software Development Plan (SDP)

SDTP. *See* Software Development Test Plan (SDTP)

SEAP. *See* Software End-Product Acceptance Plan (SEAP)

SEI. *See* Software Engineering Institute (SEI)

SEI Maturity Level, 95

SFMEA. *See* software FMEA (SFMEA)

SFMECA. *See* software failure modes and effects criticality analysis (SFMECA)

Shakespeare, William, 1, 205

Shen, V. Y., 408, 413, 415, 422, 424

Shneiderman, B., 376

Shooman, M. L., 424–425

simulations, 43, 56, 231, 248

Skylab project, 39

SLOC (source lines of code), 408

Software Analysis Methodology policy, 63, 67

Software Anomaly Report, 201, 227–229

Software Capability Evaluation method, 440

Software Change Review Board (SCRB)
    change control and, 324–325
    CRAs and, 228
    policy elements, 81–82, 86

Software Code Walk-Throughs policy, 63, 67

Software Configuration Audit Report (SCAR)
    elements of, 72–73, 77
    purpose of, 173–174
    verification and validation policies, 80

Software Configuration Change Processing policy, 81–82, 84

Software Configuration Item Identification policy, 81–82

software configuration management (SCM), 454

Software Configuration Management of Subcontractor and Vendor Products policy, 81–84

Software Configuration Management Organization policy, 81–82

Software Configuration Management Plan (SCMP)
    elements of, 69, 81–84
    features of, 147–150
    purpose of, 323
    software quality assurance and, 98
    used in postmortems, 255
    verification and validation policies, 74, 77, 79–80

Software Configuration Status Accounting policy, 81–83, 86

Software Configuration Status Report (SCSR), 82–83, 86

software design. *See also* Architecture Design Specification (ADS); Detailed Design Specification (DDS)
    ANSI/IEEE Std 1016-1987, 28–29
    boundary tests and, 262
    considerations with, 215–217
    defect metrics and, 417–419

    defined, 379
    documentation, 34, 270
    elements of, 145
    factors influencing degradation, 21
    functional design phase, 110
    fuzzy-logic model and, 52
    IDS and, 184–185
    inconsistency in, 385
    iteration during, 53
    patient monitors, 383
    product estimations, 125
    review process, 23–25, 420
    versus software requirements, 221–223
    system requirements, 22–23

Software Design Methodology policy, 63, 67

Software Design Walk-Throughs policy, 63, 66–67

Software Development Management policy, 87

Software Development Plan (SDP)
    ADR and, 246
    baselines and, 319
    elements of, 63–64, 69
    features of, 150–153
    review process and, 243
    SCMP and, 84
    SQAP and, 159–160
    typical planning document, 147
    used in postmortems, 255

Software Development Support Activities policy, 88

Software Development Test Plan (SDTP)
    DTIS and, 68, 196
    elements of, 63–65, 68
    features of, 153–157
    quality assurance and, 304
    SRS and, 189
    typical planning document, 147
    used in postmortems, 255
    verification and validation review, 76

software development tools. *See also* automated tools
    as implementation step, 33–34
    lack of comprehensive, 119
    quality measurement tools, 396
    spiral model, 44

software documentation. *See also specific document types*
    ANSI/IEEE Std 829-1983, 26
    documentation rights, 152–153
    document templates, 25
    FDA medical device failures, 440
    as implementation step, 34
    importance of up-to-date, 25
    metrics and, 444
    project, 145–203
    for prototypes, 241–242
    software defects and, 418
    software methodology and process, 53–88
    standards and conventions, 90–91
    test recording, 166
    usage of, 201–203

used in postmortems, 255
Software Documentation policy, 63, 69–70
Software End-Product Acceptance Plan (SEAP)
  elements of, 63–64, 66, 70
  features of, 156–159
  typical planning document, 147
  used in postmortems, 255
Software End-Product Release policy, 87
Software Engineering Institute (SEI), 255, 439–440
software engineers/engineering
  code walk-throughs and, 270
  cognitive dissonance and, 54
  configuration management and, 315–316
  considerations, 386–391
  contributions of, 31
  discipline specifics, 205–207
  feasibility, 308
  functional organization, 119–121
  hardware engineer as, 115–117
  measuring performance, 436–437
  productivity differences in, 438–439
  quality assurance and, 1–16, 30
  standards, 26–29, 89–90
  SVTP and, 163–164
  team organization, 121–123
  term origin, 39
  user interface and, 375–376
software failure modes and effects criticality analysis
    (SFMECA), 276, 279
software FMEA (SFMEA), 341–242
software functional baseline, 319
software librarian, 321
software life cycle
  ANSI/IEEE Std 730-1989, 26
  configuration management policies, 82
  defect metrics and, 417–419
  examples of, 223–229
  incremental model and, 40–41
  object-oriented model and, 45
  of prototypes, 235
  quality assurance and, 17–18
  refining estimates for, 110
  software development, 243–244, 250
  spiral model and, 43
  testing and, 266, 279–281
  user interaction development, 385–386
  verification and validation in, 298–303
  waterfall model and, 40
software metrics. *See also* thousands of source
    instructions (KDSI)
  algorithms, 396–398
  anomalies, 95
  Change Request/Approval, 95
  code walk-throughs, 396
  composites, 414–417
  data structures, 409–412
  defects, 19, 417–419
  limitations of, 398–399

logic structures, 412–414
maintainability metrics models, 428–431
management, 399
measurement, 395–396
policies, 92, 94–103
process maturity and, 442–447
program size, 401–409
software postmortems. *See* postmortems
software process improvement (SPI), 435–437,
    448–458
Software Process Improvement Capability
    Determination (SPICE) model, 439, 441
Software Procurement Assessment, 440
software productivity. *See* programming productivity
software project planning (SPP), 454
software project tracking and oversight (SPTO), 454
software quality assurance (SQA)
  ANSI/IEEE Std 1012-1986, 28
  CMM model and, 454
  as a discipline, 317
  in maintenance cycle, 95–104
  program components, 17–36
  program documentation, 54–56
  software engineering and, 1–16
  team organization, 303–305
  transfer of software ownership, 271
Software Quality Assurance Plan (SQAP)
  elements of, 63–64, 67, 69
  features of, 159–161
  SDP and, 152
  software quality assurance and, 98
  typical planning document, 147
  used in postmortems, 255
Software Quality Function Deployment (SQFD),
    214–215
Software Requirements Review (SRR)
  elements of, 63–66, 245
  review process, 75, 243
  SCMP and, 84
  SVVP and, 71
Software Requirements Specification (SRS)
  ADS and, 202–203
  analysis output, 145
  features of, 186–190
  policy elements, 61–66
  product release policies, 87
  purpose of, 175
  Requirements Phase Verification and Validation
    policy, 74–75
  review process and, 243
  RTM and, 78, 191
  SVTP and, 78, 161
Software Science (Halstead), 405, 422–423
software sizing, 129–132
Software Tools policy, 63, 68
Software User's Manual policy, 63, 68–69
Software Validation Phase
  IDS support for, 202–203

SVTPR and, 198
Verification and Validation policy, 72, 77
VTIS and, 197
Software Validation Test Log (SVTL), 164, 166, 168, 201
Software Validation Test Plan (SVTP)
  elements of, 72–73, 75–76, 78
  features of, 161–168
  quality assurance and, 304
  SDTP and, 153
  SRS and, 189
  typical planning document, 147
  used in postmortems, 255
  VTIS and, 197
Software Validation Test Procedures (SVTPR)
  elements of, 72–73, 77, 79
  SVTP and, 163
  testing process and, 198–201
  test recording, 166
Software Validation Test Report, 166, 201
Software Verification and Validation Anomaly Report
  anomalies and, 166–167, 171–173
  elements of, 76–77
  SCMP and, 79–80
  SVTP and, 164
Software Verification and Validation Plan (SVVP)
  configuration change processing and, 84
  elements of, 70–74
  features of, 168–175
  SDP and, 152
  Software Anomaly Report, 201
  typical planning document, 147
  used in postmortems, 255
Software Verification and Validation Report (SVVR)
  acceptance criteria, 59
  elements of, 72–73, 77
  product release policies, 87
  verification and validation policies, 80
source lines of code (SLOC), 408
span (SP), 412
SPICE model, 439, 441
Spielman, B. J., 10
spiral model
  cleanroom model and, 48
  features of, 42–45
  fuzzy-logic model and, 52
SQA. *See* software quality assurance (SQA)
SQAP. *See* Software Quality Assurance Plan (SQAP)
SQFD. *See* Software Quality Function Deployment (SQFD)
SRR. *See* Software Requirements Review (SRR)
SRS. *See* Software Requirements Specification (SRS)
S-shaped models, 427, 429
Standard for Software Quality Assurance Plans, 26–27
Standard for Software Requirements Specifications, 26–27
Standard for Software Test Documentation, 26–27

Standard for Software Verification and Validation Plans, 27–28, 299
standard operating procedures (SOPs)
  configuration management policies, 82
  DTIS compliance with, 68
  IDS verification, 203
  incorporating lessons learned, 35
  Interface Design Phase Verification and Validation policy, 74
  organizing, 54–56
  process infrastructure and, 31–32
  product release policies, 87
  SCSR and, 86
  software quality assurance and, 8–9
  SQAP and, 160
  SVTP and, 166
  used in postmortems, 256–257
  verification and validation policies, 75
  VTIS and, 78, 197
standards/standardization
  for assessment, 439–441
  coding standards, 88–90
  design inconsistency, 385
  directory structure, 59–61
  for LOC, 403–405
  of measurements, 400–401
  monitoring adherence to, 18–19
  of production and inspection methods, 2
  purpose of, 25–30, 89
  quality assurance and, 7
  screen elements, 383
  SDP and, 152
  SQAP and, 160
  terminology and, 119
standby redundancy, 354
standing alarms, 371–372
Stanton, N., 371
statements, 39, 413–414
static models of defects, 420–421, 425
static testing and analysis, 268–270
statistical process control, 431–433
statistical testing, 286–290
Stolzy, J. L., 357
stress testing
  defined, 154
  elements of, 262–264
  quality assurance and, 304
  SRS and, 190
  validation testing, 164–165, 272
strict liability (doctrine of), 12
structured analysis methods, 409
structured design, 234–236, 420
structured programming, 38–39, 260
structure testing, 304–305
style guides, graphical user interface, 385
SVTL. *See* Software Validation Test Log (SVTL)
SVTP. *See* Software Validation Test Plan (SVTP)

SVTPR. *See* Software Validation Test Procedures (SVTPR)

SVVP. *See* Software Verification and Validation Plan (SVVP)

SVVR. *See* Software Verification and Validation Report (SVVR)

System Management policy, 87

system requirements, 22–23, 146

system testing, 274–276, 278

tasks
    ADS and, 178–181
    DDS and, 182–183
    intertask dependencies, 167
    milestones and, 112–114
    SVVP reporting, 172
    task-unit approach, 134–135

Tausworthe, R. C., 113

team organization
    quality assurance, 302–305
    software engineering, 121–123
    test teams, 164, 166

terminal events, 344, 346–348

Test Administrator, 164

test cases
    generating, 284
    importance of, 259
    orthogonal array testing and, 266
    quality assurance and, 304
    region faults and, 268
    reusability of, 420
    software modifications and, 276
    statistical testing and, 287
    system testing and, 275
    for unit testing, 268
    usage models and, 288–289

testing. *See also* functional testing; physical testing; regression testing; stress testing
    acceptance testing, 126
    activities during, 259–296
    ad hoc tests, 360
    alarms, 372
    ANSI/IEEE Std 829-1983, 26
    cleanroom model and, 47, 49
    detailed integration testing, 155–156
    documentation, 196–201
    DTIS and, 68
    and evaluation, 317–318
    exception testing, 364
    as first indicator of problems, 19
    growth testing, 154, 165, 190
    historical perspectives, 17–18
    IDS and, 186
    off-the-shelf software and, 310
    quality software and, 305
    reliability processes and, 20
    software quality and, 298
    specifications and, 309

SQAP and, 160

structured programming and, 38

structure testing, 304–305

test team and, 164, 166

validation testing, 8, 272–274, 304, 306

testing phase, 417–420

test procedures, 247–248, 284

Thayer, R. H., 119

Thebaut, S. M., 413, 422, 424

Therac-25 radiation therapy machine, 9–10

thousand lines of code (KLOC), 48–49, 403, 405, 422

thousands of source instructions (KDSI), 130–131

threshold values, medical devices and, 333

throwaway prototypes, 236–239

TickIT program, 439–441

time-outs, 367

time Petri nets, 356–357

time/timing
    dynamic model of defects and, 424–425
    event-driven systems and, 278
    reliability growth models and, 425–426
    safety requirements and, 23
    software metrics, 416

token count, 405–407, 414–415

top-down methods
    elements of, 134
    as estimation method, 132–133
    prototypes as, 235
    user interaction development and, 385–386

top events, 346, 348

tort claim, faulty software and, 11–12

Total Quality Management (TQM), 214

"Towards a Theory of Program Design," 39

toxicity, as potential hazard, 331

TQM. *See* Total Quality Management (TQM)

transactional functions, 136–138, 140

transform model, 42

trend analysis, software metrics and, 400

trial-and-error extraction, 51

trigger mechanisms, 336–337

Troy, R., 253

TÜV. *See* German Electrotechnical Commission (TÜV)

UFP. *See* unadjusted function points (UFPs)

unadjusted function points (UFPs), 409

underestimates, 106, 119

undersizing, 131–132

unit of measure
    for effort, 416
    function points as, 136
    of time, 416
    for volume, 406

unit testing, 268

usability
    considerations, 376–378
    measuring, 31

quality software and, 305
versus safety, 366–367
user-interface design and, 381–382
validation support for, 273
usage model
benefits of statistical testing, 289–290
cleanroom model and, 48
defined, 287–288
steps in development, 288–289
U.S. Air Force, 297
user interaction development
considerations, 390–391
life cycle for, 385–386
role, 380–381
special considerations with, 386–391
User Interface Specification (UIS)
features of, 192–196
purpose of, 175
RTM and, 188
user-machine interface
activities, 375–393
software safety and, 365–373
user manuals
prototypes as alternatives, 235
Software User's Manual policy, 63, 68–69
verification and validation policies, 75
VTIS and, 76

validation. *See* verification and validation (V & V)
Validation Test Information Sheets (VTISs)
depicted, 167
elements of, 72–73, 76, 78
intertask dependencies, 167
RTM and, 188
safety testing and, 278
SVTP and, 163
SVTPR and, 200
testing process and, 197–198
test recording, 166
value adjustment factor (VAF), 141–142
variables
control variables, 50
input variables, 284
live variables, 410–412
variants, 251–252, 326–327
Verification and Validation Management policy, 70–73
Verification and Validation Phase, 72, 74, 172
Verification and Validation Report, 201
Verification and Validation Reporting policy, 79
Verification and Validation Task Iteration policy, 72, 74
verification and validation (V & V)
code control and, 320
documentation, 196–203

DTIS and, 68
elements of, 8–9
fuzzy-logic model and, 52
as implementation step, 34
importance of policies, 55
of input, 367–368
methods, 154–155
policies, 57–59, 70–80, 90–93
process infrastructure and, 31–32
programming teams and, 122
purpose of, 317
software activities, 297–313
waterfall model and, 40
v(G). *See* cyclomatic complexity number, v(G)
video display units (VDUs), 370–371
visual congestion, patient monitors and, 383–384
vocabulary, 406
von Schowen, A. J., 10
VTIS. *See* Validation Test Information Sheets (VTISs)

waiver requests, 103–104
walk-throughs. *See* code walk-throughs; design walk-throughs
Walters, G., 305
Ward, P. T., 42
Warnier, J. D., 42
warnings, 195–196
Wasserman, A. I., 33, 42
waterfall model
cleanroom model and, 48
COCOMO model and, 130
features of, 39–42
spiral model and, 44
wear-out, 21
Weibull model, 429
Wherry, P., 10
white-box testing, 278
Wilson, T. A., 106
Wirth, N., 39
Witterrongel, D. M., 106
Witty, R. W., 310–311
Wolverton, R. W., 129, 425
Wood, R. C., 119
Wooden, J., 145
Woodward, M. R., 414
work breakdown structure (WBS), 110–117, 125, 134
work year, 113

Yamada model, 429
Yamada-Raleigh model, 429
Yourdon, E., 39, 42, 178, 182
Yu, T. J., 413, 422, 424

zero defects, 252–253
Zhuo, F., 428